Head and Neck Oncology

Head and Neck Oncology

Editor: Agnes Carter

AMERICAN
MEDICAL PUBLISHERS
www.americanmedicalpublishers.com

AMERICAN
MEDICAL PUBLISHERS
www.americanmedicalpublishers.com

Cataloging-in-Publication Data

Head and neck oncology / edited by Agnes Carter.
p. cm.
Includes bibliographical references and index.
ISBN 979-8-88740-167-6
1. Head--Cancer. 2. Neck--Cancer. 3. Oncology. 4. Head--Cancer--Treatment.
5. Neck--Cancer--Treatment. I. Carter, Agnes.
RC280.H4 H434 2023
616.994 91--dc23

American Medical Publishers,
41 Flatbush Avenue,
1st Floor, New York,
NY 11217, USA

ISBN 979-8-88740-167-6 (Hardback)

Contents

Preface

Every book is a source of knowledge and this one is no exception. The idea that led to the conceptualization of this book was the fact that the world is advancing rapidly; which makes it crucial to document the progress in every field. I am aware that a lot of data is already available, yet, there is a lot more to learn. Hence, I accepted the responsibility of editing this book and contributing my knowledge to the community.

Head and neck cancer refers to a group of malignant diseases that originate from the oral cavity, nasal cavity, nose, paranasal sinuses, larynx, pharynx, salivary glands, or skin of the face. Some of the most prominent causes of head and neck cancer include consumption of alcohol and tobacco, betel nut, infection, gastroesophageal reflux disease, hematopoietic stem cell transplantation, and exposure to UV and certain chemicals. The most common symptoms are persistent pain in the throat, a sensation of pain or difficulty when swallowing, jaw pain, a change in voice, persistent pain in the ear, etc. Most of the head and neck cancers are caused due to squamous cell carcinomas (SCCs). Diagnosis depends on specific signs and symptoms, and the results of blood tests. Computed tomography scan and magnetic resonance imaging scans are the imaging tests that are used to diagnose these cancers. Treatment for head and neck cancer is planned as per the specific needs and general health of individual patients. Treatment and management may include surgery, chemotherapy, radiation therapy, targeted therapy, and immunotherapy. This book is a valuable compilation of topics, ranging from the basic to the most complex principles and practices in head and neck oncology. It will help the readers in keeping pace with the rapid changes in this field.

While editing this book, I had multiple visions for it. Then I finally narrowed down to make every chapter a sole standing text explaining a particular topic, so that they can be used independently. However, the umbrella subject sinews them into a common theme. This makes the book a unique platform of knowledge.

I would like to give the major credit of this book to the experts from every corner of the world, who took the time to share their expertise with us. Also, I owe the completion of this book to the never-ending support of my family, who supported me throughout the project.

Editor

1

Identification of Hub Genes Associated with Development of Head and Neck Squamous Cell Carcinoma by Integrated Bioinformatics Analysis

***Chia Ying Li*[1,2]*, Jia-Hua Cai*[3†]*, Jeffrey J. P. Tsai*[3] *and Charles C. N. Wang*[3*]**

[1] Department of Surgery, Show Chwan Memorial Hospital, Changhua, Taiwan, [2] Ph.D. Program in Tissue Engineering and Regenerative Medicine, National Chung Hsing University, Taichung, Taiwan, [3] Department of Bioinformatics and Medical Engineering, Asia University, Taichung, Taiwan

***Correspondence:**
Charles C. N. Wang
cnwang@asia.edu.tw

† These authors have contributed equally to this work

Improved insight into the molecular mechanisms of head and neck squamous cell carcinoma (HNSCC) is required to predict prognosis and develop a new therapeutic strategy for targeted genes. The aim of this study is to identify significant genes associated with HNSCC and to further analyze its prognostic significance. In our study, the cancer genome atlas (TCGA) HNSCC database and the gene expression profiles of GSE6631 from the Gene Expression Omnibus (GEO) were used to explore the differential co-expression genes in HNSCC compared with normal tissues. A total of 29 differential co-expression genes were screened out by Weighted Gene Co-expression Network Analysis (WGCNA) and differential gene expression analysis methods. As suggested in functional annotation analysis using the R clusterProfiler package, these genes were mainly enriched in epidermis development and differentiation (biological process), apical plasma membrane and cell-cell junction (cellular component), and enzyme inhibitor activity (molecular function). Furthermore, in a protein-protein interaction (PPI) network containing 21 nodes and 25 edges, the ten hub genes (S100A8, S100A9, IL1RN, CSTA, ANXA1, KRT4, TGM3, SCEL, PPL, and PSCA) were identified using the CytoHubba plugin of Cytoscape. The expression of the ten hub genes were all downregulated in HNSCC tissues compared with normal tissues. Based on survival analysis, the lower expression of CSTA was associated with worse overall survival (OS) in patients with HNSCC. Finally, the protein level of CSTA, which was validated by the Human Protein Atlas (HPA) database, was down-regulated consistently with mRNA levels in head and neck cancer samples. In summary, our study demonstrated that a survival-related gene is highly correlated with head and neck cancer development. Thus, CSTA may play important roles in the progression of head and neck cancer and serve as a potential biomarker for future diagnosis and treatment.

Keywords: head and neck squamous cell carcinoma, differential gene expression analysis, weighted gene co-expression network analysis, the differential co-expression genes, biomarkers

INTRODUCTION

Head and neck squamous cell carcinoma (HNSCC) is one of most common types of cancer in the world. HNSCC includes several malignancies that originate in the mouth, nasopharynx, oropharynx, hypopharynx, larynx, and neck (1). According to the published global cancer statistics report, there were more than an estimated 650,000 new cases and 330,000 deaths diagnosed in 2018 (2). Many lifestyle factors have been investigated, with tobacco use, alcohol consumption, human papillomavirus (HPV), and Epstein-Barr virus (EBV) infection being considered as the risk factors that are associated with the progression of HNSCC (3). However, HPV is currently the one most well-studied and frequently used biomarker in HNSCC (4–6). In the past several years, the treatments for managing head and neck cancer included the following: radiation therapy, surgery, and chemotherapy. Appropriate combinations of the three treatment modalities is selected according to the site of the cancer and the stage of the disease (1, 3). Although there are diverse treatments for HNSCC, patients have a limited survival advantage.

With the development of genomic technologies, bioinformatics has become increasingly popular for gene expression profiles analysis to study the molecular mechanisms of diseases and discover disease-specific biomarkers (7). One important method to understand the gene function and gene association from genome-wide expression is Weighted Gene Co-expression Network Analysis (WGCNA) (8). WGCNA can be used to detect co-expression modules of highly correlated genes and interested modules associated with clinical traits (9), providing great insight into predicting the functions of co-expression genes and finding genes that play key roles in human diseases (10–12). Furthermore, another powerful analysis within transcriptomics is differential gene expression analysis, which provides methods for studying molecular mechanisms underlying genome regulation and discovering quantitative changes in expression levels between experimental groups and control groups (13). Such gene expression differences can lead to the discovery of potential biomarkers for a particular disease. Therefore, using two approaches, the findings from WGCNA and differential gene expression analysis are combined to enhance the discriminating ability of highly related genes that are useful to serve as candidate biomarkers.

In this study, the mRNA expression data of HNSCC from the TCGA and GEO databases were analyzed by WGCNA and differential gene expression analysis to obtain differential co-expression genes. We further explored HNSCC development

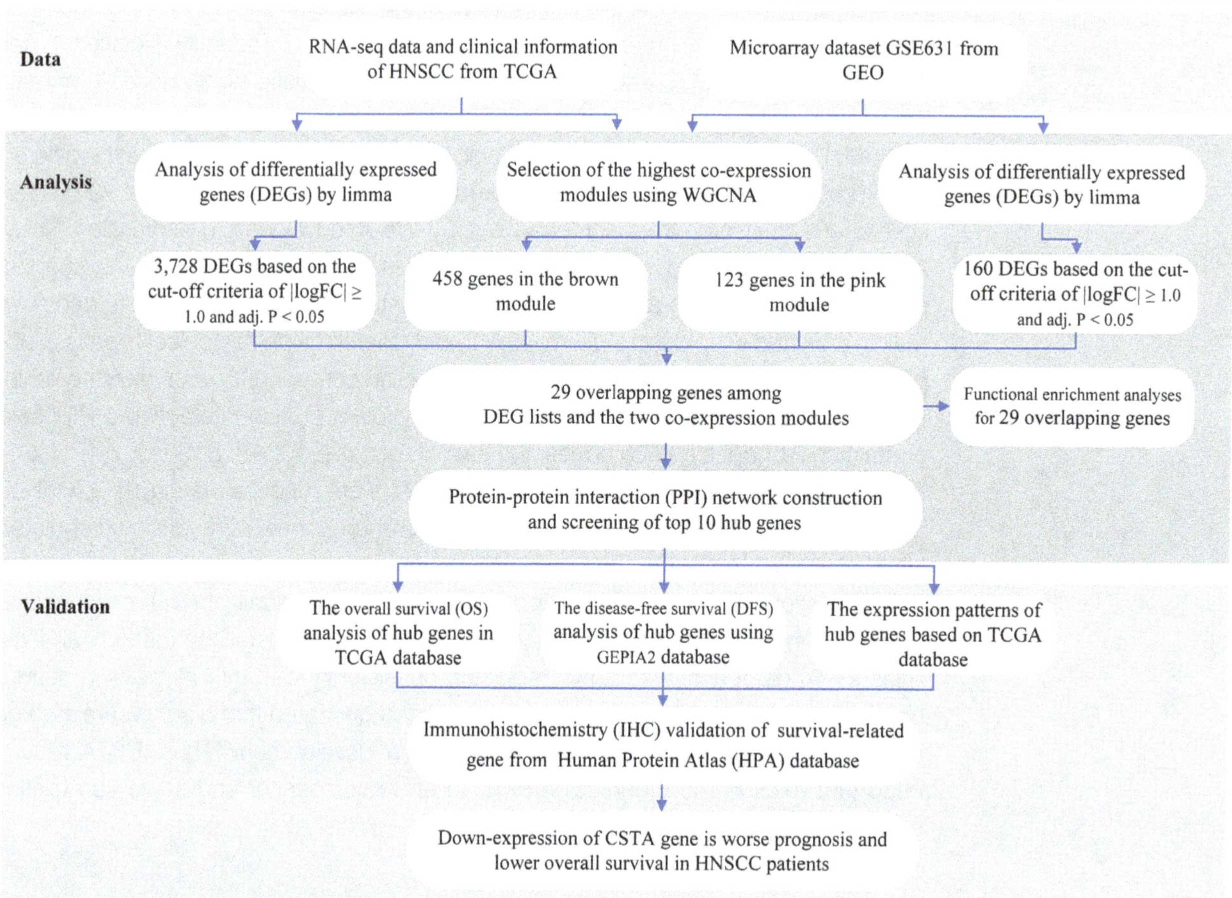

FIGURE 1 | Study design and workflow of this study.

through functional enrichment and protein-protein interaction (PPI) analysis combined with survival analysis. The study provides a potential basis to understand the cause and potential molecular events of HNSCC by analyzing differential co-expression genes for clinical diagnosis or treatment.

MATERIALS AND METHODS

The workflow of the analysis hub gene extraction curation pipeline is shown in **Figure 1**.

We elaborate on each step in the following sub-sections.

Datasets From TCGA and GEO Database

The gene expression profiles of HNSCC were downloaded from TCGA (https://portal.gdc.cancer.gov/) and GEO (https://www.ncbi.nlm.nih.gov/gds). In the TCGA database, all data on HNSCC and corresponding clinical information were freely downloaded by R package *TCGAbiolinks* (14). There were 544 NHSCC samples, including 500 head and neck cancers and 44 normal tissues, and RNAseq count data on 19,430 genes. A total of the data had been generated by using the Illumina HiSeq 2,000 platform, and were annotated to a reference transcript set of Human hg38 gene standard track. As suggested by the *edgeR* package tutorial (15), genes of low

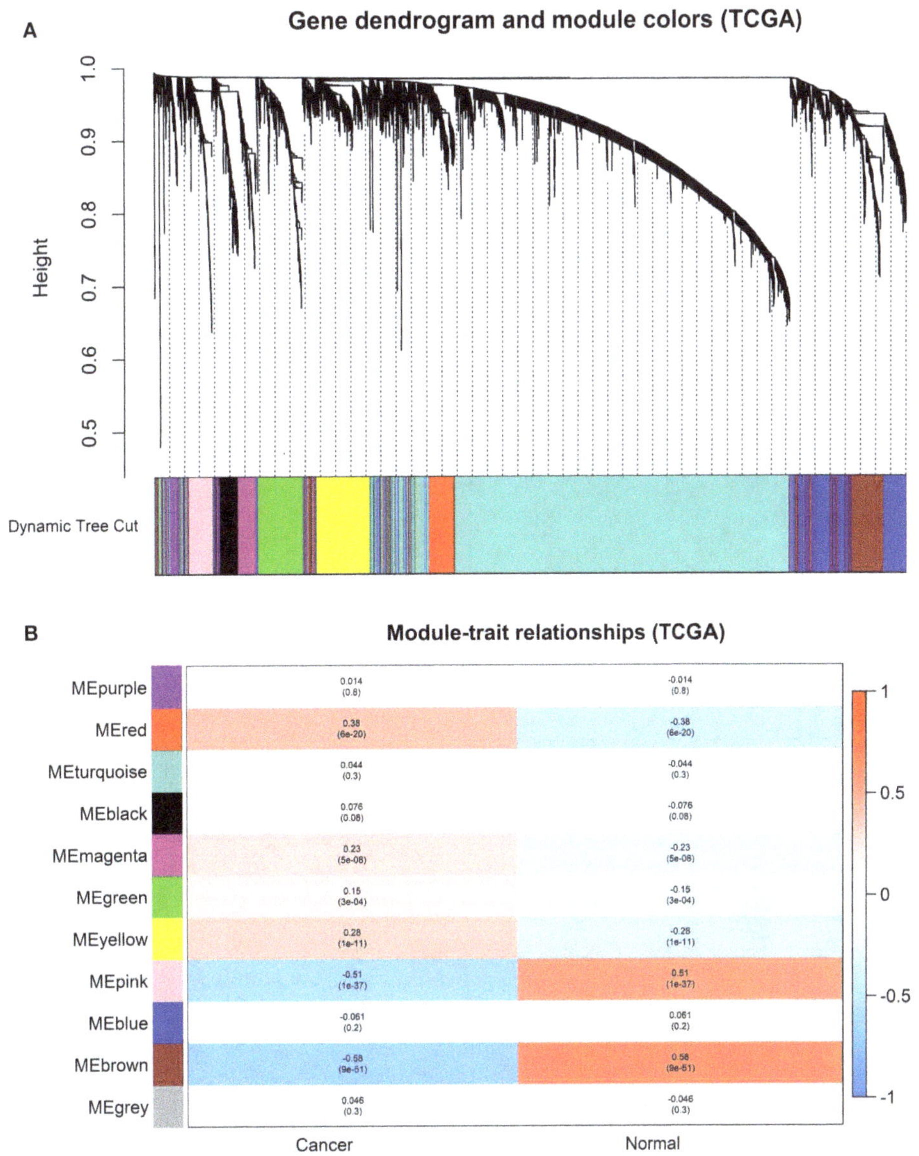

FIGURE 2 | Identification of modules associated with the clinical information in the TCGA-HNSCC dataset. **(A)** The Cluster dendrogram of co-expression network modules was ordered by a hierarchical clustering of genes based on the 1-TOM matrix. Each module was assigned different colors. **(B)** Module-trait relationships. Each row corresponds to a color module and column corresponds to a clinical trait (cancer and normal). Each cell contains the corresponding correlation and *P*-value.

read counts are usually not of interest for further analysis. So, we kept the genes with a cpm (count per million) ≥1 in this study. After filtering using function *rpkm* in *edgeR* package, which is calculated by dividing gene counts by gene length, a total of 15,367 genes with RPKM values were subject to our next analysis.

In addition, the normalized expression profiles of GSE6631, another gene expression profile of HNSCC from GEO, was obtained using R package *GEOquery* (16). GSE6631 consisted of 22 tumor samples and 22 paired normal tissues from patients with HNSCC, which were studied with the GPL8300 platform [HG_U95Av2] Affymetrix Human Genome U95 Version 2 Array. Probes were converted to the gene symbols based on a manufacturer-provided annotation file and duplicated probes for the same gene were removed by determining the median expression value of all its corresponding probes. As a result, a list of 9,203 genes were selected for the subsequent analysis.

Identification of Key Co-expression Modules Using WGCNA

Co-expression networks facilitate methods on network-based gene screening that can be used to identify candidate biomarkers and therapeutic targets. In our study, the gene expression data profiles of TCGA-HNSCC and GSE6631 were constructed to gene co-expression networks using the *WGCNA* package in R (8).

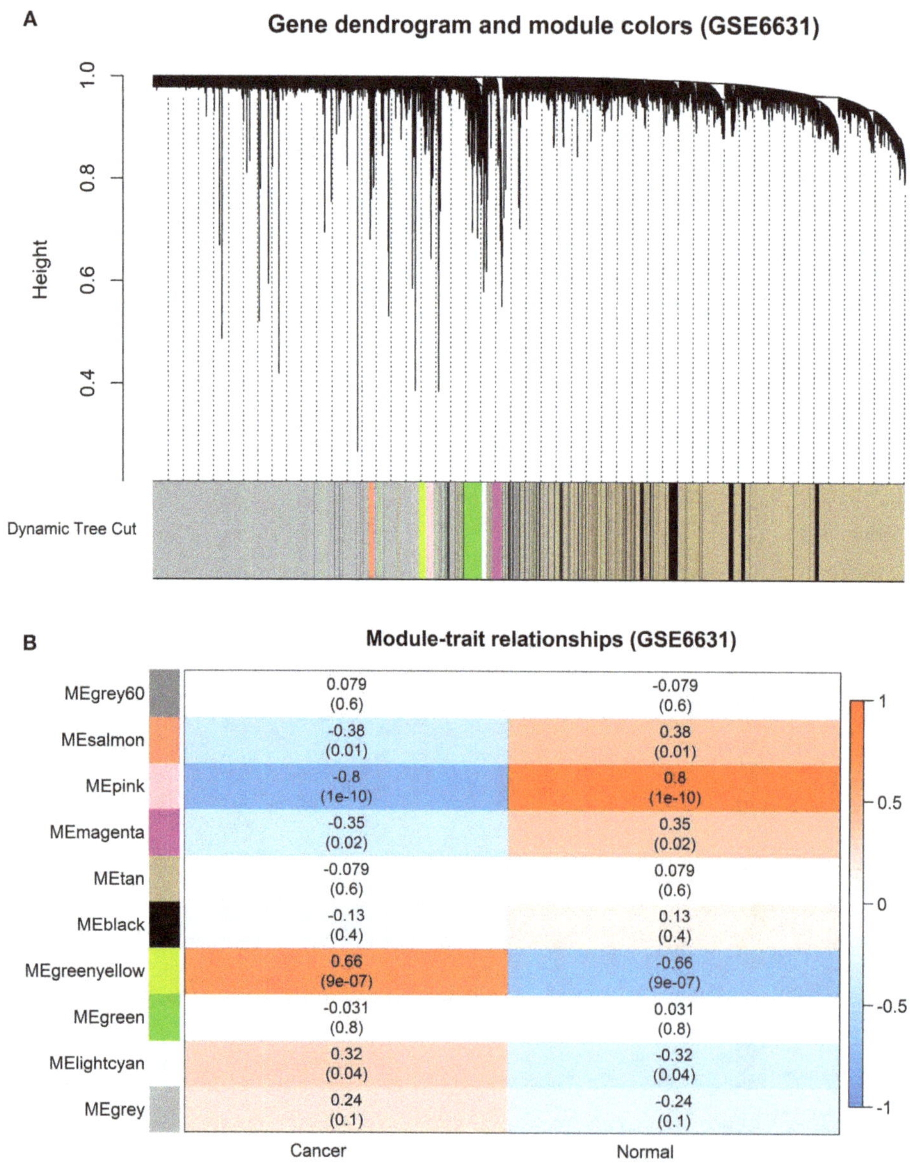

FIGURE 3 | Identification of modules associated with clinical information in the GSE6631 dataset. **(A)** The Cluster dendrogram of co-expression network modules was ordered by a hierarchical clustering of genes based on the 1-TOM matrix. Each module was assigned different colors. **(B)** Module-trait relationships. Each row corresponds to a color module and each column correlates to a clinical trait (cancer and normal). Each cell contains the corresponding correlation and *P*-value.

WGCNA was used to explore the modules of highly correlated genes among samples for relating modules to external sample traits. To build a scale-free network, soft powers $\beta = 3$ and 20 were selected using the function *pickSoftThreshold.* Next, the adjacency matrix was created by the following formula: $a_{ij} = |S_{ij}|^{\beta}$ (a_{ij}: adjacency matrix between gene i and gene j, S_{ij}: similarity matrix which is done by Pearson correlation of all gene pairs, β: softpower value), and was transformed into a topological overlap matrix (TOM) as well as the corresponding dissimilarity (1-TOM). Afterwards, a hierarchical clustering dendrogram of the 1-TOM matrix was constructed to classify the similar gene expressions into different gene co-expression modules. To further identify functional modules in a co-expression network, the module-trait associations between modules, and clinical trait information were calculated according to the previous study (17). Therefore, modules with high correlation coefficient were considered candidates relevant to clinical traits, and were selected for subsequent analysis. A more detailed description of the WGCNA method was reported in our previous study (17).

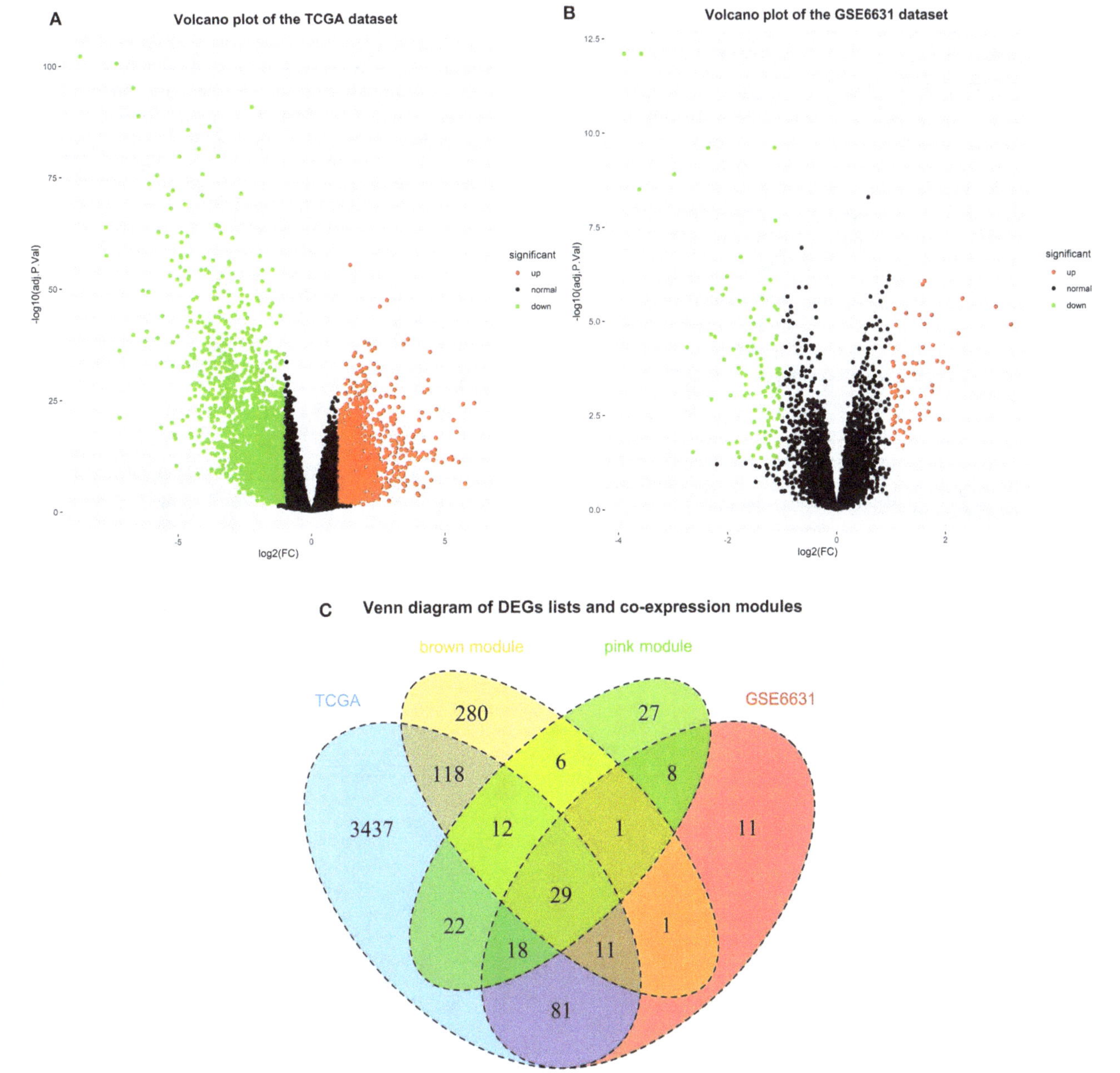

FIGURE 4 | Identification of differentially expressed genes (DEGs) among the TCGA and GSE6631 datasets of HNSCC with the cut-off criteria of $|\log FC| \geq 1.0$ and adj. $P < 0.05$. **(A)** Volcano plot of DEGs in the TCGA dataset. **(B)** Volcano plot of DEGs in the GSE6631 dataset. **(C)** The Venn diagram of genes among DEG lists and co-expression module. In total, 29 overlapping genes in the intersection of DEG lists and two co-expression modules.

Differential Expression Analysis and Interaction With the Modules of Interest

The R package *limma* (linear models for microarray data) provides an integrated solution for differential expression analyses on RNA-Sequencing and microarray data (18). In order to find the differentially expressed genes (DEGs) between HNSCC and normal tissues, *limma* was applied in the TCGA-HNSCC and GSE6631 dataset, respectively, to screen out DEGs. The *p*-value was adjusted by the Benjamini–Hochberg method to control for the false discovery Rate (FDR). Genes with the cut-off criteria of $|\text{logFC}| \geq 1.0$ and adj. $P < 0.05$ were regarded as DEGs. The DEGs of the TCGA-HNSCC and GSE6631 dataset were visualized as a volcano plot by using the R package *ggplot2* (19). Subsequently, the overlapping genes between DEGs and co-expression genes that were extracted from the co-expression network were used to identify potential prognostic genes, which were presented as a Venn diagram using the R package *VennDiagram* (20).

Functional Annotation for Genes of Interest

To explore Gene Ontology (GO) of selected genes, R package clusterProfiler package (21) was used to explore the functions among genes of interest, with a cut-off criterion of adjusted $p < 0.05$. GO annotation that contains the three sub-ontologies—biological process (BP), cellular component (CC), and molecular function (MF)—can identify the biological properties of genes and gene sets for all organisms (22).

Construction of PPI and Screening of Hub Genes

In our study, we used the STRING (Search Tool for the Retrieval of Interacting Genes) online tool, which is designed for predicting protein–protein interactions (PPI), to construct a PPI network of selected genes (23). Using the STRING database, genes with a score ≥ 0.4 were chosen to build a network model visualized by Cytoscape (v3.7.2) (24). In a co-expression network, Maximal Clique Centrality (MCC) algorithm was reported to be the most

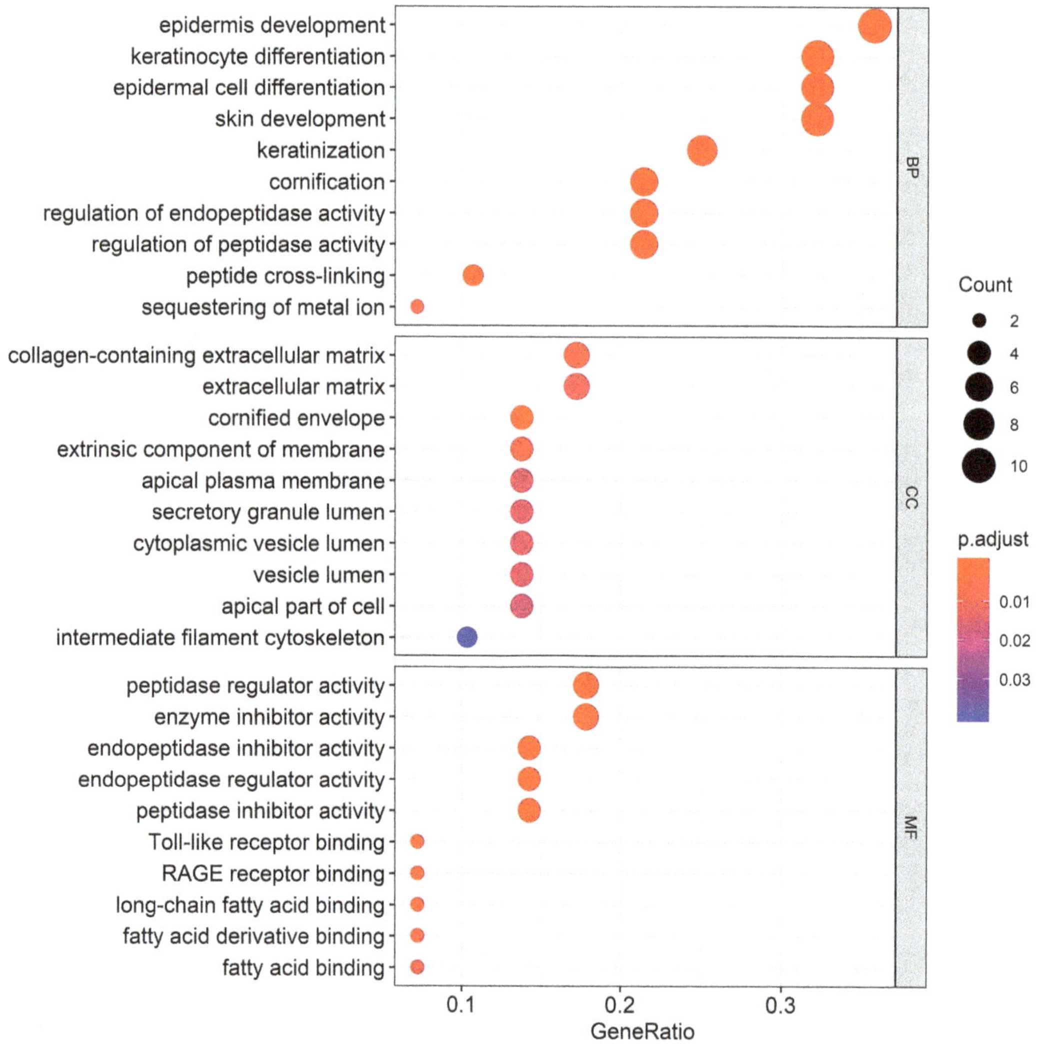

FIGURE 5 | Gene Ontology (GO) enrichment analysis for the genes in the brown module. The color represents the adjusted *p*-values (BH), and the size of the spots represents the gene number.

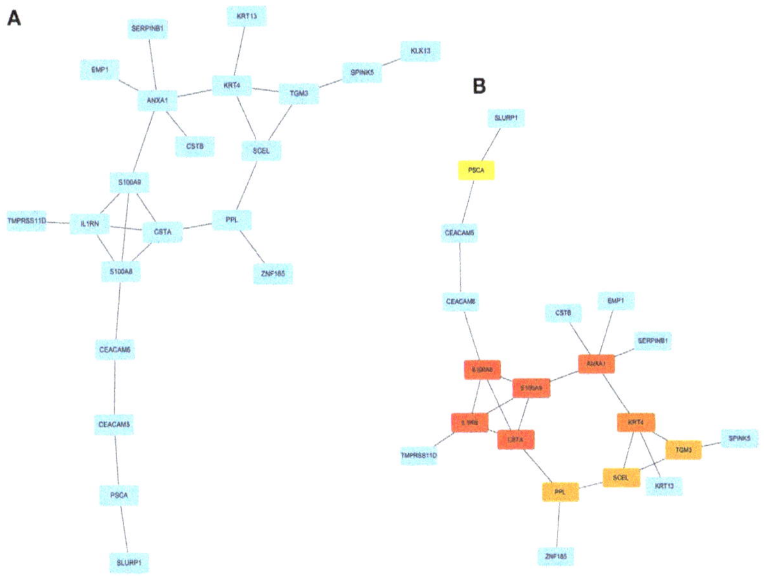

FIGURE 6 | Visualization of the protein-protein interaction (PPI) network and the candidate hub genes. **(A)** PPI network of the genes between DEG lists and two co-expression modules. The blue nodes represent the genes. Edges indicate interaction associations between nodes. **(B)** Identification of the hub genes from the PPI network using maximal clique centrality (MCC) algorithm. Edges represent the protein-protein associations. The red nodes represent genes with a high MCC sores, while the yellow node represent genes with a low MCC sore.

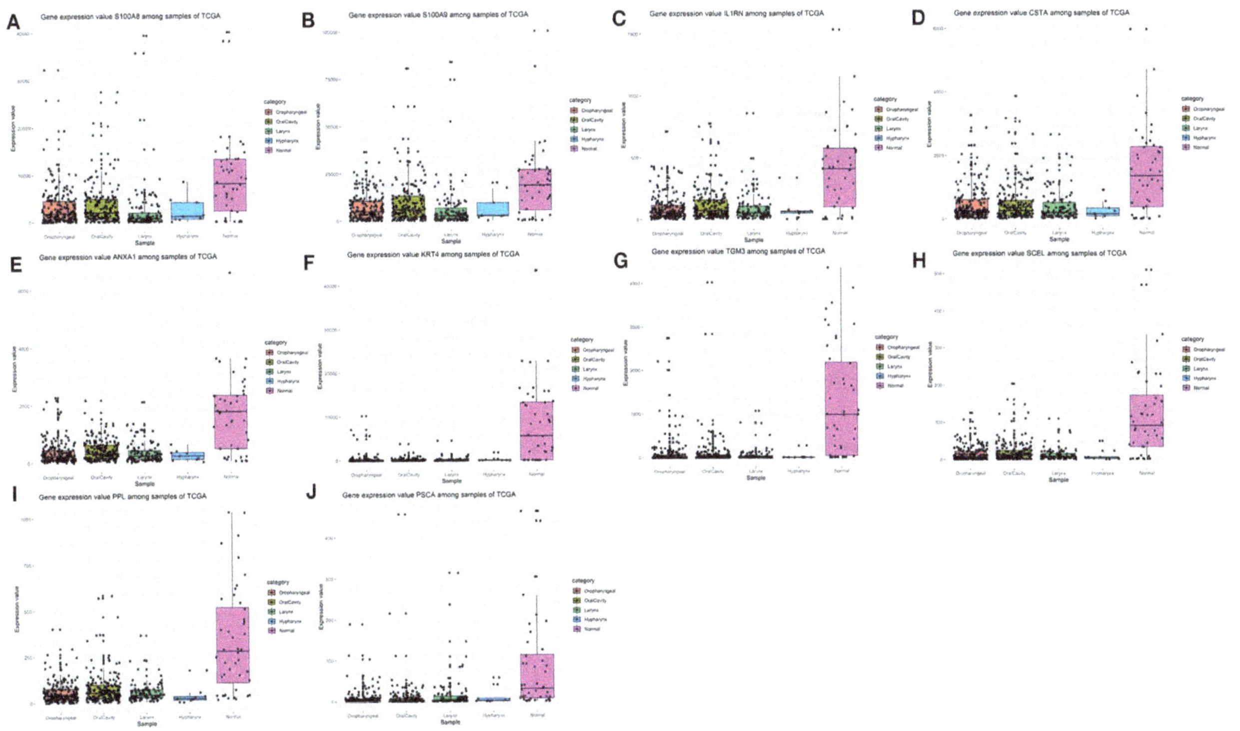

FIGURE 7 | Validation of expression levels of the ten hub genes among HNSCCs and normal tissues from the TCGA database. **(A)** Gene expression value S100A8 among samples of TCGA. **(B)** Gene expression value S100A9 among samples of TCGA. **(C)** Gene expression value IL1RN among samples of TCGA. **(D)** Gene expression value CSTA among samples of TCGA. **(E)** Gene expression value ANXA1 among samples of TCGA. **(F)** Gene expression value KRT4 among samples of TCGA. **(G)** Gene expression value TGM3 among samples of TCGA. **(H)** Gene expression value SCEL among samples of TCGA. **(I)** Gene expression value PPL among samples of TCGA. **(J)** Gene expression value PSCA among samples of TCGA.

effective method of finding hub nodes (25). The MCC of each node was calculated by CytoHubba, a plugin in Cytoscape (25). In this study, the genes with the top 10 MCC values were considered as hub genes.

Verification of the Expression Patterns and the Prognostic Values of Hub Genes

In order to confirm the reliability of the hub genes, we verified the expression patterns of the hub genes in different pathological tumors and normal tissues. The expression level of each hub gene between cancer and normal tissue was plotted as a box plot graph. Based on the data from the TCGA database, Kaplan–Meier univariate survival analysis was performed by using the *survival* package in R software to explore the relationship between overall survival (OS) and hub genes in patients. Moreover, the association between disease-frcc survival (DFS) and hub genes expressed in HNSCC patients was determined using the online tool GEPIA2 (26). In our study, only patients with completed follow-up times were selected for survival analysis and then divided into two separate groups based on the median expression value of hub genes. The survival-related hub genes with log-rank $p < 0.05$ were regarded as statistically significant.

Validation of Protein Expressions of Survival-Related Hub Genes by the HPA Database

The protein expression of the survival-related genes between HNSCC and normal tissues was determined using immunohistochemistry (IHC) from the Human Protein Atlas database (HPA, https://www.proteinatlas.org/). HPA is a valuable database that provides a large amount of transcriptomics and proteomics data in specific human tissues and cells for

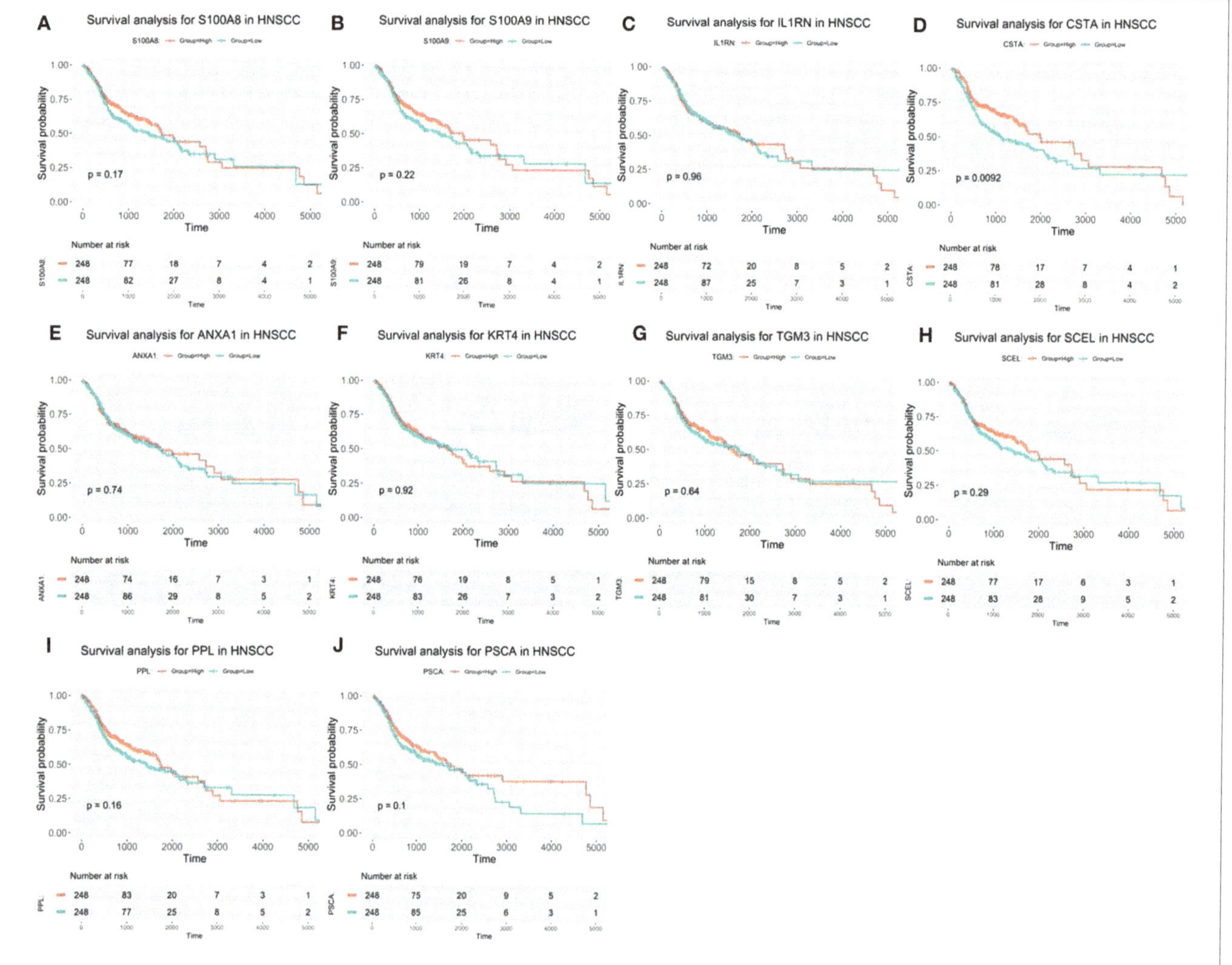

FIGURE 8 | Overall survival (OS) analysis of 10 hub genes in HNSCC patients from the GEPIA2 database. **(A)** Survival analysis for S100A8 in HNSCC. **(B)** Survival analysis for S100A9 in HNSCC. **(C)** Survival analysis for IL1RN in HNSCC. **(D)** Survival analysis for CSTA in HNSCC. **(E)** Survival analysis for ANXA1 in HNSCC. **(F)** Survival analysis for KRT4 in HNSCC. **(G)** Survival analysis for TGM3 in HNSCC. **(H)** Survival analysis for SCEL in HNSCC. **(I)** Survival analysis for PPL in HNSCC. **(J)** Survival analysis for PSCA in HNSCC. The patients were stratified into high-level group (red) and low-level group (green) according to median expression of the gene. Log-rank $P < 0.05$ was considered to be a statistically significant difference.

researchers (27). Moreover, the IHC-based protein expression pattern is the most common application of immunostaining to detect the relative location and abundance of proteins (28).

RESULTS

Construction of Weighted Gene Co-expression Modules

In order to find the functional clusters in HNSCC patients, the gene co-expression networks were constructed from the TCGA-HNSCC and GSE6631 datasets with the *WGCNA* package. With each module assigned a color, a total of 10 modules in the TCGA-HNSCC (**Figure 2A**) and nine modules in the GSE6631 (**Figure 3A**) were identified in the present study (excluding a gray module that was not assigned into any cluster). Then, we plotted the heatmap of module-trait relationships to evaluate the association between each module and two clinical traits (cancer and normal). The results of the module-trait relationships are presented in **Figure 2B, 3B**, revealing that the brown module in the TCGA-HNSCC and pink module in the GSE6631 were found to have the highest association with normal tissues (brown module: $r = 0.58, p = 9e{-}51$; pink module: $r = 0.8, p = 1e{-}10$).

Identification of Genes Between the DEG Lists and Co-expression Modules

Based on the cut-off criteria of $|\text{logFC}| \geq 1.0$ and adj. $P < 0.05$, a total of 3,728 DEGs in the TCGA dataset (**Figure 4A**) and 160 DEGs in the GSE6631 dataset (**Figure 4B**) were found to be dysregulated in tumor tissues by the *limma* package. As shown in **Figure 4C**, 458 and 123 co-expression genes were found in the brown module of TCGA dataset and the pink module in GSE6631, respectively. In total, the 29 overlapping genes were extracted for validating the genes of co-expression modules (**Figure 4C**).

Functional Enrichment Analyses for the 29 Genes

To gain further insight into the potential functions of the 29 genes that overlapped with DEG lists and two co-expression modules, gene enrichment analysis was performed by the *clusterProfiler*

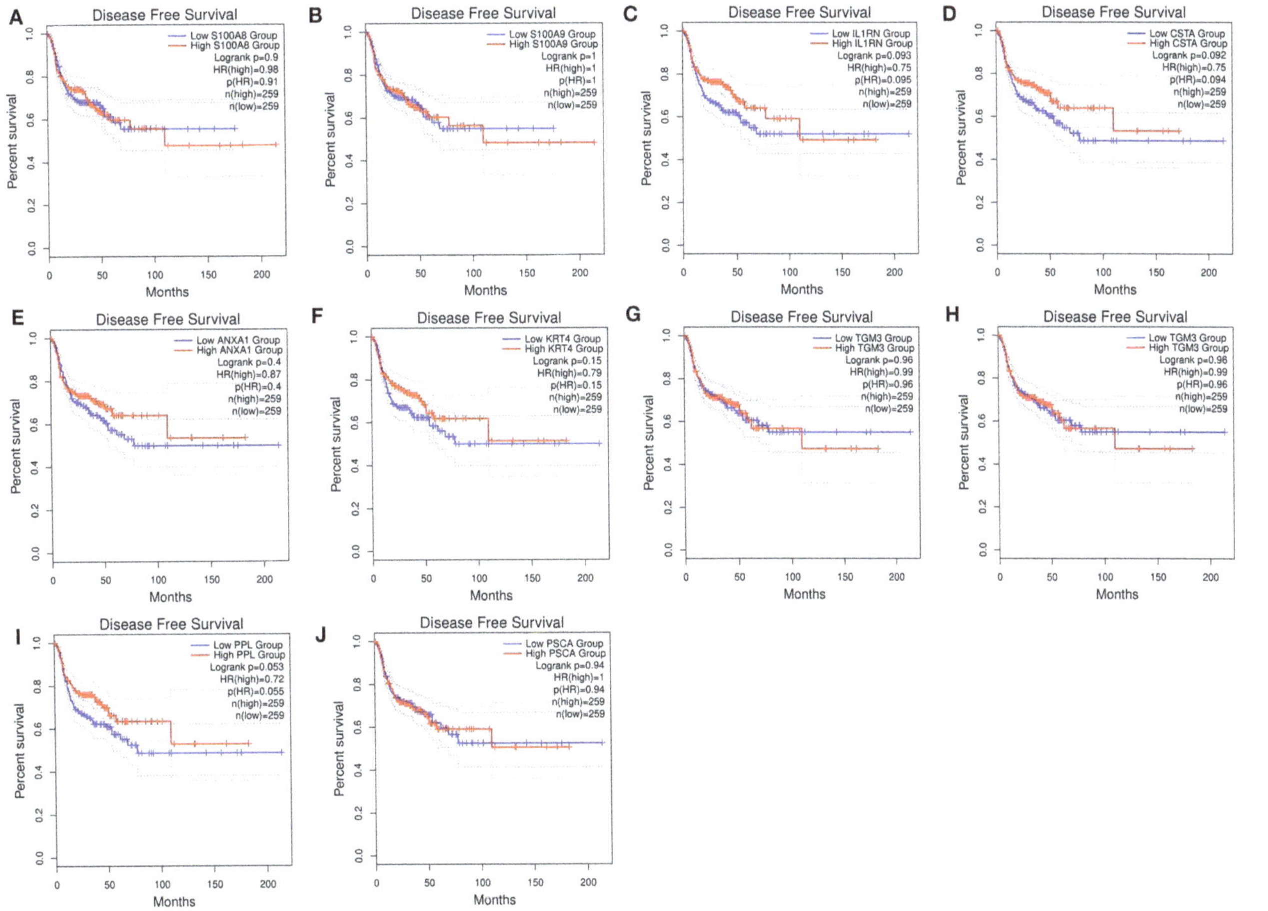

FIGURE 9 | Disease-free survival (DFS) analysis of 10 hub genes in HNSCC patients from the GEPIA2 database. **(A)** Survival analysis for S100A8 in HNSCC. **(B)** Survival analysis for S100A9 in HNSCC. **(C)** Survival analysis for IL1RN in HNSCC. **(D)** Survival analysis for CSTA in HNSCC. **(E)** Survival analysis for ANXA1 in HNSCC. **(F)** Survival analysis for KRT4 in HNSCC. **(G)** Survival analysis for TGM3 in HNSCC. **(H)** Survival analysis for SCEL in HNSCC. **(I)** Survival analysis for PPL in HNSCC. **(J)** Survival analysis for PSCA in HNSCC. The patients were stratified into high-level group (red) and low-level group (green) according to median expression of the gene. Log-rank $P < 0.05$ was considered to be a statistically significant difference.

package. After screening of GO enrichment analysis, we observed several enriched gene sets shown in **Figure 5**. The biological process (BP) of 29 genes are mainly enriched in epidermis development and epidermal cell differentiation. For the result of the cellular component (CC), it was revealed that these genes were mainly involved in apical plasma membrane, apical part of cell, and cell-cell junction. Moreover, in the molecular function (MF) analysis, peptidase regulator activity and enzyme inhibitor activity were suggested to be related to the 29 genes.

PPI Network Construction and Hub Genes Identification

The PPI network among the overlapped genes was established by using the STRING database, with 21 nodes and 25 edges (**Figure 6A**). The hub genes selected from the PPI network using the MCC algorithm of CytoHubba plugin were shown in **Figure 6B**. According to the MCC sores, the top ten highest-scored genes, including S100 calcium-binding protein A8 (S100A8), S100 calcium-binding protein A9 (S100A9), Interleukin-1 receptor antagonist (IL1RN), Cystatin A (CSTA), Annexin-A1 (ANXA1), Keratin 4 (KRT4), Transglutaminase 3 (TGM3), Sciellin (SCEL), Periplakin (PPL), and Prostate Stem Cell Antigen (PSCA), were selected as the hub genes.

Verification of the Expression Patterns, the Prognostic Values, and Protein Expression of Hub Genes

After the ten hub genes (S100A8, S100A9, IL1RN, CSTA, ANXA1, KRT4, TGM3, SCEL, PPL, and PSCA) were screened out by CytoHubba plugin, we verified the expression levels of the hub genes among the patients of the TCGA database. As shown in **Figure 7**, all of the ten hub genes were found to be significantly downregulated in HNSCC carcinoma compared with normal tissues. In addition, OS and DFS analyses of the ten hub genes were performed by Kaplan–Meier plotter using the R *survival* package (**Figure 8**) and the GEPIA2 database (**Figure 9**) for investigating the prognostic values of the hub gens in the HNSCC patients. Of the ten hub genes, the Kaplan–Meier analyses suggested that the lower expression level of CSTA was significantly associated with worse OS of the HNSCC patients ($P < 0.05$) (**Figure 8D**), while with DFS there was no significant difference observed in HNSCC patients with an expression level of CSTA ($P < 0.05$) (**Figure 9D**). Furthermore, the protein levels of the CSTA gene was significantly lower in tumor tissues compared with normal tissues based on the HPA database (**Figure 10**). All the above-mentioned observations confirmed down-expression of CSTA is associated with worse prognosis and lower overall survival in HNSCC patients.

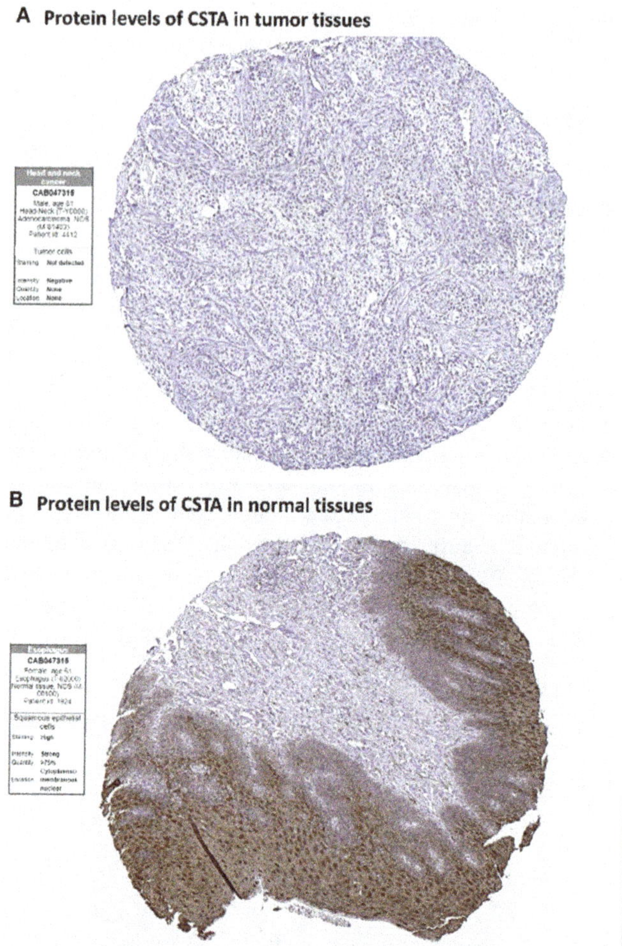

FIGURE 10 | Immunohistochemistry of the CSTA gene in HNSCC and normal tissues from the human protein atlas (HPA) database. **(A)** Protein levels of CSTA in HNSCC tissues (antibody CAB047315; staining: not detected; intensity: negative; quantity: none). **(B)** Protein levels of CSTA in normal oral mucosa tissues (antibody CAB047315; staining: high; intensity: strong; quantity: >75%).

DISCUSSION

Head and neck squamous cell carcinomas (HNSCC) are a group of cancers found in several regions, including the mouth, nose, throat, larynx, sinuses, or salivary glands. Although the treatment of head and neck cancer has improved, the prognosis of patients is generally poor due to the lack of precise molecular targets. Therefore, better biomarkers for specific prognosis and progression of HNSCC are demanded. In this study, a total of 29 significant genes with the same expression trends were identified in the TCGA and GSE6631 databases using integrated bioinformatic analysis. As suggested in functional annotation analysis by the *clusterProfiler* package, these genes were mainly enriched in epidermis development and differentiation, which are basic processes in cell proliferation. Furthermore, according to MCC scores from the CytoHubba plugin in Cytoscape, the top 10 HNSCC-related genes were screened out (namely S100A8, S100A9, IL1RN, CSTA, ANXA1, KRT4, TGM3, SCEL, PPL, and PSCA) and all their expression patterns were found be downregulated in HNSCC tissues compared with the normal controls. Among them, CSTA downexpression was significantly associated with poor overall survival in head and neck cancers. Finally, survival and immunohistochemical analysis for CSTA was carried out.

CSTA, also known as Cystatin A or stefin A, is a member of the cystatin superfamily. It is an intracellular inhibitor regulating the activities of cystatin proteinase and has an important role in desmosome-mediated cell-cell adhesion (29, 30). Furthermore, lower mRNA levels of CSTA have been reported in breast (31), prostate (32), skin (30), and esophagus tumors (33) as compared to adjacent control tissues (34, 35). In our study, CSTA was down-regulated in tumor tissues compared with normal tissues, showing a significant correlation with HNSCC. Previous studies demonstrated that higher levels of CSTA in tumor tissues have been shown to correlate with a favorable prognosis of patients with HNSCC, that was consistent with our finding of survival analysis (36–39).

As with all research, our study also had limitations about the classification of tumors to different subtypes. Although we provided a comprehensive bioinformatics analysis to identify potential diagnostic genes between cancer and normal tissues, it may not be very accurate for each patient with HNSCC subtypes. Moreover, the molecular mechanisms involved in the survival-related genes that affected the prognosis of HNSCC patients should be further validated through a series of experiments.

In summary, by integrating WGCNA with differential gene expression analysis, our study generated the significant survival-related gene CSTA that has potential for prognosis prediction in HNSCC.

AUTHOR CONTRIBUTIONS

J-HC, CW, and CL: conceptualization and methodology. CW and J-HC: software and data curation. JT and CL: validation. J-HC and CL: writing—original draft preparation. CW and JT: writing—review, editing, and supervision.

REFERENCES

1. Marur S, Forastiere AA. Head and neck squamous cell carcinoma: update on epidemiology, diagnosis, and treatment. *Mayo Clin Proc.* (2016) 91:386–96. doi: 10.1016/j.mayocp.2015.12.017
2. Bray F, Ferlay J, Soerjomataram I, Siegel RL, Torre LA, Jemal A. Global cancer statistics 2018: GLOBOCAN estimates of incidence and mortality worldwide for 36 cancers in 185 countries. *CA Cancer J Clin.* (2018) 68:394–424. doi: 10.3322/caac.21492
3. Spitz MR. Epidemiology and risk factors for head and neck cancer. *Semin Oncol.* (1994) 21:281–8.
4. Marur S, D'Souza G, *Westra* WH, Forastiere AA. HPV-associated head and neck cancer: a virus-related cancer epidemic. *Lancet Oncol.* (2010) 11:781–9. doi: 10.1016/S1470-2045(10)70017-6
5. D'Souza G, Dempsey A. The role of HPV in head and neck cancer and review of the HPV vaccine. *Prev Med.* (2011) 53 (Suppl. 1):S5–11. doi: 10.1016/j.ypmed.2011.08.001
6. Ragin CC, Modugno F, Gollin SM. The epidemiology and risk factors of head and neck cancer: a focus on human papillomavirus. *J Dent Res.* (2007) 86:104–14. doi: 10.1177/154405910708600202
7. Can T. Introduction to bioinformatics. *Methods Mol Biol.* (2014) 1107:51–71. doi: 10.1007/978-1-62703-748-8_4
8. Langfelder PS. Horvath WGCNA: an R package for weighted correlation network analysis. *BMC Bioinform.* (2008) 9:559. doi: 10.1186/1471-2105-9-559
9. Zhang B, Horvath S. A general framework for weighted gene co-expression network analysis. *Stat Appl Genet Mol Biol.* (2005) 4:17. doi: 10.2202/1544-6115.1128
10. Li J, Zhou D, Qiu W, Shi Y, Yang JJ, Chen S, et al. Application of weighted gene co-expression network analysis for data from paired design. *Sci Rep.* (2018) 8:622. doi: 10.1038/s41598-017-18705-z
11. Saris CGJ, Horvath S, van Vught WJP, van Es MA, Blauw HM, Fuller TF, et al. Weighted gene co-expression network analysis of the peripheral blood from amyotrophic lateral sclerosis patients. *BMC Genomics.* (2009) 10:405. doi: 10.1186/1471-2164-10-405
12. Yang Y, Han L, Yuan Y, Li J, Hei N, Liang H. Gene co-expression network analysis reveals common system-level properties of prognostic genes across cancer types. *Nat Commun.* (2014) 5:3231. doi: 10.1038/ncomms4231
13. Segundo-Val IS, Sanz-Lozano CS. Introduction to the Gene Expression Analysis. *Methods Mol Biol.* (2016) 1434:29–43. doi: 10.1007/978-1-4939-3652-6_3
14. Colaprico A, Silva TC, Olsen C, Garofano L, Cava C, Garolini D, et al. TCGAbiolinks: an R/Bioconductor package for integrative analysis of TCGA data. *Nucleic Acids Res.* (2016) 44:e71. doi: 10.1093/nar/gkv1507
15. Robinson MD, McCarthy DJ, Smyth GK. edgeR: a Bioconductor package for differential expression analysis of digital gene expression data. *Bioinformatics.* (2010) 26:139–40. doi: 10.1093/bioinformatics/btp616
16. Sean D, Meltzer PS. GEOquery. *Bioinformatics.* (2007) 23:1846–7. doi: 10.1093/bioinformatics/btm254
17. Wang CCN, Li CY, Cai JH, Sheu PC, J.Tsai JP, Wu MY, et al. Identification of prognostic candidate genes in breast cancer by integrated bioinformatic analysis. *J Clin Med.* (2019) 8:1160. doi: 10.3390/jcm8081160
18. Ritchie ME, Phipson B, Wu D, Hu Y, Law CW, Shi W, et al. Limma powers differential expression analyses for RNA-sequencing and microarray studies. *Nucleic Acids Res.* (2015) 43:e47. doi: 10.1093/nar/gkv007
19. Wickham H. *Ggplot2: Elegant Graphics for Data Analysis.* (2009) Dordrecht; New York, NY: Springer.
20. Chen H, and Boutros PC. VennDiagram: a package for the generation of highly-customizable Venn Euler diagrams in R. *BMC Bioinform.* (2011) 12:35. doi: 10.1186/1471-2105-12-35
21. Yu G, Wang LG, Han Y, He QY. clusterProfiler: an R package for comparing biological themes among gene clusters. *Omics.* (2012) 16:284–7. doi: 10.1089/omi.2011.0118
22. Gene Ontology Consortium. The Gene Ontology (GO) project in 2006. *Nucleic Acids Res.* (2006) 34:D322–6. doi: 10.1093/nar/gkj021
23. Szklarczyk D, Gable AL, Lyon D, Junge A, Wyder S, Huerta-Cepas J, et al. STRING v11: protein-protein association networks with increased coverage, supporting functional discovery in genome-wide experimental datasets. *Nucleic Acids Res.* (2019) 47:D607–13. doi: 10.1093/nar/gky1131
24. Shannon P, Markiel A, Ozier O, Baliga NS, Wang JT, Ramage D, et al. Cytoscape: a software environment for integrated models of biomolecular interaction networks. *Genome Res.* (2003) 13:2498–504. doi: 10.1101/gr.1239303
25. Chin CH, Chen SH, Wu HH, Ho CW, Ko MT, Lin CY. cytoHubba: identifying hub objects and sub-networks from complex interactome. *BMC Syst Biol.* (2014) 8(Suppl. 4):S11. doi: 10.1186/1752-0509-8-S4-S11

26. Tang Z, Kang B, Li C, Chen T, Zhang Z. GEPIA2: an enhanced web server for large-scale expression profiling and interactive analysis. *Nucleic Acids Res.* (2019) 47:W556–60. doi: 10.1093/nar/gkz430
27. Thul PJ, Lindskog C. The human protein atlas: a spatial map of the human proteome. *Protein Sci.* (2018) 27:233–44. doi: 10.1002/pro.3307
28. Maity B, Sheff D, Fisher RA. Immunostaining: detection of signaling protein location in tissues, cells and subcellular compartments. *Methods Cell Biol.* (2013) 113:81–105. doi: 10.1016/B978-0-12-407239-8.00005-7
29. Blaydon DC, Nitoiu D, Eckl KM, Cabral RM, Bland P, Hausser I, et al. Mutations in CSTA, encoding Cystatin A, underlie exfoliative ichthyosis and reveal a role for this protease inhibitor in cell-cell adhesion. *Am J Hum Genet.* (2011) 89:564–71. doi: 10.1016/j.ajhg.2011.09.001
30. Gupta A, Nitoiu D, Brennan-Crispi D, Addya S, Riobo NA, Kelsell DP, et al. Cell cycle- and cancer-associated gene networks activated by Dsg2: evidence of cystatin a deregulation and a potential role in cell-cell adhesion. *PLoS ONE.* (2015) 10:e0120091. doi: 10.1371/journal.pone.0120091
31. Duivenvoorden HM, Rautela J, Edgington-Mitchell LE, Spurling A, Greening DW, Nowell CJ, et al. Myoepithelial cell-specific expression of stefin A as a suppressor of early breast cancer invasion. *J Pathol.* (2017) 243:496–509. doi: 10.1002/path.4990
32. Mirtti T, Alanen K, Kallajoki M, Rinne A, Soderstrom KO. Expression of cystatins, high molecular weight cytokeratin, and proliferation markers in prostatic adenocarcinoma and hyperplasia. *Prostate.* (2003) 54:290–8. doi: 10.1002/pros.10196
33. Luo A, Kong J, Hu G, Liew CC, Xiong M, Wang X, et al. Discovery of Ca2+-relevant and differentiation-associated genes downregulated in esophageal squamous cell carcinoma using cDNA microarray. *Oncogene.* (2004) 23:1291–9. doi: 10.1038/sj.onc.1207218
34. Kos J, Lah TT. Cysteine proteinases and their endogenous inhibitors: target proteins for prognosis, diagnosis and therapy in cancer (review). *Oncol Rep.* (1998) 5:1349–61. doi: 10.3892/or.5.6.1349
35. Kos J, Krasovec M, Cimerman N, Nielsen HJ, Christensen IJ, Brunner N. Cysteine proteinase inhibitors stefin A, stefin B, and cystatin C in sera from patients with colorectal cancer: relation to prognosis. *Clin Cancer Res.* (2000) 6:505–11.
36. Ma Y, Chen Y, Li Y, Grün K, Berndt A, Zhou Z, et al. Cystatin A suppresses tumor cell growth through inhibiting epithelial to mesenchymal transition in human lung cancer. *Oncotarget.* (2018) 9:14084–98. doi: 10.18632/oncotarget.23505
37. Strojan P, Budihna M, Smid L, Svetic B, Vrhovec I, Kos J, et al. Prognostic significance of cysteine proteinases cathepsins B and L and their endogenous inhibitors stefins A and B in patients with squamous cell carcinoma of the head and neck. *Clin Cancer Res.* (2000) 6:1052–62.
38. Anicin A, Gale N, Smid L, Kos J, Strojan P. Expression of stefin A is of prognostic significance in squamous cell carcinoma of the head and neck. *Eur Arch Otorhinolaryngol.* (2013) 270:3143–51. doi: 10.1007/s00405-013-2465-5
39. Ralhan R, Desouza LV, Matta A, Tripathi SC, Ghanny S, Datta Gupta S, et al. Discovery and verification of head-and-neck cancer biomarkers by differential protein expression analysis using iTRAQ labeling, multidimensional liquid chromatography, and tandem mass spectrometry. *Mol Cell Proteomics.* (2008) 7:1162–73. doi: 10.1074/mcp.M700500-MCP200

2

Pinostilbene Hydrate Inhibits the Migration and Invasion of Human Nasopharyngeal Carcinoma Cells by Downregulating MMP-2 Expression and Suppressing Epithelial–Mesenchymal Transition Through the Mitogen-Activated Protein Kinase Signaling Pathways

Pao-Yu Tseng[1†], *Yen-Tze Liu*[2,3,4,5†], *Chia-Chieh Lin*[5], *Yi-Ching Chuang*[5], *Yu-Sheng Lo*[5], *Yi-Ting Hsi*[5], *Ming-Ju Hsieh*[3,4,5,6*] and *Mu-Kuan Chen*[1*]

[1] Department of Otorhinolaryngology, Head and Neck Surgery, Changhua Christian Hospital, Changhua, Taiwan, [2] Department of Family Medicine, Changhua Christian Hospital, Changhua, Taiwan, [3] Institute of Medicine, Chung Shan Medical University, Taichung, Taiwan, [4] Department of Holistic Wellness, Mingdao University, Changhua, Taiwan, [5] Oral Cancer Research Center, Changhua Christian Hospital, Changhua, Taiwan, [6] Graduate Institute of Biomedical Sciences, China Medical University, Taichung, Taiwan

***Correspondence:**
Ming-Ju Hsieh
170780@cch.org.tw
Mu-Kuan Chen
53780@cch.org.tw

† These authors have contributed equally to this work

Background: Nasopharyngeal carcinoma (NPC) is one of the most common head and neck cancers in East and Southeast Asia. During the past decades, advances in radiotherapy and chemotherapy had shown the improvement in tumor control with fewer side effects. Nevertheless, metastasis of NPC causes treatment failure and is often associated with poor clinical outcome and cancer mortality.

Hypothesis/Purpose: Pinostilbene hydrate (PSH) was recently demonstrated to have anti-metastatic properties on human oral cancers. However, the effects of PSH on NPC cells remain unknown.

Methods and Results: This study aims to investigate the anti-cancer ability of PSH on human NPC by wound healing, transwell assays, zymography assay, and Western blot assay to explore the possible underlying mechanisms. PSH significantly reduced the migrated distance of NPC cells in a dose-dependent manner and the abilities of cancer cell migration and invasion were markedly inhibited. The activity and the expression of MMP-2 were also significantly decreased after treatment with PSH. Furthermore, combined treatment of PSH with ERK1/2 inhibitor (U0126) caused significant elevation of the activity and the expression of MMP-2. Additionally, PSH upregulated the expression levels of E-cadherin and Claudin-1 while downregulating that of N-cadherin and vimentin on both NPC cell lines.

Conclusion: Our research illustrates that PSH inhibits the migration and invasion of human NPC cells. After exposure to PSH on NPC, the expression of MMP-2 is downregulated and EMT is suppressed through MAPK signaling pathways. These observations suggest that PSH could be a potential anti-metastatic agent for patients with NPC.

Keywords: pinostilbene hydrate, MMP-2, epithelial–mesenchymal transition, MAPK, nasopharyngeal carcinoma

INTRODUCTION

Nasopharyngeal carcinoma (NPC), a malignant epithelial tumor arising from the lining of the nasopharynx, is commonly found at the fossa of Rosenmüller. It has a distinct geographical and ethnic distribution. Many of new cases were reported in east and southeast parts of Asia (1). Worldwide, an estimated 87,000 incident cases and 51,000 deaths occur annually, accounting for about 0.6% of the global cancer burden (1). In Taiwan, the age-adjusted incidence rate of NPC per 100,000 person-years is 8.18 for men and 2.35 for women (2), in contrast to <1 in North America and Europe for both sexes (1). Many risk factors are associated with NPC, including Epstein-Barr virus (EBV) infection (3), host genetic susceptibility in endemic regions (4–6), dietary exposure to salted fish and environment factors (7, 8). Depending on the histological appearance, the World Health Organization (WHO) subtypes NPC as keratinizing squamous cell carcinoma (SCC), non-keratinizing carcinoma and basaloid SCC. Non-keratinizing carcinoma is further sub-categorized into differentiated or undifferentiated tumors (9). In regions with endemic NPC, undifferentiated carcinoma comprises over 95% of cases and the vast majority are associated with EBV infection (10, 11).

During the past decades, advances in population screening, diagnostic imaging, intensity-modulated radiotherapy (IMRT) and systemic agents have driven the improvement in disease control and survival (12, 13). The primary treatment for early stage patients is definitive radiotherapy and the addition of chemotherapy for locally advanced cases has shown a benefit in overall survival (12, 14). However, the metastatic potentiality of NPC remains the major reason of treatment failure for patients; the 5- and 8-years distant metastatic rates were reported as 14.5 and 16.4% in the era of IMRT (15). Furthermore, around 15% of cases were found to have distant metastases at initial staging in endemic NPC (16). Therefore, an effort must be made to optimize the management of tumor invasion and migration in order to achieve a better clinical outcome.

Cancer metastasis is a complex process; it involves the translocation of a cancer cell to a distant organ and the colonization of tumor cells at distant site (17). The metastatic dissemination consists of a series of sequential, interrelated steps: cancer cells invade the host stroma and surrounding tissue, enter the lymphatic channels and blood systems (intravasation), survive in the circulation and translocate to distant organs through the bloodstream, exit from the bloodstream (extravasation), survive the foreign microenvironment of distant tissues, and finally proliferate within the organ parenchyma into a macroscopic metastatic tumor (colonization) (17, 18).

Invasion of ECM is another critical process in cancer metastasis; both chemokine signaling and interactions between cancer cells and physical components of the metastatic niche are involved (17, 19). The matrix metalloproteinases (MMPs), a family of zinc-dependent endopeptidases that consist of more than 20 human MMPs, are the most prominent proteinases associated with cancer progression. Numerous studies had found the upregulated activity of MMPs in head and neck SCC and a negative association between the MMP level and the prognosis (20–24). Therefore, to understand how MMPs work in metastasis of NPC may help us to find more ways of tumor control.

People are increasing their interests in studying naturally extracted compounds or their analogs as one of anti-cancer agents. Resveratrol (*trans*-3,5,4′-trihydroxystilbene), existing in grapes, berries and red wine, is one of the well-studied agents with potential roles in both cancer prevention and treatment (25, 26). Resveratrol also showed synergistic effects with 5-fluoruracyl and cisplatin in the adjuvant therapy which increased the chemosensitization of cancers (27, 28). While resveratrol is unstable in the environment, it is very sensitive to air and light. For years, many derivatives of resveratrol were investigated and studies demonstrated that methylated resveratrol derivatives were more effective in the treatment of cancer with better bioavailability and bioactivity (29–31). Pinostilbene (3,4'-dihydroxy-5-methoxystilbene) is one of the naturally occurring methylated derivatives of resveratrol; it was reported to exert a potent neuroprotective effect against parkinsonism mimetic 6-hydroxydopamine-induced neurotoxicity in SH-SY5Y cells (31) and inhibitory effects on human colon cancer cells (32). More recently, study also found the antimetastatic effects of pinostilbene hydrate (PSH) on human oral SCC by downregulation of MMP-2 through mitogen-activated protein kinase (MAPK) signaling pathway (33). However, anti-cancer ability of PSH on NPC cells remains unknown. Here we try to evaluate the effects of PSH on NPC-039 and NPC-BM cells and discuss the possible involved mechanisms.

MATERIALS AND METHODS

Reagents

Pinostilbene hydrate (3, 4′-Dihydroxy-5-methoxy-trans-stilbene hydrate, PSH) (≥95% purity) was purchased from Sigma-Aldrich (St. Louis, MO, USA) and dissolved in pure grade dimethyl sulfoxide (DMSO). Antibodies against MMP-2, protein kinase B (PKB, also known as AKT), phospho-AKT (p-AKT), p38, phospho-p38 (p-p38), extracellular signal-regulated kinase 1/2 (ERK 1/2), phospho-ERK 1/2 (p-ERK1/2), c-Jun N-terminal

Abbreviations: NPC, Nasopharyngeal carcinoma; PSH, Pinostilbene hydrate; ERKs, Extracellular signal-regulated kinases; JNKs, c-Jun N-terminal kinases; MAPK, Mitogen-activated protein kinases.

kinase 1/2 (JNK 1/2), phospho-JNK1/2 (p-JNK1/2), E-cadherin, Claudin-1, Vimentin, and N-cadherin were purchased from cell Signaling Technology (Danvers, MA, USA) and stored at −20°C. β-actin was bought from Novus Biologicals (Littleton, CO, USA). 3-(4, 5-dimethylthiazol-2-yl)-2, 5-diphenyltetrazolium bromide (MTT) were obtained from Sigma-Aldrich (St Louis, MO, USA) and stored at 4°C. Specific ERK1/2 inhibitor (U0126) and JNK1/2 inhibitor (SP600125) were purchased from Santa Cruz Biotechnology (Santa Cruz, CA, USA) and stored at −20°C.

Cell Culture

The human NPC cell lines NPC-BM and NPC-039 were provided by doctor Jen-Tsun Lin, Hematology and Oncology, Changhua Christian Hospital. The human nasopharyngeal normal primary cell line was obtained from Celprogen (Torrance, CA). The cells were cultured in RPMI 1640 Medium (Gibco BRL, Grand Island, NY, USA) supplemented with 10% fetal bovine serum (FBS), 1% penicillin/streptomycin, 1.5 g/l sodium bicarbonate, 1 mM glutamine, and 1 mM sodium pyruvate (Sigma, St. Louis, MO) at 37°C in one atmosphere with 5% CO_2.

Cell Viability (MTT Assay)

The cell viability was determined by MTT assay. NPC-039 and NPC-BM (1×10^4 cells/well) were seeded in 24-well plates and treated with various concentrations of PSH (0, 20, 40, and 80 μM) for 24 h. Then the medium was removed and the cells were incubated with MTT reagent 500 μl (0.5 mg/mL) at 37°C in 5% CO_2 for 4 h. After removing the supernatant, DMSO was added to dissolve the formed formazan crystals. At last, the absorbance of the converted dye was measured using an enzyme-linked immunosorbent assay (ELISA) plate reader at a wavelength of 595 nm to determine the cell viability.

Wound Healing Assay

NPC-039 and NPC-BM cells were seeded on 6-well plates at 5×10^5 cells/well and incubated for 24 h. Then the cells were wounded by scratching with a 200-μl sterile pipette tip. After being washed twice, the cells were treated with PSH (0, 20, 40, and 80 μM) for 24 h. Then the cell migration was observed and photographed at the appropriate fields by using a phase-contrast microscope. The wound closure was monitored for 6 h. The cell-free area in the dish was measured by an inverted microscope (OlympusIX71, Tokyo, Japan) and the cell migrated distance was calculated by ImageJ software. Experiments were performed for at least three times.

Cell Migration and Invasion Assays

Cell migration and invasion assays were performed as previously described (33, 34). NPC-039 and NPC-BM cells were incubated with different concentrations of PSH (0, 20, 40, and 80 μM) for 24 h. For migration assay, the lower chamber was filled with 600 μL of medium supplemented with 10% FBS in advance. Then the treated cells were seeded to the upper compartment of Transwell (Greiner Bio-One, North Carolina, USA) and incubated at 37°C for 16 h. For invasion assay, the treated cells were seeded in a matrigel (25 mg/50 mL, 60 μl; BD Biosciences, MA) coated upper compartment of chamber with growth medium placed in underneath chamber and incubated for 24 h. The non-migratory cells were removed after incubation for 24 h. Finally, the membrane was fixed with methanol and stained with 10% Giemsa for 2 h. The migratory cell number was quantified by randomly counting at more than three independent visual fields under the light microscope.

Assessment of MMP-2 Activity

NPC-039 and NPC-BM cells were plated in 24-well plates and treated with different concentrations of PSH (0, 20, 40, and 80 μM) for 24 h. Then the cultured medium was collected, mixed with a loading buffer and subjected to 0.1% gelatin−8% sodium dodecyl sulfate-polyacrylamide gel electrophoresis (SDS-PAGE). After the proteins were electrophoretically separated, the gels were washed for 30 min twice in 2.5% Triton X-100 and incubated in reaction buffer (40 mM Tris-HCL, pH 8.0, 0.02% NaN_3, 10 mM $CaCl_2$) at 37°C for overnight. Subsequently, the gel was stained with Coomassie Brilliant Blue R-250 as described previously (33, 34) and the zones corresponding to proteolytic activity of MMP-2 were analyzed by ImageJ software.

Western Blot Analysis

The treated cells were harvested and lysed in ice-cold RIPA buffer to extract all proteins. The protein concentrations were detected using the bicinchoninic acid (BCA) assay. Equal amounts of proteins were separated by 10% polyacrylamide gel and transferred onto a polyvinylidene fluoride (PVDF) membrane (EMD Millipore). After blocking in 5% non-fat milk with TBS-T buffer (20 mM Tris, 137 mM NaCl, pH 7.4) at room temperature for 1 h, membranes were incubated with diluted primary antibody (dilution of 1:1,000) and β-actin at 4°C with gentle shaking for overnight. Then washing with TBS-T for three times, membranes were incubated with the appropriate horseradish peroxidase-conjugated secondary antibody at room temperature for 1 h, rewashing with TBS-T for three times, the blots were visualized using an enhanced chemiluminescence (ECL) reagent (EMD Millipore) and autoradiography. β-actin was used as a loading control. The relative photographic density was quantified by ImageQuant LAS 4000 mini Biomolecular Imager (GE Healthcare Bio-Sciences AB, Björkgatan 30 751 84 Uppsala, Sweden). The relative density was quantitated with gel documentation and analysis (AlphaImager 2000; Alpha Innotech Corporation, San Leandro, CA, USA).

Statistical Analysis

Statistical analysis was performed using SigmaStat 2.0 (Jandel Scientific, San Rafael, CA). Data were presented as the mean ± standard deviation (SD) of at least three independent experiments. Student's t-test was used for comparison among different groups. $P < 0.05$ was considered as statistically significant.

RESULTS

Effects of PSH on the Viability of Human NPC Cells

To examine the cytotoxicity of PSH on NPC cell lines, the cells were evaluated by MTT assay. The chemical structure of PSH is shown in **Figure 1A**. NPC-039, NPC-BM, and human nasopharyngeal normal primary cell lines were treated with various concentrations of PSH (0, 20, 40, and 80 μM) for 24 h. The growth-inhibitory effects were observed (**Figures 1B–D**). Comparing with the control group, PSH significantly inhibited the cell viability when NPC-039 and NPC-BM were incubated with 80 μM of PSH. No significant cytotoxic effects were observed on both cell lines when treated with other concentrations of PSH. A concentration range of 0–80 μM of PSH was then chosen for subsequent experiments.

Inhibitory Effects of PSH on Motility, Migration, and Invasion of NPC Cell Lines

To determine the role of PSH on motility of NPC cells, the wound healing assay was performed. The results showed a significant reduction in migrated distance for both cell lines after exposure to PSH (**Figures 2A–D**). PSH markedly inhibited the wound gap closure in a dose-dependent manner. To evaluate the effects of PSH in migration and invasion of NPC-039 and NPC-BM cells, transwell assays were used. As shown in **Figure 2**, the abilities of cancer cell migration (**Figures 2E,F**) and invasion (**Figures 2G,H**) were significantly decreased by PSH on both cell lines in a dose-dependent manner. These results indicated that PSH played a negative role in migration and invasion of human NPC cells.

PSH Downregulated MMP-2 Activity and Expression on NPC Cells

Degradation of ECM by extracellular proteinases is crucial to the invasion and migration of cancer cells (35, 36) and MMPs are the most famous proteinases associated with tumorigenesis. We investigated the activity of MMP-2 in PSH treated human NPC cells through the gelatin zymography assay. After exposure to PSH (0, 20, 40, and 80 μM) for 24 h, significantly reduced activity of MMP-2 in a dose-dependent manner was noticed on NPC-039 and NPC-BM cells (**Figures 3A–D**). Furthermore, the expression of MMP-2 was examined by Western blot assay. With higher dose of PSH administration on both cell lines, the expression level of MMP-2 became lower (**Figures 3E–H**). PSH significantly downregulated the activity and expression of MMP-2 in human NPC cells.

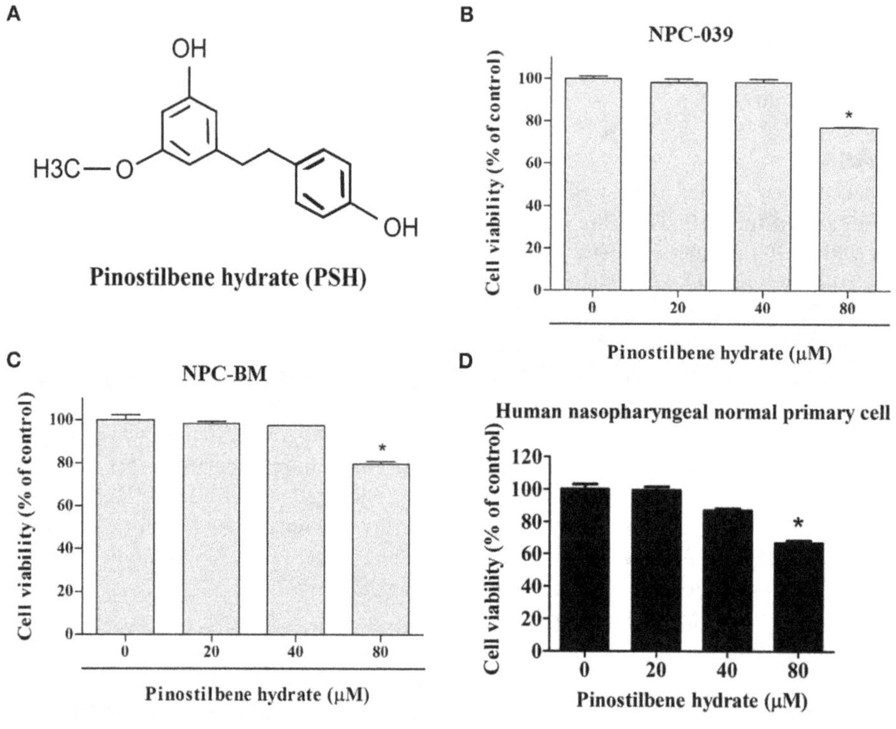

FIGURE 1 | Effects of PSH on the viability of human NPC cells. NPC-039 and NPC-BM cells were treated with various concentrations of PSH (0, 20, 40, and 80 μM) for 24 h. The cell viability was determined by MTT assay. **(A)** Chemical structure of pinostilbene hydrate (PSH). The cytotoxicity was observed on **(B)** NPC-039, **(C)** NPC-BM, and **(D)** human nasopharyngeal normal primary cell lines. PSH significantly inhibited the cell viability of NPC-039 and NPC-BM cells after treatment with 80 μM of PSH. The values are the mean ± SD of at least three independent experiments. $^{*}p < 0.05$.

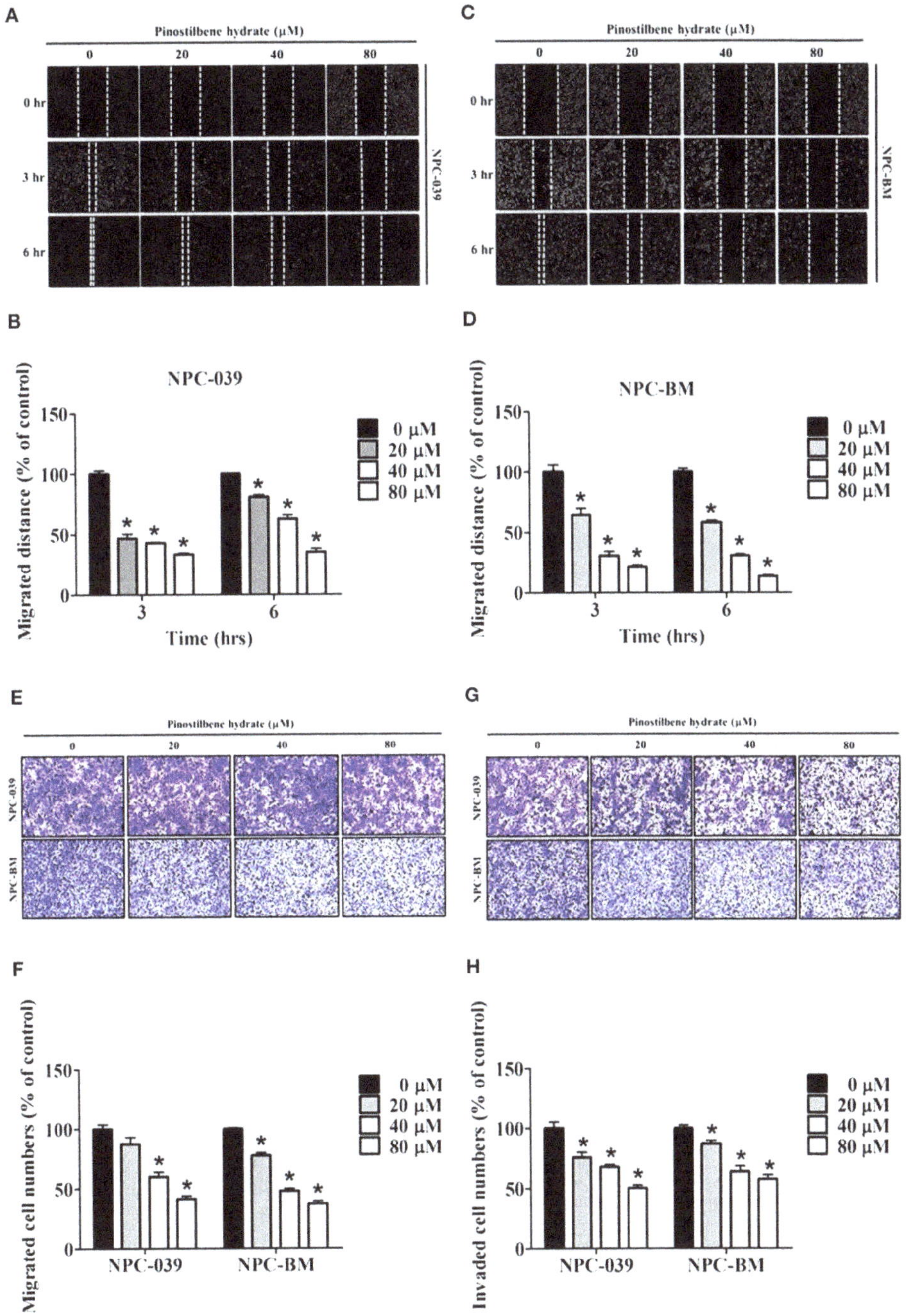

FIGURE 2 | Effects of PSH on motility, migration, and invasion of NPC cell lines. NPC cells were treated with various concentrations of PSH (0, 20, 40, and 80 μM) for 24 h. The migrated distance was determined by the wound healing assay on NPC-039 **(A,B)** and NPC-BM **(C,D)** cell lines. PSH significantly reduced the migrated distance of NPC cells when pictured at 3 and 6 h in a dose-dependent manner. To evaluate the effects of PSH in migration **(E,F)** and invasion **(G,H)** transwell assays were used. The abilities of cell migration and invasion were markedly inhibited by PSH on both cell lines in a dose-dependent manner. The values are the mean ± SD of at least three independent experiments. $^{*}p < 0.05$.

PSH Reduced the Activity of MMP-2 via the MAPK Signaling Pathways on NPC-039 and NPC-BM Cell Lines

Previous studies indicated that the MAPK pathways were involved in the regulation of MMP-2 expression on oral cancer cells (33, 37). To evaluate the associated mechanisms in NPC, we directly measured the expression and the phosphorylation of AKT, ERK1/2, JNK1/2, p38 on NPC cells in response to PSH by Western blot analysis. The findings revealed that PSH promoted the expression of p-ERK1/2 and p-JNK1/2,

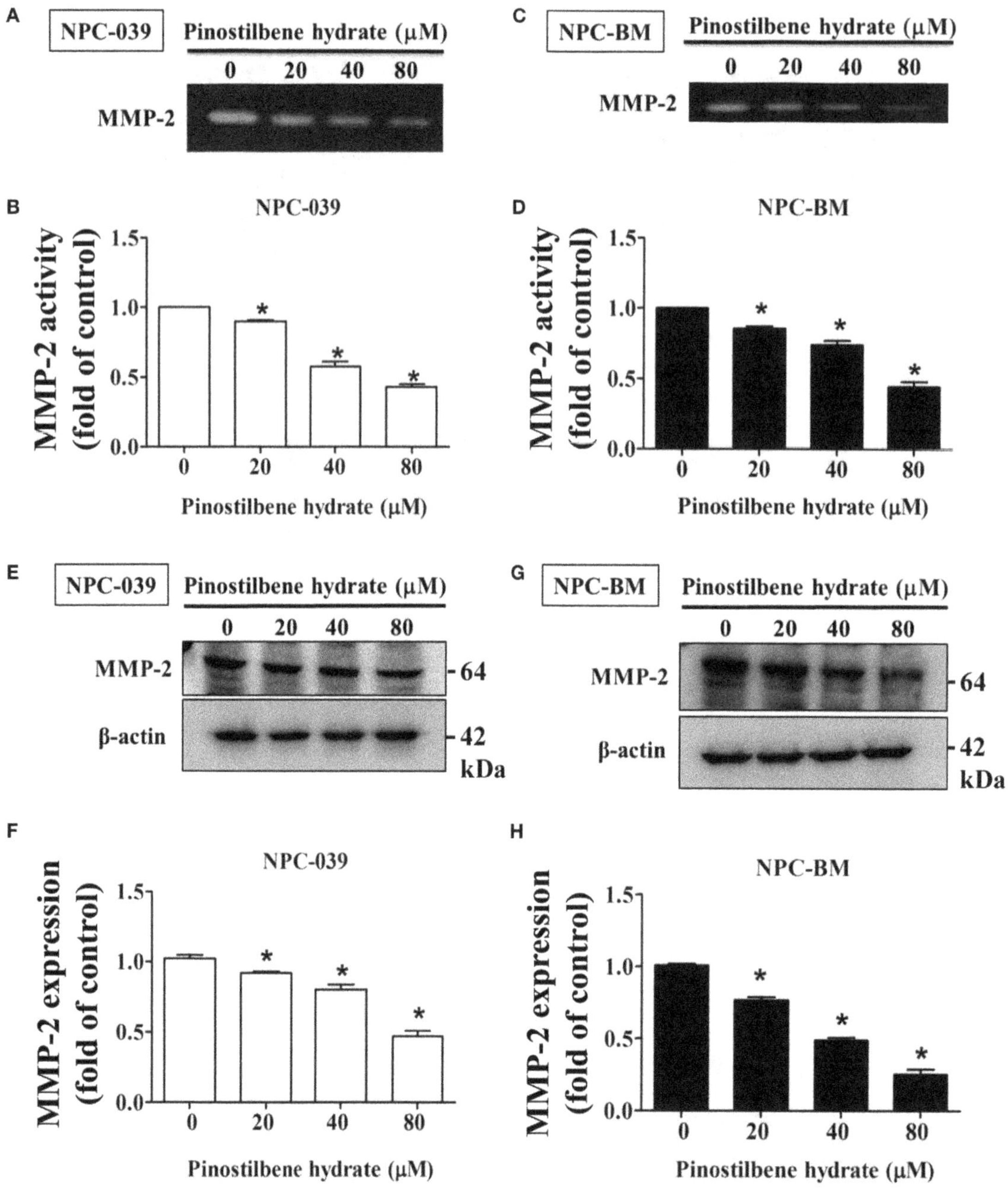

FIGURE 3 | PSH downregulated the activity and expression of MMP-2 in NPC cells. The activity of MMP-2 in PSH treated human NPC cells was examined by the gelatin zymography assay. Significant decreased activity of MMP-2 in a dose-dependent manner was noticed on NPC-039 **(A,B)** and NPC-BM cell lines **(C,D)**. **(E–H)** The expression of MMP-2 level was detected by Western blot assay. PSH significantly reduced the expression of MMP-2 in a dose-dependent manner on both cell lines. β-actin was used as a loading control. The values are the mean ± SD of at least three independent experiments. $^*p < 0.05$.

but not p-AKT and p-p38, on NPC-039 and NPC-BM cell lines in a dose-dependent manner (**Figures 4A–C**). To further clarify whether PSH regulated the activity of MMP-2 through MAPK signaling pathways, cells were pretreated with or without specific ERK1/2 inhibitor (U0126) or JNK1/2 inhibitor (SP600125) for 1 h followed by treatment with PSH (0 and 80 μM) for 24 h. The activity of MMP-2 was then determined by gelatin zymography as previously described in methods. The results showed a significant elevation in activity of MMP-2 on 80 μM PSH treated NPC cells with exposure to U0126 or SP600125 when compared with PSH treatment only (**Figures 4D–G**). In addition, a combined treatment of PSH with U0126, but not SP600125, also significantly contributed to the increased expression of MMP-2 level on both cell lines

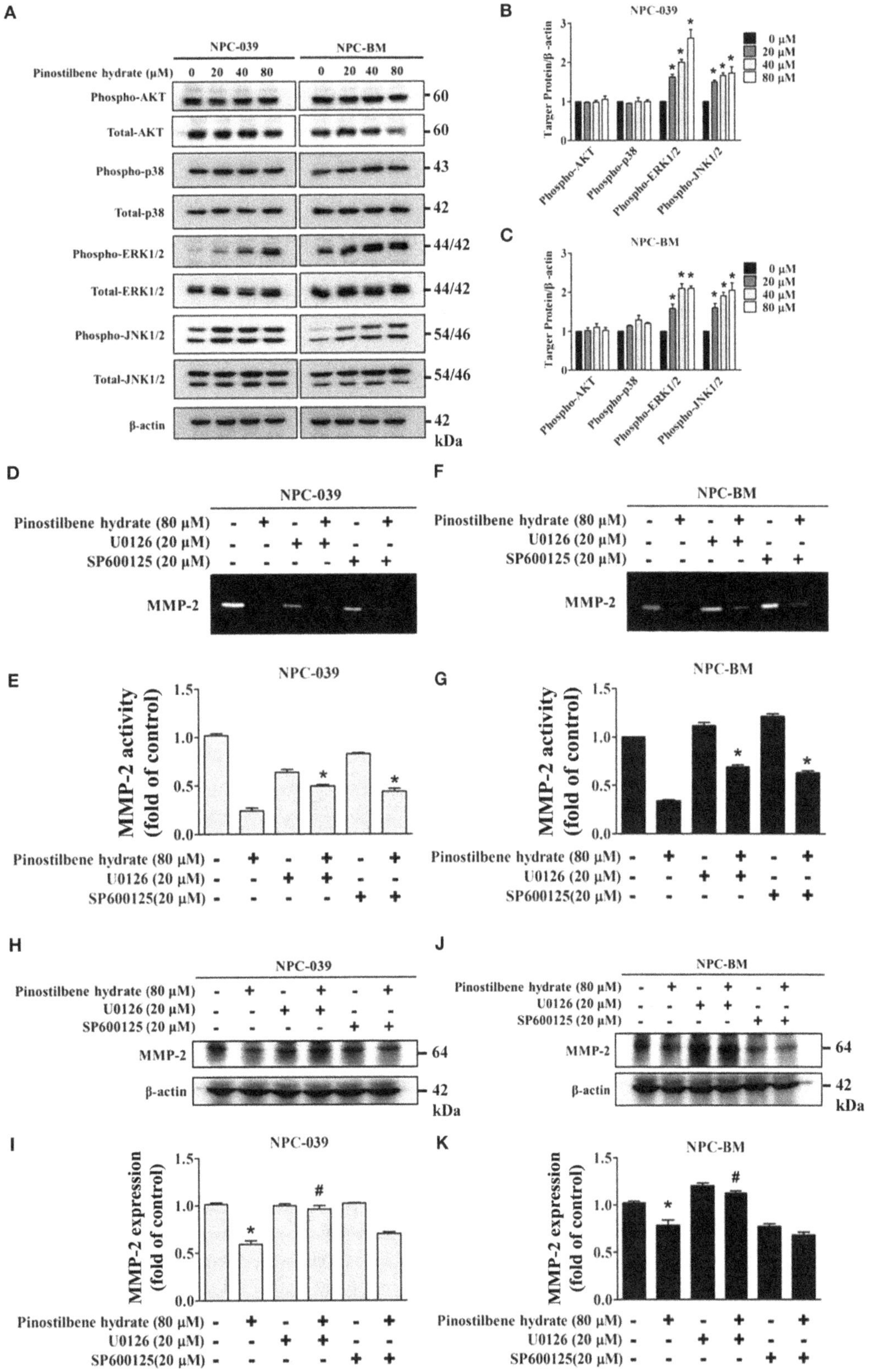

FIGURE 4 | PSH regulated the activity of MMP-2 via the MAPK signaling pathways on NPC-039 and NPC-BM cell lines. **(A)** Cells were treated with different concentrations of PSH (0–80 μM) for 24 h. The p-AKT, p-ERK1/2, p-JNK1/2, and p-p38 were analyzed by Western blot with their respective antibodies. The total

(Continued)

FIGURE 4 | protein of AKT, ERK1/2, JNK1/2, and p38 is also shown. **(B,C)** PSH significantly promoted the expression of p-ERK1/2 and p-JNK1/2 on NPC-039 and NPC-BM cell lines in a dose-dependent manner. Values represent the mean ± SD of at least three independent experiments. $^{*}P < 0.05$, compared with the control (0 μM). **(D–G)** The cells were pretreated with or without ERK1/2 inhibitor (U0126) or JNK1/2 inhibitor (SP600125) followed by treatment with PSH (0 and 80 μM) for 24 h significantly upregulated activity of MMP-2 in combined treatment of PSH with U0126 or SP600125 was noted. $^{*}P < 0.05$, compared with 80 μM PSH treated only group. **(H–K)** A co-treatment of PSH with U0126, but not SP600125, significantly contributed to the elevated expression of MMP-2 level on both cell lines. $^{*}P < 0.05$, compared with the control. $^{\#}P < 0.05$, compared with 80 μM PSH treated only group.

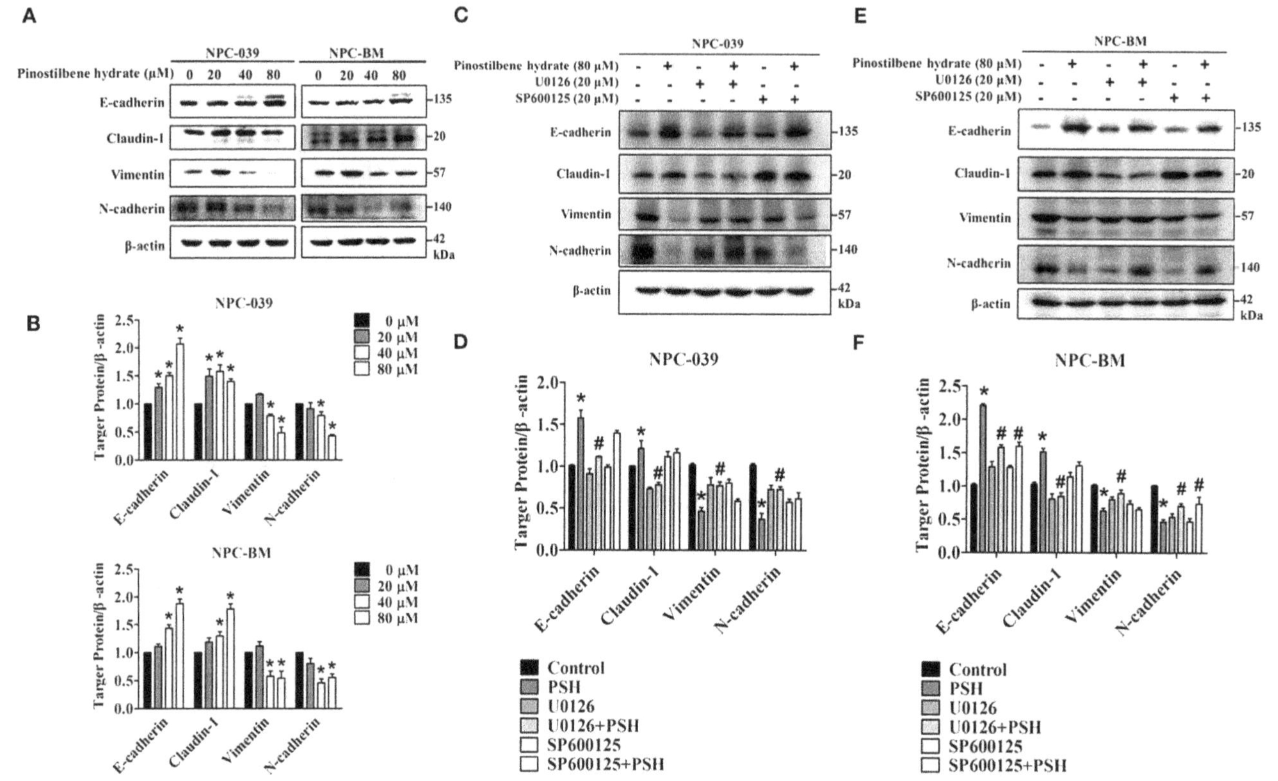

FIGURE 5 | PSH suppressed EMT on NPC cells via the MAPK signaling pathways. **(A,B)** Cells were treated with PSH (0–80 μM) for 24 h. The expression levels of epithelial marker proteins (E-cadherin, Claudin-1) and mesenchymal marker proteins (vimentin, N-cadherin) were analyzed by Western blot. PSH upregulated the expression of E-cadherin and Claudin-1 while downregulating that of N-cadherin and vimentin on both NPC cell lines. $^{*}P < 0.05$, compared with the control (0 μM). **(C,D)** Combined treatment of PSH with U0126 in NPC-039 cells showed significant increased levels of vimentin and N-cadherin with decreased levels of E-cadherin and Claudin-1 when compared with 80 μM PSH treatment only group. $^{*}P < 0.05$, compared with the control. $^{\#}P < 0.05$, compared with 80 μM PSH treated only group. **(E,F)** Relative to the group treated with 80 μM PSH alone, a co-treatment of PSH with U0126 or SP600125 in NPC-BM cell lines elevated the expression levels of mesenchymal markers and suppressed the expression of epithelial marker proteins. $^{*}P < 0.05$, compared with the control. $^{\#}P < 0.05$, compared with 80 μM PSH treated only.

(**Figures 4H–K**). Therefore, the phosphorylation of ERK1/2 was involved in the regulation of MMP-2 in NPC cells with PSH administration.

PSH Suppressed EMT in NPC Cells via the MAPK Signaling Pathways

EMT is also one important process in cancer metastasis. We thus examined the influence of PSH on EMT markers in NPC cell lines. After incubation with various concentrations of PSH (0, 20, 40, and 80 μM) for 24 h, the expression levels of epithelial marker proteins (E-cadherin, Claudin-1) and mesenchymal marker proteins (vimentin, N-cadherin) were analyzed by Western blot assay (**Figures 5A,B**). The findings indicated that PSH upregulated the expression levels of E-cadherin and Claudin-1 while downregulating that of N-cadherin and vimentin on both NPC cell lines ($^{*}P < 0.05$). To further clarify the association between PSH-suppressed EMT and MAPK signaling pathways, cells were pretreated with or without U0126 or SP600125 for 1 h followed by treatment with PSH (0 and 80 μM) for 24 h. The EMT markers were then determined again. In NPC-039 cells, co-treatment with PSH and U0126 showed significant elevated levels of vimentin and N-cadherin with decreased levels of E-cadherin and Claudin-1 as compared with 80 μM PSH treatment only (**Figures 5C,D**). Similar results were also noted in NPC-BM cells; co-treatment of PSH with U0126 or SP600125 increased the expression levels of mesenchymal marker proteins while suppressing the levels of epithelial marker proteins relative to the group treated with 80 μM PSH alone (**Figures 5E,F**). These data revealed that PSH could suppress EMT in human NPC cells through the MAPK pathways.

DISCUSSION

NPC is a radiosensitive tumor and definitive radiotherapy or chemoradiotherapy forms the main treatment for non-metastatic NPC. The introduction of IMRT and the addition of systemic agents to radiotherapy partly contribute to the improvement in disease control and survival (12, 14). However, the great potentiality of systemic dissemination in NPC patients is troublesome and the outcomes for metastatic cases are heterogeneous and can be very poor (12, 15). In previous study, the anti-metastatic effect of PSH on human oral SCC by downregulation of MMP-2 through MAPK pathways was reported (33). Here, we further examined the effects of PSH on two NPC cell lines and discussed the possible mechanisms. Our results suggested that PSH inhibited the migration and invasion of NPC cells by downregulating MMP-2 expression and suppressing EMT through the MAPK signaling pathways.

Cancer metastasis is a complicated process; both EMT and the invasion of ECM play crucial roles during the metastatic dissemination (17, 18). The MMPs are proteinases that involve the ECM invasion, cancer migration and signaling pathways that control cell growth and angiogenesis (35, 36). Among MMPs, MMP-2 and MMP-9 are collagenase that can selectively degrade type IV collagen, a major component of ECM; overexpression of MMP-2 or MMP-9 is associated with more lymph node metastases, distant metastases and poor survival in head and neck SCC (21–24). Furthermore, Wong and colleague reported that a high pro-MMP2 level was correlated with poor survival in patients with undifferentiated NPC (38). Liu et al. demonstrated an increased MMP-9 level as an unfavorable prognostic factor for NPC; patients with elevated MMP-9 level had a significantly shorter overall survival (OS) time and higher MMP-9 level was positively associated with the status of lymph node metastasis and clinical stage (39). Therefore, MMPs inhibitor had become one of molecular targeted therapy in development for treatment of NPC (40). One study had shown zoledronic acid (MMP inhibitor) combined with chemotherapy could improve progression-free survival (PFS) and OS in NPC patients with bone metastases (41).

In the present study, the cell viability of NPC-039 and NPC-BM cells were significantly decreased after exposure to 80 μM of PSH for 24 h (**Figures 1B,C**). A significant reduction in migrated distance was also observed through the wound healing assay; PSH markedly suppressed the wound gap closure in a dose-dependent manner (**Figures 2A–D**). In addition, the ability of cancer cell migration and invasion were inhibited by PSH on both NPC cell lines (**Figures 2E–H**). These results indicated that PSH played a negative role in the migration and invasion of human NPC cells and PSH could be a potential anti-metastatic drug for NPC. Various studies had shown the anti-metastatic effects of certain agent on NPC or oral cancers through the downregulation of MMP-2 or MMP-9 via the MAPK signaling pathways (33, 34, 37, 42). We thus used the gelatin zymography assay and Western blot to analyze the effects of PSH on MMPs in NPC cells. Our findings showed PSH reduced the activity and the expression of MMP-2 in a dose-dependent manner on NPC cells (**Figure 3**). We then further evaluated the mechanisms that involved PSH mediated MMP-2 expression in NPC. The levels of MAPK pathway proteins were examined after treatment with PSH. Our data revealed PSH promoted the expression of p-ERK1/2 and p-JNK1/2, but not p-AKT and p-p38, in human NPC cells (**Figures 4A–C**). Moreover, co-treatment with PSH and ERK1/2 inhibitor (U0126) or JNK1/2 inhibitor (SP600125) contributed to the upregulated activity of MMP-2 in NPC when compared with PSH treatment only group (**Figures 4D–G**). Therefore, MAPK signaling pathways were involved in PSH mediated MMP-2 regulation in NPC and blocking the ERK or JNK pathway might interfere the anti-metastatic ability of PSH to NPC cells.

EMT is also recognized as an important step in the metastasis of malignancies and the level of E-cadherin was negatively correlated with the clinical prognosis in NPC (40, 43–45). Nowadays demethylation of E-cadherin gene is considered to be a potential therapeutic strategy for patients with NPC (46). Some studies demonstrated the inhibitory effects on migration and invasion of NPC cells by suppressing EMT (47, 48). We then observed the influence of PSH on EMT markers in NPC-039 and NPC-BM cells by Western blot assay. After exposure to PSH, expression levels of the epithelial markers E-cadherin and Claudin-1 increased, while that of the mesenchymal markers N-cadherin and vimentin decreased (**Figures 5A,B**). Furthermore, combined treatment with PSH and U0126 or SP600125 showed significantly elevated levels of mesenchymal markers with decreased levels of epithelial markers relative to the group treated with PSH alone (**Figures 5C–F**). Taken together, PSH suppressed the EMT process in NPC cells; the addition of ERK 1/2 inhibitor or JNK1/2 inhibitor reversed this ability and induced NPC cells to regain EMT characteristics which restored the invasiveness of NPC cells. These data suggested that PSH might suppress EMT in human NPC cell lines through the MAPK pathways.

Our results demonstrated that PSH downregulated the activity and the expression of MMP-2 on both NPC-039 and NPC-BM cell lines. A significant reduced migrated distance under the wound healing assay and marked inhibitory effects on the migration and invasion of NPC cells were also observed. After exposure to PSH, the expression of epithelial markers increased, while that of mesenchymal markers decreased, which suggested the ability of PSH to reverse the EMT process in NPC. We also found the associations of MAPK pathways with PSH mediated MMP-2 downregulation and EMT suppression in NPC; ERK and JNK pathways were involved in these molecular mechanisms. In conclusion, PSH inhibited the migration and invasion of human NPC cells *in vitro* by downregulating MMP-2 and suppressing EMT through MAPK signaling pathways. Data obtained from our study indicated that PSH could be a potential anti-metastatic agent for patients with NPC, though more detailed studies may be needed for further application.

AUTHOR CONTRIBUTIONS

P-YT, M-JH, and M-KC: study conception and design. C-CL, Y-CC, Y-SL, and Y-TH: acquisition, analysis, and interpretation of data. P-YT, Y-TL, and M-JH: drafting/revision of the work for intellectual content and context. M-KC: final approval and overall responsibility for the published work. All authors read and approved the final manuscript.

REFERENCES

1. Ferlay J, Soerjomataram I, Dikshit R, Eser S, Mathers C, Rebelo M, et al. Cancer incidence and mortality worldwide: sources, methods and major patterns in GLOBOCAN 2012. *Int J Cancer.* (2015) 136:E359–86. doi: 10.1002/ijc.29210
2. Huang WY, Lin CL, Lin CY, Jen YM, Lo CH, Sung FC, et al. Survival outcome of patients with nasopharyngeal carcinoma: a nationwide analysis of 13 407 patients in Taiwan. *Clin Otolaryngol.* (2015) 40:327–34. doi: 10.1111/coa.12371
3. Andersson-Anvret M, Forsby N, Klein G, Henle W. Relationship between the Epstein-Barr virus and undifferentiated nasopharyngeal carcinoma: correlated nucleic acid hybridization and histopathological examination. *Int J Cancer.* (1977) 20:486–94. doi: 10.1002/ijc.2910200403
4. Bei JX, Jia WH, Zeng YX. Familial and large-scale case-control studies identify genes associated with nasopharyngeal carcinoma. *Semin Cancer Biol.* (2012) 22:96–106. doi: 10.1016/j.semcancer.2012.01.012
5. Hildesheim A, Wang CP. Genetic predisposition factors and nasopharyngeal carcinoma risk: a review of epidemiological association studies, 2000-2011: Rosetta Stone for NPC: genetics, viral infection, and other environmental factors. *Semin Cancer Biol.* (2012) 22:107–16. doi: 10.1016/j.semcancer.2012.01.007
6. Lin DC, Meng X, Hazawa M, Nagata Y, Varela AM, Xu L, et al. The genomic landscape of nasopharyngeal carcinoma. *Nat Genet.* (2014) 46:866–71. doi: 10.1038/ng.3006
7. Ward MH, Pan WH, Cheng YJ, Li FH, Brinton LA, Chen CJ, et al. Dietary exposure to nitrite and nitrosamines and risk of nasopharyngeal carcinoma in Taiwan. *Int J Cancer.* (2000) 86:603–9. doi: 10.1002/(SICI)1097-0215(20000601)86:5<603::AID-IJC1>3.0.CO;2-H
8. Guo X, Johnson RC, Deng H, Liao J, Guan L, Nelson GW, et al. Evaluation of nonviral risk factors for nasopharyngeal carcinoma in a high-risk population of Southern China. *Int J Cancer.* (2009) 124:2942–7. doi: 10.1002/ijc.24293
9. Stelow EB, Wenig BM. Update from the 4th edition of the World Health Organization classification of head and neck tumours: nasopharynx. *Head Neck Pathol.* (2017) 11:16–22. doi: 10.1007/s12105-017-0787-0
10. Nicholls JM. Nasopharyngeal carcinoma: classification and histologic appearances. *Adv Anat Pathol.* (1997) 4:71–84. doi: 10.1097/00125480-199703000-00001
11. Niedobitek G, Hansmann ML, Herbst H, Young LS, Dienemann D, et al. Epstein-Barr virus and carcinomas: undifferentiated carcinomas but not squamous cell carcinomas of the nasopharynx are regularly associated with the virus. *J Pathol.* (1991) 165:17–24. doi: 10.1002/path.1711650105
12. Chua MLK, Wee JTS, Hui EP, Chan ATC. Nasopharyngeal carcinoma. *Lancet.* (2016) 387:1012–24. doi: 10.1016/S0140-6736(15)00055-0
13. Lam WKJ, Chan JYK. Recent advances in the management of nasopharyngeal carcinoma. *F1000Res.* (2018) 7:F1000. doi: 10.12688/f1000research.15066.1
14. Blanchard P, Lee A, Marguet S, Leclercq J, Ng WT, Ma J, et al. Chemotherapy and radiotherapy in nasopharyngeal carcinoma: an update of the MAC-NPC meta-analysis. *Lancet Oncol.* (2015) 16:645–55. doi: 10.1016/S1470-2045(15)70126-9
15. Li AC, Xiao WW, Shen GZ, Wang L, Xu AA, Cao YQ, et al. Distant metastasis risk and patterns of nasopharyngeal carcinoma in the era of IMRT: long-term results and benefits of chemotherapy. *Oncotarget.* (2015) 6:24511–21. doi: 10.18632/oncotarget.4312
16. Tang LQ, Chen QY, Fan W, Liu H, Zhang L, Guo L, et al. Prospective study of tailoring whole-body dual-modality [18F]fluorodeoxyglucose positron emission tomography/computed tomography with plasma Epstein-Barr virus DNA for detecting distant metastasis in endemic nasopharyngeal carcinoma at initial staging. *J Clin Oncol.* (2013) 31:2861–9. doi: 10.1200/JCO.2012.46.0816
17. Chaffer CL, Weinberg RA. A perspective on cancer cell metastasis. *Science.* (2011) 331:1559–64. doi: 10.1126/science.1203543
18. Fidler IJ. The pathogenesis of cancer metastasis: the 'seed and soil' hypothesis revisited. *Nat Rev Cancer.* (2003) 3:453–8. doi: 10.1038/nrc1098
19. Blaha L, Zhang C, Cabodi M, Wong JY. A microfluidic platform for modeling metastatic cancer cell matrix invasion. *Biofabrication.* (2017) 9:045001. doi: 10.1088/1758-5090/aa869d
20. Kusukawa J, Sasaguri Y, Morimatsu M, Kameyama T. Expression of matrix metalloproteinase-3 in stage I and II squamous cell carcinoma of the oral cavity. *J Oral Maxillofac Surg.* (1995) 53:530–4. doi: 10.1016/0278-2391(95)90065-9
21. Hong SD, Hong SP, Lee JI, Lim CY. Expression of matrix metalloproteinase-2 and—9 in oral squamous cell carcinomas with regard to the metastatic potential. *Oral Oncol.* (2000) 36:207–13. doi: 10.1016/S1368-8375(99)00088-3
22. Riedel F, Gotte K, Schwalb J, Bergler W, Hormann K. Expression of 92-kDa type IV collagenase correlates with angiogenic markers and poor survival in head and neck squamous cell carcinoma. *Int J Oncol.* (2000) 17:1099–105. doi: 10.3892/ijo.17.6.1099
23. Shimada T, Nakamura H, Yamashita K, Kawata R, Murakami Y, Fujimoto N, et al. Enhanced production and activation of progelatinase A mediated by membrane-type 1 matrix metalloproteinase in human oral squamous cell carcinomas: implications for lymph node metastasis. *Clin Exp Metastasis.* (2000) 18:179–88. doi: 10.1023/A:1006749501682
24. Yoshizaki T, Maruyama Y, Sato H, Furukawa M. Expression of tissue inhibitor of matrix metalloproteinase-2 correlates with activation of matrix metalloproteinase-2 and predicts poor prognosis in tongue squamous cell carcinoma. *Int J Cancer.* (2001) 95:44–50. doi: 10.1002/1097-0215(20010120)95:1<44::AID-IJC1008>3.0.CO;2-M
25. Shrotriya S, Agarwal R, Sclafani RA. A perspective on chemoprevention by resveratrol in head and neck squamous cell carcinoma. *Adv Exp Med Biol.* (2015) 815:333–48. doi: 10.1007/978-3-319-09614-8_19
26. Varoni EM, Lo Faro AF, Sharifi-Rad J, Iriti M. Anticancer molecular mechanisms of resveratrol. *Front Nutr.* (2016) 3:8. doi: 10.3389/fnut.2016.00008
27. Buhrmann C, Shayan P, Kraehe P, Popper B, Goel A, Shakibaei M. Resveratrol induces chemosensitization to 5-fluorouracil through up-regulation of intercellular junctions, Epithelial-to-mesenchymal transition and apoptosis in colorectal cancer. *Biochem Pharmacol.* (2015) 98:51–68. doi: 10.1016/j.bcp.2015.08.105
28. Ma L, Li W, Wang R, Nan Y, Wang Q, Liu W, et al. Resveratrol enhanced anticancer effects of cisplatin on non-small cell lung cancer cell lines by inducing mitochondrial dysfunction and cell apoptosis. *Int J Oncol.* (2015) 47:1460–8. doi: 10.3892/ijo.2015.3124
29. Tolomeo M, Grimaudo S, Di Cristina A, Roberti M, Pizzirani D, Meli M, et al. Pterostilbene and 3′-hydroxypterostilbene are effective apoptosis-inducing agents in MDR and BCR-ABL-expressing leukemia cells. *Int J Biochem Cell Biol.* (2005) 37:1709–26. doi: 10.1016/j.biocel.2005 03.004
30. Mikstacka R, Przybylska D, Rimando AM, Baer-Dubowska W. Inhibition of human recombinant cytochromes P450 CYP1A1 and CYP1B1 by trans-resveratrol methyl ethers. *Mol Nutr Food Res.* (2007) 51:517–24. doi: 10.1002/mnfr.200600135

31. Chao J, Li H, Cheng KW, Yu MS, Chang RC, Wang M. Protective effects of pinostilbene, a resveratrol methylated derivative, against 6-hydroxydopamine-induced neurotoxicity in SH-SY5Y cells. *J Nutr Biochem.* (2010) 21:482–9. doi: 10.1016/j.jnutbio.2009.02.004
32. Sun Y, Wu X, Cai X, Song M, Zheng J, Pan C, et al. Identification of pinostilbene as a major colonic metabolite of pterostilbene and its inhibitory effects on colon cancer cells. *Mol Nutr Food Res.* (2016) 60:1924–32. doi: 10.1002/mnfr.201500989
33. Hsieh MJ, Chin MC, Lin CC, His YT, Lo YS, Chuang YC, et al. Pinostilbene hydrate suppresses human oral cancer cell metastasis by downregulation of matrix metalloproteinase-2 through the mitogen-activated protein kinase signaling pathway. *Cell Physiol Biochem.* (2018) 50:911–23. doi: 10.1159/000494476
34. Ho HY, Lin CW, Chien MH, Reiter RJ, Su SC, Hsieh YH, et al. Melatonin suppresses TPA-induced metastasis by downregulating matrix metalloproteinase-9 expression through JNK/SP-1 signaling in nasopharyngeal carcinoma. *J Pineal Res.* (2016) 61:479–92. doi: 10.1111/jpi.12365
35. Egeblad M, Werb Z. New functions for the matrix metalloproteinases in cancer progression. *Nat Rev Cancer.* (2002) 2:161–74. doi: 10.1038/nrc745
36. Kessenbrock K, Plaks V, Werb Z. Matrix metalloproteinases: regulators of the tumor microenvironment. *Cell.* (2010) 141:52–67. doi: 10.1016/j.cell.2010.03.015
37. Huang YW, Chuang CY, Hsieh YS, Chen PN, Yang SF, Shih Hsuan L, et al. Rubus idaeus extract suppresses migration and invasion of human oral cancer by inhibiting MMP-2 through modulation of the Erk1/2 signaling pathway. *Environ Toxicol.* (2017) 32:1037–46. doi: 10.1002/tox.22302
38. Wong TS, Kwong DL, Sham JS, Wei WI, Kwong YL, Yuen AP. Clinicopathologic significance of plasma matrix metalloproteinase-2 and−9 levels in patients with undifferentiated nasopharyngeal carcinoma. *Eur J Surg Oncol.* (2004) 30:560–4. doi: 10.1016/j.ejso.2004.02.007
39. Liu Z, Li L, Yang Z, Luo W, Li X, Yang H, et al. Increased expression of MMP9 is correlated with poor prognosis of nasopharyngeal carcinoma. *BMC Cancer.* (2010) 10:270. doi: 10.1186/1471-2407-10-270
40. Liu MT, Chen MK, Huang CC, Huang CY. Prognostic value of molecular markers and implication for molecular targeted therapies in nasopharyngeal carcinoma: an update in an era of new targeted molecules development. *World J Oncol.* (2015) 6:243–61. doi: 10.14740/wjon610w
41. Jin Y, An X, Cai YC, Cao Y, Cai XY, Xia Q, et al. Zoledronic acid combined with chemotherapy bring survival benefits to patients with bone metastases from nasopharyngeal carcinoma. *J Cancer Res Clin Oncol.* (2011) 137:1545–51. doi: 10.1007/s00432-011-1027-8
42. Hsin CH, Huang CC, Chen PN, Hsieh YS, Yang SF, Ho YT, et al. Rubus idaeus inhibits migration and invasion of human nasopharyngeal carcinoma cells by suppression of MMP-2 through modulation of the ERK1/2 pathway. *Am J Chin Med.* (2017) 45:1557–72. doi: 10.1142/S0192415X17500847
43. Huang GW, Mo WN, Kuang GQ, Nong HT, Wei MY, Sunagawa M, et al. Expression of p16, nm23-H1, E-cadherin, and CD44 gene products and their significance in nasopharyngeal carcinoma. *Laryngoscope.* (2001) 111:1465–71. doi: 10.1097/00005537-200108000-00025
44. Li Z, Ren Y, Lin SX, Liang YJ, Liang HZ. Association of E-cadherin and beta-catenin with metastasis in nasopharyngeal carcinoma. *Chin Med J.* (2004) 117:1232–9.
45. Galera-Ruiz H, Rios MJ, Gonzalez-Campora R, De Miguel M, Carmona MI, Moreno AM, et al. The cadherin-catenin complex in nasopharyngeal carcinoma. *Eur Arch Otorhinolaryngol.* (2011) 268:1335–41. doi: 10.1007/s00405-010-1464-z
46. Ran Y, Wu S, You Y. Demethylation of E-cadherin gene in nasopharyngeal carcinoma could serve as a potential therapeutic strategy. *J Biochem.* (2011) 149:49–54. doi: 10.1093/jb/mvq128
47. Wang D, Wu C, Liu D, Zhang L, Long G, Hu G, et al. Ginsenoside Rg3 inhibits migration and invasion of nasopharyngeal carcinoma cells and suppresses epithelial mesenchymal transition. *Biomed Res Int.* (2019) 2019:8407683. doi: 10.1155/2019/8407683
48. Yu D, An X, Fan W, Wang X, He Y, Li B. PNUTS mediates ionizing radiation-induced CNE-2 nasopharyngeal carcinoma cell migration, invasion, and epithelial-mesenchymal transition via the PI3K/AKT signaling pathway. *Onco Targets Ther.* (2019) 12:1205–14. doi: 10.2147/OTT.S188571

3

Predictive Value of Skeletal Muscle Mass in Recurrent/Metastatic Head and Neck Squamous Cell Carcinoma Patients Treated with Immune Checkpoint Inhibitors

Lorena Arribas [1,2,3,4], Maria Plana [3,5], Miren Taberna [2,3,5], Maria Sospedra [6], Noelia Vilariño [5], Marc Oliva [2,3,5], Natalia Pallarés [7], Ana Regina González Tampán [1,3], Luis Miguel Del Rio [8], Ricard Mesia [2,3,9†] and Vickie Baracos [10†]*

[1] Clinical Nutrition Unit, Catalan Institute of Oncology (ICO), L'Hospitalet de Llobregat, Barcelona, Spain, [2] Bellvitge Biomedical Research Institute (IDIBELL), L'Hospitalet de Llobregat, Barcelona, Spain, [3] Head and Neck Cancer Unit, Bellvitge University Hospital, Catalan Institute of Oncology (ICO), L'Hospitalet de Llobregat, Barcelona, Spain, [4] University of Barcelona, Barcelona, Spain, [5] Medical Oncology Department, Catalan Institute of Oncology (ICO), ONCOBELL, L'Hospitalet de Llobregat, Barcelona, Spain, [6] Unitat de Nutrició Clínica i Dietètica, Hospital Universitari Germans Trias i Pujol (HUGTiP), Barcelona, Spain, [7] Unitat de Bioestadística (UBiDi), Bellvitge University Hospital, L'Hospitalet de Llobregat, Barcelona, Spain, [8] Grupo Ascires, CETIR Grupo Médico, Barcelona, Spain, [9] Medical Oncology Department, Catalan Institute of Oncology (ICO)-Badalona, B-ARGO group, Barcelona, Spain, [10] Division of Palliative Care Medicine, Department of Oncology, University of Alberta, Cross Cancer Institute, Edmonton, AB, Canada

***Correspondence:**
Lorena Arribas
larribas@iconcologia.net

†These authors have contributed equally to this work and share senior authorship

Background: Reduced muscle mass has been associated with increased treatment complications in several tumor types. We evaluated the impact of skeletal muscle index (SMI) on prognosis and immune-related adverse events (IrAEs) in a cohort of recurrent/ metastatic (R/M) head and neck squamous cell carcinoma (HNSCC) treated with immune checkpoints inhibitors (ICI).

Methods: A single-institutional, retrospective study was performed including 61 consecutive patients of R/M HNSCC diagnosed between July 2015 and December 2018. SMI was quantified using a CT scan at L3 to evaluate body composition. Median baseline SMI was used to dichotomize patients in low and high SMI. Kaplan-Meier estimations were used to detect overall survival (OS) and progression-free survival (PFS). Toxicity was recorded using Common Terminology Criteria for Adverse Event v4.3.

Results: Patients were 52 men (85.2%) with mean of age 57.7 years (SD 9.62), mainly oral cavity (n = 21; 34.4%). Low SMI was an independent factor for OS in the univariate (HR, 2.06; 95% CI, 1.14–3.73, p = 0.017) and multivariate Cox analyses (HR, 2.99; 95% CI, 1.29–6.94; p = 0.011). PFS was also reduced in patients with low SMI (PFS HR, 1.84; 95% CI, 1.08–3.12; p = 0.025). IrAEs occurred in 29 (47.5%) patients. There was no association between low SMI and IrAEs at any grade (OR, 0.56; 95% CI, 0.20–1.54; p = 0.261). However, grades 3 to 4 IrAEs were developed in seven patients of whom three had low SMI.

Conclusions: Low SMI before ICI treatment in R/M HNSCC patients had a negative impact on OS and PFS. Further prospective research is needed to confirm the role of body composition as a predictive biomarker in ICI treatment.

Keywords: head and neck (H&N) cancer, body composition, muscle mass, immune checkpoint inhibitors, sarcopenia, immune-related adverse events (irAE)

INTRODUCTION

Among patients with head and neck squamous cell carcinoma (HNSCC), between 5% and 10% are diagnosed with metastatic disease. Additionally, despite aggressive multimodal strategies, about 60% of patients treated with radical intention for a locally advanced disease will eventually recur (1). Until the introduction of immunotherapy agents, the median survival was 10.1 months, with an 82% rate of grades 3 to 4 adverse events using the historic standard first-line EXTREME (combining platinum and 5-fluorouracil (5-FU) and cetuximab) (2). Patients with progressive disease after platinum-based chemotherapy have a poor prognosis with a 1-year survival under 5% (3). Hereby, there is an urgent need for improved therapy in the recurrent and metastatic (R/M) population.

Targeting the programmed cell death (ligand)-1 (PD-(L)1) pathway has shown significant activity, and improved overall survival (OS) in patients with previously treated R/M HNSCC, associated with fewer grades 3 or 4 toxicities than standard therapy (4, 5). These results have led to approval of two anti-PD1 agents (pembrolizumab and nivolumab) as second-line treatment for patients with R/M HNSCC who experience disease progression on or after a platinum-based therapy (6, 7). More recently, pembrolizumab has been approved in the first-line setting, alone or in combination with chemotherapy (8). Despite improving the results compared with older strategies, approximately 70% of patients do not benefit from immune checkpoint inhibitors (ICI) as they have progression as the best response, enhancing the need for predictive biomarkers (6, 8).

Patients with R/M HNSCC are at an increased nutritional risk, and malnutrition has been shown to be an independent indicator of prognosis in cancer patients (9). The nutritional deterioration of HNSCC patients is often present from diagnosis and worsens throughout onco-specific treatments (10). This deterioration does not only occur exclusively at the expense of weight alone but also because the loss of muscle mass has been shown to associate with prognosis and complications (10, 11).

Sarcopenia, defined as a reduced skeletal muscle mass that reduce muscle function, is noted in geriatric populations (12). Reduced muscle mass is also prominent in patients at any age with different chronic diseases, including cancer. This is also termed sarcopenia, and it is typically classified in relation to the risk of disease-specific outcomes, such as mortality, surgical complications, or cancer treatment (13). Sarcopenia has been reported to have a significant impact on both OS and complications in cancer patients undergoing onco-specific treatment and/or surgery (14). These results have also been described in head and neck cancer patients (15–18). Although some studies have revealed that low muscle mass may also have a role in the oncological outcomes in patients with melanoma (19, 20) or lung cancer (21, 22) treated with ICI, as far as we know, there are no current studies evaluating the impact of low muscle mass in R/M HNSCC undergoing these therapies.

We aim to evaluate the muscle mass as a predictive biomarker of OS and progression-free survival (PFS) in patients diagnosed with R/M HNSCC treated with ICI. A secondary analysis focused on the association of muscle mass on the onset of immune-related adverse events (IrAES).

MATERIALS AND METHODS

Population and Study Design

This longitudinal retrospective single-center study was approved by the local ethics committee for clinical research (PR302/18). All patients provided written informed consent. Patients diagnosed with R/M HNSCC treated with ICI, regardless of treatment line, from July 2015 and December 2018 at the Catalan Institute of Oncology, were evaluated. Patients were eligible if they had R/M HNSCC and were treated with ICI including anti-PD1 or anti-PDL1 alone or in combination with other ICI (such as anti-CTLA4) or chemotherapy and had a staging full-body computed tomography (CT) scan as part of their pre-treatment procedure (within 10 days prior to the introduction of ICI) and at evaluation of tumor response according to RECIST criteria, version 1.1 (23).

Clinical data included age, sex, smoking status, alcohol consumption, Eastern Cooperative Oncology Group Performance Status (ECOG-PS), TNM on Cancer (7th edition) (24), primary tumor site, treatment line for R/M disease, type of recurrence prior ICI, and response. Those patients, who had received the last dose of platinum 6 months before of initiation of ICI, were classified as platinum-refractory. Additional information regarding IrAEs according to the CTCAE version 4.3 2009 (25) and vital status were also collected from medical records.

Nutritional data were collected at baseline (before starting treatment). These data included body mass index (BMI calculated as [(weight (kg)/height (m^2)], serum albumin levels, and type of nutritional intervention if any.

Image Analysis

All treatment images were selected by a trained researcher to ensure they correspond to the same vertebra landmarks to allow a proper comparison of body composition. Values were obtained by a single observer blinded to the patients' data.

Images were accessed from the axial cross-sectional CT as all patients had an abdominal CT scan as part of their routine care. The third lumbar (L3) vertebra was chosen on the axial cross-section CT component of the full-body CT scans as the reference point, based on previous reports with this level to calculate the skeletal muscle index (SMI) (26, 27) using SliceOmatic© software (v5.0 Rev 8, Tomovision, Montreal, Quebec, Canada). Regional analysis at L3 strongly predicted whole-body fat and fat-free mass (r=0.86-0.94; $p < 0.001$) (26). Muscle cross-sectional area (CSA) was quantified within a Hounsfield unit (HU) range from -29 to +150HU and then normalized for height to report as SMI (cm^2/m^2). Sarcopenia was defined according to Martin L et al. (28) using specific SMI cut points for advanced cancer patients. CSA of adipose tissue were determined using tissue-specific HU range defined at this level (29).

Statistical Analysis

To define cohort characteristics, categorical variables were presented as the number of cases and percentages, whereas continuous variables were presented as the mean and standard deviation (SD) or median and interquartile range (IQR). Median baseline SMI was used to dichotomize patients in two groups: low SMI (patients with baseline SMI lower than median baseline SMI) or high SMI (patients with baseline SMI equal or higher than median baseline SMI).

It was planned to test for the effect of baseline SMI on survival. Time between treatment initiation and disease progression or death from any cause (PFS) and time between treatment initiation and death from any cause (OS) was assessed using the Kaplan-Meier estimator. One-year OS rate and 1-year PFS rate were also analyzed. The Cox proportional hazards model was used to perform univariate and multivariate survival analyses, which are reported as the hazard ratio (HR) and 95% confidence interval. Covariates with a p-value lower than 0.1 in the univariate model were included in the multivariate models. The proportionality of risks in the Cox model was verified using the Schoenfeld residuals.

To evaluate the effect of baseline variables in the development of toxicity, logistic regression models were used. Odds ratios and their corresponding 95% confidence intervals were derived from both univariate and multivariate models.

Statistical significance was set at a probability level ≤0.05. The statistical package used to treat the data and perform the statistical analysis was R software version 3.5.

RESULTS

Patient Characteristics

Table 1 shows baseline demographic and clinical characteristics of the 61 patients included in the analysis. Most patients were male (n = 52, 85.2%) with a mean age of 57.7 years (SD 9.62). Tumor location was mainly oral cavity (n = 21; 34.4%). Most of patients recurred with locoregional plus metastatic disease (n = 28; 45.9%). Four (6.5%) patients received ICI as the first treatment and 59% (n = 36) were platinum refractory.

At baseline, the mean BMI was 23.8 kg/m^2 (SD 4.56); underweight (BMI ≤18.5) was present in 9 (14.8%) patients and 26 (42.6%) were overweight (BMI ≥25) or obese (BMI ≥30). Median SMI was 42.0 cm^2/m^2 (IQR 37.5; 48.6) and was used to classify patients between high and low SMI. Nutritional support was required in 34 (55.7%) patients, 15 (44.1%) of them needed a tube feeding. Two thirds (n=41, 67.2%) of the patients were sarcopenic according to previously published cut points (30) and three of them were also obese (**Table 1S, Supporting Information**).

Significant differences were identified for patients with low *vs* high SMI in mean age (p = 0.035), baseline weight ($p < 0.001$), BMI ($P < 0.001$), and total adipose tissue (p = 0.003). Patients with high SMI were older, heavier, and with higher BMI. No other significant differences between patients with low and high SMI at baseline were found.

Effects of SMI in Overall Survival (OS) and Progression Free Survival (PFS)

Median follow-up time was 9 months (range, 3.6–21.3). Up to a third of patients (n=16; 26.2%) were alive at last follow-up. The median time to death was 4.3 months (range, 2.3–10.9). **Table 2** summarized univariate and multivariate analyses of OS, PFS, 1-year survival, and 1-year PFS.

Patients with low SMI had shorter OS (HR, 2.06; 95% CI, 1.14–3.73; p = 0.017) (**Figure 1**) and 1-year OS rate (HR, 2.64; 95% CI, 1.33–5.23; p = 0.005) in the univariate analysis. Low SMI was also associated with global PFS (global PFS HR, 1.84; 95% CI, 1.08–3.12; p = 0.025, and 1-year PFS rate HR, 1.83; 95% CI, 1.01–3.23; p = 0.036) among other factors such as age (PFS HR, 0.96; 95% CI, 0.94–0.99; p = 0.002), baseline albumin (PFS HR, 0.95; 95% CI, 0.91–0.99; p = 0.027), platinum-refractory (PFS HR, 3.04; 95% CI, 1.67–5.56; p = <0.001), and any number of prior lines for R/M disease (PFS HR, 1.94; 95% CI, 1.09–3.46; p = 0.025). The association was maintained at 1-year PFS, although the number of prior lines showed only a trend (PFS HR, 1.71; 95% CI, 0.93–3.16; p = 0.084). One-year PFS showed a clear association with age (PFS HR, 0.97; 95% CI, 0.94–1.00; p = 0.036), serum albumin (PFS HR, 0.94; 95% CI, 0.90–0.99; p = 0.025), low SMI (PFS HR, 2.53; 95% CI, 1.19–5.37; p = 0.015), and patients who received platinum within 6 months prior to ICI (PFS HR, 3.57; 95% CI, 1.50–8.51; p = 0.004).

The multivariate analyses adjusted for serum albumin, baseline SMI, and platinum-refractory confirmed low SMI as an independent predictor for OS (HR, 2.19; 95% CI, 1.19–4.05; p = 0.012) and 1-year survival (HR, 2.79; 95% CI, 1.37–5.67; p = 0.005) adjusting this analysis also for age. Type of recurrence prior ICI initiation and BMI were not included in the multivariate analysis because it did not show association for survival or PFS in the univariate analysis.

Similar results were found using previously published cut points for sarcopenia (28) for OS but not for PFS. These results showed that sarcopenia was an independent factor for OS (HR, 2.06; 95% CI, 1.01–4.23; p = 0.048) after adjusting by the same covariates than the analysis performed for low SMI. This analysis

TABLE 1 | Patient baseline characteristics (overall and according to low *vs* high skeletal muscle index) (SMI) (n=61).

	Overall (n=61)	Low SMI (n=30)	High SMI (n=31)	p-overall
Age, years				
Mean (SD)	57.7 (9.62)	55.1 (9.93)	60.3 (8.73)	0.035
Median (range)	59.0 (23-78)	55.9 (23-70)	61.3 (35-78)	0.753
Male, n (%)	52 (85.2)	24 (80.0)	28 (90.3)	0.301
Smoking status, n (%)				0.394
Current	28 (45.9)	16 (53.3)	12 (38.7)	
Former*	26 (42.6)	12 (40.0)	14 (45.2)	
Never	7 (11.5)	2 (6.7)	5 (16.1)	
Alcohol consumption#, n (%)				
Yes	36 (59.0)	19 (63.3)	17 (54.8)	0.699
Location, n (%)				0.283
Oral cavity	21 (34.4)	11 (36.7)	10 (32.3)	
Hypopharynx	8 (13.1)	5 (16.7)	3 (9.7)	
Larynx	19 (31.3)	6 (20.0)	13 (41.9)	
Oropharynx**	13 (21.3)	8 (26.7)	5 (16.1)	
Type of recurrence				0.700
Locoregional	23 (37.7)	10 (33.3)	13 (41.9)	
Distance	10 (16.4)	6 (20.0)	4 (12.9)	
Locoregional + distance	28 (45.9)	14 (46.7)	14 (45.2)	
Line of therapy, n (%)				0.865
First	22 (36.1)	10 (33.3)	12 (38.7)	
Second or above	39 (63.9)	20 (66.7)	19 (61.3)	
Type of ICI therapy, n (%)				0.786
AntiPD1	8 (13.1)	5 (16.7)	3 (9.7)	
AntiPD1+virus	1 (1.64)	0 (0.0)	1 (3.3)	
AntiPD1 + chemotherapy	3 (4.92)	2 (6.7)	1 (3.2)	
AntiPDL1	12 (19.7)	5 (16.7)	7 (22.6)	
AntiPDL1+antiCTLA4	22 (36.1)	11 (36.7)	11 (35.5)	
AntiPDL1+IOA	15 (24.6)	9 (29.0)	6 (20.0)	
ECOG-PS, n (%)				0.363
0	1 (1.64)	0 (0.0)	1 (3.2)	
1	58 (95.1)	30 (100)	28 (90.3)	
2	2 (3.28)	0 (0.0)	2 (6.5)	
Platinum within 6 months of ICI,n (%)	36 (59.0)	18 (60.0)	18 (58.1)	1.000
Weight, kg				
Mean (SD)	67.3 (15.0)	59.5 (10.9)	74.9 (14.7)	<0.001
Median [Q1; Q3]	65.2 [54.3;79.0]	58.8 [51.0;65.6]	77.5 [64.3;84.5]	<0.001
BMI, kg/m^2				
Mean (SD)	23.8 (4.56)	21.3 (3.33)	26.2 (4.32)	<0.001
Median (range)	23.6 (15.8-34.7)	21.7 (15.8-27.6)	26.8 (17.7-34.6)	<0.001
BMI categorized, kg/m^2				0.001
Underweight (<18.5)	9 (14.8)	7 (23.3)	2 (6.5)	
Normal (18.5 – 25)	26 (42.6)	17 (56.7)	9 (29.0)	
Overweight /obese (>25)	26 (42.6)	6 (20.0)	20 (64.5)	
Albumin, g/L				
Mean (SD)	42.9 (60.3)	43.0 (3.24)	42.9 (7.86)	0.933
Median [Q1; Q3]	44.0 [41.0;46.0]	43.0 [41.0;45.0]	44.0 [42.0;46.5]	0.302
SMI, cm^2/m^2				
Mean (SD)	43.6 (7.75)	37.2 (3.14)	49.8 (5.44)	<0.001
Median [Q1; Q3]	42.0 [37.5;48.6]	37.5 [35.2;39.6]	48.6 [46.1;53.0]	<0.001
TATI, cm^2/m^2				
Mean (SD)	91.4 (53.3)	71.7 (44.5)	111 (54.7)	0.003
Median [Q1; Q3]	98.8 [49.4;118]	70.8 [31.5;101]	112 [82.0;148]	0.004

Ex-smoker defined as no cigarettes for more than 6 months before diagnosis.
#Alcohol consumption defined as sustained heavy drinker (≥4 drinks per week in women and ≥5 drinks per week in men). Includes active and former drinkers.
ICI, immune checkpoint inhibitor; ECOG-PS, Eastern Cooperative Oncology Group Performance Status; BMI, body mass index; SMI, skeletal muscle index; TATI, total adipose tissue index; IOA, immuno-oncology agent.
***3 of them HPV-related.*

is provided as **Supplementary Information** (**Table 2S** and **Figure 1S**).

We sought to determine whether different BMIs were associated with any of the abovementioned outcomes. There were no statistically significant differences in OS and PFS, when examining overweight or obese patients (BMI ≥ 25 kg/m^2) compared with patients with normal BMI.

TABLE 2 | Univariate and multivariate analysis examining OS, one-year survival, global PFS and one-year PFS in association with skeletal muscle index (SMI) (n=61).

Univariate analysis	**SURVIVAL**						**PROGRESION FREE SURVIVAL**					
	Overall survival			**1-year survival**			**Global PFS**			**1-year PFS**		
	HR	***95% IC***	***P value***	***HR***	***95% IC***	***P value***	***HR***	***95% IC***	***P value***	***HR***	***95% IC***	***P value***
BMI	0.97	0.91;1.04	0.432	0.96	0.89;1.03	0.232	0.96	0.91;1.02	0.237	0.96	0.90;1.03	0.235
Age	0.98	0.96;1.01	0.177	0.98	0.95;1.00	0.077	0.96	0.94;0.99	0.002	0.96	0.94;0.99	0.002
Serum albumin	0.97	0.93;1.00	0.056	0.97	0.93;1.01	0.112	0.95	0.91;0.99	0.027	0.95	0.90;0.99	0.024
Low skeletal muscle index	2.06	1.14;3.73	0.017	2.64	1.33;5.23	0.005	1.84	1.08;3.12	0.025	1.83	1.01;3.23	0.036
Platinum-refractory	1.76	0.94;3.28	0.075	1.85	0.91;3.78	0.089	3.04	1.67;5.56	<0.001	2.95	1.57;5.55	0.001
Type of recurrence												
Distance	0.86	0.35;2.11	0.748	0.77	0.28;2.15	0.625	0.80	0.36;1.77	0.582	0.71	0.28;1.78	0.466
Locorregional + distance	1.16	0.61;2.22	0.651	1.08	0.53;2.19	0.830	1.03	0.58;1.83	0.929	1.11	0.61;2.02	0.736
Line of therapy 2 or above	1.26	0.68;2.34	0.470	1.21	0.60;2.41	0.596	1.94	1.09;3.46	0.025	1.71	0.93;3.16	0.084
Multivariate analysis*	***HR***	***95% IC***	***P value***	***HR***	***95% IC***	***P value***	***HR***	***95% IC***	***P value***	***HR***	***95% IC***	***P value***
Age				0.99	0.96;1.02	0.359	#	#	#	0.97	0.94;1.00	0.026
Serum albumin	0.96	0.93;1.00	0.052	0.96	0.93;1.00	0.082	#	#	#	0.94	0.90;0.99	0.016
Low skeletal muscle index	2.19	1.19;4.05	0.012	2.79	1.37;5.67	0.005	#	#	#	1.90	1.04;3.48	0.037
Platinum-refractory	1.74	0.92;3.30	0.090	1.73	0.84;3.56	0.138	#	#	#	3.31	1.40;7.83	0.006
Line of therapy 2 or above							#	#	#	0.68	0.30;1.53	0.349

OS, overall survival; PFS, progression free survival; BMI, body mass index; ICI, immune checkpoint inhibitors; Type of recurrence includes locorregional disease, distance disease and locorregional+distance disease; Line of therapy includes first vs second or above lines.

**Adjusted for the covariates with p-value <0.1 in the univariate analysis.*

#Multivariate models for global PFS were not computed due to the small numbers of patients in the no-event group.

Treatment Toxicity

IrAEs occurred in 29 (47.5%) patients mainly in those treated with anti-PDL1 plus IOA (n = 15; 80%) and treated with anti-PD1 plus chemotherapy (n = 2; 66.7%). Thyroiditis, skin, and liver alterations were the most common IrAEs, and the vast majority was grade 1 or grade 2. Only seven patients developed grade 3 or above toxicity, three of them with low SMI.

There was no association with low SMI and IrAEs of any grade (OR, 0.56; 95% CI, 0.20–1.54; p = 0.261).

Different factors were examined to determine their effect in the development of IrAEs. Patients with BMI ≤18.5 kg/m^2 (OR, 0.09; 95% CI, 0.00–0.63; p = 0.012), the presence of distance metastasis (OR, 4.93; 95% CI, 1.01–30.4, p = 0.048), and those patients platinum-refractory (OR, 0.33; 95% CI, 0.11–0.94, p = 0.037) were associated with toxicity of any grade. In the multivariate analysis, only being refractory to platinum (OR, 2.88; 95% CI, 1.05–8.98, p = 0.050) was a predictive factor of IrAEs occurrence. The presence of distant metastasis was not included in the multivariate analysis because only three patients with distant metastasis did not develop IrAEs.

DISCUSSION

Immunotherapy is significantly changing the therapeutic landscape for R/M HNSCC (4, 5). Its clinical efficacy varied among HNSCC patients, and there is a lack of accurate and effective predictive biomarkers. Low SMI is frequently encountered in HNSCC patients (10, 16). However, whether low SMI can be used as a predictive biomarker for ICI remains unknown, and the clinical data regarding the association between SMI and ICI efficacy are quite limited. To the best of our knowledge, this is the first study to assess the association between SMI and clinical outcomes of R/M HNSCC patients undergoing ICI therapy.

In our study, low SMI was confirmed to be an independent factor for reduced OS and 1-year survival after adjusting the model for relevant factors associated with clinical outcomes in HNSCC. These findings are in agreement with other studies performed in melanoma and lung cancer (19, 31). We did not assess mortality specific for cancer as only two patients died from another cause different from the primary cancer. Important variables such as age, serum albumin, refractoriness to platinum or the number of lines of therapy prior to ICI therapy are well-known predictive factors. However, body composition is often overlooked in clinical practice. BMI is not a good indicator of body composition as elevated BMI may hide a distribution of low muscle mass increasing the risk for adverse outcomes (19, 32). Moreover, muscle has been shown to be one of the strongest parameters associated with mortality in cancer patients (33) even when weight and BMI are included in the analysis.

There are numerous cut points values published for sarcopenia although none of them is yet definitive. Some of these cut points used OS as the outcome according to the SMI (27, 30). We have chosen Martin et al. (30) as their population is a large sample with advanced stage and includes all BMIs. Moreover, these cut points have been used in many previous publications, so readers can compare our results. As our cohort is a slightly distinct population, we also chose the median L3 SMI cut point to evaluate SMI as a predictive biomarker in R/M HNSCC.

Although the mechanism by which reduced SMI has a negative effect on the clinical efficacy of ICI remains unclear. New evidence shows that skeletal muscle cells, as an endocrine organ, may secrete specific cytokines that regulate immunity.

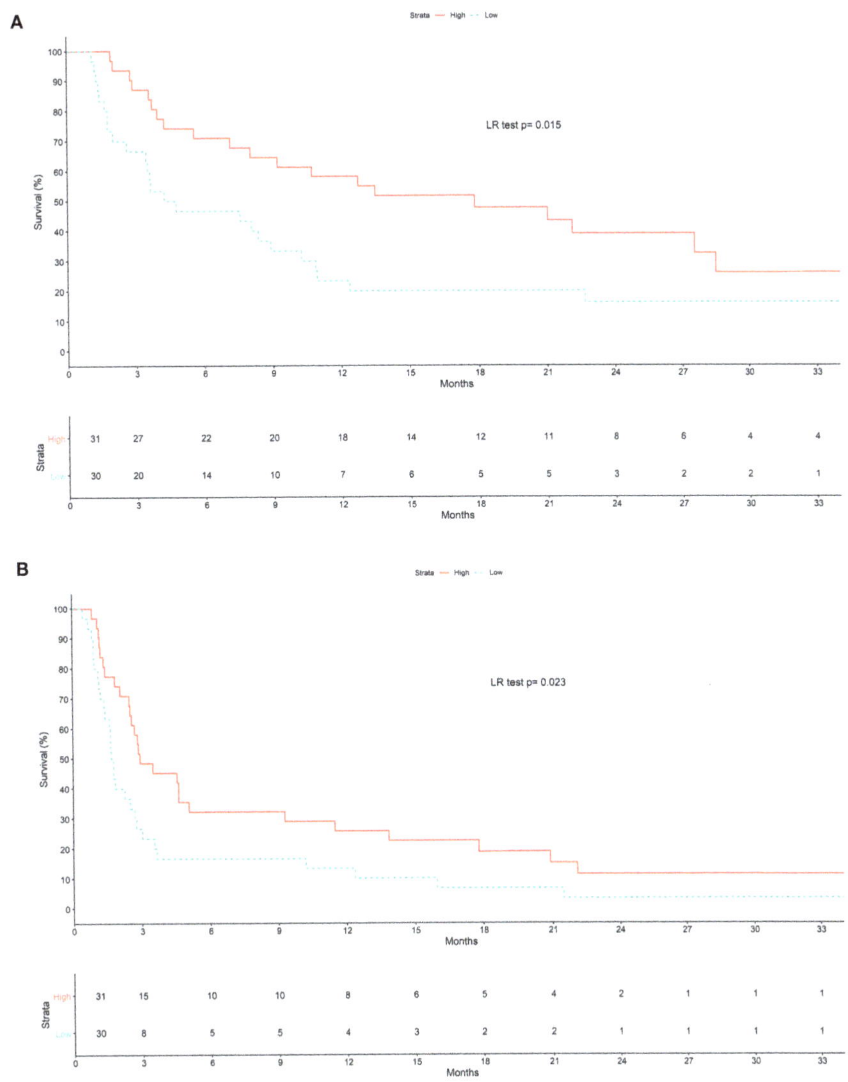

FIGURE 1 | Kaplan-Meier survival curves according to baseline SMI. **(A)** Overall survival. **(B)** Progression Free Survival.

These myokines are involved in modulating the immune response (34). Thus, a reduction in muscle mass may have a deleterious effect on the anti-tumor response mediated by the immune system, following in immunosuppression (35). A decrease in myokines due to the loss of muscle mass could suppress tumor response to ICI, resulting in the immune escape of tumor cells (36, 37). Inflammation also plays an important role in the loss of muscle mass (38). All these factors may contribute to the impairment of the antitumor immune response to ICI in HNSCC.

We did not find any statistically significant associations between BMI and clinical outcomes to ICI. Young et al. (19) identified trends toward worse outcomes in patients with high BMI and low muscle mass in patients with melanoma treated with anti-PD1. However, we included only six patients with BMI ≥ 25 kg/m^2 and low SMI.

Compared with traditional treatments (chemotherapy or radiotherapy), the incidence of toxicity in HNSCC patients treated with ICI has been reduced. We explored the effect of low SMI on the incidence of adverse event related to ICI in HNSCC patients, finding that low SMI was not significantly associated with the incidence of IrAEs. Evidence suggests that the incidence of IrAEs of any grade is associated with improved clinical outcomes (39). Unfortunately, subgroups analysis could not be further performed because of insufficient data.

Our study has some limitations that should be addressed. The main ones are the retrospective design of the study and the limited number of patients. Moreover, the CT imaging analysis was limited by the data availability; indeed, the acquisition protocol was planned according to the presence of previous examination. Finally, we did not take into account the type of ICI therapy alone or in combination.

In conclusion, our finding shows that baseline SMI is an independent factor for survival R/M HNSCC treated with ICI. SMI is not associated with the onset of IrAEs. Further prospective research is needed to confirm the role of body composition as a predictive biomarker in ICI treatment and how SMI can affect drug-specific and organ-specific adverse events caused by ICI in HNSCC patients.

ETHICS STATEMENT

The studies involving human participants were reviewed and approved by Hospital Universitari de Bellvitge Ethics Committee for Clinical Research (PR302/18). The patients/participants provided their written informed consent to participate in this study.

AUTHOR CONTRIBUTIONS

LA, MP, MT, RM, and VB were actively involved in the design of the stud writing the manuscript. LA, MP, MS, NV, AT, and LR were involved in the collection of data. NP and LA analyzed the data and all authors interpreted the data reviewed the manuscript. RM and VB supervised the study. All authors contributed to the article and approved the submitted version.

ACKNOWLEDGMENTS

The authors want to thank all the members of the clinical nutrition unit (Inmaculada Peiró, Laura Hurtós, Marta Bellver, Maryam Choulli) and the medical oncology department (Jesus Brenes, Esther Vilajosana, Victoria Gomez, Alicia Lozano, Isabel Linares, and Vanessa Tierraseca).

REFERENCES

1. Gatta G, Botta L, Sánchez MJ, Anderson LA, Pierannunzio D, Licitra L, et al. Prognoses and Improvement for Head and Neck Cancers Diagnosed in Europe in Early 2000s: The EUROCARE-5 Population-Based Study. *Eur J Cancer* (2015) 51:2130–43. doi: 10.1016/j.ejca.2015.07.043
2. Vermorken JB, Mesia R, Rivera F, Remenar E, Kawecki A, Rottey S, et al. Platinum-Based Chemotherapy Plus Cetuximab in Head and Neck Cancer. *N Engl J Med* (2008) 359:1116–27. doi: 10.1056/NEJMoa0802656
3. León X, Hitt R, Constenla M, Rocca A, Stupp R, Kovács AF, et al. A Retrospective Analysis of the Outcome of Patients With Recurrent and/or Metastatic Squamous Cell Carcinoma of the Head and Neck Refractory to a Platinum-Based Chemotherapy. *Clin Oncol (R Coll Radiol)* (2005) 17:418–24. doi: 10.1016/j.clon.2005.02.014
4. Zandberg DP, Algazi AP, Jimeno A, Good JS, Fayette J, Bouganim N, et al. Durvalumab for Recurrent or Metastatic Head and Neck Squamous Cell Carcinoma: Results From a Single-Arm, Phase II Study in Patients With ≥25% Tumour Cell PD-L1 Expression Who Have Progressed on Platinum-Based Chemotherapy. *Eur J Cancer* (2019) 107:142–52. doi: 10.1016/j.ejca.2018.11.015
5. Chow LQM, Haddad R, Gupta S, Mahipal A, Mehra R, Tahara M, et al. Antitumor Activity of Pembrolizumab in Biomarker-Unselected Patients With Recurrent and/or Metastatic Head and Neck Squamous Cell Carcinoma: Results From the Phase Ib KEYNOTE-012 Expansion Cohort. *J Clin Oncol* (2016) 34:3838–45. doi: 10.1200/JCO.2016.68.1478
6. Ferris RL, Blumenschein G, Fayette J, Guigay J, Colevas AD, Licitra L, et al. Nivolumab for Recurrent Squamous-Cell Carcinoma of the Head and Neck. *N Engl J Med* (2016) 375:1856–67. doi: 10.1056/NEJMoa1602252
7. Cohen EEW, Soulières D, Le Tourneau C, Dinis J, Licitra L, Ahn M-J, et al. Pembrolizumab Versus Methotrexate, Docetaxel, or Cetuximab for Recurrent or Metastatic Head-and-Neck Squamous Cell Carcinoma (KEYNOTE-040): A Randomised, Open-Label, Phase 3 Study. *Lancet (London England)* (2019) 393:156–67. doi: 10.1016/S0140-6736(18)31999-8
8. Burtness B, Harrington KJ, Greil R, Soulières D, Tahara M, de Castro G, et al. Pembrolizumab Alone or With Chemotherapy Versus Cetuximab With Chemotherapy for Recurrent or Metastatic Squamous Cell Carcinoma of the Head and Neck (KEYNOTE-048): A Randomised, Open-Label, Phase 3 Study. *Lancet (Lond Engl)* (2019) 394:1915–28. doi: 10.1016/S0140-6736(19)32591-7
9. Datema FR, Ferrier MB, Baatenburg de Jong RJ. Impact of Severe Malnutrition on Short-Term Mortality and Overall Survival in Head and Neck Cancer. *Oral Oncol* (2011) 47:910–4. doi: 10.1016/j.oraloncology.2011.06.510
10. Arribas L, Hurtós L, Taberna M, Peiró I, Vilajosana E, Lozano A, et al. Nutritional Changes in Patients With Locally Advanced Head and Neck Cancer During Treatment. *Oral Oncol* (2017) 71:67–74. doi: 10.1016/j.oraloncology.2017.06.003
11. Ferrão B, Neves PM, Santos T, Capelas ML, Mäkitie A, Ravasco P. Body Composition Changes in Patients With Head and Neck Cancer Under Active Treatment: A Scoping Review. *Support Care Cancer* (2020) 28:4613–25. doi: 10.1007/s00520-020-05487-w
12. Cruz-Jentoft AJ, Bahat G, Bauer J, Boirie Y, Bruyère O, Cederholm T, et al. Sarcopenia: Revised European Consensus on Definition and Diagnosis. *Age Ageing* (2019) 48:16–31. doi: 10.1093/ageing/afy169
13. Fearon K, Strasser F, Anker SD, Bosaeus I, Bruera E, Fainsinger RL, et al. Definition and Classification of Cancer Cachexia: An International Consensus. *Lancet Oncol* (2011) 12:489–95. doi: 10.1016/S1470-2045(10)70218-7
14. Shachar SS, Williams GR, Muss HB, Nishijima TF. Prognostic Value of Sarcopenia in Adults With Solid Tumours: A Meta-Analysis and Systematic Review. *Eur J Cancer* (2016) 57:58–67. doi: 10.1016/j.ejca.2015.12.030
15. Achim V, Bash J, Mowery A, Guimaraes AR, Li R, Schindler J, et al. Prognostic Indication of Sarcopenia for Wound Complication After Total Laryngectomy. *JAMA Otolaryngol Head Neck Surg* (2017) 143:1159–65. doi: 10.1001/jamaoto.2017.0547
16. Grossberg AJ, Chamchod S, Fuller CD, Mohamed ASR, Heukelom J, Eichelberger H, et al. Association of Body Composition With Survival and Locoregional Control of Radiotherapy-Treated Head and Neck Squamous Cell Carcinoma. *JAMA Oncol* (2016) 77030:1–8. doi: 10.1001/jamaoncol.2015.6339
17. Sealy MJ, Dechaphunkul T, van der Schans CP, Krijnen WP, Roodenburg JLN, Walker J, et al. Low Muscle Mass Is Associated With Early Termination of Chemotherapy Related to Toxicity in Patients With Head and Neck Cancer. *Clin Nutr* (2019) 39(2):501–9. doi: 10.1016/j.clnu.2019.02.029
18. van Rijn-Dekker MI, van den Bosch L, van den Hoek JGM, Bijl HP, van Aken ESM, van der Hoorn A, et al. Impact of Sarcopenia on Survival and Late Toxicity in Head and Neck Cancer Patients Treated With Radiotherapy. *Radiother Oncol* (2020) 147:103–10. doi: 10.1016/j.radonc.2020.03.014

19. Young AC, Quach HT, Song H, Davis EJ, Moslehi JJ, Ye F, et al. Impact of Body Composition on Outcomes From Anti-PD1 +/- Anti-CTLA-4 Treatment in Melanoma. *J Immunother Cancer* (2020) 8(2):e000821. doi: 10.1136/jitc-2020-000821
20. Cortellini A, Bozzetti F, Palumbo P, Brocco D, Di Marino P, Tinari N, et al. Weighing the Role of Skeletal Muscle Mass and Muscle Density in Cancer Patients Receiving PD-1/PD-L1 Checkpoint Inhibitors: A Multicenter Real-Life Study. *Sci Rep* (2020) 10:1456. doi: 10.1038/s41598-020-58498-2
21. Nishioka N, Uchino J, Hirai S, Katayama Y, Yoshimura A, Okura N, et al. Association of Sarcopenia With and Efficacy of Anti-PD-1/PD-L1 Therapy in Non-Small-Cell Lung Cancer. *J Clin Med* (2019) 8(4):450. doi: 10.3390/jcm8040450
22. Tsukagoshi M, Yokobori T, Yajima T, Maeno T, Shimizu K, Mogi A, et al. Skeletal Muscle Mass Predicts the Outcome of Nivolumab Treatment for Non-Small Cell Lung Cancer. *Med (Baltimore)* (2020) 99:e19059. doi: 10.1097/MD.0000000000019059
23. Therasse P, Arbuck SG, Eisenhauer EA, Wanders J, Kaplan RS, Rubinstein L, et al. New Guidelines to Evaluate the Response to Treatment in Solid Tumors. European Organization for Research and Treatment of Cancer, National Cancer Institute of the United States, National Cancer Institute of Canada. *J Natl Cancer Inst* (2000) 92:205–16. doi: 10.1093/jnci/92.3.205
24. Edge SB, Compton CC. The American Joint Committee on Cancer: The 7th Edition of the AJCC Cancer Staging Manual and the Future of TNM. *Ann Surg Oncol* (2010) 17:1471–4. doi: 10.1245/s10434-010-0985-4
25. *Common Terminology Criteria for Adverse Events (Ctcae) Version 4.0.* U.S Department of Health and Human Services, National Institutes of Heatlh, National Cancer Institute. (2009).
26. Mourtzakis M, Prado CMM, Lieffers JR, Reiman T, McCargar LJ, Baracos VE. A Practical and Precise Approach to Quantification of Body Composition in Cancer Patients Using Computed Tomography Images Acquired During Routine Care. *Appl Physiol Nutr Metab* (2008) 33:997–1006. doi: 10.1139/H08-075
27. Prado CMM, Lieffers JR, McCargar LJ, Reiman T, Sawyer MB, Martin L, et al. Prevalence and Clinical Implications of Sarcopenic Obesity in Patients With Solid Tumours of the Respiratory and Gastrointestinal Tracts: A Population-Based Study. *Lancet Oncol* (2008) 9:629–35. doi: 10.1016/S1470-2045(08)70153-0
28. Martin L, Senesse P, Gioulbasanis I, Antoun S, Bozzetti F, Deans C, et al. Diagnostic Criteria for the Classification of Cancer-Associated Weight Loss. *J Clin Oncol* (2015) 33:90–9. doi: 10.1200/JCO.2014.56.1894
29. Shen W, Punyanitya M, Wang Z, Gallagher D, St-Onge M-P, Albu J, et al. Total Body Skeletal Muscle and Adipose Tissue Volumes: Estimation From a Single Abdominal Cross-Sectional Image. *J Appl Physiol* (2004) 97:2333–8. doi: 10.1152/japplphysiol.00744.2004
30. Martin L, Birdsell L, MacDonald N, Reiman T, Clandinin MT, McCargar LJ, et al. Cancer Cachexia in the Age of Obesity: Skeletal Muscle Depletion is a Powerful Prognostic Factor, Independent of Body Mass Index. *J Clin Oncol* (2013) 31:1539–47. doi: 10.1200/JCO.2012.45.2722
31. Wang J, Cao L, Xu S. Sarcopenia Affects Clinical Efficacy of Immune Checkpoint Inhibitors in Non-Small Cell Lung Cancer Patients: A Systematic Review and Meta-Analysis. *Int Immunopharmacol* (2020) 88:106907. doi: 10.1016/j.intimp.2020.106907
32. Baracos VE, Arribas L. Sarcopenic Obesity: Hidden Muscle Wasting and its Impact for Survival and Complications of Cancer Therapy. *Ann Oncol* (2018) 29:ii1–9. doi: 10.1093/annonc/mdx810
33. Xia L, Zhao R, Wan Q, Wu Y, Zhou Y, Wang Y, et al. Sarcopenia and Adverse Health-Related Outcomes: An Umbrella Review of Meta-Analyses of Observational Studies. *Cancer Med* (2020) 9:7964–78. doi: 10.1002/cam4.3428
34. Li F, Li Y, Duan Y, Hu C-AA, Tang Y, Yin Y. Myokines and Adipokines: Involvement in the Crosstalk Between Skeletal Muscle and Adipose Tissue. *Cytokine Growth Factor Rev* (2017) 33:73–82. doi: 10.1016/j.cytogfr.2016.10.003
35. Afzali AM, Müntefering T, Wiendl H, Meuth SG, Ruck T. Skeletal Muscle Cells Actively Shape (Auto)Immune Responses. *Autoimmun Rev* (2018) 17:518–29. doi: 10.1016/j.autrev.2017.12.005
36. Lutz CT, Quinn LS. Sarcopenia, Obesity, and Natural Killer Cell Immune Senescence in Aging: Altered Cytokine Levels as a Common Mechanism. *Aging (Albany NY)* (2012) 4:535–46. doi: 10.18632/aging.100482
37. Pedersen BK, Febbraio MA. Muscle as an Endocrine Organ: Focus on Muscle-Derived Interleukin-6. *Physiol Rev* (2008) 88:1379–406. doi: 10.1152/physrev.90100.2007
38. Bano G, Trevisan C, Carraro S, Solmi M, Luchini C, Stubbs B, et al. Inflammation and Sarcopenia: A Systematic Review and Meta-Analysis. *Maturitas* (2017) 96:10–5. doi: 10.1016/j.maturitas.2016.11.006
39. Zhou X, Yao Z, Yang H, Liang N, Zhang X, Zhang F. Are Immune-Related Adverse Events Associated With the Efficacy of Immune Checkpoint Inhibitors in Patients With Cancer? A Systematic Review and Meta-Analysis. *BMC Med* (2020) 18:87. doi: 10.1186/s12916-020-01549-2

4

TERT Promoter Mutations and rs2853669 Polymorphism: Useful Markers for Clinical Outcome Stratification of Patients with Oral Cavity Squamous Cell Carcinoma

Silvia Giunco [1,2†], Paolo Boscolo-Rizzo [3,4†], Enrica Rampazzo [1], Giancarlo Tirelli [4], Lara Alessandrini [5], Roberto Di Carlo [6], Marco Rossi [7], Piero Nicolai [6], Anna Menegaldo [3], Valentina Carraro [5], Margherita Tofanelli [4], Luigia Bandolin [6], Giacomo Spinato [1,3], Enzo Emanuelli [3], Monica Mantovani [3], Marco Stellin [3], Rossana Bussani [8], Angelo Paolo Dei Tos [5], Maria Guido [9], Marzia Morello [2], Jonathan Fussey [10], Giovanni Esposito [2], Jerry Polesel [11] and Anita De Rossi [1,2]*

[1] Department of Surgery, Oncology and Gastroenterology, Section of Oncology and Immunology, University of Padova, Padova, Italy, [2] Immunology and Diagnostic Molecular Oncology Unit, Veneto Institute of Oncology (IOV), Istituto di Ricovero e Cura a Carattere Scientifico (IRCCS), Padova, Italy, [3] Department of Neurosciences, Section of Otolaryngology, University of Padova, Treviso, Italy, [4] Department of Medical, Surgical and Health Sciences, Section of Otolaryngology, University of Trieste, Trieste, Italy, [5] Department of Medicine (DIMED), Section of Pathology, University of Padova, Padova, Italy, [6] Department of Neurosciences, Section of Otolaryngology, University of Padova, Padova, Italy, [7] Unit of Oral and Maxillofacial Surgery, Treviso Regional Hospital, Treviso, Italy, [8] Department of Medical, Surgical and Health Sciences, Section of Pathology, University of Trieste, Trieste, Italy, [9] Department of Medicine (DIMED), Section of Pathology, University of Padova, Treviso, Italy, [10] Department of ENT/Head and Neck Surgery, Queen Elizabeth University Hospital Birmingham, Birmingham, United Kingdom, [11] Unit of Cancer Epidemiology, Centro di Riferimento Oncologico di Aviano (CRO) Istituto di Ricovero e Cura a Carattere Scientifico (IRCCS), Aviano, Italy

***Correspondence:**
Silvia Giunco
silvia.giunco@unipd.it

[†]These authors have contributed equally to this work and share first authorship

Objective: To date, no useful prognostic biomarker exists for patients with oral squamous cell carcinoma (OCSCC), a tumour with uncertain biological behaviour and subsequent unpredictable clinical course. We aim to investigate the prognostic significance of two recurrent somatic mutations (-124 C>T and -146 C>T) within the promoter of telomerase reverse transcriptase (*TERT*) gene and the impact of TERT single nucleotide polymorphism (SNP) rs2853669 in patients surgically treated for OCSCC.

Methods: The genetic frequencies of rs2853669, -124 C>T and -146 C>T as well as the telomere length were investigated in 144 tumours and 57 normal adjacent mucosal (AM) specimens from OCSCC patients.

Results: Forty-five tumours harboured *TERT* promoter mutations (31.3%), with -124 C>T and -146 C>T accounting for 64.4% and 35.6% of the alterations respectively. Patients with -124 C>T *TERT* promoter mutated tumours had the shortest telomeres in the AM (p=0.016) and showed higher risk of local recurrence (hazard ratio [HR]:2.75, p=0.0143), death (HR:2.71, p=0.0079) and disease progression (HR:2.71, p=0.0024) with the effect being potentiated by the co-occurrence of T/T genotype of rs2853669.

Conclusion: -124 C>T *TERT* promoter mutation as well as the T/T genotype of the rs2853669 SNP are attractive independent prognostic biomarkers in patients surgically treated for OCSCC, with the coexistence of these genetic variants showing a synergistic impact on the aggressiveness of the disease.

Keywords: oral cavity squamous cell carcinoma (OCSCC), telomerase, *TERT* promoter mutations, SNP rs2853669, telomere, prognostic biomarkers, survival

INTRODUCTION

With a worldwide estimated age-standardized incidence rate of 4.0 per 100,000 and an estimated number of new cases in 2018 of 354,864, oral cavity squamous cell carcinoma (OCSCC) is the most common carcinoma developing from the epithelial lining of the upper aero-digestive tract (UADT), thus representing an important burden on health care (1).

Based on the histopathological stage, OCSCC can exhibit an unpredictable behaviour with a fraction of patients with early-stage cancer suffering from poor prognosis (2). Patients curatively treated for OCSCC have indeed a high propensity to develop both recurrences and second field tumours (3). Thus, despite recent improvements in the management strategies of OCSCC, improvements in outcomes have been modest (4).

High-risk human papillomaviruses (HPVs), responsible for more than 50% of oropharyngeal squamous cell carcinomas (SCCs) and robust prognostic biomarkers in risk-stratifying in individuals with these malignancies (5), play only a marginal role in OCSCC (6). Thus, since not all OCSCCs are attributable to tobacco and alcohol exposure, the aetiopathogenesis of these neoplasms remains unknown in several cases and no reliable biomarker capable of stratifying the prognosis of OCSCC exists. It is, therefore, of paramount importance to identify biomarkers and molecular signatures predicting cancer relapse that may guide surveillance follow-up strategies and adjuvant treatments.

The infinite proliferation of malignant cells is a hallmark of oncogenesis and telomere/telomerase interplay dictates cell replicative capacity. Telomerase is indeed usually repressed in normal somatic cells, but it is detectable in the vast majority of tumours (7, 8). By synthesizing the telomere sequences and thus preventing cell senescence and apoptosis, the inappropriate activation of the catalytic component of the telomerase, telomerase reverse transcriptase (TERT), appears crucial for maintaining cellular replicative capacity and allowing tumour formation (9). Furthermore, through its non-canonical extra-telomeric functions, the re-activation of telomerase in cancer cells may affect cancer progression and metastasis (10, 11). These properties make TERT a potentially attractive biomarker in cancer.

Among the different mechanisms leading to the inappropriate reactivation of TERT in cancer, mutually exclusive recurrent C-to-T transitions at nucleotides 1,295,228 (-124 C>T) and 1,295,250 (-146 C>T) within the core promoter of *TERT* creating *de novo* binding sites for E-twenty-six (ETS) transcription factors and leading to increased *TERT* gene expression are particularly interesting: first, their prognostic role was consistently observed in several cancers (12), second, among SCCs of the UADT, *TERT* promoter mutations were observed to be topographically restricted to OCSCC (13), and third, unlike assessing *TERT* mRNA levels, *TERT* promoter mutations can be more easily analysed in formalin-fixed paraffin-embedded (FFPE) specimens from routinely collected biopsies.

Although a previous investigation conducted in a population of subject with OCSCC from Taiwan found that those harbouring the -124 C>T *TERT* promoter mutation had a worse prognosis, this was not statistically significant. However, current evidence suggests that the effect of *TERT* promoter mutations may be affected by a common single nucleotide polymorphism (SNP), rs2853669, within the *TERT* core promoter close to the hotspot mutation sites (14). The minor C-variant allele of the SNP disrupts a pre-existing ETS2 binding site at -245 bp in the *TERT* promoter region resulting in decreased TERT expression (15) and thus, counteracts the transactivation activity of the *TERT* promoter hotspots (14). A meta-analysis reports that among cancer patients with *TERT* promoter mutations, the rs2853669 T/T genotype confers a worse prognosis (16), but the modifying role of this SNP in the prognostic value of *TERT* promoter mutations is still controversial (12, 17–20). To date, the prognostic value of rs2853669 in OCSCC remains to be elucidated.

Thus, the main aims of this study were to investigate the prevalence and the clinical significance of *TERT* promoter mutations and the impact of the *TERT* rs2853669 SNP in a larger series of patients surgically treated for OCSCC.

MATERIALS AND METHODS

Patients and Tissue Samples

This is a multi-centre retrospective observational study conducted with the approval of the ethics committee of Treviso/Belluno provinces (Ethic vote: 346/AULSS9) and was performed in a cohort of 144 consecutive patients diagnosed with OCSCC from February 1, 2010 to September 30, 2018, who underwent up-front surgery with/without adjuvant (chemo) radiotherapy, whose samples were available for analysis. All patients gave their informed consent. The study network included three University Hospitals in Northeast Italy, located in Padova, Treviso, and Trieste.

Patients were routinely followed-up [median follow-up time: 43 months; interquartile range (IQR), 28-75 months] according to consensus guidelines with endoscopic examination of the upper aero-digestive tract every 1–3 months for the first year, 3–4 months during the second year, 4–6 months during the 3rd year, and every 6 months thereafter. A dedicated CT scan of the chest was performed annually. Additional dedicated head and neck imaging was arranged based on clinical features and local protocol.

Data for 27 OCSCC samples (tumour tissue, adjacent mucosa and patient characteristics) were available from our previous study (13). One hundred and seventeen specimens were FFPE. Estimations of tumour cell content on FFPE OCSCC sections were made by a trained pathologist. When macrodissection was necessary for enrichment in neoplastic cells, the pathologist marked tumour areas on haematoxylin and eosin-stained tissue slides; the corresponding areas were scraped from four to five serial FFPE sections of 10 µm thickness. Adjacent mucosa from 30 of 117 FFPE specimens was analysed in samples from tumours with negative/clear margins, and the stroma immediately adjacent to the neoplastic epithelium was left as a border zone. DNA from FFPE specimens was extracted using the QIAmp DNA mini kit (Qiagen, Hilden, Germany) according to the manufacturer's instructions.

TERT Promoter Analysis and Telomere Length Measurement

Genomic DNA amplification for *TERT* promoter region (260 bp) containing -124 C>T and -146 C>T mutation sites, as well as the SNP rs2853669 (-245 T>C), was performed exactly as previously described (21). The amplified products were purified with the Illustra ExoProStar (GE Healthcare, Buckinghamshire, UK) and sequenced on a 3730xl DNA analyzer (Applied Biosystems, Foster City, CA, USA). All samples were analysed in forward and reverse directions.

Telomere length was determined by multiplex PCR assay as previously described (22). Relative telomere length (RTL) values were calculated as telomere/single-copy gene ratio, as previously described (23).

Statistical Analysis

Differences in socio-demographic and clinical characteristics according to *TERT* promoter were tested through Fisher's exact test. For each patient, person-time at risk was computed from the date of diagnosis to the event date or the date of last follow-up, whichever came first. Events were defined as death for overall survival (OS), death or recurrence at any site for progression-free survival (PFS), local recurrence for mucosal control, and lymph node recurrence for regional failure. Analyses were truncated at 5 years. The association between *TERT* promoter and oncological outcomes was evaluated using the Kaplan-Meier method, and difference in survival probabilities was evaluated using the log-rank test (24). To account for competing risks, mucosal and regional control were evaluated using cumulative incidence, and differences according to strata were tested using Gray's test (25). The risk of unfavourable oncological outcome was evaluated using the Cox proportional hazards model (24); multivariable hazard ratios (HR), and corresponding 95% confidence intervals (CI), were calculated adjusting for gender, age, pathological lymph node status (pN), grading, surgical margins, and extracapsular invasion. For mucosal and regional control, HR were adjusted for competing risk according to Fine-Gray model (25).

RESULTS

Demographic and Clinical Characteristics of Patients

The clinical characteristics of the patients are summarized in **Table 1**. Globally, the study group had a median age of 65 years (IQR, 54-74 years) at presentation and included 81 (56.2%) male and 63 (43.8%) female patients (**Table 1**). The majority of patients were ever smoking (61.8%) and never drinking (58.3%). Tumour sub-sites within the oral cavity were as follows: 54.2% (78/144) in the tongue, 15.3% (22/144) in the floor of the mouth, 10.4% (15/144) in both the gingiva and the buccal mucosa, and 9.7% (14/144) in other sub-sites including the lip, the hard palate and the retromolar trigone. Pathological stage was T1-T2 in 99 cases (68.7%) and T3-T4 in 45 (31.3%); 47 (32.6%) of the cases had clinically positive regional lymph nodes and 97 cases (67.4%) were N0; collectively, 69 (47.9%) had advanced disease at diagnosis. Nearly 75% of tumours (104/139) showed G1-G2 grading and 25.2% (35/139) were G3. Close/positive surgical margins and positive extra-capsular spread were present in 21 (14.6%) and 16 (11.1%) cases, respectively (**Table 1**).

TERT Promoter Status

The distribution of *TERT* promoter mutations according to socio-demographic and clinical characteristics of patients are shown in **Table 1**. In the overall cohort, the promoter of *TERT* harboured mutations in 45/144 cases (31.3%). The *TERT* -124 C>T mutation was more common (29/144, 20.1%) than -146 C>T (16/144, 11.1%). These two mutations occurred in a mutually exclusive manner and with a heterozygous genotype. No mutations were observed in any of 57 adjacent available analysed mucosal specimens, 16 of which were surrounding mutated tumours. There was no statistically significant difference among analysed parameters with regard to *TERT* promoter mutation rate. We also genotyped 140 of 144 patients of our cohort for the rs2853669 SNP at -245 bp. A total of 86 patients (61.4%) carried the minor C-variant allele, for which 16 patients were homozygous and 70 were heterozygous. Fifty-four patients (38.6%) had the T/T genotype. Notably, patients with *TERT* promoter mutated tumours had a higher prevalence of the T/T genotype than patients with unmutated *TERT* promoter (p=0.0243) (**Table 1**).

Telomere Length

Measurement of RTL was obtained from 132 tumour tissues and 57 surrounding mucosal specimens. Values ranged between 0.42 and 4.42 (median 1.29) in tumours and between 0.62 and 2.93 (median 1.18) in surrounding mucosa; neither correlated with the age (data not shown). Telomere length in tumour cells and surrounding mucosa were not significantly associated with any

TABLE 1 | Distribution of 144 patients with oral cavity squamous cell carcinoma (OCSCC) according to socio-demographic and clinical characteristics, by *TERT* promoter mutational status.

		***TERT* promoter**			**Fisher exact test**
	N (%)	**unmutated N (%)**	**-124 C>T N (%)**	**-146 C>T N (%)**	
Overall	144	99 (68.8)	29 (20.1)	16 (11.1)	
Sex					
Female	63 (43.8)	41 (65.1)	12 (19.1)	10 (15.9)	p=0.3198
Male	81 (56.2)	58 (71.6)	17 (21.0)	6 (7.4)	
Age (years)					
<60	54 (37.5)	43 (79.6)	8 (14.8)	3 (5.6)	p=0.1415
60-69	39 (27.1)	27 (69.2)	8 (20.5)	4 (10.3)	
≥70	51 (35.4)	29 (56.9)	13 (25.5)	9 (17.7)	
Smoking status					
Never	55 (38.2)	41 (74.6)	9 (16.4)	5 (9.1)	p=0.5152
Ever	89 (61.8)	58 (65.2)	20 (22.5)	11 (12.4)	
Drinking status					
Never	84 (58.3)	58 (69.1)	17 (20.2)	9 (10.7)	p=1.000
Ever	60 (41.7)	41 (68.3)	12 (20.0)	7 (11.7)	
Cancer sub-site					
Tongue	78 (54.2)	55 (70.5)	16 (20.5)	7 (9.0)	p=0.6791
Floor of mouth	22 (15.3)	17 (77.3)	2 (9.1)	3 (13.4)	
Gingiva	15 (10.4)	9 (60.0)	3 (20. 0)	3 (20.0)	
Buccal mucosa	15 (10.4)	9 (60.0)	5 (33.3)	1 (6.7)	
Other	14 (9.7)	9 (64.3)	3 (21.4)	2 (14.3)	
pT					
T1-T2	99 (68.7)	66 (66.7)	20 (20.2)	13 (13.1)	p=0.5891
T3-T4	45 (31.3)	33 (73.3)	9 (20.0)	3 (6.7)	
pN					
N0	97 (67.4)	66 (68.0)	19 (19.6)	12 (12.4)	p=0.8553
N1-N3	47 (32.6)	33 (70.2)	10 (21.3)	4 (8.5)	
pStage					
I-II	75 (52.1)	49 (65.3)	16 (21.3)	10 (13.3)	p=0.5697
III-IV	69 (47.9)	50 (72.5)	13 (18.8)	6 (8.7)	
Grading[a]					
G1-G2	104 (74.8)	69 (66.4)	22 (21.2)	13 (12.5)	p=0.5676
G3	35 (25.2)	26 (74.3)	7 (20.0)	2 (5.7)	
RT					
No	93 (64.6)	61 (65.6)	20 (21.5)	12 (12.9)	p=0.5422
Yes	51 (35.4)	38 (74.5)	9 (17.7)	4 (7.8)	
CT					
No	124 (86.1)	84 (67.7)	26 (21.0)	14 (11.3)	p=0.9285
Yes	20 (13.9)	15 (75.0)	3 (15.0)	2 (10.0)	
Surgical margins					
Negative	123 (85.4)	86 (69.9)	23 (18.7)	14 (11.4)	p=0.5699
Close/Positive	21 (14.6)	13 (61.9)	6 (28.6)	2 (9.5)	
Extracapsular spread					
Negative	128 (88.9)	89 (69.5)	24 (18.8)	15 (11.7)	p=0.5367
Positive	16 (11.1)	10 (62.5)	5 (31.3)	1 (6.3)	
TERT-rs2853669[a]					
TT	54 (38.6)	31 (57.4)	12 (22.2)	11 (20.4)	**p=0.0243**
TC/CC	86 (61.4)	64 (74.4)	17 (19.8)	5 (5.8)	

[a]*The sum does not add up to total because of missing values; RT, radiotherapy; CT, chemotherapy.*
Bold values indicate p<0.05.

of the measured demographic or clinical characteristics (**Supplementary Table 1**). In keeping with our previous findings (13), we found that the mucosa adjacent to tumours harbouring *TERT* promoter mutations had significantly shorter telomeres than those in adjacent mucosa of cancers with unmutated *TERT* promoter (p=0.017) (**Figure 1A**). In particular, the surrounding mucosa adjacent to tumours with -124 C>T mutated *TERT* promoter showed the shortest telomeres (p=0.016; **Figure 1B**), despite these patients being younger [median (IQR), 64(58–70) years] than those with unmutated tumours [median (IQR), 67(48–74) years] or with tumours harbouring -146 C>T mutations [median (IQR), 75(71–80) years] (p for age=0.065; data not shown). Conversely, telomere length in tumour tissue did not significantly differ according to the mutational status of *TERT* promoter (p=0.1182) (**Figures 1A, B**).

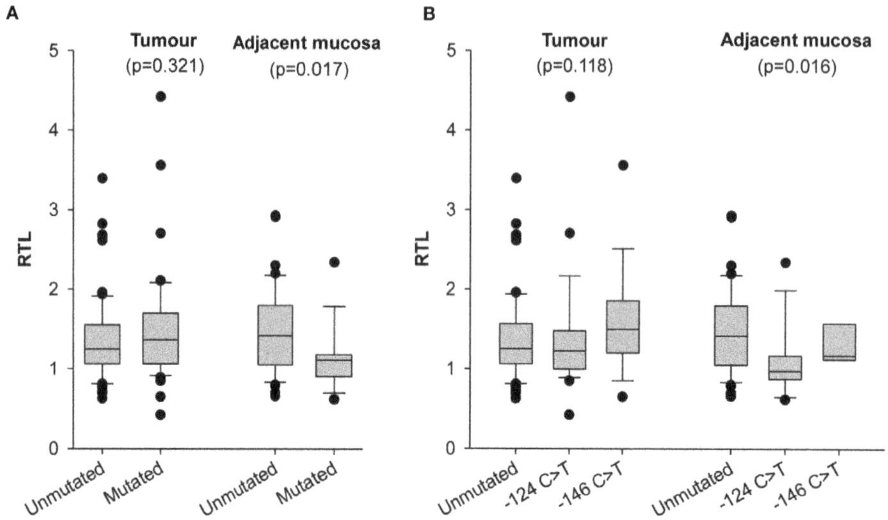

FIGURE 1 | Distribution of relative telomere length (RTL) in tumour and adjacent mucosa according to *TERT* promoter status. **(A)** samples were stratified according to absence (Unmutated) and presence of -124 C>T or -146 C>T mutations (Mutated) in the *TERT* promoter region. **(B)** samples were stratified according to *TERT* promoter status in absence (Unmutated), presence of -124 C>T and presence of -146 C>T mutations in the *TERT* promoter region.

Time-To-Event Analysis

The associations between socio-demographic and clinical characteristics of patients with clinical outcome are summarized in **Supplementary Table 2**. In a multivariate analysis adjusted for clinical variables (gender, age, pN, grading, surgical margins, and extracapsular invasion), it emerged that buccal mucosa sub-site, pathological lymph nodes, and G3 grading were significantly associated with increased risk of death (HR: 5.96, 95% CI: 1.16-30.73; p=0.0328; HR: 2.30, 95% CI: 1.12-4.75; p=0.0237; HR: 2.28, 95% CI: 1.14-4.56; p=0.0195; respectively).

In order to identify the potential impact of *TERT* promoter mutations on oncological outcome, we first investigated the association between *TERT* promoter status with PFS. Kaplan-Meier survival curve showed that the 5-year PFS for patients harbouring the -124 C>T mutation was 42.4% as opposed to 64.3% for patients without mutations, 68.2% for those harbouring the -146 C>T mutation (p=0.0069; **Figure 2B**). This association was confirmed by multivariate analysis (**Table 2**) after adjustment for clinical variables with a HR for progression of 2.71 (95% CI: 1.42-5.17; p=0.0024).

The presence of the -124 C>T mutation was also consistently associated with shorter OS, with 46.7% of patients alive after 5 years, in comparison to 73.7% and 74.5% of patients without mutations or harbouring the -146 C>T mutation, respectively (p=0.0163; **Figure 2C**). Multivariate analyses confirmed the negative effect of the -124 C>T mutation on prognosis, with a HR of death of 2.71 (95% CI: 1.30-5.66; p=0.0079) (**Table 2**). The negative impact of the -124 C>T mutation on clinical outcome was likely due to poorer mucosal control; indeed, based upon cumulative incidence estimates, patients with tumours harbouring this mutation suffered a 5-year mucosal failure rate of 38.4% in comparison to 16% and 25% in patients without mutations or harbouring the -146 C>T mutation, respectively (p=0.0136; **Figure 2A**). This association remained statistically significant in the multivariate analysis (HR: 2.75, 95% CI: 1.22-6.17; p=0.0143) (**Table 2**). These results suggest that the -124 C>T point mutation may be a risk factor for the aggressiveness of OCSCC compared to the -146 C>T mutation and unmutated *TERT* promoters which appear to be associated with a more favourable clinical outcome. Notably, the surrounding mucosa adjacent to tumours with -124 C>T mutated *TERT* promoter had the shortest telomeres (p=0.016; **Figure 1B**), and, in line with our previous studies (26, 27), adjacent mucosa with shorter telomeres (below the median value) showed a high, albeit not significant risk of tumour relapse (**Table 2**).

Kaplan-Meier survival analysis revealed that carriers of the T/T rs2853669 genotype showed significantly worse PFS (p=0.008) and OS (p=0.021) compared with C carriers (T/C+C/C genotypes) (**Supplementary Figure 1B, C**). The negative impact of the T/T genotype was confirmed in the multivariate analysis for progression (HR: 1.80, 95% CI: 1.05-3.12; p=0.0343) but not for death (HR: 1.75, 95% CI: 0.93-3.29; p=0.0837) (**Table 2**).

To evaluate if the SNP rs2853669 genotype can modulate the effect of *TERT* promoter mutations on oncological outcome, the potential role of the -124 C>T *TERT* promoter mutation as a prognostic parameter in OCSCC patients was assessed according to their rs2853669 background. Multivariate analysis revealed that the risk of mucosal failure (HR: 2.88, 95% CI: 1.01-8.25; p=0.0484), progression (HR: 5.36, 95% CI: 2.30-12.48; p<0.0001) and death (HR: 4.05, 95% CI: 1.47-11.12; p=0.0067) were significantly increased in patients with -124 C>T mutated tumours carrying the T/T genotype of the rs2853669 (**Table 2**) compared to patients without this mutation, and C carriers of the SNP.

DISCUSSION

In the present investigation, we observed that approximately one-third of OCSCC samples harboured *TERT* promoter

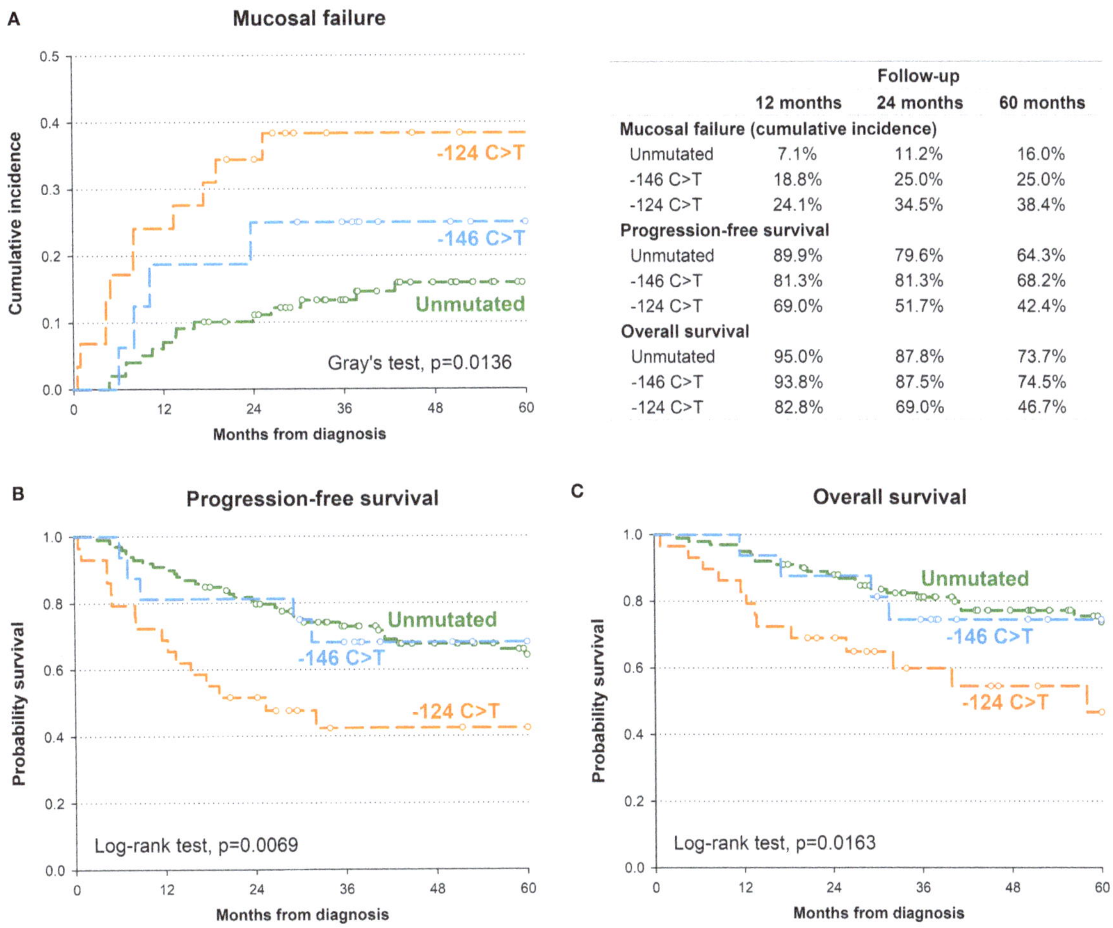

	Follow-up		
	12 months	24 months	60 months
Mucosal failure (cumulative incidence)			
Unmutated	7.1%	11.2%	16.0%
-146 C>T	18.8%	25.0%	25.0%
-124 C>T	24.1%	34.5%	38.4%
Progression-free survival			
Unmutated	89.9%	79.6%	64.3%
-146 C>T	81.3%	81.3%	68.2%
-124 C>T	69.0%	51.7%	42.4%
Overall survival			
Unmutated	95.0%	87.8%	73.7%
-146 C>T	93.8%	87.5%	74.5%
-124 C>T	82.8%	69.0%	46.7%

FIGURE 2 | Kaplan-Meier estimates of cumulative incidence of mucosal recurrence **(A)**, progression-free survival **(B)** and overall survival **(C)** by *TERT* promoter.

mutations with the -124 C>T mutation having a significant adverse impact on the outcome; particularly, when coexisting with the T/T genotype of rs2853669, -124 C>T mutation increased the risk of death by 4 times.

In the literature, the frequency of *TERT* promoter mutations in OCSCC varies significantly among studies ranging from 30.4 to 75% (13, 28–34). This variability could be attributable to different patient population characteristics or methodological approaches. In our cohort, we found 31.3% (45 of 144) of OCSCC samples harboured *TERT* promoter mutations, which was in line with other studies (13, 28, 30, 33, 34). In agreement with other studies on OCSCC (20, 28–32), the two mutations have different frequency, with a higher prevalence of -124 C>T (29 of 144) compared to -146 C>T (16 of 144).

With respect to oncological outcomes, an important finding emerging from this study is that the two somatic *TERT* promoter mutations displayed different behaviour. Indeed, while patients with the -124 C>T *TERT* promoter mutation had a higher risk of mucosal failure and poorer DFS and OS, patients with tumours harbouring the -146 C>T mutation had an improved clinical outcome, similar to those with unmutated *TERT* promoter. The recruitment of the transcription factor GABPA, a member of ETS family, specifically to mutant *TERT* promoters mediates long-range chromatin interaction and enrichment of active histone marks, and hence drives *TERT* transcription (35). Although both the -124 C>T and -146 C>T mutations generate identical sequences, enable binding of GABPA transcription factors, and are equally efficient in increasing *TERT* transcription *in vitro* (36), previous reports demonstrated that these mutations are not functionally identical. Indeed, a peculiar pathway of activation by non-canonical NF-κB signalling was only described for the -146 C>T mutation (37, 38). In addition, *in vivo*, the -124 C>T mutation was associated with higher *TERT* expression/telomerase activity compared to -146 C>T (39, 40). A significant body of evidence has demonstrated that high levels of tumour TERT expression and/or telomerase activity are significantly associated with aggressiveness of disease, advanced clinical stage, and poor OS and/or DFS in several types of tumours, including UADT SCC (13, 26, 27, 41). The mechanism(s) by which high TERT expression ultimately facilitates cancer progression and constitutes a prognostic factor are not completely elucidated, and seems not be attributable only to TERT's ability to maintain telomere length. Indeed, accumulating evidence suggests that

TABLE 2 | Hazard ratio (HR) and corresponding 95% confidence interval (CI)a for mucosal failure, regional failure, progression, and death according to strata of TERT promoter status, rs2853669 genotype and telomere length.

	Pts	Mucosal failure			Regional failure			Progression			Death		
		n	HR (95% CI) [b]	Wald χ^2	n	HR (95% CI)	Wald χ^2	n	HR (95% CI)	Wald χ^2	n	HR (95% CI)	Wald χ^2
TERT promoter													
unmutated	99	15	Ref		13	Ref		32	Ref		23	Ref	
-146C>T	16	4	2.46 (0.82-7.36)	p=0.1077	2	1.10 (0.21-5.73)	p=0.9127	5	1.35 (0.50-3.65)	p=0.5561	4	1.64 (0.53-5.08)	p=0.3891
-124C>T	29	11	2.75 (1.22-6.17)	**p=0.0143**	5	1.51 (0.48-4.73)	p=0.4822	16	2.71 (1.42-5.17)	**p=0.0024**	13	2.71 (1.30-5.66)	**p=0.0079**
TERT-rs2853669 (Dominant model)[c]													
CT/CC	86	15	Ref		12	Ref		25	Ref		18	Ref	
TT	54	14	1.36 (0.67-2.74)	p=0.3989	8	0.88 (0.37-2.11)	p=0.7820	28	1.80 (1.05-3.12)	**p=0.0343**	22	1.75 (0.93-3.29)	p=0.0837
TERT promoter – rs2853669													
unmut/-146C>T – CT/CC	69	10	Ref.		9	Ref.		19	Ref.		12	Ref.	
unmut/-146C>T – TT	42	8	1.33 (0.54-3.28)	p=0.5421	6	0.97 (0.35-2.69)	p=0.9476	18	1.50 (0.77-2.90)	p=0.2339	15	1.87 (0.86-4.08)	p=0.1156
-124C>T – CT/CC	17	5	2.69 (0.87-8.31)	p=0.0850	3	1.82 (0.47-7.06)	p=0.3857	6	1.79 (0.69-4.64)	p=0.2290	6	2.80 (0.98-8.00)	p=0.0539
-124C>T – TT	12	6	2.88 (1.01-8.25)	**p=0.0484**	2	1.06 (0.17-6.73)	p=0.9521	10	5.36 (2.30-12.48)	**p<0.0001**	7	4.05 (1.47-11.12)	**p=0.0067**
RTL (tumor)													
≤1.29[d]	66	15	Ref		8	Ref		25	Ref		21	Ref	
>1.29	66	13	0.92 (0.39-2.16)	p=0.8518	9	1.17 (0.36-3.87)	p=0.7946	23	1.04 (0.57-1.89)	p=0.8950	16	0.90 (0.45-1.78)	p=0.7564
RTL (surrounding mucosa)[e]													
>1.18[d]	26	3	Ref		3	Ref		5	Ref		3	Ref	
≤1.18	25	6	2.38 (0.48-11.73)	p=0.2869	1	0.07 (0.00-3.15)	p=0.1726	8	1.23 (0.37-4.14)	p=0.7366	8	2.21 (0.53-9.31)	p=0.2789

[a]*Estimated from Cox proportional hazard model, adjusting for gender, age, pN, grading, surgical margins, and extracapsular invasion.*
[b]*Adjusted for competing risk according to Fine-Gray model;*
[c]*Results for the best genetic model on OS;*
[d]*Cut-off were defined according to median value;*
[e]*Analysis restricted to patients with negative surgical margins; Pts, patients; RTL, relative telomere length.*
Bold values indicate p<0.05.

TERT may also contribute to carcinogenesis *via* telomere length-independent mechanisms, including enhancement of proliferation, resistance to apoptosis, inflammation, invasion and metastasis altogether contributing towards a more aggressive phenotype of cancer cells (10, 11, 42–50). Therefore, it is conceivable that the -124 C>T *TERT* promoter mutation, inducing higher expression of TERT in the tumour, results in the increased severity of disease as we observed in our cohort of OCSCC patients. Corroborating our results, Arantes et al. (33) found that the -124 C>T *TERT* promoter mutation was associated with increased risk of tumour relapse and death in a cohort of 88 Brazilian patients with SCC of the UADT. However, other studies in different tumour types have reported contradicting clinical effects of *TERT* promoter mutations, ranging from poorer survival associated with the -146 C>T *TERT* promoter mutation to unchanged clinical outcome (28, 29, 32, 51–54). Given that the two mutations create an identical sequence corresponding to a *de novo* binding site for ETS transcription factors, these alternative results may depend on the genetic context, including the SNP background in which *TERT* mutations arise.

For the common polymorphism rs2853669 T>C, which disrupts a pre-existing ETS2 binding site within the *TERT* core promoter, controversial clinical impacts have been reported (12, 17–20). Our study demonstrates for the first time that the rs2853669 T/T genotype influences the clinical outcome of OCSCC patients, being significantly associated with increased risk of disease progression. Importantly, the coexistence of the T/T genotype of rs2853669 and the -124 C>T *TERT* promoter mutation is associated with a significantly poorer prognosis including mucosal failure, disease progression and death. The effect of the rs2853669 SNP may be related to higher telomerase activity and *TERT* expression conferred by the T/T genotype (15) that can also additionally intensify the transactivation activity of *TERT* promoter mutations (14). Thus, we can speculate that high *TERT* levels conferred by the -124 C>T *TERT* promoter mutation and/or rs2853669 T/T genotype may promote tumour progression, probably as a consequence of the extra-telomeric non-canonical functions of telomerase. Unfortunately, we did not have enough tumour material to contemporaneously analyse *TERT* promoter status and TERT expression/activity, and further studies should be undertaken to extend and validate these findings.

A secondary finding of our study was the absent of *TERT* promoter mutations in the matched adjacent mucosa. This partly differs from a previous study by Chang et al. (29), and may be due to the reduced number of adjacent normal mucosal specimens available in our cohort. Nonetheless, the finding that metastatic and recurrent head and neck squamous cell carcinomas have more *TERT* promoter mutations compared to primary tumours (31) suggests that the acquisition of these mutations is a late event in carcinogenesis, and may explain the lack of *TERT* promoter mutations in the tumour's adjacent mucosa.

Interestingly, we confirmed that telomeres in mucosa adjacent to *TERT* promoter mutated tumours were significantly shorter than those adjacent to tumours retaining unmutated *TERT* promoter (13), and additionally we found that the mucosa adjacent to -124 C>T mutated tumours had the shortest telomeres. As critically short telomeres are a hallmark of genomic instability associated to carcinogenesis and may be considered a marker of field cancerization (26, 27), is not surprising that patients harbouring the -124 C>T *TERT* promoter mutation showed a significantly increased risk of tumour relapse. These data, for the first time, support a prognostic role for tumour relapse of the -124 C>T *TERT* promoter mutation in patients with OCSCC likely related to the very short telomeres in the mucosa surrounding the tumour in which the mutation arises.

In conclusion, we found that the -124 C>T *TERT* promoter mutation, as well as the T/T genotype of the rs2853669 SNP, may be a risk factor for the aggressiveness of OCSCC, and the coexistence of these genetic variations might represent a greater risk of adverse outcome. Supported by the fact that the clinical significance of this mutation is consistent with the biological properties of TERT, that *TERT* promoter mutations were found to stratify the prognosis in several other cancers, are easy to identify using tissue from routinely collected biopsies and address the unmet clinical need of having a validated prognostic marker for OCSCC, our observations raise the possibility that the -124 C>T *TERT* promoter mutation in combination with the SNP rs2853669 T/T genotype may serve as a valuable prognostic marker in this cancer, with the ability to guide therapeutic and follow-up strategies.

ETHICS STATEMENT

The studies involving human participants were reviewed and approved by the Treviso/Belluno provinces (protocol code 346/AULSS9, March 10, 2015), Italy. The patients/participants provided their written informed consent to participate in this study.

AUTHOR CONTRIBUTIONS

Conceptualization: ADR, PBR. and SG. Methodology: SG. Statistical analysis: JP. Investigation: SG, PBR, ER, GT, LA, RDC, MR, PN, AM, VC, MT, LB, GS, EE, MMa, MS, RB, APDT, MG, MMo, and GE. Resources: ADR. Writing-original draft preparation: SG and PBR. Writing-review and editing: SG, PBR, JF, and ADR. Supervision: ADR. Project administration: PBR and SG. All authors contributed to the article and approved the submitted version.

REFERENCES

1. *Cancer Today*. Available at: http://gco.iarc.fr/today/home (Accessed December 10, 2020).
2. Arora A, Husain N, Bansal A, Neyaz A, Jaiswal R, Jain K, et al. Development of a New Outcome Prediction Model in Early-Stage Squamous Cell Carcinoma of the Oral Cavity Based on Histopathologic Parameters With Multivariate Analysis: The Aditi-Nuzhat Lymph-Node Prediction Score (ANLPS) System. *Am J Surg Pathol* (2017) 41:950–60. doi: 10.1097/PAS.0000000000000843
3. Brands MT, Smeekens EAJ, Takes RP, Kaanders JHAM, Verbeek ALM, Merkx MAW, et al. Time Patterns of Recurrence and Second Primary Tumors in a Large Cohort of Patients Treated for Oral Cavity Cancer. *Cancer Med* (2019) 8:5810–19. doi: 10.1002/cam4.2124
4. van Dijk BA, Brands MT, Geurts SM, Merkx MA, Roodenburg JL. Trends in Oral Cavity Cancer Incidence, Mortality, Survival and Treatment in the Netherlands. *Int J Cancer* (2016) 139:574–83. doi: 10.1002/ijc.30107
5. Paderno A, Morello R, Piazza C. Tongue Carcinoma in Young Adults: A Review of the Literature. *Acta Otorhinolaryngol Ital* (2018) 38:175–80. doi: 10.14639/0392-100X-1932
6. Castellsagué X, Alemany L, Quer M, Halec G, Quirós B, Tous S, et al. HPV Involvement in Head and Neck Cancers: Comprehensive Assessment of Biomarkers in 3680 Patients. *J Natl Cancer Inst* (2016) 108:djv403. doi: 10.1093/jnci/djv403
7. Blackburn EH, Greider CW, Szostak JW. Telomeres and Telomerase: The Path From Maize, Tetrahymena and Yeast to Human Cancer and Aging. *Nat Med* (2006) 12:1133–8. doi: 10.1038/nm1006-1133
8. Shay JW, Wright WE. Role of Telomeres and Telomerase in Cancer. *Semin Cancer Biol* (2011) 21:349–53. doi: 10.1016/j.semcancer.2011.10.001
9. Hanahan D, Weinberg RA. Hallmarks of Cancer: The Next Generation. *Cell* (2011) 144:646–74. doi: 10.1016/j.cell.2011.02.013
10. Ségal-Bendirdjian E, Geli V. Non-Canonical Roles of Telomerase: Unraveling the Imbroglio. *Front Cell Dev Biol* (2019) 7:332. doi: 10.3389/fcell.2019.00332
11. Martínez P, Blasco MA. Telomeric and Extra-Telomeric Roles for Telomerase and the Telomere-Binding Proteins. *Nat Rev Cancer* (2011) 11:161–76. doi: 10.1038/nrc3025
12. Hafezi F, Perez Bercoff D. The Solo Play of TERT Promoter Mutations. *Cells* (2020) 9:749. doi: 10.3390/cells9030749
13. Boscolo-Rizzo P, Giunco S, Rampazzo E, Brutti M, Spinato G, Menegaldo A, et al. TERT Promoter Hotspot Mutations and Their Relationship With TERT Levels and Telomere Erosion in Patients With Head and Neck Squamous Cell Carcinoma. *J Cancer Res Clin Oncol* (2020) 146:381–9. doi: 10.1007/s00432-020-03130-z
14. Park CK, Lee SH, Kim JY, Kim JE, Kim TM, Lee ST, et al. Expression Level of Htert is Regulated by Somatic Mutation and Common Single Nucleotide Polymorphism at Promoter Region in Glioblastoma. *Oncotarget* (2014) 5:3399–407. doi: 10.18632/oncotarget.1975
15. Hsu CP, Hsu NY, Lee LW, Ko JL. Ets2 Binding Site Single Nucleotide Polymorphism at the Htert Gene Promoter-Effect on Telomerase Expression and Telomere Length Maintenance in Non-Small Cell Lung Cancer. *Eur J Cancer* (2006) 42:1466–74. doi: 10.1016/j.ejca.2006.02.014
16. Shen N, Lu Y, Wang X, Peng J, Zhu Y, Cheng L. Association Between Rs2853669 in TERT Gene and the Risk and Prognosis of Human Cancer: A Systematic Review and Meta-Analysis. *Oncotarget* (2017) 8:50864–72. doi: 10.18632/oncotarget.15140
17. Rachakonda P, Hosen I, de Verdier PJ, Fallah M, Heidenreich B, Ryk C, et al. TERT Promoter Mutations in Bladder Cancer Affect Patient Survival and Disease Recurrence Through Modification by a Common Polymorphism. *Proc Natl Acad Sci USA* (2013) 110:17426–31. doi: 10.1073/pnas.1310522110
18. Ko E, Seo HW, Jung ES, Kim BH, Jung G. The TERT Promoter SNP Rs2853669 Decreases E2F1 Transcription Factor Binding and Increases Mortality and Recurrence Risks in Liver Cancer. *Oncotarget* (2016) 7:684–99. doi: 10.18632/oncotarget.6331
19. Simon M, Hosen I, Gousias K, Rachakonda S, Heidenreich B, Gessi M, et al. TERT Promoter Mutations: A Novel Independent Prognostic Factor in Primary Glioblastomas. *Neuro Oncol* (2015) 17:45–52. doi: 10.1093/neuonc/nou158
20. Batista R, Cruvinel-Carloni A, Vinagre J, Peixoto J, Catarino TA, Campanella NC, et al. The Prognostic Impact of TERT Promoter Mutations in Glioblastomas Is Modified by the Rs2853669 Single Nucleotide Polymorphism. *Int J Cancer* (2016) 139:414–23. doi: 10.1002/ijc.30057
21. Indraccolo S, Lombardi G, Fassan M, Pasqualini L, Giunco S, Marcato R, et al. Genetic, Epigenetic, and Immunologic Profiling of MMR-Deficient Relapsed Glioblastoma. *Clin Cancer Res* (2019) 25:1828–37. doi: 10.1158/1078-0432.CCR-18-1892
22. Gianesin K, Noguera-Julian A, Zanchetta M, Del Bianco P, Petrara MR, Freguja R, et al. Premature Aging and Immune Senescence in HIV-Infected Children. *AIDS* (2016) 30:1363–73. doi: 10.1097/QAD.0000000000001093
23. Rampazzo E, Bertorelle R, Serra L, Terrin L, Candiotto C, Pucciarelli S, et al. Relationship Between Telomere Shortening, Genetic Instability, and Site of Tumour Origin in Colorectal Cancers. *Br J Cancer* (2010) 102:1300–5. doi: 10.1038/sj.bjc.6605644
24. Kalbfleisch JD, Prentice RL. The Statistical Analysis of Failure Time Data. *New York: Wiley* (2002) 95–147. doi: 10.1002/9781118032985
25. Fine JP, Gray RJ. A Proportional Hazard Model for the Subdistribution of a Competing Risk. *J Am Stat Ass* (1999) 94:496–509. doi: 10.2307/2670170
26. Boscolo-Rizzo P, Rampazzo E, Polesel J, Giunco S, Menegaldo A, Mantovani M, et al. Predictive and Prognostic Significance of Telomerase Levels/Telomere Length in Tissues and Peripheral Blood in Head and Neck Squamous Cell Carcinoma. *Sci Rep* (2019) 9:17572. doi: 10.1038/s41598-019-54028-x
27. Boscolo-Rizzo P, Rampazzo E, Perissinotto E, Piano MA, Giunco S, Baboci L, et al. Telomere shortening in mucosa surrounding the tumor: biosensor of field cancerization and prognostic marker of mucosal failure in head and neck squamous cell carcinoma. *Oral Oncol* (2015) 51:500–7. doi: 10.1016/j.oraloncology.2015.02.100
28. Vinothkumar V, Arunkumar G, Revathidevi S, Arun K, Manikandan M, Rao AK, et al. TERT Promoter Hot Spot Mutations are Frequent in Indian Cervical and Oral Squamous Cell Carcinomas. *Tumour Biol* (2016) 37:7907–13. doi: 10.1007/s13277-015-4694-2
29. Chang K, Wang CI, Pickering CR, Huang Y, Tsai CN, Tsang NM, et al. Prevalence of Promoter Mutations in the TERT Gene in Oral Cavity Squamous Cell Carcinoma. *Head Neck* (2017) 39:1131–7. doi: 10.1002/hed.24728
30. Annunziata C, Pezzuto F, Greggi S, Ionna F, Losito S, Botti G, et al. Distinct Profiles of TERT Promoter Mutations and Telomerase Expression in Head and Neck Cancer and Cervical Carcinoma. *Int J Cancer* (2018) 143:1153–61. doi: 10.1002/ijc.31412
31. Morris LGT, Chandramohan R, West L, Zehir A, Chakravarty D, Pfister DG, et al. The Molecular Landscape of Recurrent and Metastatic Head and Neck Cancers: Insights From a Precision Oncology Sequencing Platform. *JAMA Oncol* (2017) 3:244–55. doi: 10.1001/jamaoncol.2016.1790
32. Yilmaz I, Erkul BE, Ozturk Sari S, Issin G, Tural E, Terzi Kaya Terzi N, et al. Promoter Region Mutations of the Telomerase Reverse Transcriptase (TERT) Gene in Head and Neck Squamous Cell Carcinoma. *Oral Surg Oral Med Oral Pathol Oral Radiol* (2020) 130:63–70. doi: 10.1016/j.oooo.2020.02.015
33. Arantes LMRB, Cruvinel-Carloni A, de Carvalho AC, Sorroche B, Carvalho AL, Scapulatempo-Neto C, et al. TERT Promoter Mutation C228T Increases Risk for Tumor Recurrence and Death in Head and Neck Cancer Patients. *Front Oncol* (2020) 10:1275. doi: 10.3389/fonc.2020.01275
34. Mundi N, Prokopec SD, Ghasemi F, Warner A, Patel K, MacNeil D, et al. Genomic and Human Papillomavirus Profiling of an Oral Cancer Cohort Identifies TP53 as a Predictor of Overall Survival. *Cancers Head Neck* (2019) 4:5. doi: 10.1186/s41199-019-0045-0
35. Akıncılar SC, Khattar E, Boon PL, Unal B, Fullwood MJ, Tergaonkar V. Long-Range Chromatin Interactions Drive Mutant TERT Promoter Activation. *Cancer Discov* (2016) 6:1276–91. doi: 10.1158/2159-8290.CD-16-0177
36. Bell RJ, Rube HT, Kreig A, Mancini A, Fouse SD, Nagarajan RP, et al. Cancer. The Transcription Factor GABP Selectively Binds and Activates the Mutant TERT Promoter in Cancer. *Science* (2015) 348:1036–9. doi: 10.1126/science.aab0015
37. Li Y, Zhou QL, Sun W, Chandrasekharan P, Cheng HS, Ying Z, et al. Non-Canonical NF-κb Signalling and ETS1/2 Cooperatively Drive C250T Mutant TERT Promoter Activation. *Nat Cell Biol* (2015) 17:1327–38. doi: 10.1038/ncb3240

38. Xu X, Li Y, Bharath SR, Ozturk MB, Bowler MW, Loo BZL, et al. Structural Basis for Reactivating the Mutant TERT Promoter by Cooperative Binding of P52 and ETS1. *Nat Commun* (2018) 9:3183. doi: 10.1038/s41467-018-05644-0
39. Huang DS, Wang Z, He XJ, Diplas BH, Yang R, Killela PJ, et al. Recurrent TERT Promoter Mutations Identified in a Large-Scale Study of Multiple Tumour Types Are Associated With Increased TERT Expression and Telomerase Activation. *Eur J Cancer* (2015) 51:969–76. doi: 10.1016/j.ejca.2015.03.010
40. Heidenreich B, Rachakonda P, Hosen I, Volz F, Hemminki K, Weyerbrock A, et al. TERT Promoter Mutations and Telomere Length in Adult Malignant Gliomas and Recurrences. *Oncotarget* (2015) 6:10617–33. doi: 10.18632/oncotarget.3329
41. Giunco S, Rampazzo E, Celeghin A, Petrara MR, De Rossi A. Telomere and Telomerase in Carcinogenesis: Their Role as Prognostic Biomarkers. *Curr Pathobiol Rep* (2015) 3:315–28. doi: 10.1007/s40139-015-0087-x
42. Mukherjee S, Firpo EJ, Wang Y, Roberts JM. Separation of Telomerase Functions by Reverse Genetics. *Proc Natl Acad Sci U.S.A.* (2011) 108: E1363–71. doi: 10.1073/pnas.1112414108
43. Park JI, Venteicher AS, Hong JY, Choi J, Jun S, Shkreli M, et al. Telomerase Modulates Wnt Signalling by Association With Target Gene Chromatin. *Nature* (2009) 460:66–72. doi: 10.1038/nature08137
44. Haendeler J, Hoffmann J, Rahman S, Zeiher AM, Dimmeler S. Regulation of Telomerase Activity and Anti-Apoptotic Function by Protein-Protein Interaction and Phosphorylation. *FEBS Lett* (2003) 536:180–6. doi: 10.1016/s0014-5793(03)00058-9
45. Dudognon C, Pendino F, Hillion J, Saumet A, Lanotte M, Ségal-Bendirdjian E. Death Receptor Signaling Regulatory Function for Telomerase: hTERT Abolishes TRAIL-Induced Apoptosis, Independently of Telomere Maintenance. *Oncogene* (2004) 23:7469–74. doi: 10.1038/sj.onc.1208029
46. Celeghin A, Giunco S, Freguja R, Zangrossi M, Nalio S, Dolcetti R, et al. Short-Term Inhibition of TERT Induces Telomere Length-Independent Cell Cycle Arrest and Apoptotic Response in EBV-Immortalized and Transformed B Cells. *Cell Death Dis* (2016) 7:e2562. doi: 10.1038/cddis.2016.425
47. Giunco S, Zangrossi M, Dal Pozzolo F, Celeghin A, Ballin G, Petrara MR, et al. Anti-Proliferative and Pro-Apoptotic Effects of Short-Term Inhibition of Telomerase *In Vivo* and in Human Malignant B Cells Xenografted in Zebrafish. *Cancers (Basel)* (2020) 12:2052. doi: 10.3390/cancers12082052
48. Ghosh A, Saginc G, Leow SC, Khattar E, Shin EM, Yan TD, et al. Telomerase Directly Regulates NF-κb-Dependent Transcription. *Nat Cell Biol* (2012) 14:1270–81. doi: 10.1038/ncb2621
49. Liu H, Liu Q, Ge Y, Zhao Q, Zheng X, Zhao Y. hTERT Promotes Cell Adhesion and Migration Independent of Telomerase Activity. *Sci Rep* (2016) 6:22886. doi: 10.1038/srep22886
50. Boscolo-Rizzo P, Da Mosto MC, Rampazzo E, Giunco S, Del Mistro A, Menegaldo A, et al. Telomeres and Telomerase in Head and Neck Squamous Cell Carcinoma: From Pathogenesis to Clinical Implications. *Cancer Metastasis Rev* (2016) 35:457–74. doi: 10.1007/s10555-016-9633-1
51. Qu Y, Dang S, Wu K, Shao Y, Yang Q, Ji M, et al. TERT Promoter Mutations Predict Worse Survival in Laryngeal Cancer Patients. *Int J Cancer* (2014) 135:1008–10. doi: 10.1002/ijc.28728
52. Geng J, Liu Y, Guo Y, Wang H, Tai J, Jin Y, et al. Correlation Between TERT C228T and Clinic-Pathological Features in Pediatric Papillary Thyroid Carcinoma. *Sci China Life Sci* (2019) 62:1563–71. doi: 10.1007/s11427-018-9546-5
53. You H, Wu Y, Chang K, Shi X, Chen XD, Yan W, et al. Paradoxical Prognostic Impact of TERT Promoter Mutations in Gliomas Depends on Different Histological and Genetic Backgrounds. *CNS Neurosci Ther* (2017) 23:790–7. doi: 10.1111/cns.12724
54. Del Bianco P, Stagni C, Giunco S, Fabozzi A, Elefanti L, Pellegrini S, et al. TERT Promoter Mutations Differently Correlate With the Clinical Outcome of MAPK Inhibitor-Treated Melanoma Patients. *Cancers (Basel)* (2020) 12:946. doi: 10.3390/cancers12040946

5

Myb Immunohistochemical Staining and Fluorescence *in situ* Hybridization in Salivary Rare Basaloid Lesions

Binbin Li [1,2,3], Weiping Jie [1,2,3] and Huiying He [4*]

[1] Department of Oral Pathology, Peking University School and Hospital of Stomatology, Beijing, China, [2] Research Unit of Precision Pathologic Diagnosis in Tumors of the Oral and Maxillofacial Regions, Chinese Academy of Medical Sciences, Beijing, China, [3] National Clinical Research Center for Oral Diseases, Peking University School and Hospital of Stomatology, Beijing, China, [4] Department of Pathology, School of Basic Medical Sciences, Third Hospital, Peking University Health Science Center, Beijing, China

***Correspondence:**
Huiying He
hehylibb@aliyun.com

Objective: Salivary rare basaloid lesions, including cribriform type basal cell adenoma (cBCA), BCA with incomplete capsule (iBCA), sialoblastoma (SB), and intercalated duct hyperplasia (IDH), could easily be misdiagnosed as adenoid cystic carcinoma (AdCC). We aim to identify an approach for differential diagnosis and to establish an optimal workflow concerning the diagnosis of these lesions.

Material and methods: A panel of antibodies (MYB, β-catenin, CD117, SOX10, ki67, P63, calponin) and fluorescence *in situ* hybridization (FISH)-MYB were utilized to distinguish above salivary basaloid diseases from AdCC.

Results: Histologically, the striking diagnostic features of cBCA, iBCA, SB, and IDH are composed of basaloid tumor cells, well-defined encapsulation, or lack of destructive invasion. Immunohistochemically, Myb immune-labeling could effectively make a distinction among cBCA, iBCA, SB, and IDH from AdCC, except in SB. cBCA and iBCA typically expressed β-catenin in the nuclei of tumor cells. There was no statistical significance in the ki67 index between SB and AdCC, but their indices were significantly higher than those of iBCA and IDH ($p < 0.05$, $p < 0.05$, respectively). P63 and calponin immune-expression were observed in the basaloid or myoepithelial cells. CD117 were observed positively in cBCA, iBCA, SB, and AdCC, except in IDH. SOX10 were observed positively in all cases. No cases had fusion of MYB and NFIB detectable by FISH, except in AdCC.

Conclusion: Considering their sensitivity and specificity, FISH-Myb and an immunohistochemical panel of MYB/β-catenin/ki67 would be an optimal choice for the differential diagnosis of these basaloid lesions.

Clinical relevance: Some salivary basaloid tumor or tumor-like lesions have overlapping features with AdCC. Through this present research, we suggested that the panel IHC of MYB, βcatenin, and ki67 combined with FISH-Myb should be an optimal choice for differential diagnosis among those lesions.

Keywords: MYB, immunohistochemistry, fluorescence *in situ* hybridization, salivary basaloid lesions, adenoid cystic carcinoma

INTRODUCTION

Salivary rare basaloid tumor or tumor-like lesions share some features resembling adenoid cystic carcinoma (AdCC), even exhibiting a typical cribriform pattern like that of AdCC. This creates diagnosis pitfalls, especially in fine-needle aspiration testing (FNAT). iBCA and cBCA are usually treated with a conservative treatment strategy (partial or superficial parotidectomy), which is very different from the radical choice of AdCC (radical surgical excision with or without postoperative radiation). No surgical intervention is required for IDH. Most SBs are cured by primary surgical resection. Therefore, it is very important to make a differential diagnosis between them. In addition, these lesions may be less familiar to non-head and neck specialists due to the low incidence. Since exact diagnosis is crucial for an appropriate treatment choice, it is necessary to study the following AdCC mimicking lesions using the specific protein and molecular markers.

Usually, typical basal cell adenoma (BCA) is well-circumscribed and composed of basaloid cells with eosinophilic cytoplasm (1). In practice, there are two types of BCA, cribriform BCA (cBCA) and BCA with incomplete encapsulation (iBCA), which are easily misdiagnosed as AdCC. Because AdCC is mainly characterized by a cribriform growth pattern, the cribriform components apparent in cBCA would mislead pathologists to the diagnosis of AdCC. Our primary study and a recent study both proved that AdCC and cBCA were two distinct tumor entities (2, 3). Some studies suggested that β-catenin mutation was present in up to 52% of BCAs. Thus, the corresponding nuclear expression of β-catenin can be detected in BCA and would be a specific marker to identify cBCA or iBCA from AdCC (4). At the same time, few BCAs have incomplete capsules or could have focal capsule invasion, which are easily mistaken as malignant presentation. In this circumstance it is important to differentiate iBCA from AdCC, despite the capsule of micro-invasion.

Apart from iBCA and cBCA, sialoblastoma (SB), and intercalated duct hyperplasia (IDH) could occasionally resemble AdCC too. SB was ever named as congenital hybrid basal cell adenoma-adenoid cystic carcinoma (5), which suggested that its morphology overlapped with BCA or AdCC. In some instances the cribriform pattern was evident in SB, and it was problematic to distinguish between them. IDH is a salivary ductal proliferation resembling intercalated ducts, which was newly identified as a separate entity in the WHO new classification of Head and Neck Tumors 2017. It is considered as a reactive and hyperplastic process, or a precursor condition for some salivary gland tumors, such as BCA (6). It typically exhibited an idiopathic, focal hypertrophic lesion of intraoral mucous glands with limited growth possibilities (7). Due to its unencapsulation, IDH may also be misdiagnosed as AdCC.

Recent genomic study identified new markers that may be helpful in future investigations. Researchers have shown that the specific translocation *t* (6;9) involving v-myb avian myeloblastosis viral oncogene homolog (MYB) and nuclear factor 1B-type (NFIB) was the most relevant genetic alternation in AdCC (8). MYB immuno-staining was proved to be a useful ancillary test for distinguishing AdCC from other benign and malignant salivary gland neoplasms (9, 10). On the other hand, the transcriptional factor sex-determining region Y (SRY)-related HMG box-containing factor 10 (SOX10), normally only expressed during salivary gland differentiation, was found markedly upregulated in a majority of AdCC cases (11). In addition, it was reported that most AdCCs (90%) exhibited strong and diffuse expression of CD117 (12). Thus, a panel of specific immunomarkers that include MYB, SOX-10, and CD117 could be believed as very effective for the diagnosis of AdCC.

Of course, the typical AdCC is generally recognized by biopsy in HE staining. However, iBCA, cBCA, SB, and IDH are extremely rare lesions, and are much more confusing in microscopic diagnosis. Based on above research progress, genetic abnormalities, and protein expressions may be helpful in their distinction from AdCC. Taken together, it is worth identifying an approach with relatively high sensitivity and high specificity in the histologic diagnosis of salivary basaloid lesions. This study first used a combination of histologic, immunohistochemical, and a FISH test to evaluate MYB, CD117, SOX10, βcatenin, ki67, p63, and calponin in the differential diagnosis of cBCA, iBCA, SB, and IDH from AdCC. It was shown that both SB and AdCC had MYB positive immune-expression, but only AdCC had Myb rearrangement examined by FISH. The positive reaction ofβ-catenin in nuclear was specific in iBCA and cBCA. P63 and calponin immune-expression were observed in the basaloid or myoepithelial cells. CD117 were observed positively in cBCA, iBCA, SB, and AdCC, except in IDH. SOX10 were observed positively in all the cases. The ki67 indices of SB and AdCC were significantly higher than those of iBCA and IDH. Taking account of both sensitivity and specificity, we recommend FISH-Myb and an immunohistochemical panel of MYB/β-catenin/ki67 as an optimal choice for the differential diagnosis of these basaloid lesions.

MATERIALS AND METHODS

Patients

Approved by Institutional Review Board and formally numbered PKUSSIRB-201631121, 64 cases, including 23 cBCAs, 11 iBCAs, 3 SBs, 7 IDHs, and 20 AdCCs (as controls), were collected from the files of Peking University School and Hospital of Stomatology. The criteria for eligibility of AdCC were (i) histologically typical AdCC confirmed by two pathologists (Dr. Li and Dr. He) (ii) presence of adjacent tissue invasion, including muscle, gland, vessel, nerve, and bone infiltration or lung metastasis.

The investigated parameters consisted of gender, age distributions, anatomic location, histologic characteristics, treatment, and postoperative outcomes. Follow-up information was obtained from the medical records or by telephone interview.

Histological Examination

All specimens were fixed in neutral buffered 10% formalin, processed and embedded in paraffin. 4 μm sections were stained with hematoxylin and eosin, and then observed under light microscope.

Immunohistochemical Reaction

All slides were performed with the following seven antibodies by the standard streptavidin-biotin-peroxidase complex technique. The MYB antibody was bought from ABCAM Co. (clone EP769Y, dilution 1:500, ABCAM, Cambridge, MA). CD117 (clone EP10), SOX10 (clone EP268), βcatenin (clone UMAB15), ki67(clone UMAB107), p63 (clone 4A4), and calponin (clone EP63) were obtained from Zymed Co. (Zymed, Carlsbad, CA). The staining was scored qualitatively and assessed on intensity (1+ to 3+) and staining pattern (nuclear, cytoplasm or membrane). Only 2+ or 3+ intensity staining was interpreted as positive.

FISH Test

A commercially available Myb dual-color break-apart probe (ZTV-Z-2143-200, ZytoVision, Bremerhaven, Germany) was utilized for FISH. Before hybridization, 4 μm slides were baked at 65°C overnight, deparaffinized by washing with xylene and ethanol, and rehydrated with deionized water at 90°C for 30 min. Pretreated slides were incubated with a proteinase K solution (100 mg/mL; Sigma-Aldrich, UK) for 10–30 min. Slides and probes were then co-denatured at 73°C for 5 min and hybridized overnight at 37°C using an automated ThermoBrite codenaturation oven (Abbott Molecular) according to the manufacturer's instructions. After hybridization, slides were immersed in a post-hybridization solution, 2xSSC/0.3% NP40 at 73°C for 2 min, and subsequently in 2xSSC/0.1%NP40 at room temperature for 1 min. Slides were dehydrated, dried, and counterstained with 4,6-diamino-2-phenylindole (DAPI; Vysis, USA).

All the FISH slides were reviewed and confirmed by two pathologists, and microscopically scored, respectively.

Statistical Analysis

SPSS 17.0 software was used to perform statistical analysis and draw diagrams. Statistical comparisons of ki67 between all the groups were made using analysis of variance (ANOVA). The LSD *post-doc* assay was used when equal variance was assumed. Otherwise, Dunnetts T3 test was used. Correlation analysis was used to analyze the relation between MYB immuno-analysis and chromosome rearrangement. Differences of $P < 0.05$ were considered significant.

RESULTS

Clinical Features

For all the 44 cases mimicking AdCC, the mean age was 45 years and the male/female ratio was 12/32. Most iBCAs (95%) occurred in the parotid glands. All cBCA and SB occurred in the parotid gland.

All the selected benign salivary diseases have a slow growth process and were well-demarcated. Localized swelling was the main symptom in all cases. All patients underwent complete surgical excision of these lesions and there had been no recurrence at the time when this study was written up (Dec. 2018). The median follow-up time was 87 months.

In particular, three cases of SB were infants or children, including two cases in 1-year-olds, and one case in a 12-years-old. The duration of follow-up for these three patients was 80, 119, and 92 months, respectively (**Table 1**).

Histologic Findings

Generally, all the tumor types included in this study were composed mainly of basal-like cells. These small-to-medium basaloid cells consisted of a series of columnar, cuboidal, or polygonal cells. Cells had hyperchromatic nuclei with little cytoplasm, similar to the basal cells in stratified squamous epithelium. Although these basaloid cells shared similar cellular morphology, the tumors demonstrated different histologic patterns, immunoprofiles, and specific disease behavior.

At low magnification, cBCA was well-demarcated and uniform in parenchyma. These tumors had cribriform patterns with pseudocyst formation containing amorphous and basophilic material, resembling AdCC (**Figure 1A**). At higher magnification, the outermost layers of cells surrounding each cell nest were usually cuboidal with peripheral palisading. Although both BCA and AdCC are thought to arise from the same basal stem cell, BCA had a more distinct pattern with micro-encapsulated areas that were not apparent in AdCC. BCA also displayed a clear separation of epithelium from stroma, which was never seen in AdCC.

For iBCA, the tumor cells may invade the capsule, or there may be no clear boundary between the tumor mass and normal glands (**Figure 1B**). Sometimes, the mass had no definite capsule, but was surrounded by a fibrous pseudocapsule. There existed a limited extension of tumor into normal glandular parenchyma, but this was not a sign of malignancy.

IDH was often accompanied by other benign or malignant lesions. It was usually ill-defined, and lacked destructive invasion, anaplasia, or mitotic activity, and the lobular pattern of normal salivary glands was preserved (**Figure 1C**).

SB showed nests of basaloid cells with a palisading pattern at the periphery, and maturation toward the center. Neither brisk mitotic activity nor necrosis was present (**Figure 2A**). The characteristic morphology and specific age of onset of this tumor were the key points of diagnosis.

In contrast, the AdCCs under study were all typically cribriform, and exhibited invasion such as that into muscle, gland, nerve, or bone. Multiple microcytic spaces divided the nests into numerous cylinders, yielding a "honeycomb" configuration (**Figure 2B**). The nuclei were atypical and appeared hyperchromatic and pleomorphic with increased mitotic activity. The stroma in AdCC appeared more hyalinized and richer than other lesions noted above. Moreover, the separation between the stroma and parenchyma was obvious.

Cytomorphologic Descriptions

Although cancer cells in AdCC were in some instances more pleomorphic and hyperchromatic than cells in benign diseases, cytologic features alone did not serve to distinguish AdCC from its mimics. All the mimics showed overlapping cytological features with AdCC. The nuclei of the mimics were regular in shape and uniformly basophilic. Ductal structures were lined

TABLE 1 | Clinical characteristics of all the basaloid lesions.

Tumor	Median age (years)	Sex (Female/male)	Locations	Current status	Median follow-up duration (months)
cBCA (n = 23)	48	16/7	parotid	Alive/No recurrence	110
iBCA (n = 11)	47	9/2	parotid	Alive/No recurrence	43
SB (n = 3)	5	1/2	parotid	Alive/No recurrence	97
IDH (n = 7)	48	6/1	Parotid5/submandibular2	Alive/No recurrence	75
Total (n = 44)	45	32/12	Parotid (95%)	Alive/No recurrence	87

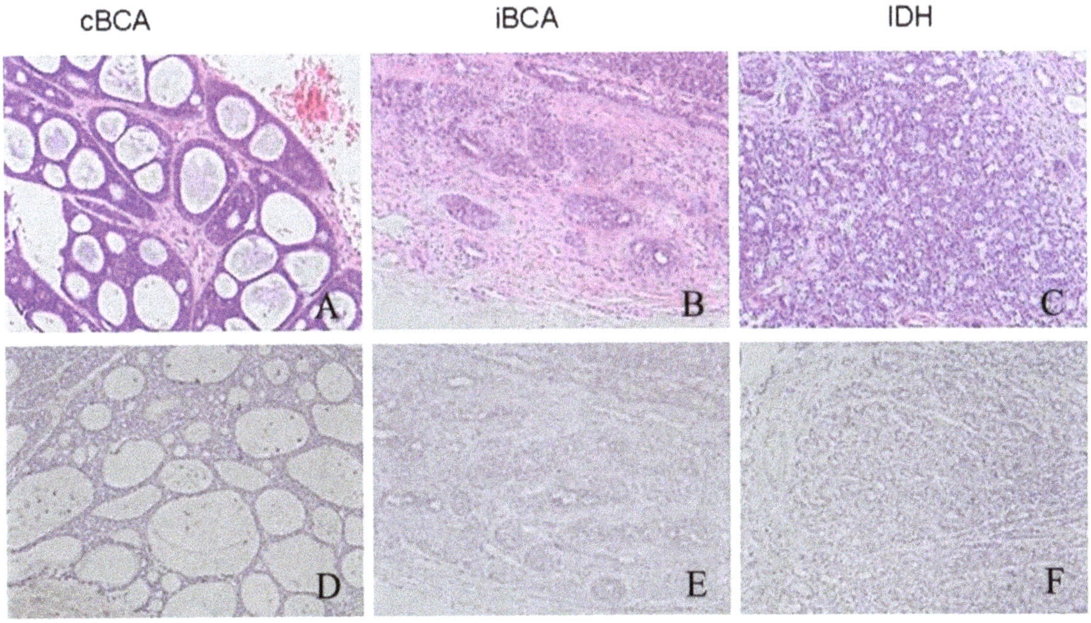

FIGURE 1 | Histology (upper line) and MYB immune-expression (lower line) in cBCA, iBCA, and IDH. cBCA was well-defined and had cribriform patterns with pseudocyst formation **(A)**. Both iBCA and IDH had no definite capsule and presented no clear boundary between the tumor mass and the surrounding tissues **(B,C)**. But iBCA showed typical BCA characteristics of peripheral palisading in parenchyma. No immunoreactivity for MYB antigen was found in these three lesions **(D–F)**.

by cuboidal cells which had uniform nuclei with condensed chromatin. An inner layer of cuboidal cells was surrounded by the outer layer of cells, which exhibited myoepithelial differentiation. Nuclear atypia was absent or minimal, and the mitotic figures were rare.

Immunohistochemistry

The overall results are listed in **Table 2**. iBCA, cBCA, and IDH showed no MYB antigen immunoreactivity (**Figures 1D–F**). However, two cases of SB were MYB positive (**Figure 2C**). As a contrast, all AdCC exhibited strong diffuse nuclear expression of MYB in myoepithelial and partial glandular tumor cells (**Figure 2D**).

Immunomarkers of p63 disclosed the presence of both basaloid and myoepithelial differentiation, while calponin marker indicated only myoepithelial differentiation here. Most tumor cells in all cases were p63-positive in parenchyma. The calponin antigen was detected in the polygonal myoepithelia and was especially prominent in the outer layer of cribriforming.

All tumors showed varied patterns of β-catenin expression: positive iBCA and cBCA staining localized in the nuclei and membrane (7 iBCA and 17cBCA), or nuclear+cytoplasm+membrane staining (4 iBCA and 6 cBCA). However, AdCC showed β-catenin immunoreactivity only in the membrane. Two cases of SB showed positivity only in the membrane, and in one case there was nuclear+cytoplasm+membrane positivity. Four cases of IDH were found to be nuclear+membrane positive, while three cases of IDH showed positivity solely in the membrane (**Figure 3**).

CD117 generally showed a positive trabecular pattern. Five cases of iBCA and three cases of cBCA were positive for CD117. Two cases of SB were positive for CD117. IDH was CD117 negative. CD117 was expressed in 14 cases of AdCC. Sox10 was expressed in all cases.

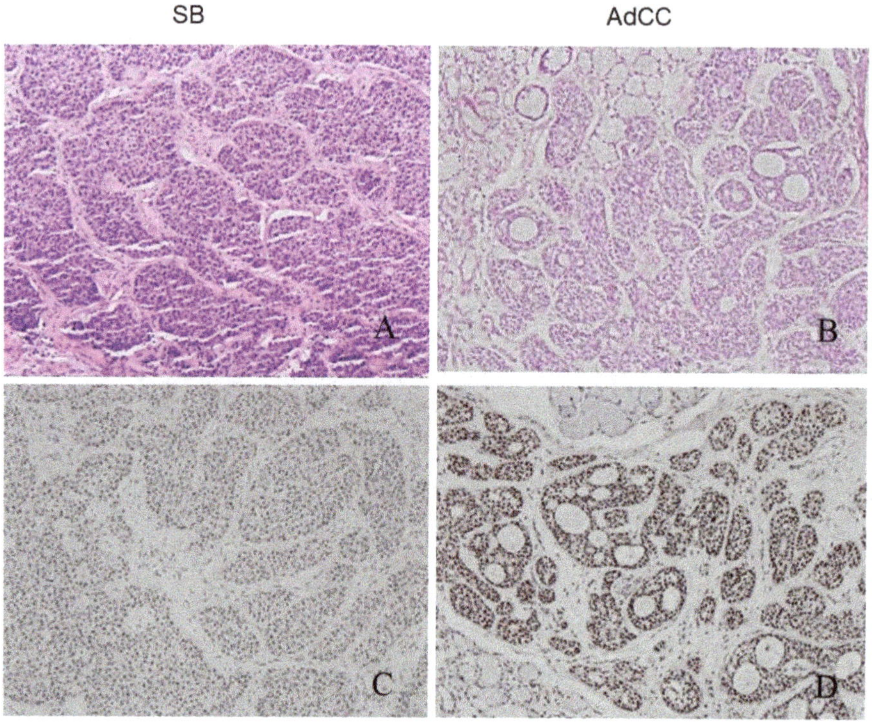

FIGURE 2 | Histology (upper line) and MYB immune-expression (lower line) in SB and AdCC. SB composed of basaloid epithelial nests with a palisading pattern **(A)**. AdCCs in this study were all typically cribriform, and exhibited invasion into normal gland **(B)**. MYB immunostains were strongly and diffusely positive in myoepithelial cells and partial glandular tumor cells of two SBs **(C)** and all the AdCC in this study **(D)**.

TABLE 2 | Immunohistochemical and FISH results of all the basaloid lesions.

Tumor	Myb	βcatenin	CD117	SOX10	ki67 (%)	P63	calponin	FISH-MYB
cBCA	-	+(including nuclear)	+(5/23)	+	0.30%	+	+	-
iBCA	-	+(including nuclear)	+(3/11)	+	2.80%	+	+	-
SB	+	+	+(3/3)	+	37.30%	+	+	-
IDH	-	+	-	+	1.00%	+	+	-
AdCC	+	+(only membrane)	+(14/20)	+	28.25%	+	+	+

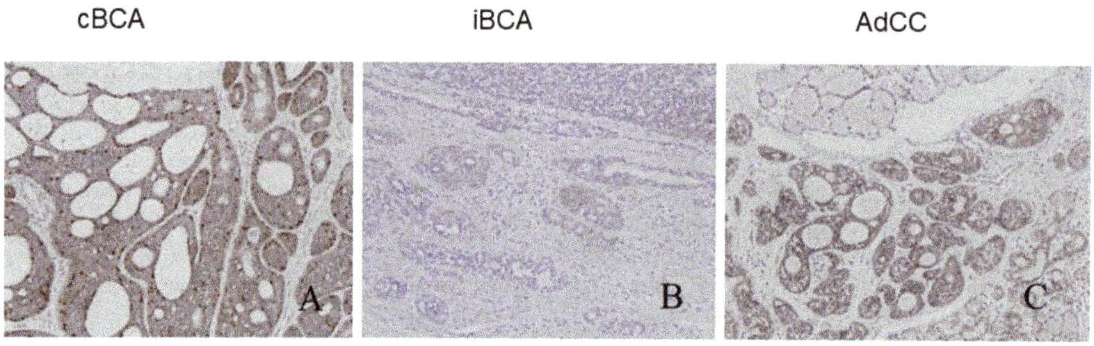

FIGURE 3 | βcatenin immune-expression in cBCA, iBCA, and AdCC. The positive staining of iBCA and cBCA localized in nuclear+membrane or nuclear+cytoplasm+membrane **(A,B)**. AdCC had immuno-activity of β-catenin only in the membrane **(C)**.

The average expression ratio of ki67 in cBCA, iBCA, SB, IDH, and AdCC was 0.3, 2.8, 37.3, 1.0, and 28.25%, respectively. The ki67 indices of SB and AdCC were significantly higher than that of cBCA, iBCA, and IDH ($p < 0.05$, $p < 0.05$, $p < 0.05$, respectively). The ki67 positive index in SB and AdCC was not significantly different.

Evaluation of *Myb* Rearrangement by FISH

None of these lesions under study, including cBCA, iBCA, IDH, and SB, showed *Myb* rearrangement by FISH. One case of cBCA and one case of iBCA did not yield enough evaluable signals due to long storage of blocks and poor probe penetration of nuclei (**Figures 4A–C**). Fourteen cases of 19 AdCC (73.68%) were found to harbor Myb rearrangement (**Figure 4D**). One case of AdCC showed no signal due to poor specimen preparation.

Noticeably, the MYB immunoprofile was significantly related to FISH results ($p = 0.00$, Pearson correlation).

DISCUSSION

Morphologic studies of salivary basaloid lesions have of late received attention (13). This study focused on the differential diagnosis of AdCC and basaloid lesions which mimic AdCC. Our data suggested that an immunoprofile incorporating MYB, ki67, and β-catenin together with FISH was advantageous for diagnosis, and these markers should be considered as first line markers. Alternative markers, including CD117, SOX10, p63, and calponin, were not as specific as MYB, ki67, and β-catenin.

Although AdCC grows comparatively slowly, it should be considered as at least a moderately differentiated cancer because of its predilection for perineural invasion, local recurrence, and distant metastasis even many years after the initial surgery (14). Therefore, its overall prognosis is poor. The recurrent *t* (6; 9) (q22-23; p23-24) translocation has been identified in AdCC (15), resulting in scrutiny of Myb in the diagnosis of AdCC. The poor prognosis of this tumor may be associated with MYB expression (16). However, the MYB expression showed no correlation with traditional prognostic factors such as TNM stage or tumor grade (17). As for the location in which MYB is expressed, it has been reported that MYB immunolabeling is confined mainly in the peripheral myoepithelial cells and has not been identified in ductal cells of tumors with either a tubular or cribriform pattern (16). We chose typical cribriform AdCC as a control and found that these tumors all showed strong MYB expression in both myoepithelial and partial glandular tumor cells. There were also controversies in the choice of immunohistochemistry and FISH to evaluate for MYB antigen or fusion of Myb and NFIB. Poling et al. found that MYB-immunohistochemistry was more sensitive and specific than Myb-FISH (18). Using the FISH technique, West et al. found a balanced translocation between Myb and NFIB was present in 49% of AdCC, while there was no apparent translocation of *Myb* in 35% of the cases (16). Sixteen percent of cases have an abnormal FISH pattern

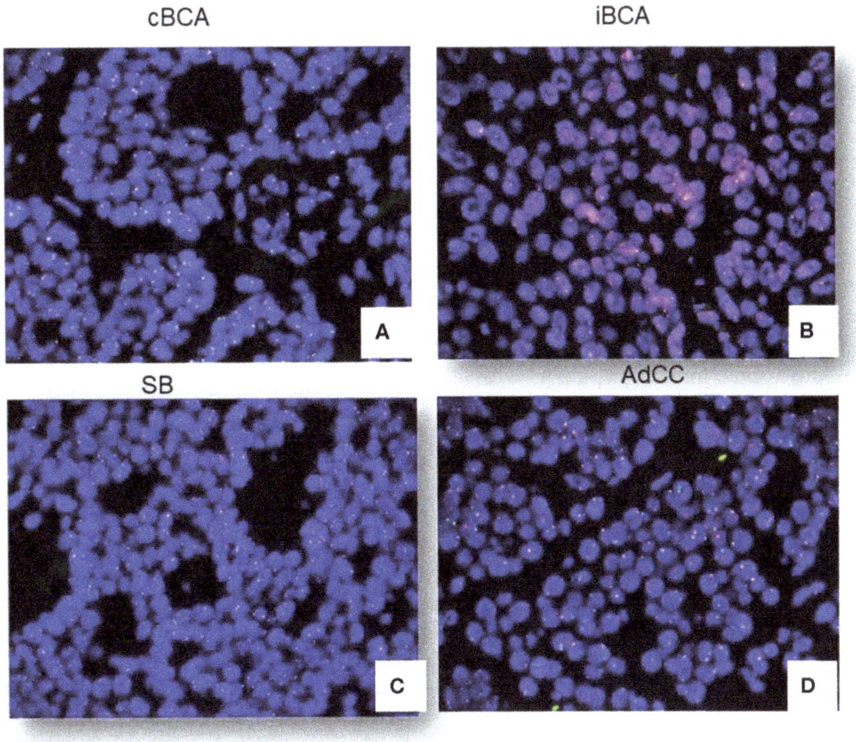

FIGURE 4 | FISH signals in cBCA, iBCA, SB, and AdCC. No cases of cBCA, iBCA, or SB showed Myb rearrangement **(A–C)**. 73.68% of AdCC showed positive signals by FISH **(D)**.

suggestive of a translocation of Myb but not necessarily involving NFIB (Myb 3′, Myb 5′, and NFIB all come together, extra 5′Myb without association with NFIB, and Myb split without association with NFIB). In our study, MYB expression was not observed in iBCA, cBCA, or IDH. MYB immunostain appeared to be a sensitive marker for differentiating AdCC from salivary gland lesions with a similar histology, except SB. However, the positive-MYB SB in immunohistochemistry showed no Myb rearrangement by FISH, while 73.68% of AdCC were found to harbor a Myb rearrangement. This strongly suggested that MYB immunostaining is a specific and cost-effective method in the diagnosis of AdCC, but further confirmation by FISH was recommended.

SB is an extremely rare tumor, and <100 cases have been reported worldwide (19). In most of the reported cases, SB occurred in the parotid, and these cases had all been diagnosed at birth. Our cases of SB involved the parotid gland, but the age of onset was a little older than infancy. There were a few youth cases of 13-years-olds reported in literature (20). The histologic features of these cases were microscopically similar to those in gland embryonic development at the 3rd month. Some pathologists believe IDH is the precursor of BCA. In the current study we found that MYB immuno-expression and the ki67 index overlapped with AdCC. As Myb is the key finding in the diagnosis of AdCC, it is critical to ensure diagnosis by FISH. None of the tumors evaluated in our study showed evidence of fusion of Myb and NFIB by FISH, except AdCC. 73.68% of AdCC showed Myb-NFIB fusion. There was a significant positive correlation of the MYB immunoprofile and Myb rearrangement. As such, we conclude FISH is a reliable diagnostic approach for differentiating basaloid lesions from AdCC.

β-catenin was useful in this study for distinguishing BCA from AdCC, including cBCA and iBCA. Its nuclear expression was typical and specific for BCA. Sato et al. demonstrated that Wnt/β-catenin signal alteration plays a role in the pathogenesis of BCA (4). Our data showed that all the selected AdCCs in our study had membrane immuno-activity of β-catenin. One case of SB was nuclear+cytoplasm+membrane positive, and four cases of IDH were nuclear+membrane positive. The above situations are infrequent but should be kept in mind in differential diagnosis.

Ki67 is widely used as a proliferation marker (21). Generally, benign neoplasms have lower ki67 indices, typically <10%. Although the average positive rates of ki67 in SB and AdCC were 37.3 and 28.25%, respectively, there was no statistic difference between them. This may serve as a reminder that the ki67 index should be taken into consideration in order to make an accurate diagnosis.

CD117 expression in AdCC varies considerably. As a proto-oncogene encoding a transmembrane receptor type tyrosine kinase, early reports suggested that CD117 expression appeared to be restricted to AdCC (22). However, our present study found that it may be expressed in most ductal cells, even including benign salivary gland diseases such as most iBCA, and a small number of cBCA and SB. IDH showed no reactivity to CD117. Therefore, CD117 was of little value in the diagnosis of AdCC. SOX-10 was all positive in our series of cases. Although SOX-10 is a marker for sero-mucinous differentiation (23), our findings demonstrated that it is not a specific marker for AdCC.

Taken together, we first used a combination of histologic, immunohistochemical and FISH test to evaluate MYB, CD117, SOX10, βcatenin, ki67, p63, and calponin in the differential diagnosis of cBCA, iBCA, SB, and IDH from AdCC. Considering their sensitivity and specificity, FISH-Myb and an immunohistochemical panel of MYB/β-catenin/ki67 would be an optimal choice for the differential diagnosis of these basaloid lesions.

ETHICS STATEMENT

The studies involving human participants were reviewed and approved by Peking University School and Hospital of Stomatology. Written informed consent for participation was not required for this study in accordance with the national legislation and the institutional requirements.

AUTHOR CONTRIBUTIONS

BL: design, IHC test, and writing. WJ: follow-up and data analyse. HH: FISH, writing, and submission. All authors contributed to the article and approved the submitted version.

REFERENCES

1. Ogawa I, Nikai H, Takata T, Miyauchi M, Ito H, Ijuhin N. The cellular composition of basal cell adenoma of the parotid gland: an immunohistochemical analysis. *Oral Surg Oral Med Oral Pathol.* (1990) 70:619–26. doi: 10.1016/0030-4220(90)90411-K
2. Tian Z, Li L, Zhang CY. Differences in MYB expression and gene abnormalities further confirm that salivary cribriform basal cell tumors and adenoid cystic carcinoma are two distinct tumor entities. *J Oral Pathol Med.* (2016) 45:698–703. doi: 10.1111/jop.12414
3. Li BB, Zhou CX, Jia SN. Basal cell adenoma of salivary glands with a focal cribriform pattern: clinicopathologic and immunohistochemical study of 19 cases of a potential pitfall for diagnosis. *Ann Diagn Pathol.* (2014) 18:5–9. doi: 10.1016/j.anndiagpath.2013.09.002
4. Sato M, Yamamoto H, Hatanaka Y, Nishijima T, Jiromaru R, Yasumatsu R, et al. Wnt/β-catenin signal alteration and its diagnostic utility in basal cell

adenoma and histologically similar tumors of the salivary gland. *Pathol Res Pract.* (2018) 214:586–92. doi: 10.1016/j.prp.2017.12.016

5. Dardick I, Daley TD, McComb RJ. Sialoblastoma in adults: distinction from adenoid cystic carcinoma. *Oral Surg Oral Med Oral Pathol Oral Radiol Endod.* (2010) 109:109–16. doi: 10.1016/j.tripleo.2009.07.049
6. Chiosea S, Seethala R, Williams MD. Intercalated hyperplasia. In: EI-Naggar AK, Chan JKC, Grandis JR, Takata T, Slootweg PJ, editors. *World Health Organization Classification of Head and Neck Tumours. 4th Edn.* Lyon: IARC Press (2017). p. 197. doi: 10.1007/s12105-017-0785-2
7. Luna MA. Salivary gland hyperplasia. *Adv Anat Pathol.* (2002) 9:251–5. doi: 10.1097/00125480-200207000-00005
8. Wysocki PT, Izumchenko E, Meir J. Adenoid cystic carcinoma: emerging role of translocations and gene fusions. *Oncotarget.* (2016) 7:66239–54. doi: 10.18632/oncotarget.11288
9. Pusztaszeri MP, Sadow PM, Ushiku A. MYB immunostaining is a useful ancillary test for distinguishing adenoid cystic carcinoma from pleomorphic adenoma in fine-needle aspiration biopsy specimens. *Cancer Cytopathol.* (2014) 122:257–65. doi: 10.1002/cncy.21381
10. Bell D, Roberts D, Karpowicz M, Hanna EY, Weber RS, El-Naggar AK. Clinical significance of Myb protein and downstream target genes in salivary adenoid cystic carcinoma. *Cancer Biol Ther.* (2011) 12:569–73. doi: 10.4161/cbt.12.7.17008
11. Ivanov SV, Panaccione A, Nonaka D. Diagnostic Sox10 gene signatures in salivary adenoid cystic and breast basal-like carcinomas. *Br J Cancer.* (2013) 109:444–51. doi: 10.1038/bjc.2013.326
12. Jain A, Shetty DC, Rathore AS, Kumar K. Characterization and localization of c-kit and epidermal growth factor receptor in different patterns of adenoid cystic carcinoma. *J Cancer Res Ther.* (2016) 12:834–9. doi: 10.4103/0973-1482.177504
13. Seethala RR. Basaloid/blue salivary gland tumors. *Mod Pathol.* (2017) 30:S84–95. doi: 10.1038/modpathol.2016.190
14. Stenman G, Licitra L, Said-AI-Naief N, van Zante A, Yarbrough WG. Adenoid cystic carcinoma. In: EI-Naggar AK, Chan JKC, Grandis JR, Takata T, Slootweg PJ, editors. *World Health Organization Classification of Head and Neck Tumours. 4th Edn.* Lyon: IARC Press (2017). p. 164–5.
15. Stenman G, Persson F, Andersson MK. Diagnostic and therapeutic implications of new molecular biomarkers in salivary gland cancers. *Oral Oncol.* (2014) 50:683–90. doi: 10.1016/j.oraloncology.2014.04.008
16. West RB, Kong C, Clarke N. MYB expression and translocation in adenoid cystic carcinomas and other salivary gland tumors with clinicopathologic correlation. *Am J Surg Pathol.* (2011) 35:92–9. doi: 10.1097/PAS.0b013e3182002777
17. Broz M, Steiner P, Salzman R, Hauer L, Starek I. The incidence of MYB gene breaks in adenoid cystic carcinoma of the salivary glands and its prognostic significance. *Biomed Pap Med Fac Univ Palacky Olomouc Czech Repub.* (2016) 160:417–22. doi: 10.5507/bp.2016.027
18. Poling JS, Yonescu R, Subhawong AP, Sharma R, Argani P, Ning Y, et al. MYB labeling by immunohistochemistry is more sensitive and specific for breast adenoid cystic carcinoma than MYB labeling by FISH. *Am J Surg Pathol.* (2017) 41:973–9. doi: 10.1097/PAS.0000000000000878
19. Vidyadhar M1, Amanda C, Thuan Q, Prabhakaran K. Sialoblastoma. *J Pediatr Surg.* (2008) 43:e113. doi: 10.1016/j.jpedsurg.2008.04.035
20. Saravakos P, Hartwein J, Fayyazi A. Sialoblastoma of the parotid gland in a 13-years-old girl with multiple recurrences and long-term follow-up. *Head Neck.* (2016) 38:e13–5. doi: 10.1002/hed.24084
21. Ben-Izhak O, Akrish S, Nagler RM. Ki67 and salivary cancer. *Cancer Invest.* (2008) 26:1015–23. doi: 10.1080/07357900802088968
22. Holst VA, Marshall CE, Moskaluk CA, Frierson HF Jr. KIT protein expression and analysis of c-kit gene mutation in adenoid cystic carcinoma. *Mod Pathol.* (1999) 12:956–60.
23. Panaccione A, Zhang Y, Ryan M, Moskaluk CA, Anderson KS, Yarbrough WG, et al. MYB fusions and CD markers as tools for authentication and purification of cancer stem cells from salivary adenoid cystic carcinoma. *Stem Cell Res.* (2017) 21:160–6. doi: 10.1016/j.scr.2017.05.002

6

SMAD4 Somatic Mutations in Head and Neck Carcinoma are Associated with Tumor Progression

Li-Han Lin [1]*, Kuo-Wei Chang* [2,3]*, Hui-Wen Cheng* [1] *and Chung-Ji Liu* [3,4*]

[1] *Department of Medical Research, MacKay Memorial Hospital, Taipei, Taiwan,* [2] *Department of Stomatology, Taipei Veterans General Hospital, Taipei, Taiwan,* [3] *School of Dentistry, Institute of Oral Biology, National Yang-Ming University, Taipei, Taiwan,* [4] *Department of Oral and Maxillofacial Surgery, Taipei MacKay Memorial Hospital, Taipei, Taiwan*

Correspondence:
Chung-Ji Liu
liucjliu3229@gmail.com

As the incidence and the mortality rate of head and neck squamous cell carcinoma (HNSCC) is increasing worldwide, gaining knowledge about the genomic changes which happen in the carcinogenesis of HNSCC is essential for the diagnosis and therapy of the disease. *SMAD4* (DPC4) is a tumor suppressor gene. It is located at chromosome 18q21.1 and a member of the SMAD family. Which mediates the TGF-β signaling pathway, thereby controlling the growth of epithelial cells. In the study presented here, we analyzed tumor samples by multiplex PCR-based next-generation sequencing (NGS) and found deleterious mutations of *SMAD4 in* 4.1% of the tumors. Knock-down experiments of endogenous and exogenous SMAD4 expression demonstrated that SMAD4 is involved in the migration and invasion of HNSCC cells. Functional analysis of a missense mutation in the MH1 domain of SMAD4 may be responsible for the loss of function in suppressing tumor progression. Missense *SMAD4* mutations, therefore, could be useful prognostic determinants for patients affected by HNSCCs. This report is the first study where NGS analysis based on multiplex-PCR is used to demonstrate the imminent occurrence of missense *SMAD4* mutations in HNSCC cells. The gene analysis that we performed may support the identification of *SMAD4* mutations as a diagnostic marker or even as a potential therapeutic target in head and neck cancer. Moreover, the analytic strategy proposed for the detection of mutations in the *SMAD4* gene may be validated as a platform to assist mutation screening.

Keywords: head and neck cancer, loss of heterozygosity, *SMAD4*, somatic mutation, survival

INTRODUCTION

Head and neck squamous cell carcinomas (HNSCC), which include oral squamous cell carcinomas, are the sixth most prevalent malignancy worldwide (1, 2). The pathogenesis of HNSCC is affected by many molecular factors, among them e.g., mutations in *TP53*, and genes related to *PIK3CA and* Notch family signaling (3–9). The role which these factors are playing in the progression of the tumors remains unclear to a wide extent (3, 4, 6, 10, 11). Although the knowledge on head and neck carcinogenesis has improved a lot in the past 40 years and many innovations in surgery as well as chemo- and radiotherapy have been made, the survival rates for many HNSCC types have not improved considerably (2). Recent developments in high-throughput, next-generation parallel sequencing technologies are facilitating sensitive detection, and quantification of genetic alterations. New insights in the molecular basis of HNSCC progression have been provided by whole-exome sequencing (WES) (8, 12, 13). The analysis of WES data which was obtained from The Cancer Genome Atlas (TCGA) (6, 14) pointed to novel genes with significant mutations and underlined the complex molecular pathogenesis of HNSCC, which includes a high degree of heterogeneity between tumors (15).

SMAD4 is a transcription factor of the SMAD family which takes part in TGF-β signaling. SMAD4 stands for SMA- and MAD-related protein 4, other names are SMAD family member 4, Deleted in Pancreatic Cancer-4 (DPC4) and Mothers against decapentaplegic homolog 4, SMAD4 is present in all metazoans and is highly conserved between species (16). As the main effector of TGF-β signaling, SMAD4 has been found to be non-functional in more than half of adenocarcinomas of the pancreatic duct (17–19), and to varying degrees, in several other types of cancers (20–24). In many studies that have been conducted in the past 20 years it was found that the loss of SMAD4 function alone does not initiate a tumor, but it may promote the progression of tumors which have been initiated by other molecular defects, like the activation of KRas activation in the case of pancreatic duct adenocarcinoma and the inactivation of APC in colorectal cancer (20, 24). The loss of SMAD4 is playing a crucial role in the response to DNA damage with the consequence of increased genomic instability. This is very prominent in skin cancer and suggests a distinct role of SMAD4 in the progression of various types of tumors (25).

Screening large genes with multiples exons for mutations by traditional Sanger sequencing is slow, labor intensive and costly. Next-generation sequencing (NGS) in contrast allows the direct analysis of mutations in monogenic diseases at low cost without pre-screening. Novel DNA variants that have been identified by NGS still may be corroborated by Sanger sequencing before reporting them.

In this study, we performed NGS analysis based on multiplex PCR NGS for the investigation of *SMAD4* mutations in HNSCC.

We found that mutations of *SMAD4*, as well as its expression level, are linked to the progression of HNSCC and affect patient survival. Moreover, we investigated the role of deleterious *SMAD4* mutations to elucidate their role in HNSCC neoplasms.

MATERIALS AND METHODS

Patients

This study was approved by the Institutional Review Board of Mackay Memorial Hospital (approval number: 15MMHIS104). All patients provided written informed consent. Tumor samples were obtained from 122 patients undergoing HNSCC surgery (**Supplementary Table 1**). Cells were isolated from tissue sections by laser capture microdissection (LCM) following established protocols (3, 4). Additionally, 10 mL of whole blood was collected in the morning after fasting in Vacutainer tubes containing EDTA as the anticoagulant (Becton Dickson, Franklin Lakes, NJ, USA) from each patient. None of the patients included in this study had received radiotherapy or adjuvant chemotherapy before surgery. DNA was extracted from blood and cancerous tissue as reported previously (26).

SMAD4 Mutation Analysis by PCR-Based NGS

Individual primer sets for 10 long PCR reactions were designed with Primer3 (version 0.4.0) (ELIXIR, funded by the European Commission) to amplify the entire coding sequence (exons 2–12) for human *SMAD4* (**Supplementary Table 2** and **Supplementary Figure 1A**). Amplicon concentrations were determined with the Qubit dsDNA HS Assay kit on a Qubit 2.0 fluorometer (Life Technologies, Carlsbad, CA, USA). PCR reactions were carried out using the KAPA LongRange HotStart kit (Kapa Biosystems, Wilmington, MA, USA). For library generation, long PCR products of each sample were pooled and then purified using Agencourt Ampure XP beads (Beckman Coulter, Pasadena, CA, USA). Indexed libraries of the pooled PCR products were prepared using the Illumina Nextera XT library preparation kit and then sequenced on the Illumina MiSeq system, following the manufacturer's instructions. Variant call format files were generated using the MiSeq Reporter software (version 2.3.32). The variants were further filtered on the basis of the following criteria: (1) DP <30, (2) genotype quality <30, (3) number of mismatches within a 40-bp window ≤3, (4) mutant allele frequency of at least 10% in tumors and <1% in normal cells, and (5) MAF in the 1000 Genomes Project and dbSNP137 > 1%. The Integrative Genomics Viewer (IGV) was used to determine the read counts of the target amplicons and to confirm the detected variants. The mutation spectrum and lollipop figures for *SMAD4* were generated with the OncoPrinter and MutationMapper tools available at cBioPortal (27, 28).

Mutation Point Validation

To validate the somatic mutations which were identified in the multiplex PCR-based NGS results, conventional Sanger sequencing was applied. Individual primer sets were designed in Primer3 (version 0.4.0), they have been listed in **Supplementary Table 3**. For Sanger sequencing, PCR reactions were performed with a standard hot start kit. Amplicons were sequenced with the ABI BigDye Terminator Cycle Sequencing kit on an ABI 3730xl DNA analyzer (Applied Biosystems, Foster City, CA, USA).

Immunohistochemistry

SMAD4 protein was visualized in tissue sections by immunohistochemistry, following previously reported protocols (29). In brief, 5-μm-thick tissue sections were dewaxed, rehydrated, and then incubated with monoclonal mouse anti-human SMAD4 antibody (sc-7966, 1:100 dilution; Santa Cruz Biotechnology, Santa Cruz, CA, USA) in a humidification chamber at 4°C overnight. After rinsing with PBS, standard immunohistochemical staining was done using streptavidin-biotin complex system (Dako Corp.) with aminoethylcarbazole as the chromogen and subsequently counterstained with hematoxylin and mounted with Clearmount

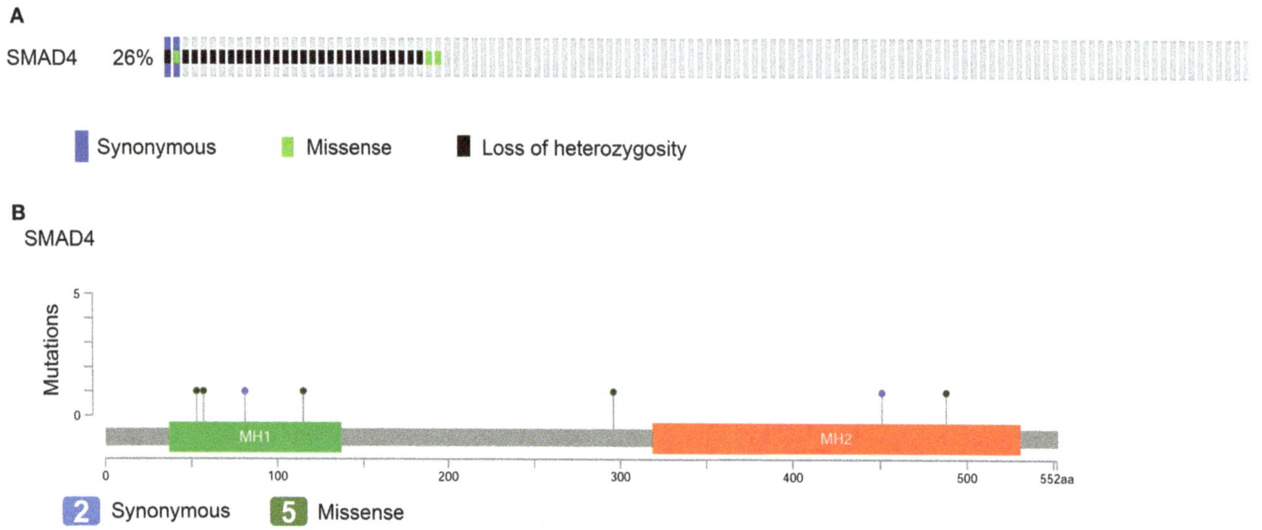

FIGURE 1 | *SMAD4* mutations in patients with HNSCC. **(A)** Frequency of *SMAD4* LOH, mutations, or both. Each column represents one patient. Colored boxes designate LOH status and mutation types. **(B)** Distribution of mutations in the sequence coding for *SMAD4*. Colored ovals represent mutation types, colored boxes represent domains. Colored boxes represent mutation types.

(Zymed Laboratories, Inc.). The primary antibody used was a Preimmune mouse IgG was used as a negative control. Normal epithelium adjacent to the tumor served as the internal positive control. Tumors containing ≥50% and <50% positive cancer cells were classified to have high and low SMAD4 expression (30).

Cell Culture, Reagents, and Phenotypic Assays

In this study, the HNSCC cell lines SAS, OECM-1, HSC3, FaDu, SCC25, OC3, and OC4 were used. Normal human oral keratinocytes (NOKs); served as controls. The cells were cultured as described previously (31). Our cell lines were authenticated by Mission Biotech (Nangang, Taipei, Taiwan) on August 8, 2017, using the Promega StemElite ID System and analyzed on ABI PRISM 3730 Genetic Analyzer with GeneMapper (version 3.7). si-*SMAD4* and scramble control (si-control) oligonucleotides were purchased from Santa Cruz Biotech (Santa Cruz). For transfection, TransFectin Lipid Reagent (BioRad Lab., Hercules, CA, USA) was used. sh-SMAD4 vectors (TRCN0000010321) and a sh-Luc control vector (TRCN0000072249), packaged in lentiviruses, were purchased from National RNAi Core (Academia Sinica, Taipei, Taiwan). The cells were infected and selected using puromycin (Sigma-Aldrich) at 5.0 μg/mL for 7 days to establish stable subclones. Phenotypic events, including proliferation, migration, and invasion, were analyzed as previously described (10, 32).

Analysis of SMAD4 Mutations in HNSCC Cell Lines

All coding exons of *SMAD4* in SAS, OECM-1, HSC3, FaDu, SCC25, OC3, and OC4 cells were amplified by PCR and then sequenced using the ABI BigDye Terminator Cycle Sequencing kit on an ABI 3730xl DNA analyzer (Applied Biosystems). The variants with MAF > 1% in the 1000 Genomes Project and dbSNP137 were filtered.

Constructs

The *SMAD4* cDNA sequence was amplified from the cDNA of SAS cells with the primers *SMAD4*_Forward and *SMAD4*_Reverse, introducing BamHI and EcoRI sites for directional cloning. The PCR product then was subcloned into the pBabe puro vector. The p.H132Y, p.P296T, and p.A488V mutations were introduced into *SMAD4* cDNA with the Q5 Site-Directed Mutagenesis kit (New England BioLabs, Ipswich, MA, USA) with the primers H132Ymut, P296Tmut, and A488Vmut. We named the resulting mutants p.H132Y, p.P296T, and p.A488V, respectively. **Supplementary Table 3** lists the primers used in this section.

Loss of Heterozygosity Analysis at the *SMAD4* Locus

Three polymorphic markers close to the *SMAD4* locus (D18S363, D18S474, and D18S46) were used to analyze the loss of heterozygosity status (LOH) of *SMAD4*. These markers are described in **Supplementary Table 3**. As templates, samples of genomic DNA (~100 ng) were extracted from HNSCCs and matching normal tissues. The PCR reaction (20 μL) contained 5× Phusion HF buffer, 200 μM of each dNTP, 0.25 μM of each marker, and 0.3 μl (0.6 units) of Phusion High-Fidelity DNA Polymerase (Thermo Fisher Scientific, Vilnius, Lithuania). Amplification was performed under the following conditions: 98°C for 5 min, followed by 35 cycles at 98°C for 20 s, 60°C for 15 s, and 72°C for 30 s. The final extension was at 72°C for 7 min. The PCR product (0.5 μL) was mixed with 0.5 μL of GeneScan-600 LIZ dye Size Standard (Applied Biosystems) in 10 μL of Hi-Di formamide (Applied Biosystems), denatured for 3 min at 95°C, and then cooled on ice. The samples were separated by capillary electrophoresis with an ABI PRISM 96-capillary 3730xl DNA Analyzer (Applied Biosystems) and the results were analyzed using GeneMapper (version 3.7; Applied Biosystems). LOH was evaluated using the following formula: LOH = (height of tumor allele 2/height of tumor allele 1)/(height of normal allele 2/height of normal allele 1). As described previously (33). When the height of the tumor alleles decreased by >40%, the calculated LOH became >1.49 or <0.5; thus, we considered this ratio to indicate LOH positivity (**Supplementary Figure 1B**). Homozygous cases were considered non-informative for LOH.

Western Blotting

Western Blot analysis was performed as previously described (29). Equal amounts of protein (30 μg) were loaded per lane. As primary antibodies anti-SMAD4 (diluted 1:500, Santa Cruz) and anti-GAPDH (diluted 1:5,000, Santa Cruz) antibodies were employed. For detection, an HRP-conjugated horse anti-mouse IgG was used as the secondary antibody (diluted 1:5,000; Cell signaling; Cell Signaling Technology, Danvers, MA, USA).

Statistical Analysis

Data are presented as the mean ± SEM. Chi-square and *t*-tests were used. Overall survival (OS) was defined as the time between

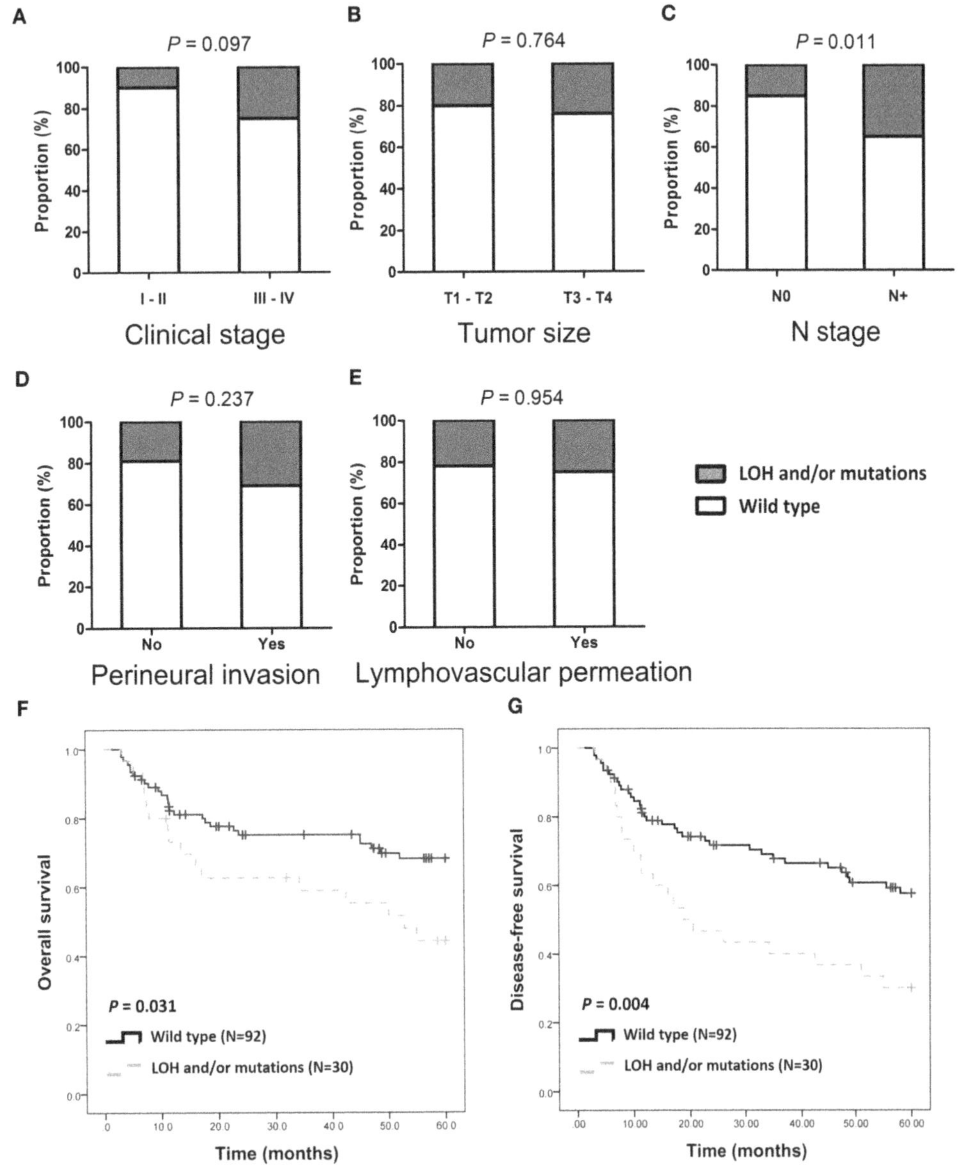

FIGURE 2 | *SMAD4* LOH and mutations and clinical/pathological parameters. **(A–E)** Histograms are showing the association of *SMAD4* LOH with mutation status and clinical stages **(A)**, tumor size **(B)**, N stage **(C)**, perineural invasion **(D)**, and lymphovascular permeation **(E)**. **(F,G)** Kaplan–Meier analysis according to *SMAD4* LOH and mutation status for OS **(F)** and DFS **(G)**.

the date of first diagnosis and the date of death or final follow-up. Disease-free survival (DFS) was defined as the time from the date of first diagnosis until the date of first recurrence or death. Patients without evidence of disease recurrence were censored at the final follow-up or death. Kaplan–Meier analysis was used to compare OS and DFS between the two groups. The multivariate Cox Proportional Hazards Model was used to assess the association of both OS and DFS with *SMAD4* LOH, mutation status, and immunoexpression. Statistical significance was assumed to be indicated by $^{*}P < 0.05$, $^{**}P < 0.01$, and $^{***}P < 0.001$ respectively. Cross-comparisons showing no statistically significant differences were not considered in further analysis.

RESULTS

Somatic Mutations and LOH in *SMAD4*

For the evaluation of the performance of SMAD4 in clinical assessments, 122 HNSCC samples were analyzed by multiplex PCR-based NGS and LOH analysis. We identified seven somatic mutations in the samples by NGS; of these, two were synonymous and five were missense mutations (**Figures 1A,B**, **Supplementary Table 4**). No hotspot region was found for *SMAD4* mutations. The missense mutation p.Ala488Val, previously has been reported by Lee et al. (chr18:48604641) (34). Three polymorphic biomarkers (D18S474, D18S46, and D18S363) which are surrounding the *SMAD4* locus were used to analyze LOH status. Percent LOH was 15.57% (19/122), 13.93% (17/122), and 13.11% (16/122) in D18S363, D18S46, and D18S474, respectively. In 28 (22.95%) patients, LOH was detected in at least one of the three markers (**Figure 1A**), whereas LOH was noted in two or all three markers in 17 (13.93%) patients.

Of the 122 patients, 32 (26.2%) had SMAD4 LOH, mutations, or both, and the remaining 90 demonstrated no mutations or LOH (**Figure 1A**). The frequency of *SMAD4* LOH was higher in patients with lymph node metastasis, mutations, or both compared to those where no metastasis was observed ($P = 0.011$, **Figure 2C**). No significant differences were observed in the clinical stage, tumor size, perineural invasion, or lymphovascular permeation (**Figures 2A–E**, **Supplementary Table 5**). The Kaplan–Meier analysis indicated that patients with *SMAD4* LOH, mutations, or both had a significantly poorer OS and DFS than those with wild-type *SMAD4* ($P = 0.031$ and 0.004, respectively; **Figures 2F,G**, respectively). Both univariate and adjusted multivariate Cox regression analyses revealed poor OS and DFS in patients with *SMAD4* LOH, mutations, or both (OS hazard ratio [HR]: 1.95, $P = 0.034$; OS adjusted HR: 2.08, $P = 0.024$; DFS HR: 2.08, $P = 0.008$, DFS adjusted HR: 1.97, $P = 0.016$; **Table 1**).

SMAD4 Expression in HNSCC Patients

SMAD4 was detected in the cytoplasm and in the nuclei of basal and parabasal cells in normal oral epithelium which was adjacent to tumors (**Figure 3A**, top left). In tumor tissues, SMAD4 immunoreactivity varied from weak (**Figure 3A**, middle) to intense (**Figure 3A**, right). Low SMAD4 expression significantly correlated with the clinical stage ($P = 0.004$), tumor size ($P = 0.020$), and lymph node metastasis ($P = 0.041$; **Figures 3B–G** and **Supplementary Table 6**). No differences were observed in SMAD4 expression in association with the LOH and mutation status, perineural invasion, and lymphovascular permeation. The Kaplan–Meier analysis revealed significantly poorer OS and DFS in patients when SMAD4 expression was low, compared to those with high SMAD4 expression ($P = 0.033$ and $P = 0.026$, respectively; **Figures 3H,I**, respectively). DFS was shorter in patients with when SMAD4 expression was low, as revealed by both univariate and adjusted multivariate Cox regression analysis. (HR: 4.43, $P = 0.043$ and HR: 4.54, $P = 0.046$, respectively; **Table 1**). Univariate Cox regression analysis showed that OS was poorer in patients with low SMAD4 expression (HR: 4.30, $P = 0.047$). However, after the multivariate Cox regression analysis, the correlation between SMAD4 expression and OS became only slightly significant (HR: 4.09, $P = 0.063$).

Association Between SMAD4 Knockdown and Increased HNSCC Invasiveness

The protein levels of SMAD4 in NOKs and HNSCC cells were determined by Western Blotting. As shown in **Figure 4A**, four of the seven (57.1%) tested HNSCC cell lines had decreased or no protein expression of SMAD4, compared to NOKs. Interestingly, in SAS and OC3 cells the endogenous SMAD4 expression relative to the NOKs was elevated. No SMAD4 protein could be detected in FaDu cells (**Figure 4A**). These findings are in agreement with the already described homozygous deletion of *SMAD4* in FaDu cells (35). The remaining two HNSCC cell lines (OC3 and HSC3 cells) were sequenced and two missense mutations were found (**Supplementary Table 7**) No mutation or LOH was found in OC4, OECM1, SAS, or SCC25 cells. OC3 and HSC3 which have missense mutation were excluded from further phenotype studies.

To further elucidate the oncogenic role of *SMAD4* in HNSCC, we established stable *SMAD4*-knockdown SAS and SCC25 subclones. The knockdown effect was confirmed through Western blotting (**Figure 4B**). Cell proliferation was not affected by the knockdown of *SMAD4* (**Figures 4C,F**), but HNSCC cell migration and invasion were significantly increased (**Figures 4D,E,G,H**). To corroborate this result, we transfected SAS and SCC25 cells with si-*SMAD4* oligonucleotides (**Supplementary Figure 2**). Western blotting confirmed the si-*SMAD4* knockdown effect on *SMAD4* expression (**Supplementary Figure 2A**). Migration and invasion of HNSCC cells were significantly increased during the transient knockdown, but their proliferation behavior did not change (**Supplementary Figures 2B–D**). These results indicate that the mobility and invasiveness of HNSCC cells were enhanced by the knockdown of *SMAD4*.

Association Between Mutations of *SMAD4* With Increased Invasiveness in HNSCC

To characterize the effects of *SMAD4* on the phenotype, the full-length coding region of *SMAD4* was amplified from SAS cells and cloned to generate the *SMAD4* construct. In the tumor

TABLE 1 | Univariate and Multivariate analysis of disease-free survival rate in HNSCC patients.

Variables	HR (95%CI)	*P*	Adjusted HR (95%CI)	*P*
Overall survival				
SMAD4 LOH and mutations				
Wild type	Reference		Reference	
LOH and/or mutations	1.95 (1.05–3.62)	0.034*	2.08 (1.10–3.92)	0.024*
SMAD4 expression				
High	Reference		Reference	
Low	4.30 (1.02–18.15)	0.047*	4.09 (0.93–18.00)	0.063
Disease-free survival				
SMAD4 LOH and mutations				
Wild type	Reference		Reference	
LOH and/or mutations	2.08 (1.21–3.57)	0.008*	1.97 (1.14–3.42)	0.016*
SMAD4 expression				
High	Reference		Reference	
Low	4.43 (1.05–18.69)	0.043*	4.54 (1.03–20.12)	0.046*

Adjusted for age, gender, and clinical stage.
HR, hazard ratio; CI, confidence interval.

samples, three missense mutations were found (p.His132Tyr, p.Pro296Thr, and p.Ala488Val, **Supplementary Table 4**). These mutations are localized in the MH1, Linker, and MH2 domains, respectively (**Figure 5A**). By Sanger sequencing, we confirmed them as somatic mutations (**Supplementary Figure 1C**). We further made constructs for these mutations to be able to express these mutant proteins for further study. FaDu and OECM1 cells (which have no or only low*SMAD4* expression) were transfected with the *SMAD4* vector and the mutant constructs. Western blotting was used to detect *SMAD4* expression levels (**Figures 5B,C**). The exogenous *SMAD4* expression reduced the migration and invasion of FaDu and OECM1 cells (**Figures 5E,F,H,I**). When the mutant p.H132Y was transfected, the phenotypes repressed by *SMAD4* overexpression was abolished. The proliferation rates of the transfected cell lines were not affected (**Figures 5D,G**). However, transfection with p.P296T and p.A488V mutant constructs did not abolish the rescuing effects of *SMAD4* overexpression on invasion and migration in HNSCC cells.

DISCUSSION

Varying rates of *SMAD4* mutations have been detected in a wide range of cancers by large-scale exome sequencing. Compared with 35% of pancreatic cancer and 12% of colon cancer cases (20, 36–38), *SMAD4* mutation in other types of cancers has occurred at lower rates. In COSMIC cohort studies, point mutations of *SMAD4* were identified in 0.21, 2.24, 2.46, and 8.86% of kidney, lung, esophagus, and biliary tract cancers, respectively (24, 38–44). In general, 2.5 to 4% of the HNSCC tumors demonstrate the somatic mutation of *SMAD4*, making *SMAD4* the fourth mutated gene in different types of cancers (8). In the study presented here, somatic *SMAD4* mutations were found in 4.1% of HNSCC tumors we analyzed. This study is the first where somatic *SMAD4* mutations in HNSCC were detected by multiplex PCR-based NGS. Besides, IGV was used to reconfirm all mutations. Sanger sequencing confirmed three specific non-sense mutations. Thus, despite *SMAD4* is a large gene that is coding for a 552-amino acid polypeptide with a molecular weight of 60.439 Da, the current NGS-based strategy can be a reliable method for *SMAD4* screening. No hotspot for mutations in the *SMAD4* gene has been reported previously and we have not detected any was it observed in our study (8); therefore, allele-specific approaches that are targeting only common mutations (45, 46) are not suitable for the exploration of *SMAD4* mutations in HNSCC. We have designed the multiplex PCR assay to generate *SMAD4* amplicon libraries for sequencing. This includes protein-coding regions as well as conserved splice sites. Because this approach is highly scalable, it may provide advantages over Sanger sequencing regarding its potential application in routine clinical diagnostics, also because the labor required for analyzing individual samples for somatic *SMAD4* mutations is low.

SMAD proteins have two evolutionarily conserved regions separated by a linker region, MAD homology 1 and 2 (MH1 and MH2, respectively). The MH1 domain at the N/terminus is responsible for sequence-specific DNA binding (47, 48), the roles of the MH2 domain are heteromerization and transactivation (49, 50). Besides, the MH2 region partially interferes with the DNA-binding function of the MH1 region (47, 50, 51). Mutations in the domain between L43 and R135 may reduce the ability of *SMAD4* to bind DNA considerably, as a β-hairpin protein motif within this region is responsible for the interaction with DNA. Our results demonstrate that the whole MH1 domain is very sensitive to changes in its overall primary structure and that tumorigenic mutations within the area of L43 and R135 interfere with its capability to bind DNA (52). Kim et al. were the first to document a non-sense mutation of *SMAD4* (GAA526TAA) in two cell lines derived from the same HNSCC patient (53). Reiss et al. reported a homozygous deletion which includes the *SMAD4* gene locus in FaDu cells (54). Others have furthermore identified the *SMAD4* mutation in this HNSCC cell line (35, 55). The results of our Western Blotting experiments verified that this mutation

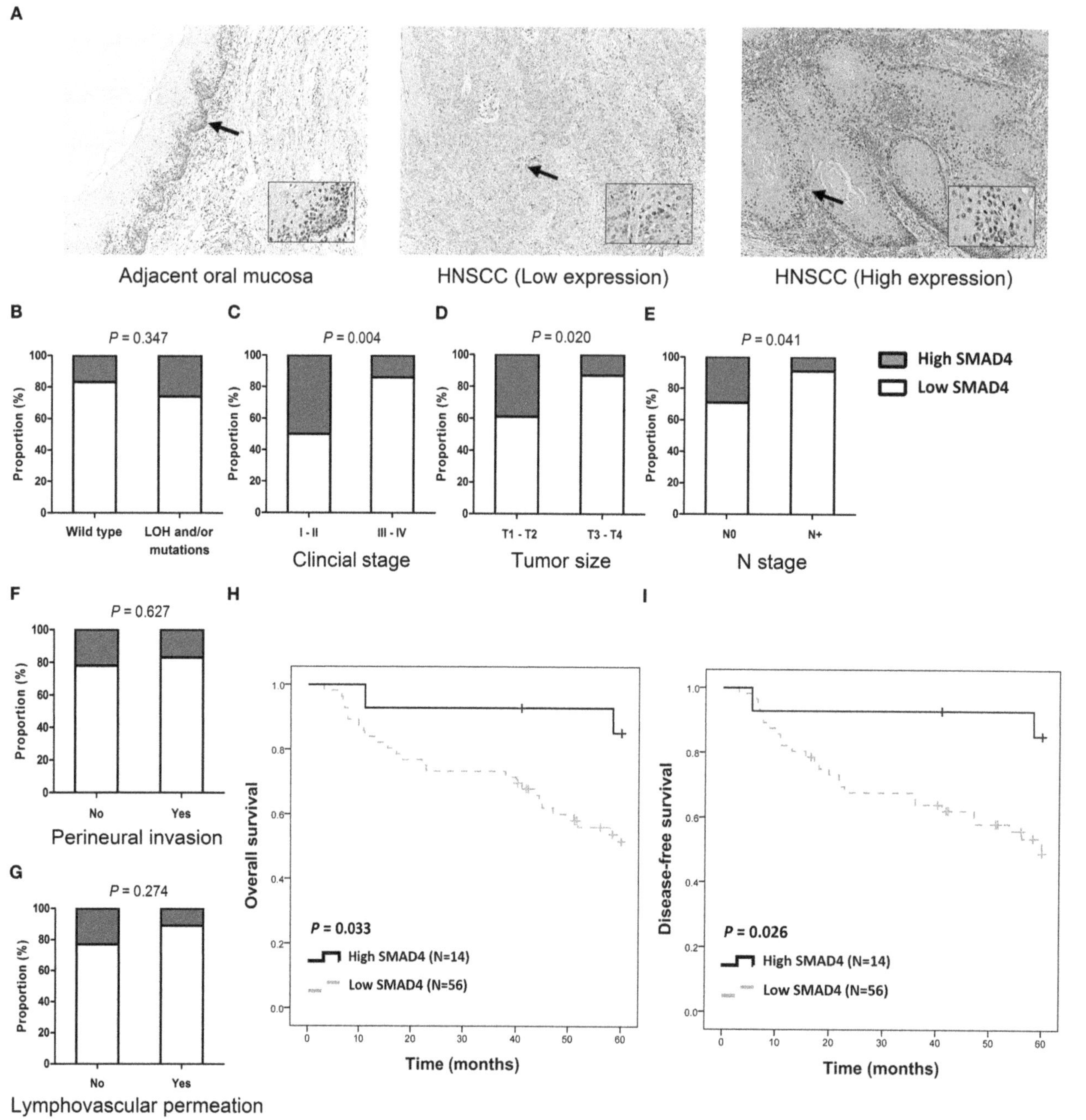

FIGURE 3 | SMAD4 immunoexpression and clinicopathological parameters. **(A)** Immunohistochemistry for SMAD4 in adjacent normal-appearing mucosa (left) and HNSCC tumor tissue (middle and right), as indicated. Tumor tissue showing low (middle), and high (right) SMAD4 staining. Arrows indicate enlarged area. Inset images enlarged by 300% relative to original image. **(B–G)** Histograms showing the association of SMAD4 immunoexpression with *SMAD4* LOH and mutation status **(B)**, clinical stage **(C)**, tumor size **(D)**, N stage **(E)**, perineural invasion **(F)**, and lymphovascular permeation **(G)**. **(H,I)** Kaplan–Meier analysis according to SMAD4 immunoexpression for OS **(H)** and DFS **(I)**.

which results in a nonsense mutation causes the complete loss of *SMAD4* expression. This finding is consistent with previous observations that the majority of missense mutations outside of codons 330–370 inactivate SMAD4 through the degradation of the protein (56). These data are pointing out the important role *SMAD4* is playing in HNSCC carcinogenesis (35). In this study, p.P296T and p.A488V mutant constructs did not abolish the rescuing effects of *SMAD4* overexpression on the migration and invasion in HNSCC cells, suggesting that these mutations may have other functions, warranting further research.

The loss of SMAD4 protein contributes to an increase in genomic instability in the tumor epithelia. This effect, together with blocking the growth inhibition and apoptosis which normally are induced by TGF-β but enhancing of

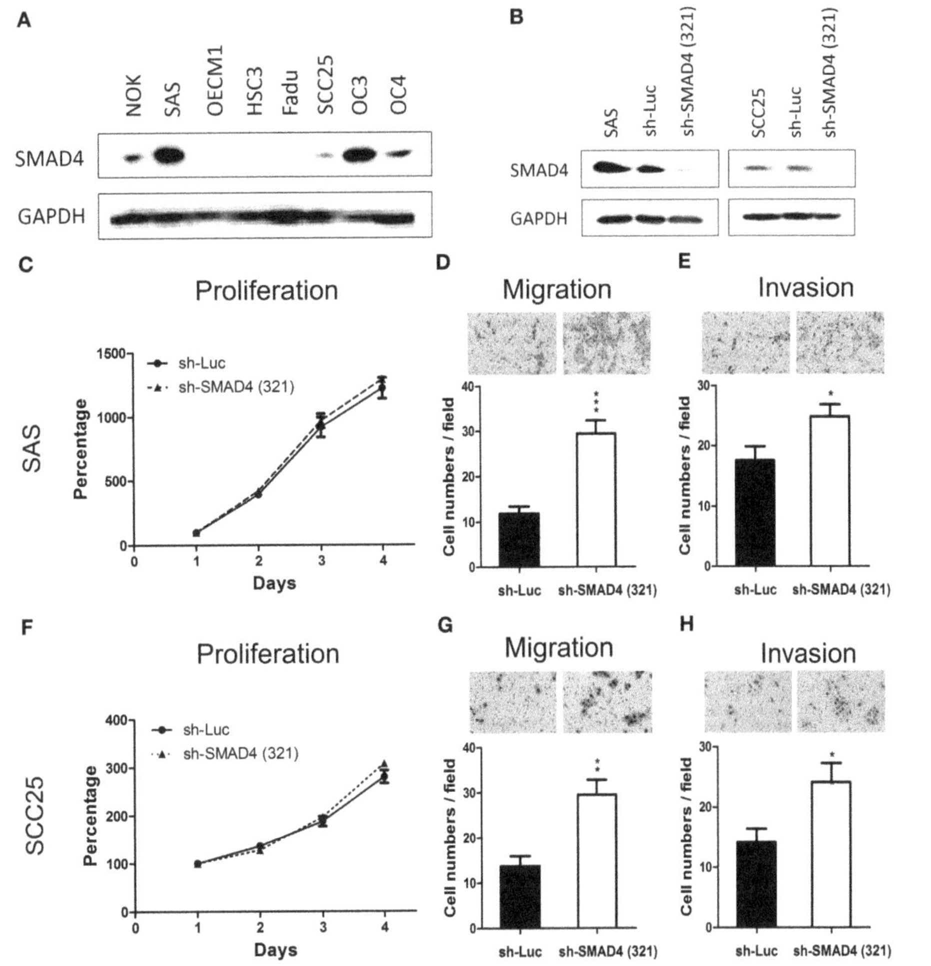

FIGURE 4 | Association of *SMAD4* knockdown with oncogenic phenotypes in HNSCC cells. **(A)** Western blotting for SMAD4 expression in NOK cells and the seven HNSCC cell lines investigated. In SAS and SCC25 cells, *SMAD4* expression levels are higher compared to other cell lines. **(B)** Western blotting on extracts from sh-Luc cell subclone (control) and sh-SMA1D4 (321) cell subclone, which was established from the construct TRCN0000010321. **(C–E)** SAS and **(F–H)** SCC25 cells: proliferation (**C,F**, respectively), migration (**D,G**, respectively), and invasion (**E,H**, respectively).

TGF-β-mediated inflammation, could give way to the expansion of genetic defects cells during HNSCC tumorigenesis (57). *SMAD4* expression may be a determinant of sensitivity/resistance to EGFR/MAPK or EGFR/JNK inhibition in HPV-negative HNSCC tumors (58). However, the studies on SMAD4 loss have reported highly inconsistent results (30, 59, 60). Hernandez et al. developed a *SMAD4* fluorescence *in situ* hybridization assay to measure chromosomal *SMAD4* loss at the single-cell level in primary HNSCC samples and in and patient-derived xenografted (PDX) HNSCC tumors (61). They found a heterozygous loss of *SMAD4* in 35% of primary HNSCCs and 41.3% of PDX tumors. Moreover, in 4.3% of the PDX tumors, the loss of *SMAD4* was homozygous. Hernandez et al. also revealed intertumor and intratumor heterogeneities of *SMAD4* chromosomal loss in HNSCCs (60, 61). In the study presented here, LCM was used to purify the cancerous tissue because LCM makes it possible to approximate the true gene profile of pure cancer cell subpopulations in the context of their actual tissue environment (3, 4). Combining LCM and NGS may be used to detect changes in the karyotype of neoplastic lesions of the oral epithelium.

Analyzing a region of chromosome 18q which has been found to be frequently lost in pancreatic cancers led to the identification of *SMAD4* and the elucidation of its role in tumorigenesis (44), which was supported by the observation that germ-line *SMAD4* mutations cause juvenile polyposis (JP), a condition which is characterized by the formation of intestinal polyps at young age and a cumulative lifetime risk for gastrointestinal cancer of 50% (62). Breast cancers with mutations in the *SMAD4* gene (63) are as sensitive to PARP inhibitors as *BRCA*-mutant breast or ovarian cancers. Similar challenges exist for lung cancers with *SMAD4* (64), but a phenotype where *SMAD4* has been lost has not yet been observed.

A convenient tool to confirm the oncogenic effects of mutated genes in question is the controlled expression of mutant constructs. The current study revealed that mutant *SMAD4* can promote HNSCC tumorigenesis via cell migration and invasion. These data are concordant with the results of our clinical analysis,

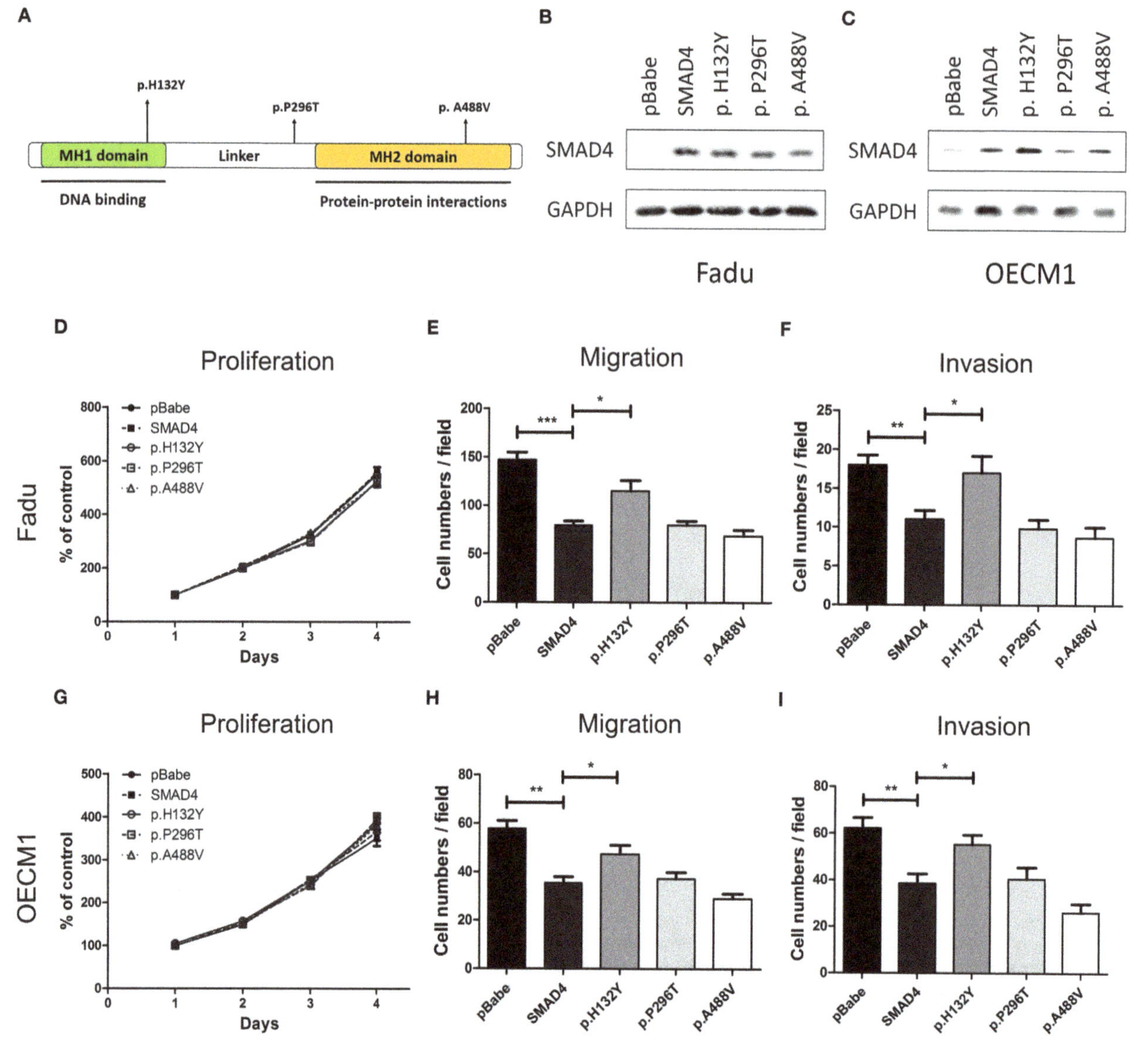

FIGURE 5 | Association of SMAD4 expression with oncogenic phenotypes in HNSCC cells. **(A)** Illustration of various *SMAD4* constructs. Vertical arrows indicate the position of various mutations that were generated for this study. **(B,D–F)** FaDu and **(C,G–I)** OECM1 cells. Results of the Western blotting analysis. The cells were transfected with the vectors, and Western blotting was performed using an anti-SMAD4 antibody to detect the expression of exogenous SMAD4 proteins (**B,C**, respectively): Proliferation (**D,G**, respectively), migration (**E,H**, respectively), and invasion (**F,I**, respectively).

demonstrating more aggressive behavior and the potential for nodal metastasis of tumors with *SMAD4* mutations. The mechanisms that cause diverse *SMAD4* mutations, particularly missense mutations, confer loss-of-function to *SMAD4*.

In HNSCC, the region on chromosome 18q where *SMAD4* is located is frequently lost at the genetic level in HNSCC (65). In esophageal cancer, the loss of SMAD4 correlates with the invasion depth and the pathologic stage (59) as well as with regional metastases and with decreased survival (30).In animal models for HNSCC, *SMAD4* haploid insufficiency promoted tumor development (57). The loss of *SMAD4* is contributing to increased genomic instability in the tumor epithelia. Defects in the signaling of *SMAD* family proteins are associated with an increased tendency for metastatic spread and regional or distant recurrence of HNSCC (66). Thus, inactivation of TGF-β/SMAD signaling is frequently observed in HNSCC, and the inactivation of these signaling pathways might adversely affect patient outcomes. However, the location at which *SMAD4* is downregulated in human HNSCCs and the causal role of *SMAD4* LOH HNSCC development and progression remain unknown. We are the first to demonstrate that LOH and lower expression of SMAD4 can cause regional nodal metastasis and reduce the OS and DFS of HNSCC.

The inactivation of SMAD4 signaling is also associated with poorer prognosis in patients with adenocarcinoma of the pancreas and cancers of the esophagus (23, 43, 67). When *SMAD4* expression is lost in colorectal cancers (CRCs), it is associated with advanced stage disease, the presence of lymph node metastasis, and poor prognosis (38, 67, 68). However, Kouvidou et al. failed to illustrate this relationship in colon cancer (69). Bacman et al. observed that missing nuclear expression of *SMAD4* does not correlate with tumor grade or with the clinical outcome in colon cancer (70). Similar to CRCs, poor HNSCC-related patient outcomes are associated with 18q LOH (71, 72). SMAD4 depletion in an HNSCC cell line induces cetuximab resistance and results in worse survival in an orthotopic mouse model *in vivo*. JNK and MAPK activation as mediators of cetuximab resistance and provide the foundation for the concomitant EGFR and JNK/MAPK inhibition as a potential strategy for overcoming cetuximab resistance in HNSCCs with SMAD4 loss (58). However, in other studies, 18q loss did not appear to affect the survival of patients with HNSCCs (73, 74). This study indicates that LOH with *SMAD4* mutations may significantly decrease the survival of patients with HNSCCs.

Our analysis results demonstrated an inverse correlation between somatic *SMAD4* mutations and the downregulation of *SMAD4* in HNSCCs, following other studies. Furthermore, the results of our studies demonstrate that *SMAD4* loss due to mutations and downregulation results in increased tumor progression and recurrence rates. Moreover, *SMAD4* mutation and loss, as well as low *SMAD4* expression, worsened the OS. These factors may have led to the substantial differences between our and TCGA database's mutation profiles. Although the disparities warrant further resolution, the presented findings are congruent with those reported for other malignancies (75–77).

To summarize, HNSCC is highly heterogeneous at both the cellular and the genetic levels. The current findings show clearly that *SMAD4* expression is suppressing the progression of HNSCC. Somatic mutations in *SMAD4* and its expression determine the recurrence of HNSCC and go along with poor prognosis. Therefore, the proposed analysis of the genetic status may facilitate the identification of mutations in the *SMAD4* gene as a novel diagnostic marker or therapeutic target in HNSCC and other head and neck cancers.

ETHICS STATEMENT

The studies involving human participants were reviewed and approved by MacKay Memorial Hospital. The patients/participants provided their written informed consent to participate in this study.

AUTHOR CONTRIBUTIONS

C-JL: study design. C-JL, L-HL, and K-WC: data analysis. H-WC and L-HL: lab work. C-JL and K-WC: paper preparation.

ACKNOWLEDGMENTS

This manuscript was edited by Wallace Academic Editing.

SUPPLEMENTARY MATERIAL

Supplementary Figure 1 | Identification of *SMAD4* mutations in HNSCC. **(A)** Schematic of five amplicons (blue arrows) covering exons 2–12 of *SMAD4* for sequencing. **(B)** Representative fluorescent electropherograms for LOH marker D18S363 (left), D18S474 (middle), and D18S46 (right). Samples of genomic DNA that were extracted from tumors and matching normal tissues were used as templates. **(C)** Representative Sanger sequencing analysis of mutations p.His132Tyr, p.Pro296Thr, and p.Ala488Val. Upper panels, blood samples; lower panels, cancer samples. The arrows depict wild-type or mutated nucleotides.

Supplementary Figure 2 | Effect of si-*SMAD4* transfection in HNSCC cells. **(A)** Western blotting for OC4 (left) and OECM1 (right) treated with 20 and 40-nM si-*SMAD4* or control oligonucleotides for 48 h: **(B)** proliferation, **(C)** migration, and **(D)** invasion.

Supplementary Table 1 | Clinicopathological characteristics of the HNSCC patients ($n = 122$).

Supplementary Table 2 | List of long PCR primers used for amplification of *SMAD4* gene.

Supplementary Table 3 | List of PCR primers used for PCR, sequencing, and construction, site directed mutagenesis, and *SMAD4* LOH.

Supplementary Table 4 | List of *SMAD4* mutations in HNSCC tumors.

Supplementary Table 5 | Clinical parameters and *SMAD4* LOH and/or mutations in HNSCC patients ($n = 122$).

Supplementary Table 6 | Clinical parameter and *SMAD4* expression in OSCC patients ($n = 70$).

Supplementary Table 7 | List of *SMAD4* mutations in HNSCC cell lines.

REFERENCES

1. Ferlay J, Soerjomataram I, Dikshit R, Eser S, Mathers C, Rebelo M, et al. Cancer incidence and mortality worldwide: sources, methods and major patterns in GLOBOCAN 2012. *Int J Cancer.* (2015) 136:E359–86. doi: 10.1002/ijc.29210
2. Gupta S, Kong W, Peng Y, Miao Q, Mackillop WJ. Temporal trends in the incidence and survival of cancers of the upper aerodigestive tract in Ontario and the United States. *Int J Cancer.* (2009) 125:2159–65. doi: 10.1002/ijc.24533
3. Liu CJ, Lin SC, Chen YJ, Chang KM, Chang KW. Array-comparative genomic hybridization to detect genomewide changes in microdissected primary and metastatic oral squamous cell carcinomas. *Mol Carcinog.* (2006) 45:721–31. doi: 10.1002/mc.20213
4. Liu CJ, Liu TY, Kuo LT, Cheng HW, Chu TH, Chang KW, et al. Differential gene expression signature between primary and metastatic head

and neck squamous cell carcinoma. *J Pathol.* (2008) 214:489–97. doi: 10.1002/path.2306
5. Lin SC, Chen YJ, Kao SY, Hsu MT, Lin CH, Yang SC, et al. Chromosomal changes in betel-associated oral squamous cell carcinomas and their relationship to clinical parameters. *Oral Oncol.* (2002) 38:266–73. doi: 10.1016/S1368-8375(01)00054-9
6. Cancer Genome Atlas Research N, Weinstein JN, Collisson EA, Mills GB, Shaw KR, Ozenberger BA, et al. The cancer genome atlas pan-cancer analysis project. *Nat Genet.* (2013) 45:1113–20. doi: 10.1038/ng.2764
7. Chang KW, Sarraj S, Lin SC, Tsai PI, Solt D. P53 expression, p53 and Ha-ras mutation and telomerase activation during nitrosamine-mediated hamster pouch carcinogenesis. *Carcinogenesis.* (2000) 21:1441–51. doi: 10.1093/carcin/21.5.441
8. Agrawal N, Frederick MJ, Pickering CR, Bettegowda C, Chang K, Li RJ, et al. Exome sequencing of head and neck squamous cell carcinoma reveals inactivating mutations in NOTCH1. *Science.* (2011) 333:1154–7. doi: 10.1126/science.1206923
9. Croce CM. Oncogenes and cancer. *N Engl J Med.* (2008) 358:502–11. doi: 10.1056/NEJMra072367
10. Liu CJ, Tsai MM, Hung PS, Kao SY, Liu TY, Wu KJ, et al. miR-31 ablates expression of the HIF regulatory factor FIH to activate the HIF pathway in head and neck carcinoma. *Cancer Res.* (2010) 70:1635–44. doi: 10.1158/0008-5472.CAN-09-2291
11. Gaykalova DA, Mambo E, Choudhary A, Houghton J, Buddavarapu K, Sanford T, et al. Novel insight into mutational landscape of head and neck squamous cell carcinoma. *PLoS ONE.* (2014) 9:e93102. doi: 10.1371/journal.pone.0093102
12. Stransky N, Egloff AM, Tward AD, Kostic AD, Cibulskis K, Sivachenko A, et al. The mutational landscape of head and neck squamous cell carcinoma. *Science.* (2011) 333:1157–60. doi: 10.1126/science.1208130
13. Pickering CR, Zhang J, Yoo SY, Bengtsson L, Moorthy S, Neskey DM, et al. Integrative genomic characterization of oral squamous cell carcinoma identifies frequent somatic drivers. *Cancer Discov.* (2013) 3:770–81. doi: 10.1158/2159-8290.CD-12-0537
14. Cancer Genome Atlas N. Comprehensive genomic characterization of head and neck squamous cell carcinomas. *Nature.* (2015) 517:576–82. doi: 10.1038/nature14129
15. Kandoth C, McLellan MD, Vandin F, Ye K, Niu B, Lu C, et al. Mutational landscape and significance across 12 major cancer types. *Nature.* (2013) 502:333–9. doi: 10.1038/nature12634
16. Massague J. TGFbeta signalling in context. *Nat Rev Mol Cell Biol.* (2012) 13:616–30. doi: 10.1038/nrm3434
17. Wilentz RE, Iacobuzio-Donahue CA, Argani P, McCarthy DM, Parsons JL, Yeo CJ, et al. Loss of expression of Dpc4 in pancreatic intraepithelial neoplasia: evidence that DPC4 inactivation occurs late in neoplastic progression. *Cancer Res.* (2000) 60:2002–6. Retrieved from: https://cancerres.aacrjournals.org/content/60/7/2002
18. Gu G, Dubauskaite J, Melton DA. Direct evidence for the pancreatic lineage: NGN3+ cells are islet progenitors and are distinct from duct progenitors. *Development.* (2002) 129:2447–57. Retrieved from: https://dev.biologists.org/content/129/10/2447.long
19. Kawaguchi Y, Cooper B, Gannon M, Ray M, MacDonald RJ, Wright CV. The role of the transcriptional regulator Ptf1a in converting intestinal to pancreatic progenitors. *Nat Genet.* (2002) 32:128–34. doi: 10.1038/ng959
20. Miyaki M, Iijima T, Konishi M, Sakai K, Ishii A, Yasuno M, et al. Higher frequency of Smad4 gene mutation in human colorectal cancer with distant metastasis. *Oncogene.* (1999) 18:3098–103. doi: 10.1038/sj.onc.1202642
21. Liao X, Hao Y, Zhang X, Ward S, Houldsworth J, Polydorides AD, et al. Clinicopathological characterization of SMAD4-mutated intestinal adenocarcinomas: a case-control study. *PLoS ONE.* (2019) 14:e0212142. doi: 10.1371/journal.pone.0212142
22. Ding Z, Wu CJ, Chu GC, Xiao Y, Ho D, Zhang J, et al. SMAD4-dependent barrier constrains prostate cancer growth and metastatic progression. *Nature.* (2011) 470:269–73. doi: 10.1038/nature09677
23. Haeger SM, Thompson JJ, Kalra S, Cleaver TG, Merrick D, Wang XJ, et al. Smad4 loss promotes lung cancer formation but increases sensitivity to DNA topoisomerase inhibitors. *Oncogene.* (2016) 35:577–86. doi: 10.1038/onc.2015.112
24. Zhao M, Mishra L, Deng CX. The role of TGF-beta/SMAD4 signaling in cancer. *Int J Biol Sci.* (2018) 14:111–23. doi: 10.7150/ijbs.23230
25. Yang L, Mao C, Teng Y, Li W, Zhang J, Cheng X, et al. Targeted disruption of Smad4 in mouse epidermis results in failure of hair follicle cycling and formation of skin tumors. *Cancer Res.* (2005) 65:8671–8. doi: 10.1158/0008-5472.CAN-05-0800
26. Hung PS, Chang KW, Kao SY, Chu TH, Liu CJ, Lin SC. Association between the rs2910164 polymorphism in pre-mir-146a and oral carcinoma progression. *Oral Oncol.* (2012) 48:404–8. doi: 10.1016/j.oraloncology.2011.11.019
27. Gao J, Aksoy BA, Dogrusoz U, Dresdner G, Gross B, Sumer SO, et al. Integrative analysis of complex cancer genomics and clinical profiles using the cBioPortal. *Sci Signal.* (2013) 6:pl1. doi: 10.1126/scisignal.2004088
28. Cerami E, Gao J, Dogrusoz U, Gross BE, Sumer SO, Aksoy BA, et al. The cBio cancer genomics portal: an open platform for exploring multidimensional cancer genomics data. *Cancer Discov.* (2012) 2:401–4. doi: 10.1158/2159-8290.CD-12-0095
29. Chen YF, Yang CC, Kao SY, Liu CJ, Lin SC, Chang KW. MicroRNA-211 enhances the oncogenicity of carcinogen-induced oral carcinoma by repressing TCF12 and increasing antioxidant activity. *Cancer Res.* (2016) 76:4872–86. doi: 10.1158/0008-5472.CAN-15-1664
30. Natsugoe S, Xiangming C, Matsumoto M, Okumura H, Nakashima S, Sakita H, et al. Smad4 and transforming growth factor beta1 expression in patients with squamous cell carcinoma of the esophagus. *Clin Cancer Res.* (2002) 8:1838–42. Retrieved from: https://clincancerres.aacrjournals.org/content/8/6/1838.long
31. Lin SC, Lin LH, Yu SY, Kao SY, Chang KW, Cheng HW, et al. FAT1 somatic mutations in head and neck carcinoma are associated with tumor progression and survival. *Carcinogenesis.* (2018) 39:1320–30. doi: 10.1093/carcin/bgy107
32. Hung PS, Tu HF, Kao SY, Yang CC, Liu CJ, Huang TY, et al. miR-31 is upregulated in oral premalignant epithelium and contributes to the immortalization of normal oral keratinocytes. *Carcinogenesis.* (2014) 35:1162–71. doi: 10.1093/carcin/bgu024
33. Demopoulos K, Arvanitis DA, Vassilakis DA, Siafakas NM, Spandidos DA. MYCL1, FHIT, SPARC, p16(INK4) and TP53 genes associated to lung cancer in idiopathic pulmonary fibrosis. *J Cell Mol Med.* (2002) 6:215–22. doi: 10.1111/j.1582-4934.2002.tb00188.x
34. Lee S, Cho YS, Shim C, Kim J, Choi J, Oh S, et al. Aberrant expression of Smad4 results in resistance against the growth-inhibitory effect of transforming growth factor-beta in the SiHa human cervical carcinoma cell line. *Int J Cancer.* (2001) 94:500–7. doi: 10.1002/ijc.1494
35. Qiu W, Schonleben F, Li X, Su GH. Disruption of transforming growth factor beta-Smad signaling pathway in head and neck squamous cell carcinoma as evidenced by mutations of SMAD2 and SMAD4. *Cancer Lett.* (2007) 245:163–70. doi: 10.1016/j.canlet.2006.01.003
36. Rozenblum E, Schutte M, Goggins M, Hahn SA, Panzer S, Zahurak M, et al. Tumor-suppressive pathways in pancreatic carcinoma. *Cancer Res.* (1997) 57:1731–4.
37. Yatsuoka T, Sunamura M, Furukawa T, Fukushige S, Yokoyama T, Inoue H, et al. Association of poor prognosis with loss of 12q, 17p, and 18q, and concordant loss of 6q/17p and 12q/18q in human pancreatic ductal adenocarcinoma. *Am J Gastroenterol.* (2000) 95:2080–5. doi: 10.1111/j.1572-0241.2000.02171.x
38. Chang YC, Chang JG, Liu TC, Lin CY, Yang SF, Ho CM, et al. Mutation analysis of 13 driver genes of colorectal cancer-related pathways in Taiwanese patients. *World J Gastroenterol.* (2016) 22:2314–25. doi: 10.3748/wjg.v22.i7.2314
39. Martin D, Abba MC, Molinolo AA, Vitale-Cross L, Wang Z, Zaida M, et al. The head and neck cancer cell oncogenome: a platform for the development of precision molecular therapies. *Oncotarget.* (2014) 5:8906–23. doi: 10.18632/oncotarget.2417
40. India Project Team of the International Cancer Genome C. Mutational landscape of gingivo-buccal oral squamous cell carcinoma reveals new recurrently-mutated genes and molecular subgroups. *Nat Commun.* (2013) 4:2873. doi: 10.1038/ncomms3873
41. Kim KT, Kim BS, Kim JH. Association between FAT1 mutation and overall survival in patients with human papillomavirus-negative head and

neck squamous cell carcinoma. *Head Neck.* (2016) 38(Suppl. 1):E2021–9. doi: 10.1002/hed.24372

42. Chen SJ, Liu H, Liao CT, Huang PJ, Huang Y, Hsu A, et al. Ultra-deep targeted sequencing of advanced oral squamous cell carcinoma identifies a mutation-based prognostic gene signature. *Oncotarget.* (2015) 6:18066–80. doi: 10.18632/oncotarget.3768
43. Blackford A, Serrano OK, Wolfgang CL, Parmigiani G, Jones S, Zhang X, et al. SMAD4 gene mutations are associated with poor prognosis in pancreatic cancer. *Clin Cancer Res.* (2009) 15:4674–9. doi: 10.1158/1078-0432.CCR-09-0227
44. Hahn SA, Schutte M, Hoque AT, Moskaluk CA, da Costa LT, Rozenblum E, et al. DPC4, a candidate tumor suppressor gene at human chromosome 18q21.1. *Science.* (1996) 271:350–3. doi: 10.1126/science.271.5247.350
45. Nakaya K, Yamagata HD, Arita N, Nakashiro KI, Nose M, Miki T, et al. Identification of homozygous deletions of tumor suppressor gene FAT in oral cancer using CGH-array. *Oncogene.* (2007) 26:5300–8. doi: 10.1038/sj.onc.1210330
46. Chosdol K, Misra A, Puri S, Srivastava T, Chattopadhyay P, Sarkar C, et al. Frequent loss of heterozygosity and altered expression of the candidate tumor suppressor gene 'FAT' in human astrocytic tumors. *BMC Cancer.* (2009) 9:5. doi: 10.1186/1471-2407-9-5
47. Kim J, Johnson K, Chen HJ, Carroll S, Laughon A. Drosophila Mad binds to DNA and directly mediates activation of vestigial by Decapentaplegic. *Nature.* (1997) 388:304–8. doi: 10.1038/40906
48. Zawel L, Dai JL, Buckhaults P, Zhou S, Kinzler KW, Vogelstein B, et al. Human Smad3 and Smad4 are sequence-specific transcription activators. *Mol Cell.* (1998) 1:611–7. doi: 10.1016/S1097-2765(00)80061-1
49. Shi Y, Hata A, Lo RS, Massague J, Pavletich NP. A structural basis for mutational inactivation of the tumour suppressor Smad4. *Nature.* (1997) 388:87–93. doi: 10.1038/40431
50. Dai JL, Turnacioglu KK, Schutte M, Sugar AY, Kern SE. Dpc4 transcriptional activation and dysfunction in cancer cells. *Cancer Res.* (1998) 58:4592–7.
51. Hata A, Lo RS, Wotton D, Lagna G, Massague J. Mutations increasing autoinhibition inactivate tumour suppressors Smad2 and Smad4. *Nature.* (1997) 388:82–7. doi: 10.1038/40424
52. Jones JB, Kern SE. Functional mapping of the MH1 DNA-binding domain of DPC4/SMAD4. *Nucleic Acids Res.* (2000) 28:2363–8. doi: 10.1093/nar/28.12.2363
53. Kim SK, Fan Y, Papadimitrakopoulou V, Clayman G, Hittelman WN, Hong WK, et al. DPC4, a candidate tumor suppressor gene, is altered infrequently in head and neck squamous cell carcinoma. *Cancer Res.* (1996) 56:2519–21.
54. Reiss M, Santoro V, de Jonge RR, Vellucci VF. Transfer of chromosome 18 into human head and neck squamous carcinoma cells: evidence for tumor suppression by Smad4/DPC4. *Cell Growth Differ.* (1997) 8:407–15.
55. Ikediobi ON, Davies H, Bignell G, Edkins S, Stevens C, O'Meara S, et al. Mutation analysis of 24 known cancer genes in the NCI-60 cell line set. *Mol Cancer Ther.* (2006) 5:2606–12. doi: 10.1158/1535-7163.MCT-06-0433
56. Thiagalingam S, Lengauer C, Leach FS, Schutte M, Hahn SA, Overhauser J, et al. Evaluation of candidate tumour suppressor genes on chromosome 18 in colorectal cancers. *Nat Genet.* (1996) 13:343–6. doi: 10.1038/ng0796-343
57. Bornstein S, White R, Malkoski S, Oka M, Han G, Cleaver T, et al. Smad4 loss in mice causes spontaneous head and neck cancer with increased genomic instability and inflammation. *J Clin Invest.* (2009) 119:3408–19. doi: 10.1172/JCI38854
58. Ozawa H, Ranaweera RS, Izumchenko E, Makarev E, Zhavoronkov A, Fertig EJ, et al. SMAD4 loss is associated with cetuximab resistance and induction of MAPK/JNK activation in head and neck cancer cells. *Clin Cancer Res.* (2017) 23:5162–75. doi: 10.1158/1078-0432.CCR-16-1686
59. Fukuchi M, Masuda N, Miyazaki T, Nakajima M, Osawa H, Kato H, et al. Decreased Smad4 expression in the transforming growth factor-beta signaling pathway during progression of esophageal squamous cell carcinoma. *Cancer.* (2002) 95:737–43. doi: 10.1002/cncr.10727
60. Xie W, Aisner S, Baredes S, Sreepada G, Shah R, Reiss M. Alterations of Smad expression and activation in defining 2 subtypes of human head and neck squamous cell carcinoma. *Head Neck.* (2013) 35:76–85. doi: 10.1002/hed.22924
61. Hernandez AL, Wang Y, Somerset HL, Keysar SB, Aisner DL, Marshall C, et al. Inter- and intra-tumor heterogeneity of SMAD4 loss in head and neck squamous cell carcinomas. *Mol Carcinog.* (2019) 58:666–73. doi: 10.1002/mc.22958
62. Zbuk KM, Eng C. Hamartomatous polyposis syndromes. *Nat Clin Pract Gastroenterol Hepatol.* (2007) 4:492–502. doi: 10.1038/ncpgasthep0902
63. Zhong D, Morikawa A, Guo L, Colpaert C, Xiong L, Nassar A, et al. Homozygous deletion of SMAD4 in breast cancer cell lines and invasive ductal carcinomas. *Cancer Biol Ther.* (2006) 5:601–7. doi: 10.4161/cbt.5.6.2660
64. Nagatake M, Takagi Y, Osada H, Uchida K, Mitsudomi T, Saji S, et al. Somatic *in vivo* alterations of the DPC4 gene at 18q21 in human lung cancers. *Cancer Res.* (1996) 56:2718–20.
65. Snijders AM, Schmidt BL, Fridlyand J, Dekker N, Pinkel D, Jordan RC, et al. Rare amplicons implicate frequent deregulation of cell fate specification pathways in oral squamous cell carcinoma. *Oncogene.* (2005) 24:4232–42. doi: 10.1038/sj.onc.1208601
66. Xie W, Bharathy S, Kim D, Haffty BG, Rimm DL, Reiss M. Frequent alterations of Smad signaling in human head and neck squamous cell carcinomas: a tissue microarray analysis. *Oncol Res.* (2003) 14:61–73. doi: 10.3727/000000003108748612
67. Jia X, Shanmugam C, Paluri RK, Jhala NC, Behring MP, Katkoori VR, et al. Prognostic value of loss of heterozygosity and sub-cellular localization of SMAD4 varies with tumor stage in colorectal cancer. *Oncotarget.* (2017) 8:20198–212. doi: 10.18632/oncotarget.15560
68. Xie W, Rimm DL, Lin Y, Shih WJ, Reiss M. Loss of Smad signaling in human colorectal cancer is associated with advanced disease and poor prognosis. *Cancer J.* (2003) 9:302–12. doi: 10.1097/00130404-200307000-00013
69. Kouvidou C, Latoufis C, Lianou E, Kouvatseas G, Kakouri E, Anagnostakis D, et al. Expression of Smad4 and TGF-beta2 in colorectal carcinoma. *Anticancer Res.* (2006) 26:2901–7. Retrieved from: http://ar.iiarjournals.org/content/26/4B/2901
70. Bacman D, Merkel S, Croner R, Papadopoulos T, Brueckl W, Dimmler A. TGF-beta receptor 2 downregulation in tumour-associated stroma worsens prognosis and high-grade tumours show more tumour-associated macrophages and lower TGF-beta1 expression in colon carcinoma: a retrospective study. *BMC Cancer.* (2007) 7:156. doi: 10.1186/1471-2407-7-156
71. Pearlstein RP, Benninger MS, Carey TE, Zarbo RJ, Torres FX, Rybicki BA, et al. Loss of 18q predicts poor survival of patients with squamous cell carcinoma of the head and neck. *Genes Chromosomes Cancer.* (1998) 21:333–9. doi: 10.1002/(SICI)1098-2264(199804)21:4<;333::AID-GCC7>;3.0.CO;2-#
72. Kelker W, Van Dyke DL, Worsham MJ, Christopherson PL, James CD, Conlon MR, et al. Loss of 18q and homozygosity for the DCC locus: possible markers for clinically aggressive squamous cell carcinoma. *Anticancer Res.* (1996) 16:2365–72.
73. Choi HR, Roberts DB, Johnigan RH, Sturgis EM, Rosenthal DI, Weber RS, et al. Molecular and clinicopathologic comparisons of head and neck squamous carcinoma variants: common and distinctive features of biological significance. *Am J Surg Pathol.* (2004) 28:1299–310. doi: 10.1097/01.pas.0000138003.46650.dc
74. Ng IO, Xiao L, Lam KY, Yuen PW, Ng M. Microsatellite alterations in squamous cell carcinoma of the head and neck—clustering of loss of heterozygosity in a distinct subset. *Oral Oncol.* (2000) 36:484–90. doi: 10.1016/S1368-8375(00)00040-3
75. Morris LG, Kaufman AM, Gong Y, Ramaswami D, Walsh LA, Turcan S, et al. Recurrent somatic mutation of FAT1 in multiple human cancers leads to aberrant Wnt activation. *Nat Genet.* (2013) 45:253–61. doi: 10.1038/ng.2538
76. Wang L, Lyu S, Wang S, Shen H, Niu F, Liu X, et al. Loss of FAT1 during the progression from DCIS to IDC and predict poor clinical outcome in breast cancer. *Exp Mol Pathol.* (2016) 100:177–83. doi: 10.1016/j.yexmp.2015.12.012
77. Yu J, Li H. The expression of FAT1 is associated with overall survival in children with medulloblastoma. *Tumori.* (2017) 103:44–52. doi: 10.5301/tj.5000570

7

Choosing the Right Treatment Option for the Right R/M HNSCC Patient: Should we Adhere to PFE for First-Line Therapy?

*Katharina Lübbers, Mykola Pavlychenko, Theresa Wald, Susanne Wiegand, Andreas Dietz, Veit Zebralla and Gunnar Wichmann**

Department of Otorhinolaryngology, Head and Neck Surgery, University Hospital Leipzig, Leipzig, Germany

Correspondence:
Gunnar Wichmann
Gunnar.Wichmann@medizin.uni-leipzig.de

Background: The landmark EXTREME trial established cisplatin, 5-fluorouracil and cetuximab (PFE) as first-line chemotherapy (1L-ChT) for recurrent/metastatic head and neck squamous cell carcinoma (R/M HNSCC). We were interested in outcome differences of R/M HNSCC in 1L-ChT and factors influencing outcome in certain subgroups, especially patients receiving PFE, and the value of PFE compared to other 1L-ChT regimens to provide real world evidence (RWE).

Methods: For this retrospective monocentric study, 124 R/M HNSCC patients without curative surgical or radiotherapy options receiving at least one cycle of 1L-ChT were eligible. We analyzed their outcome using Kaplan-Meier plot and Cox regression to identify predictors for prolonged survival.

Results: Subgroups benefiting significantly from PFE were patients suffering from an index HNSCC outside the oropharynx. The PFE regimen proved to be superior to all other 1L-ChT regimens in clinical routine. Significant outcome differences between PFE treatment within or outside controlled trials were not seen.

Conclusion: This retrospective analysis provides RWE for factors linked to improved outcome. Subgroup analyses highlight the lasting value of PFE among the growing spectrum of 1L-ChT. Importantly, fit smokers with high level alcohol consumption benefit from PFE; considering the patient's lifestyle factors, PFE should not be ignored in decision-making.

Keywords: head and neck cancer, head and neck squamous cell carcinoma, palliative chemotherapy, first-line therapy, recurrent/metastatic head and neck squamous cell carcinoma, multivariate Cox proportional hazard regression, outcome research, p16+ oropharyngeal cancer

INTRODUCTION

Squamous cell carcinoma of the head and neck (HNSCC) is an entity with growing importance, in clinical but also in research settings. According to the EUROCARE-5 trial (1), there were 238,608 cases recorded from 1999 to 2007 in Europe. Five-years overall survival (OS) for all HNSCC entities was 42.2% (95% confidence interval, 95%CI: 41.5–42.9%), ranging from 25.5% for oropharynx to

61.1% for larynx cancer. At initial diagnosis of HNSCC, 54.0% of all HNSCC were classified as UICC IV due to regional or distant metastasis. According to the NCCN Guidelines for Head and Neck Cancer (2018) (2), curative therapy is considered appropriate until UICC IVB, whereas detection of distant metastasis (M1 defining stage IVC) means loss of curative treatment options advising switch to systemic treatment and palliative care (with the only exception of resectable solitary M1). The same applies to recurrent locally advanced HNSCC after radiotherapy without resectability. While there are certain therapy algorithms for HNSCC in curable stages, only a few approved options for first-line chemotherapy and other systemic first-line therapies (altogether summarized under the abbreviation 1L-ChT) are available in case of R/M HNSCC following the NCCN guidelines from 2018. Since publication of the landmark EXTREME trial (3), treatment with up to six cycles of cisplatin, 5-fluorouracil and cetuximab (PFE), became standard 1L-ChT in R/M HNSCC. After the KEYNOTE-048 trial (4), this standard was recommended being replaced by a stratified 1L-ChT according to programmed death ligand 1 (PD-L1) expression assessed by combined positivity score (CPS). According to immune histopathology, PFE remains a standard of care for patients with a CPS <1, whereas patients with a CPS ≥ 20 should be treated with pembrolizumab mono and patients with CPS ≥ 1 and <20 should receive cisplatin/5-fluoruracil/pembrolizumab (5).

Prior trials often used PFE as control arm (6–9), but new 1L-ChT options superior to PFE have not yet been identified or been established based on lower toxicity. In the course of precision medicine and decision-making for stratified therapy regimens leading to a more individualized or even personalized treatment, new therapy options became eligible for specific groups of patients as second-line therapy (2L-ChT) or 1L-ChT for patients not eligible for PFE (frail patients and/or insufficient kidney or liver function). We were interested in the outcome of PFE *versus* the other 1L-ChT and predictors for good outcome after PFE therapy and consequentially aimed on defining groups of patients that still benefit the most from PFE as part of a widened spectrum of therapy options.

MATERIALS AND METHODS

Study Population and Patient Samples

Eligible for the study were patients with pathological confirmed R/M HNSCC treated in the University Hospital Leipzig with data recorded in the Microsoft Access® tumor database (TDB) of the ENT department, comprising data of all patients diagnosed with a malignant disease since 1990, and data taken from the hospital's electronic health records. **Figure 1** shows the selection of patients for analyses according to the CONSORT recommendations. Among 346 R/M HNSCC patients presented to the multidisciplinary tumor board (MDTB; see below), 130 R/M HNSCC without curative treatment option were subjected to systemic therapy and received at least one cycle 1L-ChT. To prevent any inconsistency based on minor R/M HNSCC subgroups, patients with primary HNSCC localized in the nasopharynx (ICD10-C11), or nasal cavity (ICD-10-C30 and C31) were excluded from the present analyses resulting in a sample of 124 patients (**Table 1**). Pathological reports were available for all 124 patients. All resected specimen underwent pathological examination, and hematoxylin–eosin (HE) staining revealed squamous cell carcinoma histology. A sub-cohort of patients participated in a study approved by our Ethics Committee (votes 201-10-12072010 and 202-10-12072010).

Clinical Work-Up for R/M HNSCC

As recommended (2), clinical work-up for R/M HNSCC included clinical examination, ultrasound sonography, contrast-enhanced CT for head and neck and thorax, eventually PET-CT/PET-MRI, followed by a panendoscopy accompanied by taking biopsies before decision-making for treatment in the MDTB. Patient and tumor characteristics, diagnostic procedures, treatment and clinical follow-up were recorded in our Microsoft Access® tumor database (TDB) and OncoFlow® (10, 11).

CT and PET-CT Imaging

According to clinical guidelines, all patients received a head and neck and a CT scan of the chest during staging. In 2006, a PET-CT became available. An experienced board-certified nuclear-medicine physician and a radiologist analyzed PET-CTs. Sites of tumor involvement were identified visually by enhanced, non-physiologically [^{18}F]-FDG uptake.

Decision-Making Process in the MDTB

The decision-making process in the MDTB followed ASCO and NCCN guidelines (2) and principles published earlier (10–13). Briefly, a radiologist and a nuclear medicine specialist presented all radiological imaging. The MDTB consisting of head and neck and maxillofacial surgeons, a pathologist, an oncologist, a radiation oncologist, and other clinical staff involved in the treatment of head and neck cancer patients discussed the results of diagnostic procedures. Considering the general health and comorbidity of the patient the pre-therapeutic MDTB regarding the guidelines (2) recommended the type of 1L-ChT according to inclusion criteria of open randomized controlled trials (RCTs) or according to fitness for current therapy standards, PFE or other 1L-ChT. For the subgroup of patients receiving 1L-ChT other than PFE, the most relevant RCTs were CeFCiD (NCT02268695), RESGEX (NCT02052960) and ADVANTAGE (NCT00705016) (6–8).

Immunohistochemistry for P16 and HPV Genotyping

Before decision-making in MDTB and starting therapy, biopsies were taken under general anesthesia and underwent pathological examination. Pathological reports were available for all 124 patients. Besides hematoxylin–eosin (HE) staining, molecular analyses of p16 by immunohistochemistry utilizing the CINtec kit (Roche) were done in oropharynx squamous cell carcinomas (OPSCC) of RCT participants and performed in OPSCC routinely since 2013. Double-stained, p16-positive/Ki67-

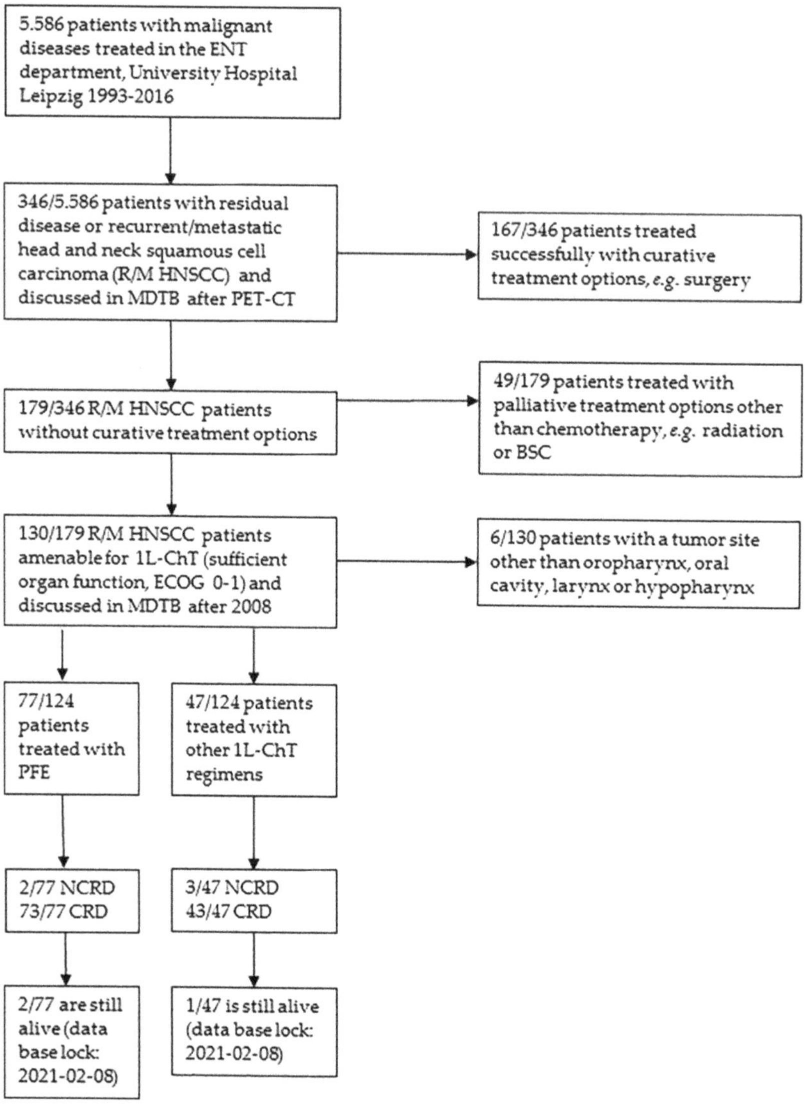

FIGURE 1 | CONSORT diagram showing the selection criteria of recurrent/metastatic head and neck squamous cell carcinoma (R/M HNSCC) patients of the two cohorts compared. ECOG, Eastern Cooperative Oncology Group performance score; BSC, Best Supportive Care; MDTB, multi-disciplinary tumor board; NCRD, non cancer-related death; CRD, cancer-related death.

positive cells or a cutoff level of ≥70% p16-positive OPSCC cells were considered p16+. DNA of p16+ OPSCC was extracted and analyzed for high-risk human papillomavirus utilizing the INNO-LiPA HPV Genotyping Extra kit (Innogenetics) as described earlier (14).

Statistical Analysis

Overall survival (OS) was the time from initial diagnosis of HNSCC to cancer-related (CRD) or non-cancer-related death (NCRD) censoring patients alive at the end of follow-up (data base lock: 08.02.2021). Survival after 1L-ChT ($OS_{1L\text{-}ChT}$) was the time from diagnosis that led to 1L-ChT until death by any cause, censoring patients alive at the end of follow-up or data base lock. We performed a statistical analysis in SPSS 25®. We used *Chi-square* tests, paired and heteroscedastic *t*-tests, receiver-operating characteristics (ROC) curves and Fisher's exact test to investigate the association of clinical characteristics and the outcome of patients receiving PFE or other 1L-ChT. Kaplan–Meier cumulative survival plots and log-rank tests were used to investigate the impact of particular characteristics on $OS_{1L\text{-}ChT}$. We analyzed all parameters achieving P <0.2 in univariate models in multivariate Cox proportional hazard regression (MCR) models. After checking collinearity, independent predictors for the $OS_{1L\text{-}ChT}$ have been identified in MCR applying the step-wise-forward method. For internal validation and to reduce over-optimism based on the effects of random sampling errors, we utilized bootstrapping (1,000 iterations). We considered P <0.05 being significant.

TABLE 1 | Clinical and epidemiological characteristics, diagnostic procedures and treatment as well as various survival measures for 5-years outcome of recurrent/metastatic head and neck squamous cell carcinoma (R/M HNSCC) patients of the two subgroups, PFE and other 1L-ChT.

Characteristics		**Number of Patients (%)**						
		Total	***N* = 124**	**PFE**	***N* = 77**	**other 1L-ChT**	***N* = 47**	***P*-value***
Age at inital diagnosis, years	<50	29	(23.4)	16	(20.8)	13	(27.7)	0.272
	50–60	48	(38.7)	35	(45.5)	13	(27.7)	
	60–70	40	(32.3)	22	(28.6)	18	(38.3)	
	>70	7	(5.6)	4	(5.2)	3	(6.4)	
	median (IQR)	56.7	(50.2-63.7)	56.6	(50.2–63.1)	58.4	(49.4–64.1)	0.592
Age at 1L-ChT, years	<50	19	(15.3)	11	(14.3)	8	(17.0)	0.199
	50–59	50	(40.3)	36	(46.8)	14	(29.8)	
	60–69	45	(36.3)	26	(33.8)	19	(40.4)	
	>70	10	(8.1)	4	(5.2)	6	(12.8)	
	median (IQR)	58.8	(53.2–65.6)	58.1	(53.1–65.5)	61.0	(54.1–66.4)	0.279
ECOG	0–1	123	(99.2)	77	(100.0)	46	(97.9)	0.199
	2	1	(0.8)	0		1	(2.1)	
Sex	Male	105	(84.7)	67	(63.8)	38	(80.9)	0.355
	Female	19	(15.3)	10	(13.0)	9	(19.1)	
Alcohol, status	Missing	7	(5.6)	5	(6.5)	2	(4.3)	0.991
	Never	15	(12.1)	9	(11.7)	6	(12.8)	
	Former	13	(10.5)	8	(10.4)	5	(10.6)	
	Current	89	(71.8)	55	(71.4)	34	(72.3)	
Alcohol, (g/d)	Missing	7	(5.6)	5	(6.5)	2	(4.3)	0.999
	0 g/d	15	(12.8)	9	(11.7)	6	(12.8)	
	<30 g/d	36	(30.8)	22	(28.6)	14	(29.8)	
	30–60 g/d	29	(24.8)	18	(23.4)	11	(23.4)	
	>60 g/d	37	(31.6)	23	(29.9)	14	(29.8)	
Tobacco smoking, status	Missing	5	(4.0)	4	(5.2)	1	(2.1)	0.490
	Never	13	(10.5)	6	(7.8)	7	(14.9)	
	Former	24	(19.4)	15	(19.5)	9	(19.1)	
	Current	82	(66.1)	52	(67.5)	30	(63.8)	
Tobacco smoking history, pack years	Missing	7	(5.6)	4	(5.2)	3	(6.4)	0.489
	<30 py	59	(47.6)	35	(45.5)	24	(51.1)	
	>30 py	58	(46.8)	38	(49.4)	20	(42.6)	
Localization	L-/HPSCC	31	(25.0)	17	(22.1)	14	(29.8)	0.053
	OSCC	45	(36.3)	23	(29.9)	22	(46.8)	
	OPSCC	42	(33.9)	32	(41.6)	10	(21.3)	
	other	6	(4.6)	5	(6.5)	1	(2.1)	
p16 status	p16 positive	17	(13.7)	13	(16.9)	4	(8.5)	0.188
	p16 negative	107	(86.3)	64	(83.1)	43	(91.5)	
HPV status	HPV positive	15	(12.1)	12	(15.6)	3	(6.4)	0.127
	HPV negative	109	(87.9)	65	(84.4)	44	(93.6)	
Initial UICC	Missing	1	(0.8)	1	(1.3)		–	0.227
	I	14	(11.3)	7	(9.1)	7	(14.9)	
	II	11	(8.9)	4	(5.2)	7	(14.9)	
	III	12	(9.7)	6	(7.8)	6	(12.8)	
	IVA	52	(41.9)	33	(42.9)	19	(40.4)	
	IVB	15	(12.1)	12	(15.6)	3	(6.4)	
	IVC	19	(15.3)	14	(18.2)	5	(10.6)	
Duration of disease, months	median (IQR)	15.1	(7.2–33.1)	10.7	(6.4–30.4)	21.8	(9.8–37.3)	0.186
Extent of disease	LRR	39	(31.5)	19	(24.7)	20	(42.6)	**0.038**
	M1	85	(68.5)	58	(75.3)	27	(57.4)	
Previous treatments	None	10	(8.1)	9	(11.7)	1	(2.1)	0.104
	One	66	(53.2)	44	(57.1)	22	(46.8)	
	Two	40	(32.3)	19	(24.7)	21	(44.7)	
	Three	6	(4.8)	4	(5.2)	2	(4.3)	
	Four	2	(1.6)	1	(1.3)	1	(2.1)	
Type of prior treatment	No prior ChT	56	(45.2)	36	(46.8)	20	(42.6)	0.652
	• none	*10*	*(17.9)*	*9*	*(25.0)*	*1*	*(5.0)*	
	• PORT	*28*	*(50.0)*	*20*	*(55.6)*	*8*	*(40.0)*	
	• RT	*8*	*(14.3)*	*4*	*(11.1)*	*4*	*(20.0)*	

(Continued)

TABLE 1 | Continued

Characteristics		Number of Patients (%)						
		Total	***N*** **= 124**	**PFE**	***N*** **= 77**	**other 1L-ChT**	***N*** **= 47**	***P*-value***
	• OP	*10*	*(17.9)*	*3*	*(8.3)*	*7*	*(35.0)*	
	Prior ChT	68	(54.8)	41	(53.2)	27	(57.4)	
	• CRT	*14*	*(20.6)*	*9*	*(22.0)*	*5*	*(18.5)*	
	• PORCT	*54*	*(79.4)*	*32*	*(78.0)*	*22*	*(81.5)*	
RCT enrollment	No	56	(45.2)	43	(55.8)	13	(27.7)	**0.002**
	Yes	68	(54.8)	34	(44.2)	34	(72.3)	
	• 1L trial	*68*	*(100.0)*	*34*	*(50.0)*	*34*	*(50.0)*	
	• 2L trial	*13*	*(19.1)*	*11*	*(32.4)*	*2*	*(5.9)*	
Prior cisplatin	Yes	61	(49.2)	36	(46.8)	25	(53.2)	0.487
	No	63	(50.8)	41	(53.2)	22	(46.8)	
Further	no	97	(78.2)	56	(72.7)	41	(87.2)	0.058
therapies	2L-/3L-ChT	27	(21.8)	21	(27.3)	6	(12.8)	
OS status	alive	3	(2.4)	2	(2.6)	1	(2.1)	0.577
	NCRD	5	(4.0)	2	(2.6)	3	(6.4)	
	CRD	116	(93.5)	73	(94.8)	43	(91.5)	

**P value from Pearson's Chi-square (χ^2) tests. PFE, Cisplatin/5-fluoruracil/cetuximab—EXTREME regimen; IQR, Interquartile range; 1L-ChT, first-line chemotherapy; py, pack years; L-/HPSCC, laryngeal/hypopharyngeal squamous cell carcinoma; OSCC, oral squamous cell carcinoma; OPSCC, oropharyngeal squamous cell carcinoma; UICC, tumor stages according to the Union International Contre le Cancer; LRR, locoregional recurrence; M1, distant metastasis; ChT, chemotherapy; PORT, postoperative radiation; RT, primary radiation; OP, surgical therapy; CRT, combined chemo-radio-therapy; PORCT, postoperative chemo-radio-therapy; RCT, randomized controlled trial; 1L trial, first-line controlled trial; 2L trial, second-line controlled trial; 2L-/3L-ChT, second-/third-line chemotherapy; OS, Overall Survival; NCRD, Non-cancer-related death; CRD, cancer-related death.*
P values from Pearson's Chi-square tests < 0.05 are in bold.

RESULTS

Patients' Characteristics

Of 124 R/M HNSCC patients, 77 received PFE (**Table 1**). The frequency of PFE was numerically higher in patients younger than 60 years (68.1% *vs.* 54.5%; X^2 = 2.4, P = 0.122). Other 1L-ChT regimens applied to 47 patients not receiving PFE were PFE plus docetaxel (TPFE; *n* = 15) according to the CeFCiD trial (6) and other cisplatin-based regimens (*n* = 21 in total, every subgroup *n* <5); 11/47 patients received in 1L-ChT docetaxel plus cetuximab (*n* = 3) or a monotherapy with methotrexate (*n* = 1) or immunotherapy with either cetuximab (*n* = 3) or nivolumab (*n* = 4). ECOG performance status in subgroups receiving PFE or other 1L-ChT did not differ significantly (**Table 1**).

Patients' Clinical Course Before and After 1L-ChT

The median time from the initial diagnosis of HNSCC to 1L-ChT was 15.1 months for the total cohort. There was no significant correlation between the time to 1L-ChT and the lifestyle-associated risk factors or patients' age. Patients receiving surgery followed by postoperative radio-chemotherapy (PORCT; n = 52) had a prolonged median time from curative treatment to 1L-ChT of 30.6 months (95%CI: 21.5–40.2) compared to 10.4 months (95% CI: 0.3–20.4) of patients with other types of curative treatment (radiation, surgery, surgery followed by postoperative radiation; n = 62). Median time from initial diagnosis of HNSCC to death/lost to follow-up (OS) was 25.5 months; median time from start of 1L-ChT to death/lost to follow up ($mOS_{1L\text{-}ChT}$) was 8.4 months; 21/124 (16.9%) died within 3 months after starting 1L-ChT (14.3% after PFE, 21.3% after other 1L-ChT regimen). Of 124 patients progressing after 1L-ChT, 27/124 (21.8%) were fit enough to receive either a 2L-ChT or further therapies, 21/77 (27.3%) after PFE, 6/47 (12.8%) after other cisplatin-based regimen. None of the patients treated without cisplatin-based 1L-ChT including all 1L-immunotherapies were fit enough for any 2L-ChT.

$OS_{1L\text{-}ChT}$ After PFE Compared to Other 1L-ChT Regimen

In Kaplan–Meier plots utilizing log-rank tests, a difference of 3 months in $mOS_{1L\text{-}ChT}$ was identified between patients being treated with PFE and those being treated with other 1L-ChT ($mOS_{1L\text{-}ChT}$ (95%CI): 9.8 months (8.1–11.5) *vs.* 6.8 months (3.9–9.7); P = 0.066; **Figure 2A**).

$OS_{1L\text{-}ChT}$ after PFE in RCT *Versus* Clinical Routine

In the group of patients not enrolled in first-line RCT ("real world patients"), a significant benefit from PFE was noticed [$mOS_{1L\text{-}ChT}$ (95%CI): 9.3 (3.3–15.3) months *vs.* 4.1 (1.8–6.4) months, P = 0.016; **Figures 2B** and **4**]. In RCT, other 1L-ChT combined *vs.* PFE showed a similar OS [$mOS_{1L\text{-}ChT}$ (95%CI): 7.0 (3.0–11.0) months *vs.* 9.8 (8.7–11.9) months; P = 0.701; **Figure 2C**]. $OS_{1L\text{-}ChT}$ after PFE outside controlled trials [$mOS_{1L\text{-}ChT}$ (95%CI): 9.3 (3.3–11.3) months) was not significantly different from $mOS_{1L\text{-}ChT}$ in RCTs (9.8 (8.7–10.9) months; P = 0.728; **Figure 2D**]. Of seven long-term survivors within the subgroup of patients treated with PFE in clinical routine (**Figure 2D**), 4/7 were current drinkers, only 1/7 drank >30 g/d alcohol, and 5/7 were current smokers. The median age (56.9 years) was comparable to the median age in the total PFE subgroup (56.6 years, **Table 1**). Five of them (71.4%) had been treated with cisplatin prior to PFE, compared to 46.8% in the total PFE cohort (**Table 1**).

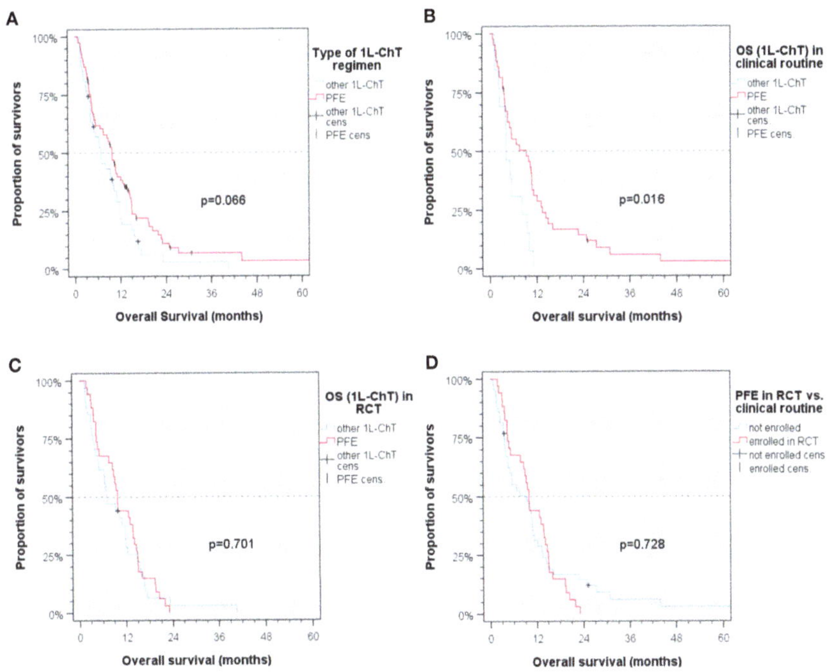

FIGURE 2 | Kaplan–Meier plots for cumulative overall survival ($OS_{1L\text{-}ChT}$) measured from diagnosis of incurable recurrent/metastatic head and neck squamous cell carcinoma receiving first-line chemotherapy as indicated; **(A)** $OS_{1L\text{-}ChT}$ after PFE according to the EXTREME protocol *vs.* other 1L-ChT regimens; **(B)** $OS_{1L\text{-}ChT}$ of patients receiving outside randomized controlled trials (RCT) PFE *vs.* other 1L-ChT regimens; **(C)** $OS_{1L\text{-}ChT}$ of patients receiving PFE *vs.* other 1L-ChT within RCT; **(D)** $OS_{1L\text{-}ChT}$ of patients receiving PFE in RCT *vs.* outside RCT; *P* values shown are from 2-sided log-rank tests.

$OS_{1L\text{-}ChT}$ After Other 1L-ChT Regimen

In this subgroup, the enrollment in RCT was predictive for improved $OS_{1L\text{-}ChT}$ only in these 34 *vs.* 13 patients ($mOS_{1L\text{-}ChT}$ (95%CI): 9.3 (4.7–13.9) *vs.* 4.1 (1.8–6.4); $P = 0.013$). The small number of patients with other 1L-ChT ($n = 47$), however, did not allow to identify further predictors for $OS_{1L\text{-}ChT}$ in this subgroup.

Predictive Factors for $OS_{1L\text{-}ChT}$ After PFE

Kaplan–Meier plots showed the number of pretreatments to be important for therapy outcome in general. Patients initially diagnosed in the metastatic or very advanced stage or after two or more pretreatments had significantly shorter $OS_{1L\text{-}ChT}$ than those receiving 1L-ChT after one pretreatment ($mOS_{1L\text{-}ChT}$ (95% CI): 6.8 (4.2–9.4) *vs.* 9.9 (7.6–12.2) months; $P = 0.038$). Stratified by PFE *vs.* other 1L-ChT, there was still a statistical trend for this finding (**Figure 4**). Patients progressing after cisplatin-based ChT treated with PFE 1L-ChT had prolonged $mOS_{1L\text{-}ChT}$ (9.9 *vs.* 6.8 months; $P = 0.082$; **Figure 4**). Cisplatin-based ChT as part of multimodal pretreatment in the curative setting was equally predictive for $OS_{1L\text{-}ChT}$ in univariate Cox regression model.

Kaplan–Meier analysis linked outcome and age: the $mOS_{1L\text{-}ChT}$ in the age groups (a) ≤49 years (7.6 months, 95%CI: 0.2–15.0), (b) 50–59 years (9.3 months, 95%CI: 7.6–11.0), and (c) ≥60 years (6.8 months, 95%CI: 4.6–9.0) was insignificantly different ($P = 0.192$). Stratified by PFE *vs.* other 1L-ChT, the statistical trend proved to be true and revealed patients aged 50–59 years having the longest $OS_{1L\text{-}ChT}$ independent from the type of 1L-ChT applied ($mOS_{1L\text{-}ChT}$ (95%CI): 9.8 (7.7–11.9) after PFE *vs.* 8.2 (0.0–17.6) months after other 1L-ChT regimen; $P = 0.560$). There were only 11 *vs.* 8 patients aged ≤ 49 years, the $mOS_{1L\text{-}ChT}$ after PFE *vs.* other 1L-ChT was 10.3 (95%CI: 1.6–19.0) months *vs.* 3.3 (95%CI: 0.0–8.0) months (Δ 7.0 months; $P = 0.754$). However, there was a statistical trend in patients ≥ 60 years (30 *vs.* 25 patients) for improved $mOS_{1L\text{-}ChT}$ after PFE *vs.* other 1L-ChT of 7.5 (95%CI: 1.6–13.4) months *vs.* 6.4 (95%CI: 3.6–9.2) months (Δ 1.1 months; $P = 0.082$; **Figure 4**). Among PFE-treated patients, we did not see an inferior $OS_{1L\text{-}ChT}$ of patients older than 65 years compared to younger patients (21 *vs.* 56 patients; $OS_{1L\text{-}ChT}$ (95%CI): 9.9 (1.3–18.5) *vs.* 9.3 (6.9–11.7); $P = 0.467$). Even with a slightly different cut-off point of 60 years (30 *vs.* 47 patients then), we did not see a significant difference neither ($OS_{1L\text{-}ChT}$ (95% CI): 7.5 (1.6–13.4) *vs.* 9.9 (8.0–11.8); $P = 0.974$). However, the heterogeneity in response to PFE in older patients is demonstrated by the enlarged 95%CI.

Regarding different localizations of the primary site of the R/M HNSCC, a statistical trend for oropharyngeal cancer *vs.* HNSCC outside oropharynx was found in Kaplan–Maier analyses ($mOS_{1L\text{-}ChT}$ (95%CI): 6.8 (2.9–10.7) months *vs.* 9.5 (6.6–12.4) months; $P = 0.281$; **Figure 3A**). Analyzing the PFE subgroup (n = 77), this difference was more than 3 months ($OS_{1L\text{-}ChT}$ (95%CI): 7.6 (2.5–12.7) *vs.* 10.7 (9.2–12-2); $P = 0.097$, **Figure 3B**). The p16-status was critical for $OS_{1L\text{-}ChT}$. As p16-positive (p16+) OPSCC had $mOS_{1L\text{-}ChT}$ of 9.3 (95%CI: 4.6–14.0) months comparable with non-oropharyngeal cancer (9.5 (6.6–12.4) months; $P = 0.784$), p16-negative OPSCC had impaired

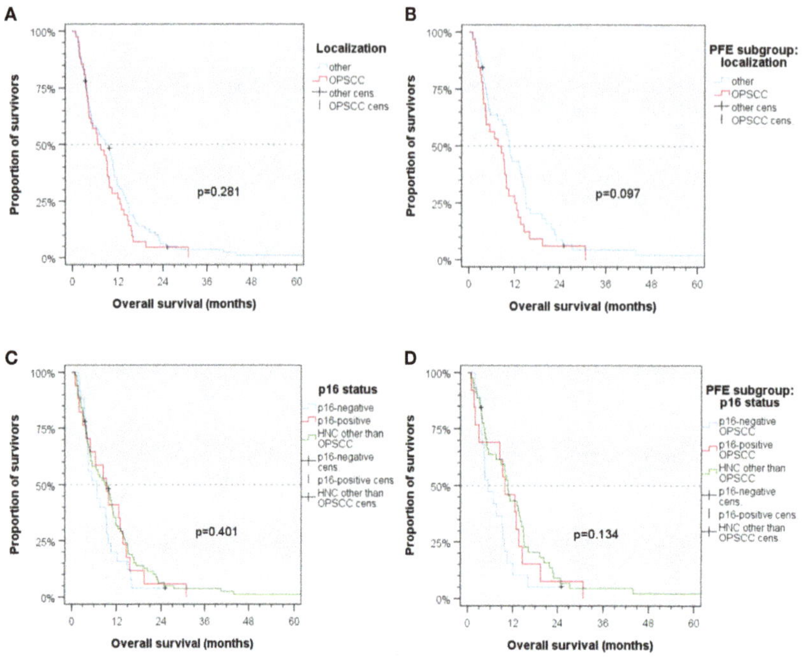

FIGURE 3 | Kaplan–Meier plots for cumulative overall survival ($OS_{1L\text{-}ChT}$) measured from diagnosis of incurable recurrent/metastatic head and neck squamous cell carcinoma **(A, C)** in the total cohort and **(B, D)** PFE treated patients. **(A)** $OS_{1L\text{-}ChT}$ for OPSCC *vs.* index HNSCC outside the oropharynx; **(B)** $OS_{1L\text{-}ChT}$ after PFE for OPSCC *vs.* HNSCC outside the oropharynx; **(C)** $OS_{1L\text{-}ChT}$ in p16-negative OPSCC *vs.* p16-positive OPSCC *vs.* HNSCC outside the oropharynx; **(D)** $OS_{1L\text{-}ChT}$ after PFE in p16-negative *vs.* p16-positive *vs.* HNSCC outside the oropharynx; *P* values shown are from 2-sided log-rank tests.

$mOS_{1L\text{-}ChT}$ of 6.7 (95%CI: 2.9–10.5) months (**Figure 3C**). Stratified by type of 1L-ChT, we saw impaired $OS_{1L\text{-}ChT}$ in p16-negative OPSCC patients even if PFE treated (**Figure 3D**). Considering HPV-driven OPSCC (*n* = 15 p16+ HR-HPV-DNA+ OPSCC out of *n* = 17 p16+ OPSCC) did not result in deviating measures but reduced differences due to enlarged 95% CI and increased *P* values, besides use of sole p16-IHC in clinical routine the reason for reporting results for p16+ OPSCC in **Figures 3–5**.

Patients with index HNSCC outside the oropharynx had a significant benefit from PFE *vs.* other 1L-ChT regimens [$OS_{1L\text{-}ChT}$ (95%CI): 10.7 (9.2–12.2) *vs.* 6.5 (3.8–9.2) months; *P* = 0.043; Δ 4.2 months; **Figure 4**]. Patients by the time of 1L-ChT

Predictor	Characteristic	*n* (%)	Events (%)	PFE - mOS1L-ChT (95% CI), months	other 1L-ChT - mOS1L-ChT (95% CI), months	*P*-value (log-rank)	Δ OS1L-ChT, months	*HR* (95% CI)	*P*-value
Sex	**Male**	67 (87.0)	65 (97.0)	9.4 (7.4 - 11.4)	5.5 (3.2 - 7.8)	0.132	3.9	0.73 (0.49 - 1.10)	0.135
Tobacco smoking	**≥ 30 packyears**	38 (49.4)	38 (100.0)	5.5 (1.6 - 9.4)	4.2 (2.0 - 6.4)	0.091	1.3	0.62 (0.35 - 1.09)	0.096
	Current smoker	67 (87.0)	66 (98.5)	9.1 (6.0 - 12.2)	5.1 (2.6 - 7.6)	0.100	4.0	0.72 (0.48 - 1.07)	0.103
Risk accumulation	**Tobacco and alcohol**	59 (76.6)	58 (98.3)	9.3 (6.0 - 12.6)	4.2 (2.7 - 5.7)	0.130	5.1	0.72 (0.47 - 1.11)	0.134
Alcohol consumption	**Current consumption**	55 (71.4)	54 (98.2)	9.4 (7.2 - 11.6)	5.5 (2.2 - 8.8)	0.178	3.9	0.74 (0.48 - 1.15)	0.182
Localization	**HNSCC outside Oropharynx**	45 (58.4)	44 (97.8)	10.7 (9.2 - 12.2)	6.5 (3.8 - 9.2)	**0.043**	4.2	0.63 (0.40 - 0.99)	**0.046**
	p16+ OPSCC and HNSCC outside Oropharynx	58 (75.3)	57 (98.3)	10.7 (9.3 - 12.2)	6.4 (3.9 - 8.9)	**0.039**	4.3	0.65 (0.43 - 0.98)	**0.041**
	OSCC	23 (29.9)	23 (100.0)	10.7 (9.3 - 12.1)	4.1 (2.4 - 5.8)	0.060	6.6	0.56 (0.30 - 1.04)	0.064
Extent of disease	**M1**	58 (75.3)	56 (96.6)	9.8 (7.7 - 11.9)	4.8 (3.3 - 6.3)	0.127	5.0	0.70 (0.44 - 1.11)	0.130
Enrollment in 1L-RCT	**Not enrolled**	43 (55.8)	41 (95.3)	9.3 (3.3 - 15.3)	4.1 (1.8 - 6.4)	**0.016**	5.2	0.45 (0.23 - 0.88)	**0.019**
Type of pretreatment	**Platinum-based ChT**	36 (46.8)	34 (94.4)	9.9 (8.3 - 11.5)	6.8 (0.0 - 13.8)	0.082	3.1	0.62 (0.36 - 1.07)	0.086
Number of pretreatments	**One pretreatment**	44 (57.1)	42 (95.5)	10.8 (6.6 - 15)	6.5 (1.3 - 11.7)	0.177	4.3	0.70 (0.41 - 1.18)	0.181
Age by the time of 1L-ChT	**≥ 60 years**	30 (61.0)	30 (100.0)	7.5 (1.6 - 13.4)	6.4 (3.6 - 9.2)	0.082	1.1	0.60 (0.34 - 1.07)	0.085

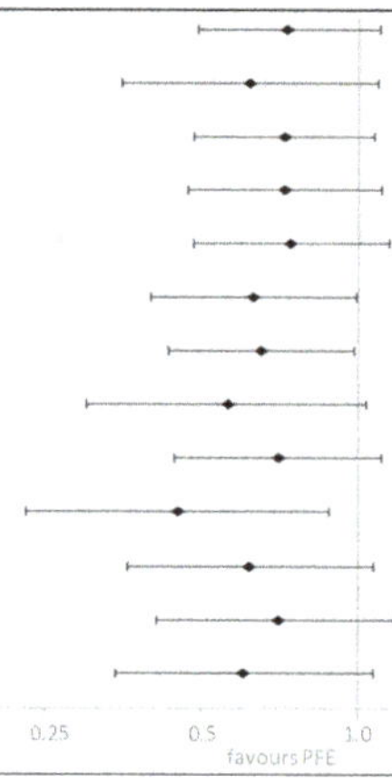

FIGURE 4 | Subgroups of incurable recurrent/metastatic head and neck squamous cell carcinoma benefitting from PFE administered according to the EXTREME protocol by prolonged $OS_{1L\text{-}ChT}$, demonstrated by Kaplan–Meier estimates applying log-rank tests and univariate Cox proportional hazard regression. *P* values of significant predictors <0.05 are in bold.

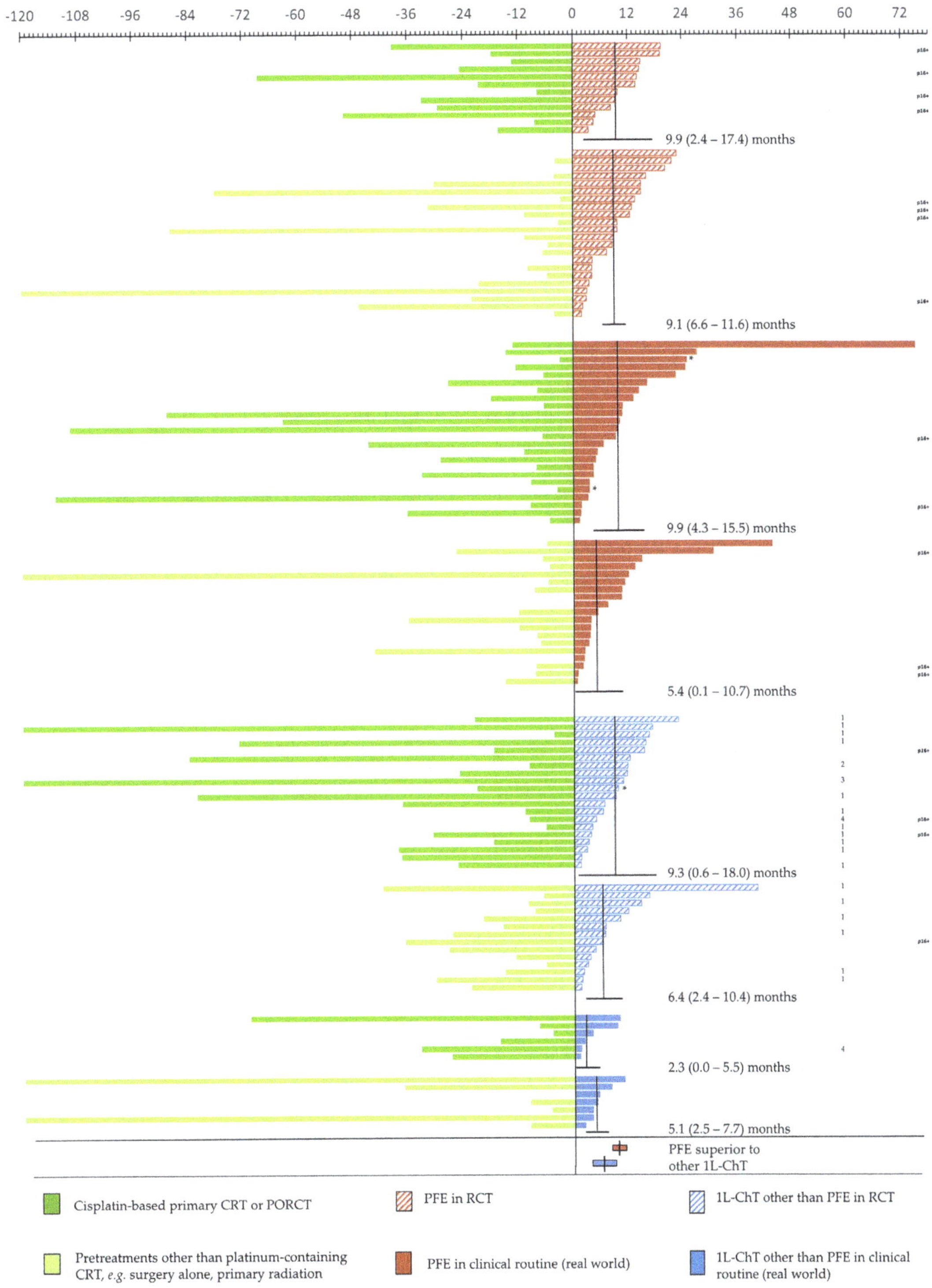

FIGURE 5 | Individual outcome of 124 patients with incurable recurrent/metastatic head and neck squamous cell carcinoma (R/M HNSCC) receiving various first-line chemotherapy regimens are depicted according to overall survival measured from diagnosis of R/M HNSCC til death ($OS_{1L\text{-}ChT}$). Patients are shown sorted stratified according to 1L-ChT, either EXTREME-regimen (PFE, red; *n* = 77) or other 1L-ChT (blue; *n* = 47) and treatment either within randomized controlled trial (RCT; shaded) or in clinical routine ("real world setting", full). Type of prior treatment in curative attempt is indicated in dark green (cisplatin-based chemo-radiation (CRT) or post-operative radio-chemotherapy (PORCT)) *vs.* light green (other or no pretreatment); time from initial diagnosis of HNSCC until diagnosis of incurable disease requiring 1L-ChT is shown in the left panel, $OS_{1\text{-}ChT}$ in the right panel according to the upper scale showing time in months. The horizontal lines indicate $mOS_{1\text{-}ChT}$ (95% confidence interval). Median and 95%CI of $OS_{1l\text{-}ChT}$ of PFE *vs.* other 1L-ChT in the total cohorts are shown in the lower rows. *censored: alive at last follow-up (*n* = 3); 1, CeFCiD (6); 2, ADVANTAGE (7); 3 RESGEX (8); 4, TPExtreme (9); p16+, p16+ OPSCC.

diagnosed with distant metastasis (M1) demonstrated an improved benefit from PFE compared to patients with loco-regional recurrence (**Figure 4**). However, we performed sensitivity analyses and excluded all patients that were diagnosed already in a locally very advanced and metastatic stage without any curative option and therefore receiving 1L-ChT as first treatment (n = 10). Kaplan–Meier estimates showed a $mOS_{1L\text{-}ChT}$ after PFE *vs.* other 1L-ChT of 9.4 (95%CI: 7.8–10.9) months *vs.* 6.5 (95%CI: 4.1–9.2) months for the remaining 114 patients (P = 0.163). This compares well to the $OS_{1L\text{-}ChT}$ for the total cohort.

The lifestyle-factors tobacco and alcohol showed an impact on outcome (**Figure 4**). There were patients with both risk factors (current or former alcohol consumption and tobacco smoking; n = 93) and those without or solely one risk factor (n = 26; five patients without information). Both groups demonstrated a benefit from PFE, patients with two risk factors had an impaired $mOS_{1L\text{-}ChT}$ but showed a higher benefit from PFE in Kaplan–Meier estimates [$mOS_{1L\text{-}ChT}$ (95% CI): 9.3 (6.0–12.6) *vs.* 4.2 (2.7–5.7) months; P = 0.130; **Figure 4**]. We found a significant correlation of double-positive risk factor-anamnesis with two baseline characteristics: young patients (≤60 years at 1L-ChT; *Pearson's r* = 0.272; P = 0.003) and male patients (*Pearson's r* = 0.288, P = 0.002) did more often belong to the group with both risk factors.

Multivariate Cox Proportional Hazard Regression for Outcome

The MCR model for OS in the total cohort achieving highest significance (X^2 = 21.7, P = 0.001) included five independent risk factors: the number of pretreatments and pack years smoking history, alcohol consumption status, index HNSCC of the oropharynx, and type of 1L-ChT (**Figure 6**). Bootstrapping revealed these factors to be predictive for $OS_{1L\text{-}ChT}$. The stepwise forward method for building the MCR failed to detect any predictive value of the patient's age by the time of 1L-ChT, TNM at first diagnosis or even enrollment in a first-line RCT for $OS_{1L\text{-}ChT}$. Interestingly, having a p16+ OPSCC was also not predictive for improved outcome, and MCR including either p16 positivity or p16 negativity as covariate had reduced significance compared to MCR including OPSCC as covariate; therefore OPSCC summarizing p16+ and p16- OPSCC remained in the MCR.

In MCR model for the PFE subgroup (n = 77; X^2 = 15.0, P = 0.002), three risk factors were found to be predictive for $OS_{1L\text{-}ChT}$ after PFE. Cisplatin-based CRT/PORCT prior to PFE (*HR* (95% CI): 0.67 (0.42–1.09); P = 0.106) was beneficial, index OPSCC (*HR* (95%CI): 1.61 (0.97–2.68); P =0.066) and alcohol consumption ≥ 30 g/d (*HR* (95%CI): 2.04 (1.22–3.41); P = 0.007) predicted impaired $OS_{1L\text{-}ChT}$.

Identification of PFE Long-Term Survivors

Figure 5 shows individual $OS_{1L\text{-}ChT}$ in R/M HNSCC stratified according to PFE *vs.* other 1L-ChT either in treatment within RCT or in clinical routine providing "real world evidence". According to identification of prior cisplatin-based CRT or PORCT as significant $OS_{1L\text{-}ChT}$ predictor, we further stratified these groups by cisplatin-based CRT or PORCT *vs.* other pretreatments. The improved outcome of certain PFE-treated R/M HNSCC patients allowed further investigations in the subgroup surviving more than 11.3 months, the upper bound of 95%CI for $mOS_{1L\text{-}ChT}$ in PFE-treated patients. These 28 individuals had a median age (57.3 years) comparable to the total cohort of PFE patients (n = 77, 56.6 years). They were quite similar to the total PFE cohort respective to sex (17.9% female), type of prior treatment (50% cisplatin-based CRT/PORCT) besides slightly lower median exposure to risk factors (22 pack years in 64.3% current smokers, as well as 64.3% current alcohol consumers; **Table 1**). Even the 12 RWE-PFE patients with $OS_{1L\text{-}ChT}$ above 95%CI $OS_{1L\text{-}ChT}$ in the CRT/PORCT and "other" subgroups (10.7 and 15.5 months, respectively) had a similar median age at the time of initial diagnosis of HNSCC (57.4 years) compared to median age in the PFE subgroup (56.6 years, **Table 1**). Eleven of these 12 patients received PFE at first recurrence, one (8.3%) was treated with PFE at second recurrence. As one curative treatment prior to any 1L-ChT is

Predictor	Characteristic	n (%)	events (%)	HR (95% CI)	*P*-value	*P*-value bootstrapping
Number of pretreatments	**One pretreatment [A]**	66 (53.2)	64 (96.7)	0.582 (0.391 - 0.865)	**0.007**	**0.007**
Type of 1L-ChT	**PFE [B]**	77 (62.1)	75 (97.4)	0.720 (0.476 - 1.064)	0.107	0.087
Alcohol consumption	**≥ 60g/d [C]**	37 (29.8)	37 (100.0)	1.470 (0.937 - 2.313)	0.095	0.058
Tobacco smoking	**≥ 30 packyears [D]**	58 (46.8)	58 (100.0)	1.621 (1.041 - 2.451)	**0.027**	**0.027**
Localization and p16-status	**p16-negative OPSCC [E]**	25 (20.2)	24 (96.0)	1.425 (0.868 - 2.34)	0.161	0.153

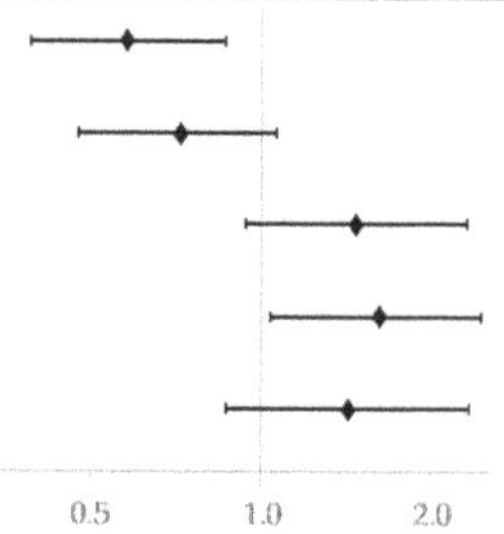

FIGURE 6 | Predictors in multivariate Cox proportional hazard regression (HR) and 2-sided *P*-values from internal validation using bootstrapping applying 1,000 iterations. Significant independent predictors P <0.005 are in bold. [A] Reference: 1L-ChT at initial diagnose or ≥2 pretreatments; [B] Reference: other 1L-ChT regimen; [C] Reference: <60 g/d; [D] Reference: <30 pack years; *E* Reference: HNSCC outside oropharynx.

an independent predictor for improved $OS_{1L\text{-}ChT}$ in the total cohort, this might be causative involved in their prolonged $OS_{1L\text{-}ChT}$. However, only 2/12 (16.7%) of RWE-PFE long-term survivors had a current alcohol consumption >30 g/d, pointing to the absent detrimental impact of maintained alcohol consumption on $OS_{1L\text{-}ChT}$ in most of RWE-PFE long-term survivors. Interestingly, smoking history and adhering to tobacco smoking may also play a role as only seven of these 12 long-term survivors (58.3%) were current smokers, and the median cumulative nicotine exposure was 25 pack years and somewhat lower compared to the total PFE cohort (**Table 1**). The proportion of p16+ OPSCC was higher in RCT; their $OS_{1L\text{-}ChT}$, however, was not superior compared with R/M HNSCC localized outside the oropharynx (**Figure 3C**).

Identification of Long-Term Survivors in Other 1L-ChT Regimens

As enrollment in RCT was predictive for improved $OS_{1L\text{-}ChT}$ only in 34 *vs.* 13 patients (see *$OS_{1L\text{-}ChT}$ after other 1L-ChT regimen*) we were interested in long-term survivors in this subgroup. According to numbers in the right panel of **Figure 5**, PFE-based regimens containing an additional (investigational) drug, for instance docetaxel (TPFE) in the CeFCiD trial [labeled 1 (6)], cilengitide in the ADVANTAGE trial [labeled 2 (7)], or replaced cetuximab by glycosylation-modified cetuximab in the RESGEX trial [labeled 3 (8)], long-term survivors were only seen after PFE-based 1L-ChT. However, the outcome observed in such intensified PFE-based 1L-ChT did not improve outcome in general at least in our cohort as it is obvious that a huge heterogeneity exists in this regard.

DISCUSSION

According to several lines of evidence, our monocentric study comprises a sufficient number of R/M HNSCC receiving 1L-ChT to show outcome differences dependent on a number of well-defined covariates. The $mOS_{1L\text{-}ChT}$ in our sample is comparable to the survival times found in prior trials (6, 7, 15). Therefore, the subgroups with and without benefit from PFE identified in our study confirm the existence of certain subgroups already described (3). Uni- and multivariate analyses demonstrated that the number of pretreatments, consumption of alcohol and/or tobacco smoking as well as localization of the index cancer and patients' age have a certain effect on $OS_{1L\text{-}ChT}$. When treated with PFE in particular, predictive covariates are mostly the same. However, our study provides evidence that prior intensified treatments making use of cisplatin-based CRT and especially cisplatin-based PORCT do not negatively affect survival in PFE but rather improve $OS_{1L\text{-}ChT}$. Indeed, prior cisplatin-based CRT or PORCT appeared to be an additional independent predictor for significant prolonged $OS_{1L\text{-}ChT}$. These findings from multivariate Cox regression analyses may contribute to the ongoing discussion about a potential negative impact of treatment escalation in the curative setting on further therapies and the possibility to re-challenge R/M HNSCC with cisplatin when progressing after cisplatin-based curative treatment. As the median time from curative treatment with surgery followed by cisplatin-based PORCT to 1L-ChT (n = 52) was 30.6 months (95%CI: 21.5–40.2) and substantially longer (P = 0.005) compared to 10.6 months (95%CI: 5.0–16.3) of patients without prior treatment or other types of prior curative treatment, and these cisplatin-pretreated R/M HNSCC patients had the highest benefit from PFE, treatment escalation in presence of risk factors in the curative setting improves outcome and does not reduce $OS_{1L\text{-}ChT}$ if PFE is used. As, additionally, a 2L-ChT could be applied in a higher frequency after PFE as compared to other 1L-ChT, treatment escalation in the curative setting *via* cisplatin-based PORCT whenever high risk for relapse/recurrent disease (more than two disease-positive neck nodes, extracapsular extension of neck nodes, positive or narrow resection margins below 5 mm) is detected appears to be warranted.

Our results confirm OS data for PFE including subgroup analyses obtained in the landmark phase-III RCT EXTREME (3). Comparing outcome of PFE with PF, Vermorken et al. (3) showed in univariate models that patients ≥ 65 years demonstrate a minor benefit from PFE compared to younger patients. Our retrospective study comprises only 21 *vs.* 15 R/M HNSCC patients ≥65 years receiving PFE *vs.* other 1L-ChT regimen. We have not seen an inferiority of PFE in this subgroup compared to patients <65 years. By performing this analysis with a slightly different cut-off point of 60 years (30 *vs.* 15 patients), we found no evidence for an inferiority of PFE neither.

The recently published ELAN-FIT trial by Guigay et al. (16) showed a $mOS_{1L\text{-}ChT}$ of 14.7 months (95%CI: 11.0–18.2) after PFE for patients aged 70 and older and ECOG performance status 0 or 1. The impact of age and its influence on PFE efficacy and risk will be probably important in future trials. However, we found no evidence in our cohort for calendar age alone being the most relevant eligibility criterion for PFE, provided good general health (ECOG 0 or 1). PFE is only approved for ECOG 0 and 1 patient presenting, so the MDTB made the decision for either offering participation in a 1L-ChT RCT or 1L-ChT treatment in the routine setting only provided good general health as reflected by ECOG 0 or 1. Consequently, our sample mainly included "fit" patients in our retrospective trial to ensure comparability. As Guigay et al. (17) showed, "unfit" patients may be eligible for PFE or comparable regimens after a comprehensive geriatric assessment. By performing RCTs after a geriatric assessment, there could be more evidence about the impact of calendar age *vs.* biological age on treatment eligibility and potential benefit in older patients.

Referring to Guigay et al. (9), the TPExtreme (TPE; docetaxel, cis- or carboplatin, cetuximab) 1L-ChT regimen is beneficial when followed by ICB in 2L-ChT. As retrospectively found, TPE outperformed PFE only in this treatment sequence. Due to our small sample of 124 patients collected over years and only two TPE patients unfit to receive 2L-ChT after recurrence, there are no such patients in our cohort.

Patients in the PFE subgroup had a longer $mOS_{1L\text{-}ChT}$ –independently on the following 2L-ChT— than patients treated with other 1L-ChT in our analysis. As all studies demonstrated the lasting value of PFE, we recommend—against the often suggested alternative use of TPE as unproblematic replacement for PFE to avoid potential dihydropyrimidine dehydrogenase-(DPD-) toxicity—rather DPD testing according to established guidelines (18) so that R/M HNSCC patients still can benefit from PFE. As only one RCT demonstrated an improved OS of R/M HNSCC in the minor subgroup of patients treated sequentially first with TPE followed by ICB over PFE followed by ICB in a retrospective analysis (17), it might be too soon to change 1L-ChT of R/M HNSCC in absence of a positive phase III RCT demonstrating superiority of TPE over PFE. Moreover, we were unable to see a benefit from TPE as only 2/124 patients received TPE, and both (indicated with four in **Figure 5**) had a rather impaired outcome below the $mOS_{1L\text{-}ChT}$. Without replication of the findings by Guigay et al. (9) in such a phase-III RCT the TPExtreme-ICB treatment sequence so far remains experimental at best.

Today, no published data for the efficacy of PFE for R/M HNSCC progressing under 1L-ICB are available. The question if patients failing on curative treatment involving ICB thereafter progressing and requiring 1L-ChT should preferentially be treated with PFE is not yet completely clear. However, we expect that PFE can benefit a substantial proportion of such R/M HNSCC.

Regarding the influence of HPV-status on $OS_{1L\text{-}ChT}$, we have seen an impaired $OS_{1L\text{-}ChT}$ in patients suffering from a p16-negative OPSCC compared to patients with a p16+ OPSCC or index HNSCC outside the oropharynx. This is in line with former findings (19, 20). Based on the study by Mehra et al. (19) showing an improved OS in p16+/HPV+ R/M HNSCC patients, Vermorken et al. (20) performed a retrospective analysis of data from the EXTREME trial (3) and found a p16+/HPV-prevalence and p16+/HPV-related $OS_{1L\text{-}ChT}$ similar to our findings. There is an ongoing discussion about the influence of HPV on survival in R/M HNSCC. In contrast to Mehra et al. and Vermorken et al., Szturz et al. (21) found in a meta-analysis of four prospective RCT that HPV-related (p16+ or HPV-DNA+) tumors barely responded to EGFR-directed monotherapy, whereas improved response rates were only observed in HPV-negative cases. Since we did not observe detrimental effects by p16 positivity on $OS_{1L\text{-}ChT}$ no matter if EXTREME or other regimens were applied, but $OS_{1L\text{-}ChT}$ was strongly reduced in oropharyngeal R/M HNSCC and even further reduced in p16-negative cases, our study highlights the importance of further investigations in this field. The poorest $OS_{1L\text{-}ChT}$ in oropharyngeal R/M HNNSCC could be linked to the proximity to essential cervical structures including arteries and their infiltration. Therefore, R/M HNSCC with rather reduced infiltrating growth patterns and without vascular infiltration may have prolonged $OS_{1L\text{-}ChT}$ independent from being HPV-related. Additionally, distance of the R/M HNSCC from vital vessels might prolong the time to life-threatening destruction of indispensable organs and critical bleeding events including arterial blowout leading to death.

During the time period analyzed in this retrospective study, therapy guidelines for R/M HNSCC have changed. Nowadays, and according to KEYNOTE-048 trial (4), immune checkpoint blockade (ICB) by pembrolizumab is declared new standard of care for patients with CPS >20 or ICB-PF combination for patients with CPS >1 to ≤20. According to KEYNOTE-048 investigators, PFE remains standard of care for CPS ≤1. Consequently, PFE may be 1L-ChT standard for this subgroup and 2L-ChT option for patients progressing after ICB. However, as we confirm data from the EXTREME trial (3), especially male patients, subgroups accumulating more lifestyle-associated risk factors, and those with their index HNSCC outside oropharynx still benefit the most from PFE. KEYNOTE-048 subgroup analyses (4) addressed this issue showing that patients <65 years and ≥65 years do not differ in benefit from pembrolizumab ± chemotherapy. There was no significant difference between never and former/current smokers. It may be interesting to conduct further analyses to see if there are any differences in OS depending on patients' characteristics described here (**Figure 5**).

Unlike ICB in the KEYNOTE-048 trial, ICB with durvalumab (PD-L1 inhibitor) ± tremelimumab (CTLA-4-inhibitor) in the KESTREL phase III trial failed to meet the primary endpoint of improved OS compared to PFE. As AstraZeneca reported this result just recently [2021-02-05 (22)] and a peer-reviewed paper on KESTREL is still not published, it might be too soon to rank any ICB in general over PFE. At least, PFE should be considered standard for all 1L-ChT not belonging to the CPS >1 subgroup of R/M HNSCC patients.

Argiris et al. (23) showed an improved response rate and progression-free survival by adding the anti-VEGF antibody bevacizumab to chemotherapy. This may provide evidence for a benefit by targeted therapies other than EGFR- or PD-L1-inhibitors combined with PF. However, acute toxicity appeared to be increased if PF and bevacizumab were used in 1L-ChT, and the gain in OS compared to PF rather limited (18).

Discussing their KEYNOTE-048 results and referring to retrospective trials (24, 25), post-pembrolizumab sensitization of R/M HNSCC to a subsequent therapy with PFE was mentioned by Burtness et al. (4). This highlights the potential importance of 2L-PFE applied after 1L-ICB in the future. In the light of ICB applied within multimodal treatment regimen in the curative setting, *e.g.* during induction-chemotherapy for larynx-organ preservation or ICB as component of adjuvant therapies after curative resection and in postoperative maintenance, we are convinced that PFE will have a dominant role as 1L-ChT also in the future (26, 27). In context of earlier investigations highlighting improved outcome after increased utilization of PORCT in treatment of L/HSCC (23), prolonged $OS_{1L\text{-}ChT}$ through PFE after cisplatin-based PORCT may at least partially have contributed to the welcome impact of indication shift towards increased use of cisplatin-based PORCT according to Bernier and Cooper (12, 13) on heightened OS time (28).

In our study, 14.3% of the patients died within 3 months after starting PFE. These figures compare well to 17.1% found by Vermorken et al. (3). The majority of early deaths observed in our cohort occurred outside RCTs (72.7% *vs.* 27.3% of all fatalities during PFE treatment). Treatment in clinical routine apart from adherence to the complete checklist of eligibility criteria as required to enter any of the RCT as well as survivorship bias may have potentially contributed to this situation. However, outcome in RCT *vs.* "real world" was not significantly different overall. Reproducibility of survival benefit of certain subgroups independent from RCT participation shows that RCT results are representative for the outcome achieved by PFE even in clinical routine. Subgroup analyses of the seven long-term survivors within the subgroup of RWE-PFE treated patients allude to the impact of risk factors on survival. Those seven patients barely drank alcohol but received PFE after cisplatin-based CRT/PORCT. The overall well-comparable or even slightly improved outcome in RWE compared to RCT PFE-treated R/M HNSCC patients demonstrates an unprecedented translation of findings from RCT into routine results with high concordance.

Only a minority of R/M HNSCC patients treated in other 1L-ChT RCT demonstrated superior $OS_{1l\text{-}ChT}$ from a further intensified PFE-based regimen, whereas most had inferior $OS_{1l\text{-}ChT}$ compared to PFE (**Figure 5**). However, the only long-term survivors detected among other 1L-ChT received an intensified PFE-based regimen. Unfortunately, the frequency of patients without benefit from treatment escalation was found to be higher than those with prolonged $OS_{1L\text{-}ChT}$. Increased toxicity as reported also in (6) and (7) may have essentially contributed to this finding by causing detrimental effects. Further investigations to distinguish long-term survivors and those unsuitable for treatment escalation beyond the use of PFE appear to be warranted.

There are limitations of our study. Our retrospective monocentric study involved 124 R/M HNSCC patients including 77 treated with PFE. However, this case number was sufficiently large enough to elucidate some independent predictors for outcome and to confirm the existence of the earlier described subgroups of R/M HNSCC patients. Moreover, we did not find any significant survival differences between patients receiving PFE in- or outside the numerous first-line RCT arguing for a representative mixture of patients that at least in our clinic remained stable over two decades, a consistency in decision-making for usage of PFE in 1L-ChT for R/M HNSCC, and improved outcome achieved through PFE. Therefore, the effects detected in our sample demonstrate stability over time and confirm the initial findings from the EXTREME trial (3) being representative for good outcome after PFE in general. A strength of our study is the complete follow-up and the multivariate analyses including bootstrapping for internal validation of independent predictors to avoid over-optimism in interpretation of our findings.

CONCLUSIONS

This retrospective study highlights the lasting value of the triplet cisplatin, 5-fluoruracil, cetuximab (PFE) not only as comparator treatment within randomized controlled trials (RCT) but also—and independent on the age of R/M HNSCC patients—in clinical routine. Interestingly, we found no evidence for a negative impact of prior intensified treatments making use of primary or postoperative cisplatin-based chemo-radiotherapy on overall survival following first-line chemotherapy but rather improved outcome in this subgroup achieved by PFE independent from participation in RCT or applied in the "real world" setting. Demonstrating again the high value of PFE in first-line chemotherapy, this effective treatment should not be replaced by treatments that failed to demonstrate superiority in RCT. PFE should hence remain standard for first-line chemotherapy at least in patients not belonging to the well-defined subgroups of recurrent/metastatic head and neck squamous cell carcinoma eligible for pembrolizumab or PF plus pembrolizumab according to KEYNOTE-048 (4).

ETHICS STATEMENT

The studies involving human participants were reviewed and approved by The Institutional Human Ethics Committee of the University Leipzig (votes 201-10-12072010 and 202-10-12072010). The patients/participants provided their written informed consent to participate in this study.

AUTHOR CONTRIBUTIONS

Conceptualization, GW. Data curation, KL, MP, TW, and GW. Formal analysis, KL and GW. Investigation, KL and GW. Methodology, GW. Project administration, GW. Resources, AD and GW. Validation, GW. Visualization, KL and GW. Writing – original draft, KL and GW. Supervision, SW, AD, VZ, and GW. Writing – review and editing, KL, MP, TW, SW, AD, VZ, and GW. All authors contributed to the article and approved the submitted version.

ACKNOWLEDGMENTS

We thank all patients who participated in clinical studies and agreed with analyzing their data and all contributors who added data to the tumor database of our department. The authors acknowledge support from the German Research Foundation (DFG) and University Leipzig within the program of Open Access Publishing.

REFERENCES

1. Gatta G, Botta L, Sánchez MJ, Anderson LA, Pierannunzio D, Licitra L. Prognoses and Improvement for Head and Neck Cancers Diagnosed in Europe in Early 2000s: The EUROCARE-5 Population-Based Study. *Eur J Cancer* (2015) 51:2130–43. doi: 10.1016/j.ejca.2015.07.043
2. Colevas AD, Yom S, Pfister D, Spencer S, Adelstein D, Adkins D, et al. NCCN Guidelines Insights: Head and Neck Cancers, Version 1.2018. *J Natl Compr Canc Netw* (2018) 16:479–90. doi: 10.6004/jnccn.2018.0026
3. Vermorken JB, Mesia R, Rivera F, Remenar E, Kawecki A, Rottey S, et al. Platinum-Based Chemotherapy Plus Cetuximab in Head and Neck Cancer. *N Engl J Med* (2008) 359:1116–27. doi: 10.1056/NEJMoa0802656
4. Burtness B, Harrington KJ, Greil R, Soulières D, Tahara M, Castro G, et al. Pembrolizumab Alone or With Chemotherapy *Versus* Cetuximab With Chemotherapy for Recurrent or Metastatic Squamous Cell Carcinoma of the Head and Neck (KEYNOTE-048): A Randomised, Open-Label, Phase 3 Study. *Lancet* (2019) 394:1915–28. doi: 10.1016/S0140-6736(19)32591-7
5. Pfister DG, Spencer S, Adelstein D, Adkins D, Anzai Y, Brizel DM, et al. Head and Neck Cancers, Version 2.2020, NCCN Clinical Practice Guidelines in Oncology. *J Natl Compr Canc Netw* (2020) 18:873–98. doi: 10.6004/jnccn.2020.0031
6. Klinghammer K, Gauler T, Dietz A, Grünwald V, Stöhlmacher J, Knipping S, et al. Cetuximab, Fluorouracil and Cisplatin With or Without Docetaxel for Patients With Recurrent and/or Metastatic Squamous Cell Carcinoma of the Head and Neck (CeFCiD): An Open-Label Phase II Randomised Trial (AIO/IAG-KHT Trial 1108). *Eur J Cancer* (2019) 122:53–60. doi: 10.1016/j.ejca.2019.08.018
7. Vermorken JB, Peyrade F, Krauss J, Mesía R, Remenar E, Gauler TC, et al. Cisplatin, 5-Fluorouracil, and Cetuximab (PFE) With or Without Cilengitide in Recurrent/Metastatic Squamous Cell Carcinoma of the Head and Neck: Results of the Randomized Phase I/II ADVANTAGE Trial (Phase II Part). *Ann Oncol Off J Eur Soc Med Oncol* (2014) 25:682–8. doi: 10.1093/annonc/mdu003
8. Keilholz U, Kawecki A, Dietz A, Zurawski B, Schenker M, Kukielka-Budny B, et al. Efficacy and Safety of CetuGEX in Recurrent/Metastatic Squamous Cell Carcinoma of the Head and Neck (RM-HNSCC): Results From the Randomized Phase II RESGEX Study. *J Clin Oncol Off J Am Soc Clin Oncol* (2018) 36:59. doi: 10.1200/JCO.2018.36.5_suppl.59
9. Guigay J, Fayette J, Mesia R, Saada-Bouzid E, Lafond C, Geoffrois L, et al. TPExtreme Randomized Trial: Quality of Life (QoL) and Survival According to Second-Line Treatments in Patients With Recurrent/Metastatic Head and Neck Squamous Cell Carcinoma (R/M HNSCC). *J Clin Oncol Off J Am Soc Clin Oncol* (2020) 38:6507. doi: 10.1200/JCO.2020.38.15_suppl.6507
10. Meier J, Boehm A, Kielhorn A, Dietz A, Bohn S, Neumuth T. Design and Evaluation of a Multimedia Electronic Patient Record "Oncoflow" With Clinical Workflow Assistance for Head and Neck Tumor Therapy. *Int J Comput assisted Radiol Surg* (2014) 9:949–65. doi: 10.1007/s11548-014-0988-x
11. Oeser A, Gaebel J, Dietz A, Wiegand S, Oeltze-Jafra S. Information Architecture for a Patient-Specific Dashboard in Head and Neck Tumor Boards. *Int J Comput assisted Radiol Surg* (2018) 13(8):1283–90. doi: 10.1007/s11548-018-1741-7
12. Bernier J, Domenge C, Ozsahin M, Matuszewska K, Lefèbvre J-L, Greiner RH, et al. Postoperative Irradiation With or Without Concomitant Chemotherapy for Locally Advanced Head and Neck Cancer. *N Engl J Med* (2004) 350:1945–52. doi: 10.1056/NEJMoa032641
13. Cooper JS, Pajak TF, Forastiere AA, Jacobs J, Campbell BH, Saxman SB, et al. Postoperative Concurrent Radiotherapy and Chemotherapy for High-Risk Squamous-Cell Carcinoma of the Head and Neck. *N Engl J Med* (2004) 350:1937–44. doi: 10.1056/NEJMoa032646
14. Freitag J, Wald T, Kuhnt T, Gradistanac T, Kolb M, Dietz A, et al. Extracapsular Extension of Neck Nodes and Absence of Human Papillomavirus 16-DNA Are Predictors of Impaired Survival in P16-Positive Oropharyngeal Squamous Cell Carcinoma. *Cancer* (2020) 126:1856–72. doi: 10.1002/cncr.32667
15. Vermorken JB, Herbst RS, Leon X, Amellal N, Baselga J. Overview of the Efficacy of Cetuximab in Recurrent and/or Metastatic Squamous Cell Carcinoma of the Head and Neck in Patients Who Previously Failed Platinum-Based Therapies. *Cancer* (2008) 112:2710–9. doi: 10.1002/cncr.23442
16. Guigay J, Auperin A, Mertens C, Even C, Geoffrois L, Cupissol D, et al. Personalized Treatment According to Geriatric Assessment in First-Line Recurrent and/or Metastatic (R/M) Head and Neck Squamous Cell Cancer (HNSCC) Patients Aged 70 or Over: ELAN (ELderly heAd and Neck Cancer) FIT and UNFIT Trials. *Ann Oncol* (2019) 30:v450. doi: 10.1093/annonc/mdz252.002
17. Guigay J, Le Caer H, Ortholan C, Aupérin A, Michel C, Mertens C. Treatment of Inoperable Elderly Head and Neck Cancer Patients. *Curr Opin Oncol* (2019) 31:152–9. doi: 10.1097/CCO.0000000000000526
18. Wörmann B, Arnold D, Blohmer J. *Positionspapier: Dihydropyrimidin-Dehydrogenase (DPD) -Testung Vor Einsatz Von 5-Fluorouracil, Capecitabin Und Tegafur. Oncol Res Treat* (2020) 43:628–36. doi: 10.1159/000510258
19. Mehra R, Egloff AM, Li S, Yang D, Wang L, Zhu F, et al. Analysis of HPV and ERCC1 in Recurrent or Metastatic Squamous Cell Carcinoma of the Head and Neck (R/M SCCHN). *J Clin Oncol Off J Am Soc Clin Oncol* (2013) 31:6006. doi: 10.1200/jco.2013.31.15_suppl.6006
20. Vermorken JB, Psyrri A, Mesía R, Peyrade F, Beier F, de BB, et al. Impact of Tumor HPV Status on Outcome in Patients With Recurrent and/or Metastatic Squamous Cell Carcinoma of the Head and Neck Receiving Chemotherapy With or Without Cetuximab: Retrospective Analysis of the Phase III EXTREME Trial. *Ann Oncol Off J Eur Soc Med Oncol* (2014) 25:801–7. doi: 10.1093/annonc/mdt574
21. Szturz P, Seiwert TY, Vermorken JB. How Standard Is Second-Line Cetuximab in Recurrent or Metastatic Head and Neck Cancer in 2017? *J Clin Oncol Off J Am Soc Clin Oncol* (2017) 35:2229–31. doi: 10.1200/JCO.2016.71.8072
22. *Update on KESTREL Phase III Trial of Imfinzi With or Without Tremelimumab in the 1st-Line Treatment of Recurrent or Metastatic Head and Neck Cancer* (2021). Available at: https://www.astrazeneca.com/media-centre/press-releases/2021/update-on-kestrel-phase-iii-trial-for-imfinzi.html.
23. Argiris A, Li S, Savvides P, Ohr JP, Gilbert J, Levine MA, et al. Phase III Randomized Trial of Chemotherapy With or Without Bevacizumab in Patients With Recurrent or Metastatic Head and Neck Cancer. *J Clin Oncol* (2019) 37(34):3266–74. doi: 10.1200/JCO.19.00555
24. Aspeslagh S, Matias M, Palomar V, Dercle L, Lanoy E, Soria J-C, et al. In the Immuno-Oncology Era, Is Anti-PD-1 or Anti-PD-L1 Immunotherapy Modifying the Sensitivity to Conventional Cancer Therapies? *Eur J Cancer* (2017) 87:65–74. doi: 10.1016/j.ejca.2017.09.027
25. Saleh K, Daste A, Martin N, Pons-Tostivint E, Auperin A, Herrera-Gomez RG, et al. Response to Salvage Chemotherapy After Progression on Immune Checkpoint Inhibitors in Patients With Recurrent and/or Metastatic Squamous Cell Carcinoma of the Head and Neck. *Eur J Cancer* (2019) 121:123–9. doi: 10.1016/j.ejca.2019.08.026
26. Wiegand S, Wichmann G, Dietz A. Perspectives of Induction With Chemo and/or Immune Check Point Inhibition in Head and Neck Organ Preservation Treatment. *Front Oncol* (2019) 9:191. doi: 10.3389/fonc.2019.00191
27. Dietz A, Wiegand S, Kuhnt T, Wichmann G. Laryngeal Preservation Approaches: Considerations for New Selection Criteria Based on the DeLOS-II Trial. *Front Oncol* (2019) 9:625. doi: 10.3389/fonc.2019.00625
28. Boehm A, Lindner F, Wichmann G, Bauer U, Wittekind C, Knoedler M, et al. Impact of Indication-Shift of Primary and Adjuvant Chemo Radiation in Advanced Laryngeal and Hypopharyngeal Squamous Cell Carcinoma. *Eur Arch Otorhinolaryngol* (2015) 272:2017–25. doi: 10.1007/s00405-014-3134-z

8

Anticancer Effect and Mechanism of Hydroxygenkwanin in Oral Squamous Cell Carcinoma

Yi-Chao Huang [1,2], *Po-Chuan Lee* [1], *Jane Jen Wang* [3] *and Yi-Chiung Hsu* [1*]

[1] *Department of Biomedical Sciences and Engineering, National Central University, Taoyuan, Taiwan,* [2] *Department of Medical Laboratory, Taoyuan Armed Forces General Hospital, Taoyuan, Taiwan,* [3] *The Department of Nursing, School of Nursing, National Taipei University of Nursing and Health Sciences, Taipei, Taiwan*

***Correspondence:**
Yi-Chiung Hsu
syicncu@g.ncu.edu.tw

The incidence and mortality of oral squamous cell carcinoma (OSCC) are high, and the number of oral cancers had risen in the world. However, chemotherapy drugs have numerous side effects. There is an urgent requirement to develop a novel drug that can be used to treat oral cancer. Hydroxygenkwanin (HGK) is a nature flavonoid extracted from *Daphne genkwa Sieb. et Zucc. (Thymelaeaceae).* Previous studies had demonstrated that HGK exhibits anticancer effect, but the effect is still unclear in oral cancer. HGK inhibited cell growth dose-dependently in SAS and OCEM1 cells. The functional enrichment analysis showed the significant pathway in cellular movement, cell cycle and cellular growth and proliferation. We further demonstrated the HGK induced the cell cycle arrest by flow cytometry and inhibited colony formation ability and cell movement. The western blot showed that HGK induced cell cycle arrest through p21 activation and caused intrinsic cell apoptosis pathway. HGK inhibited the cell invasion and migration through down-regulation vimentin. HGK might be an effective natural product for oral cancer therapy.

Keywords: oral cancer, RNA sequencing, apoptosis, cell cycle, migration, invasion

INTRODUCTION

Oral cancer is a lethal disease worldwide with a 5-year survival rate of around 50% and oral squamous cell carcinoma (OSCC) accounts for 90% of all oral cancer types found in the mouth, tongue, and lips (1). The oral cancer is highly related to the exposure of risk factors such as betel nut chewing, smoking, alcohol drinking, and virus infection (2). From 2004 to 2015, the oral cancer incidence keeps increasing in Taiwan. Surgery, radiotherapy, and chemotherapy are the three main treatments intended to stop or eliminate the spread of oral cancer (3). However, chemotherapy compounds would cause normal cells damage. In order to reduce the side effect of treatment in oral cancer, identification of the new potentially anticancer compounds is necessary. Hydroxygenkwanin (HGK) is purification from *Daphne genkwa* plant. *Daphne genkwa* (*yuanhua* in Chinese), is one kind of Daphne plants (*Thymelaeaceae*) distributed in Europe, Taiwan and China. *Daphne genkwa* is a commonly used traditional Chinese medicine (TCM) known to have purgative and diuretic effects (4). The daphnane diterpenoid from the flowers of *Daphne genkwa*, has been demonstrated a potential anti-cancer effect in human non-small cell lung cancer (NSCLC) cells and anti-gioma (5, 6). The *Genkwa flos* flavonoids significantly decreased arthritis through antioxidant and hemorheological modulatory mechanisms in animal study (7). However, the systematic studies of HGK, the compound from *Daphnis Genkwa Flo*, in oral cancer is limited. We systematically study the gene expression profile in OECM1 and SAS cells treated with HGK. Furthermore, we investigate the anti-cancer mechanism of HGK in oral cancer cells.

MATERIALS AND METHODS

Cell Culture

HGK was purchased from Shanghai BS Bio-Tech Co., Ltd (Shanghai, China) and was dissolved in dimethyl sulfoxide (DMSO) (Merck, Darmstadt, Germany) as a stock solution of 100 mM and stored at −20°C before use. SAS is a human tongue squamous cell carcinoma from the Japanese Collection of Research Bioresources (Tokyo, Japan) (2). OECM1, a human gingival squamous carcinoma cells, derived according to previous study (2). Two cell lines were authenticated by short tandem repeat analysis and cultured in Dulbecco's modified Eagle's medium (DMEM) supplemented with 10% fetal bovine serum (FBS), 1.2 g/L sodium bicarbonate, 0.5 mM sodium pyruvate, and 2.5 mM L-glutamine. Chemical compounds, culture medium and FBS were purchased from Life Technologies (Grand Island, NY, USA).

Phenotypic Examination

Phenotypes including cell proliferation (MTT assay), clonogenic ability, migration, and invasion assay were done as described previously (2, 8).

RNA Sequencing

The total RNA samples are first treated with DNase I to degrade any possible DNA contamination. Then the mRNA is enriched by using the oligo (dT) magnetic beads. Mixed with the fragmentation buffer, the mRNA is fragmented into short fragments. Then the first strand of cDNA is synthesized by using random hexamer-primer. Buffer, dNTPs, RNase H and DNA polymerase I are added to synthesize the second strand. The double strand cDNA is purified with magnetic beads. End reparation and 3′-end single nucleotide A (adenine) addition is then performed. Finally, sequencing adaptors are ligated to the fragments. The fragments are enriched by PCR amplification. During the QC step, Agilent 2100 Bioanaylzer and ABI Step One Plus Real-Time PCR System are used to qualify and quantify of the sample library. The library products are ready for sequencing via Illumina HiSeq 4000 or other sequencer when necessary.

Differential Expression Analysis

Primary sequencing data that produced by Illumina Hiseq 4000 (San Diego, CA), called as raw reads, is subjected to quality control (QC) to determine if a resequencing step is needed (Using Trimmomativ v0.33). After QC, raw reads are filtered into clean reads which will be aligned to the reference sequences (mm10 for mouse) by Bowtie2 v2.2.6. QC of alignment

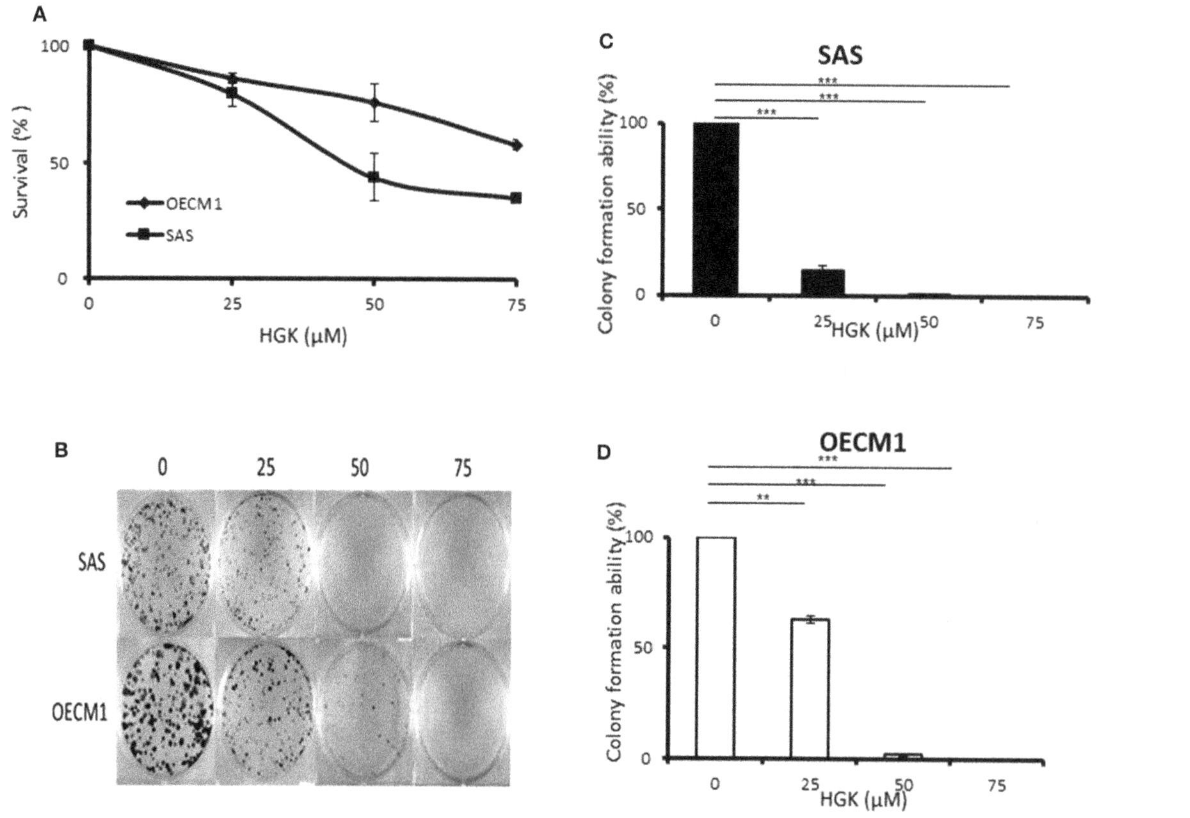

FIGURE 1 | Effects of HGK on the cell survival assay and colony formation of SAS and OECM1 cells. SAS and OECM1 cells were treated with HGK for 24 h in different concentrations (0, 25, 50, 75 μM). **(A)** MTT assay **(B)** The images showing colony formation assay in two cancer cells treated with HGK. **(C)** The quantitative analysis of colony numbers in SAS cells **(D)** in OECM1 cells. $^{**}P < 0.01$ and $^{***}P < 0.001$.

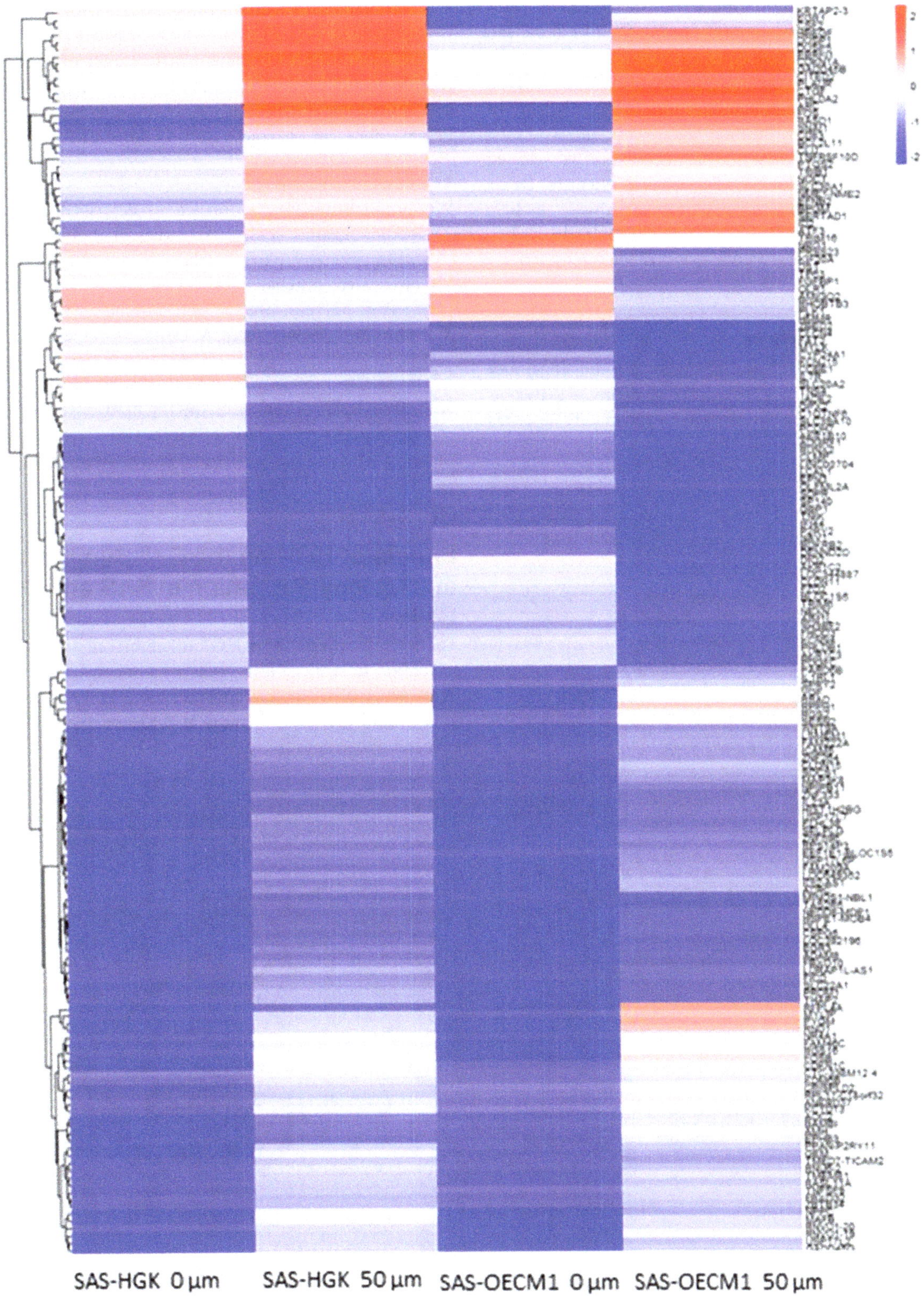

FIGURE 2 | Heatmap showing differential gene expression level with 50 µM HGK treatment for 24 h. Red indicating upregulation, and blue representing downregulation.

is performed to determine if resequencing is needed. The alignment data is utilized to calculate distribution of reads on reference genes and mapping ratio. Once all of the clean reads mapped to reference sequences, we're using "RSEM (RNA-seq by Expectation Maximization)" for calculating read raw count and normalized quantification from each sample. As we got the read quantification data, we could continue various different comparisons. The statistical tool we selected is "EBSeq v1.16.0" which may be used to identify DEGs (differential expressed genes). The RNAseq data were publicly available on NCBI's Sequence Read Archive (SRA) database (Bio-project: PRJNA559691).

Functional Enrichment

The pathway enrichment were analyzed by the Ingenuity Pathway Analysis (IPA) (QIAGEN company, Redwood City, CA, USA), and Gene set enrichment analysis (GSEA) (9).

TABLE 1 | Molecular and cellular functions analysis of differential gene expression in HGK-treated oral cancer cells.

Name	*p*-value range	#Molecules
Cellular movement	2.32E-04–2.39E-15	68
Cell death and survival	2.34E-04–7.60E-12	74
Cell cycle	2.35E-04–1.09E-11	87
Cellular growth and proliferation	2.35E-04–1.09E-11	78
DNA replication	2.80E-11–2.80E-11	22

Cell Cycle Analysis

Cell cycle analysis was performed as previously described (10). Briefly, cells were fixed in −20°C absolute ethanol for 4 h and resuspended in PBS having 20 µg/ml ribonuclease A. After incubating at 37°C for 30 min, propidium iodide 100 µg/ml was added to samples. Cell cycle was examined by flow cytometry (BD FACSCalibur TM system, Becton-Dickinson).

Western Blotting

Western blotting was performed as described previously (2). Antibodies against poly (ADP-ribose) polymerase (PARP) (Asp214), caspase 9, phosphor-H2A.X (ser139), E-cadherin, and Vimentin were purchased from Cell Signaling (Temecula, CA, USA). Anti-p21 and β-actin were purchased from Santa Cruz Biotechnology (Santa Cruz, CA, USA).

Statistics

Student's *t*-test was completed by the Statistical Package for the Social Sciences version 12.0 (SPSS, Inc). Differences between the variables were considered significant for *p*-values < 0.05.

RESULTS

Effects of HGK on the Cell Survival Assay and Colony Formation in SAS and OECM1 Cells

To determine the ability of HGK to inhibit cell growth and colony formation in two cell lines, cells were incubated in the absence or presence of increasing concentrations of HGK for 24 h. The growth and colony formation of SAS and OECM1 cells were reduced after exposure to 25–75 µM HGK for 24 h (**Figure 1**).

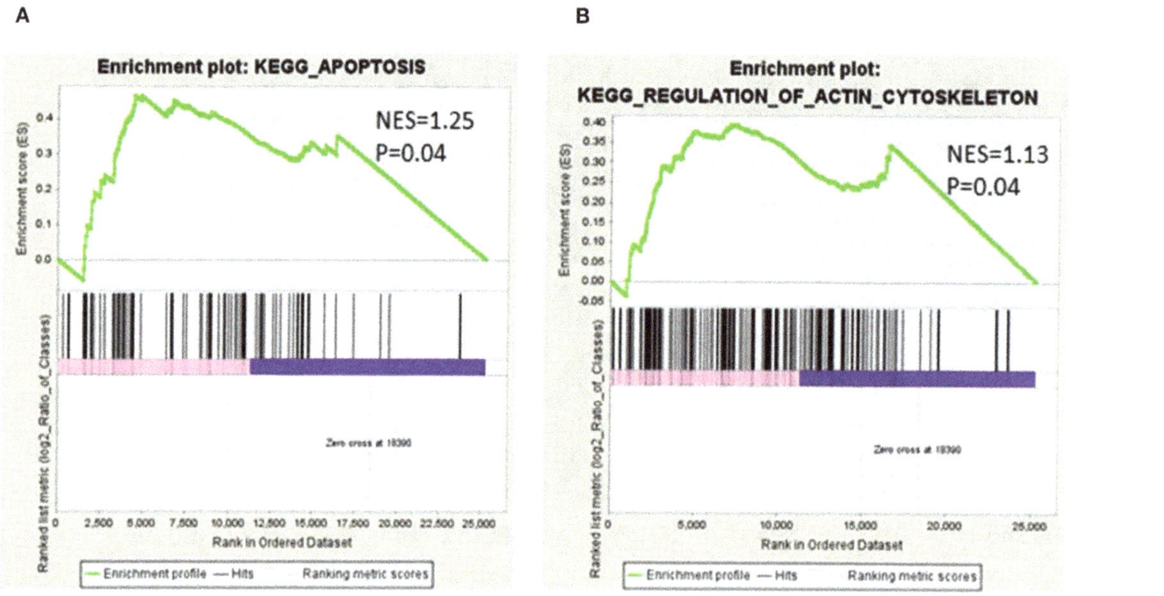

FIGURE 3 | Gene Set Enrichment Analysis (GSEA) enrichment plot involved in **(A)** apoptosis **(B)** in regulation of actin cytoskeleton.

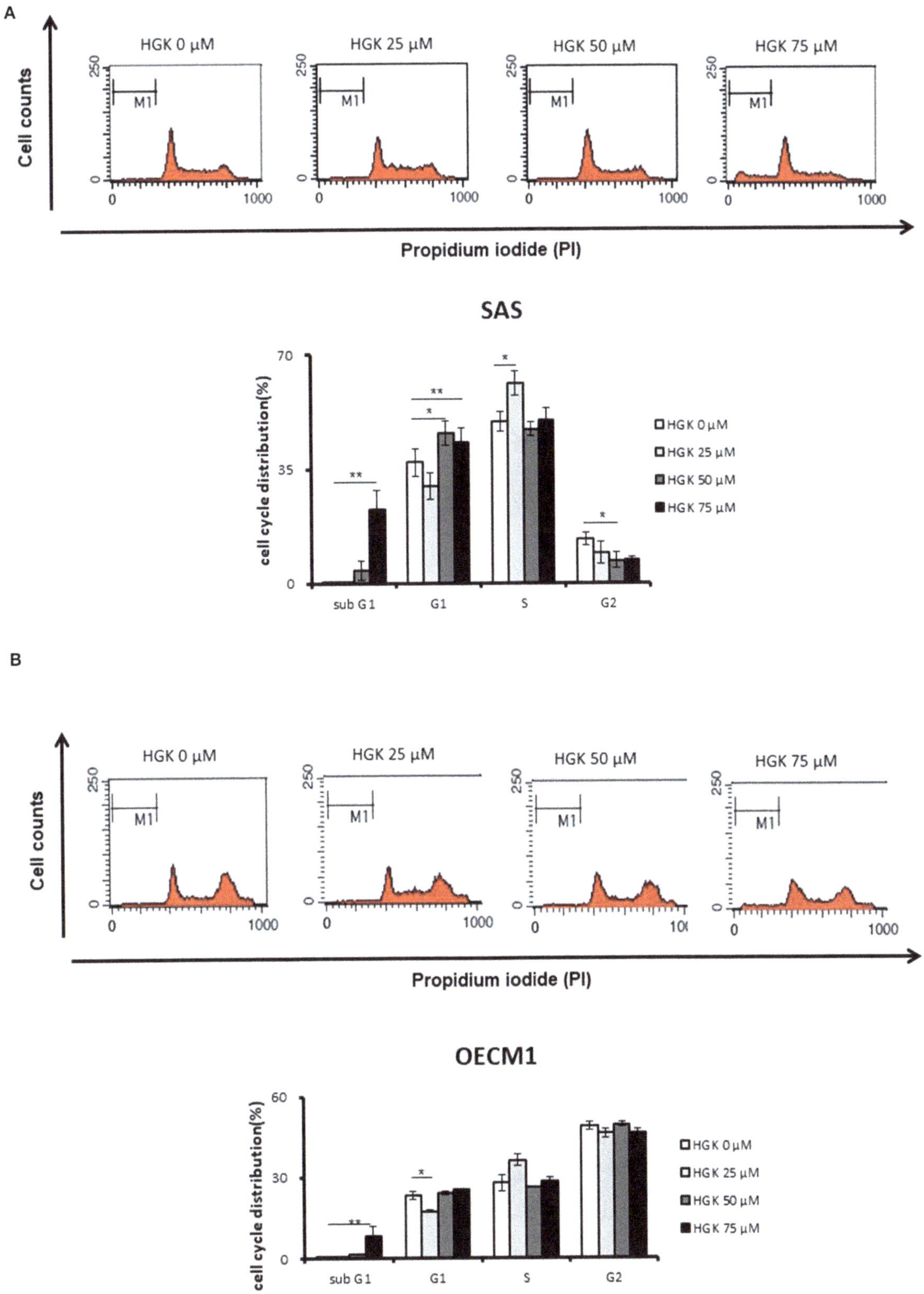

FIGURE 4 | Effects of HGK on the cell cycle progression in SAS and OECM1 cells. SAS cells **(A)** and OECM1 cell **(B)** were treated with 0, 25, 50, 75 μM for 24 h. The results are shown as the mean ± S.E. of three independent experiments. $^{*}P < 0.05$ and $^{**}P < 0.01$.

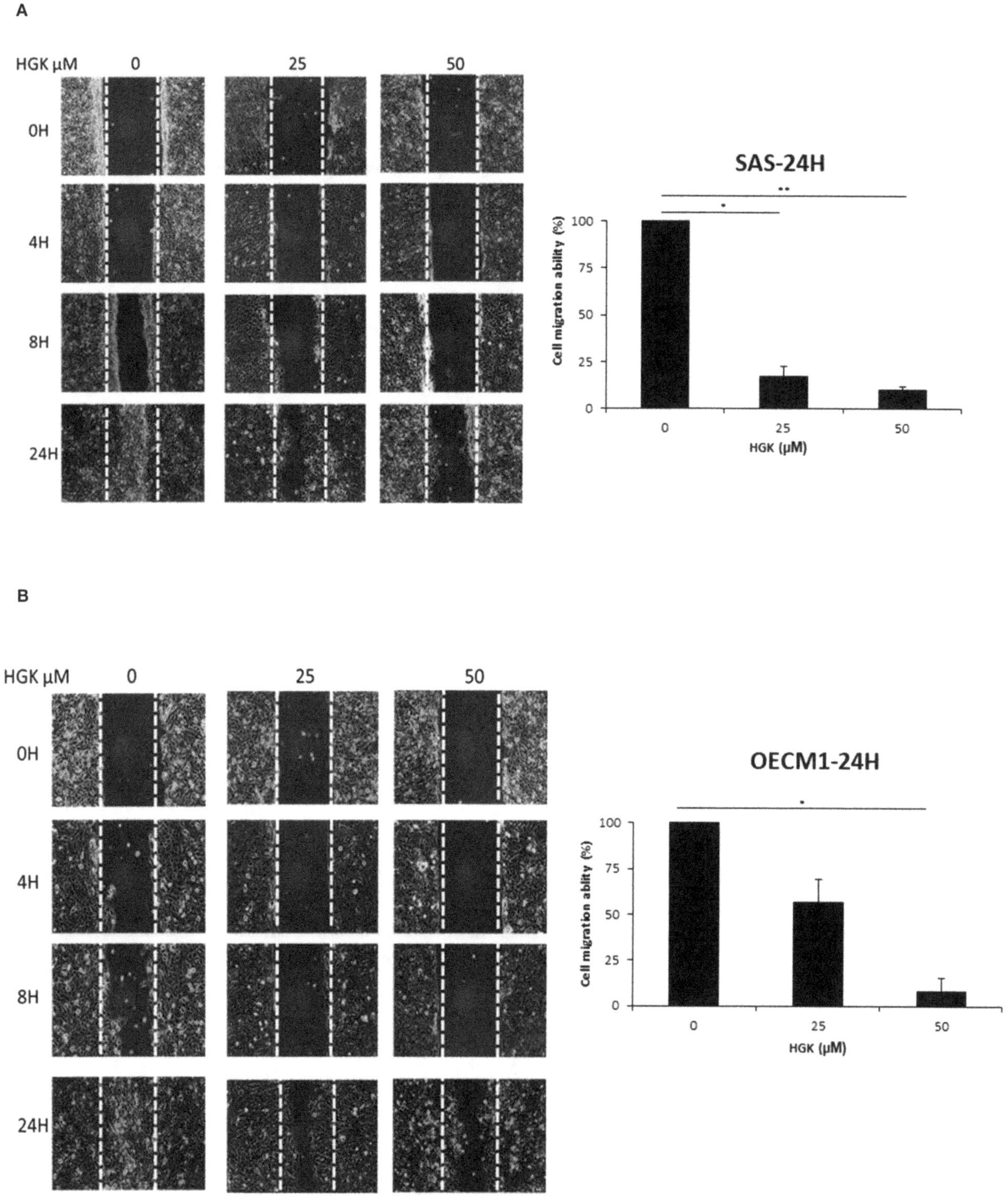

FIGURE 5 | Effects of HGK on cell migration in SAS **(A)** and OECM1 **(B)** cells. SAS and OECM1 cells were treated with 0, 25, 50, 75 μM HGK for 24 h. The results are shown as the mean ± S.E. of three independent experiments. $^{*}P < 0.05$ and $^{**}P < 0.01$.

The inhibition activity of HGK on cell survival assay and colony formation of SAS cells was more potent than on OECM1 cells.

Functional Enrichment Analysis of Differential Gene Expression Genes After HGK Treatment

We identified the differential gene expression genes from RNAseq data. A filtering criterion of FPKM value is more than 1 (11), and log2 fold change was greater than two in both SAS and OECM1 datasets. The sign of change must be consistent in both cell lines. A total of 274 genes were significant in the SAS dataset and 969 genes in the OECM1 dataset (**Table S1**). 170 genes were consistent change in both cell lines (**Figure 2**). **Table 1** showed the most significant molecular and cellular function of differential expression genes after HGK treatment in SAS and OECM1 cells. The final consistency 170 genes were listed in the **Table S2**. The cellular functions affected by HGK were involved in the cellular movement, cell cycle and cell proliferation (**Table 1**). GSEA shows a statistically significant difference between biological samples association with apoptosis and regulation of actin cytoskeleton functions

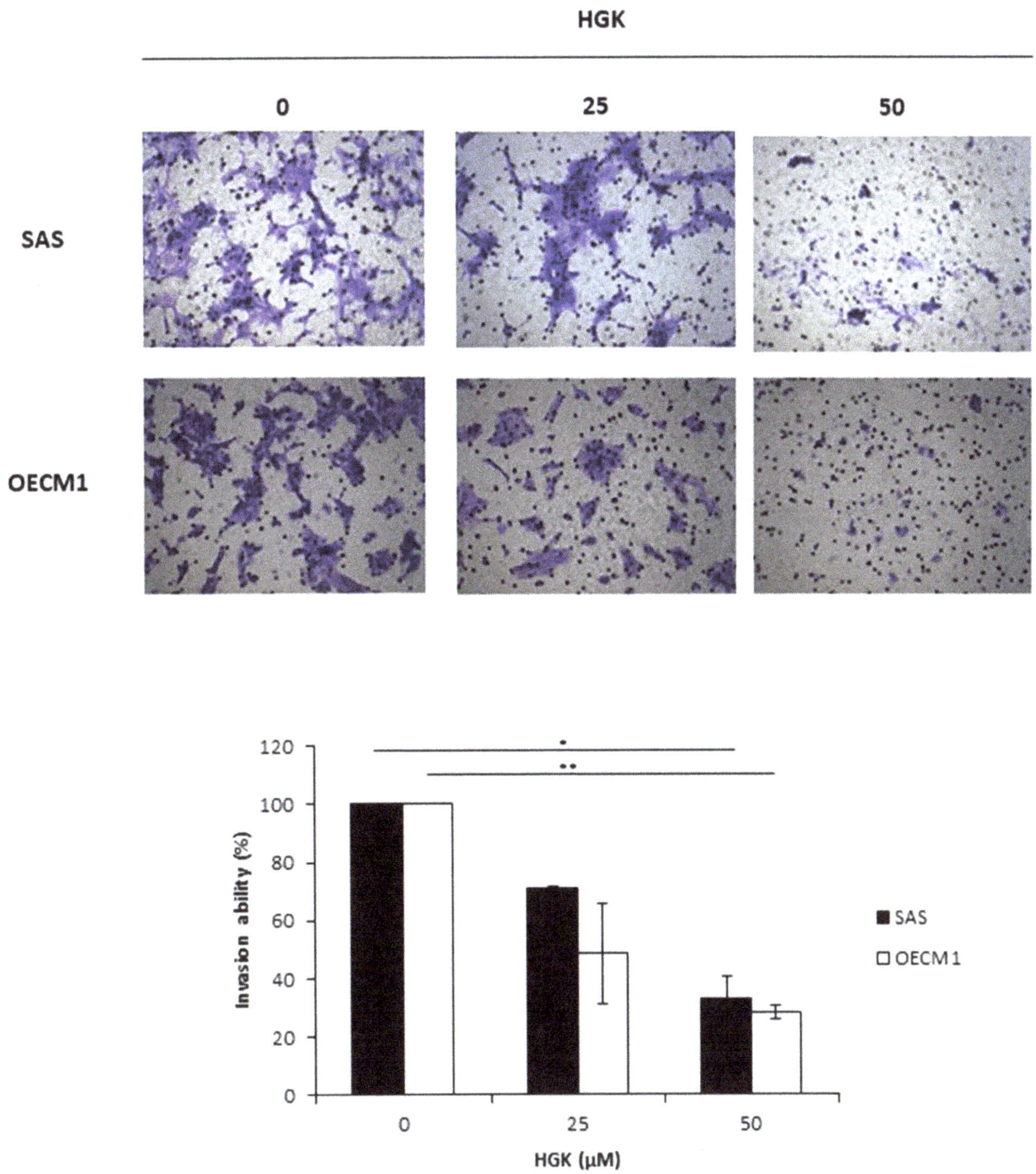

FIGURE 6 | Effects of HGK on cell invasion in SAS and OECM1 cells. SAS and OECM1 cells were treated with 0, 25, 50, 75 μM HGK for 24 h. The results are shown as the mean ± S.E. of three independent experiments. *$P < 0.05$ and **$P < 0.01$.

(**Figure 3**). Differential expression and pathway analysis in HGK treatment oral cancer cells indicated the cell cycle, cell survival and cell movement pathways were potential mechanisms.

Effects of HGK on the Cell Cycle Progression in SAS and OECM1 Cells

We further examine the HGK biological function according to the results of functional enrichment. For investigation of the effect of HGK on cell cycle progression, cells were stained by propidium iodide (PI) and measured by flow cytometry at 24 h following 25–75 μM HGK drug treatments. In **Figure 4**, as compare to control (0 μM), HGK dose dependently increased the percentage of sub G_0/G_1 phase SAS and OECM1 cells, and reduced the cells in G2/M phases of SAS cells but not OECM1 cells. 50 and 75 μM HGK increased the percentage of G_0/G_1 phase SAS cells, but 25 μM HGK reduced both of the cells in G_0/G_1 phases and concomitantly increased the percentage of S phase cells (**Figure 4**).

Effects of HGK on Cell Motion in SAS and OECM1 Cells

To investigate the HGK effect on SAS and OECM1 cell migration, we used wound healing assay. The cell migration was obviously reduced in SAS and OECM1 cells at 8 and 24 h after 25 and 50 μM HGK treatment (**Figure 5**). To investigate the HGK effect on SAS and OECM1 cell invasion, we used transwell invasion assay. As shown in **Figure 6**, the invasion was significantly reduced in 25 and 50 μM HGK treated- SAS and OECM1 cells.

Effects of HGK on Cell Cycle, Apoptosis, and EMT Regulatory Proteins in SAS and OECM1 Cells

In a previous result, we confirmed that HGK increased the percentage of SAS cells but not OECM1 cells in G0/G1 phase. In order to identify the molecular involved in the HGK effect of the G0/G1 phase, SAS and OECM1 cells were treated with 50 and 75 μM HGK for 24 h, and the cells were harvested for Western blotting. We observed the up-regulation of p21 in SAS cells after HGK treatment, but downregulation of p21 in OECM1 cells (**Figure 7**). p21 acts at the checkpoint in the cell cycle at the G1 phase. Western blot indicated that cell cycle regulated p21 might play an important role in in HGK-induced cell cycle arrest. HGK dose dependently increased the percentage of sub G_0/G_1 phase SAS and OECM1 cells (**Figure 4**). We further examined the apoptosis effect by using of H2AX Phosphorylation (12) and cleaved PARP cleaved caspase 9 (13). Western blot analyses of pH2AX, cl-PARP and cleaved caspase 9 in both HGK treated-SAS and OECM1 cells. The epithelial–mesenchymal transition (EMT) provides cells with migration and invasion abilities (14). We measured the e-cadherin (epithelial marker), and vimentin (mesenchymal markers) in HGK-treated cells. Vimentin showed significantly decreased between the HGK-treated and control groups, but not significant up-regulation of E-cadherin (**Figure 7**).

DISCUSSION

Natural compound and their related moieties played an important role in drug discovery and development (15). HGK

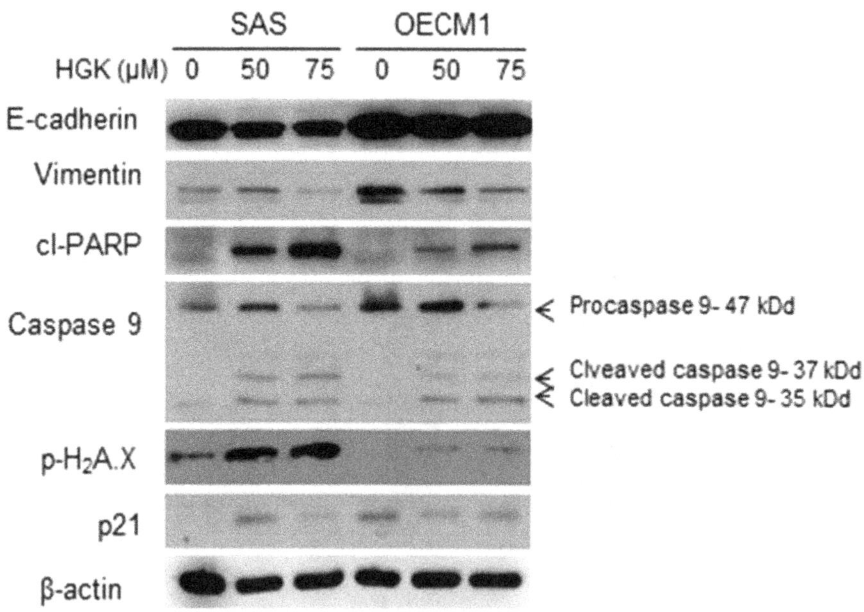

FIGURE 7 | Western blot analysis of cell cycle, apoptosis, and EMT regulatory proteins after treatment with HGK in SAS and OECM1 cells. β-actin was used as the internal marker.

was obtained from novel flavonoid extracted from *Daphne genkwa* and induced cancer cell toxicity, cell cycle arrest, apoptosis and EMT signaling pathways in different types of OSCC cell lines (OECM1 and SAS). We demonstrated that HGK significantly dose-dependently inhibited the rate of cell growth in OECM1 and SAS cells. SAS cells were higher sensitivity to HGK than OECM1 cells (**Figure 1**). The SAS cell line was high malignancy and metastasis derived from a poorly differentiated squamous cell carcinoma. The OECM-1 cell line was less malignancy established from a Taiwanese patient (16). Next-generation sequencing technologies are being widely applied in biomedical research (17). Systems for transcriptome profiling provided the insight into the specific biological pathways. Increases in G0/G1 phase cell cycle arrest with increasing doses of HGK treatments in SAS cells, but not OECM1 (**Figure 4**). Increase of the sub-G1 phase with various doses of HGK in both SAS and OECM1 cells. Western blot results showed that HGK activated the protein levels of p21in SAS cells, but decrease in OECM1 cells (**Figure 7**). The results were consistent with cell cycle analysis. The G1-S transition in cell cycle is driven mainly by cyclin-dependent kinase (CDK) 2 that is controlled by abundance of CDK inhibitors: p21 (18). p21 was a key cell cycle regulator that arrests cells in the G1 and G2 phases. Therefore, p21 proteins were involved in HGK-induced the cell cycle arrest in SAS cells. HGK induce the cell death of OSCC cells by apoptosis. The mechanisms of apoptosis are involving two main apoptotic pathways: the extrinsic and the intrinsic pathway (19). HGK induced cell apoptosis through the intrinsic pathway by activation of cleave Caspase 9, and cleave PARP (**Figure 7**). Histone H2AX phosphorylation was sensitive marker for DNA double-strand breaks (20). We demonstrated that HGK induce DNA damage in both two cell lines. Moreover, H2AX phosphorylation also an essential role in cell cycle arrest regulated by p21 and cell growth (21). HGK induced cell cycle arrest not only through p21 activation but also H2AX phosphorylation. Decrease of E-cadherin and gain of vimentin promoted tumor migration, leading to higher metastatic risk of head and neck squamous cell carcinoma patients (22). E-cadherin was an important therapeutic target for designing anti-tumor drugs (6). **Figure 7** showed that SAS1 and OECM1 cells did not loss the E-cadherin expression. Therefore, HGK inhibited the cell invasion and migration through down-regulation vimentin, not increase in E-cadherin.

In this study, we provided the bioinformatics analysis and biological functions experiments of HGK-treated oral cancer cells. Our results showed HGK had anti-cancer activities through multiple mechanisms including inhibition of cellular movement, cell cycle arrest and blocking cell proliferation in oral cancer cells. In conclusion, this study provided evidence that HGK was a potential natural anti-tumor compound for squamous cell carcinoma. However, further pharmacological and investigations *in vivo* are required.

AUTHOR CONTRIBUTIONS

Y-CHu and P-CL performed the experiments and analyzed the data. Y-CHu, Y-CHs, and JW drafted the manuscript. Y-CHs contributed to conception and design of the study. All authors have read and approved the final manuscript.

REFERENCES

1. Markopoulos AK. Current aspects on oral squamous cell carcinoma. *Open Dent J.* (2012) 6:126–30. doi: 10.2174/1874210601206010126
2. Chen CY, Chiou SH, Huang CY, Jan CI, Lin SC, Hu WY, et al. Tid1 functions as a tumour suppressor in head and neck squamous cell carcinoma. *J Pathol.* (2009) 219:347–55. doi: 10.1002/path.2604
3. Hsu YY, Bai CH, Wang CC, Chen WL, Wu WT, Lai CH. Health disparities of employees in taiwan with major cancer diagnosis from 2004 to 2015: a nation- and population-based analysis. *Int J Environ Res Public Health.* (2019) 16:E1982. doi: 10.3390/ijerph16111982
4. Li S, Chou G, Hseu Y, Yang H, Kwan H, Yu Z. Isolation of anticancer constituents from flos genkwa (*Daphne genkwa* Sieb.et Zucc.) through bioassay-guided procedures. *Chem Cent J.* (2013) 7:159. doi: 10.1186/1752-153X-7-159
5. Kang JI, Hong JY, Lee HJ, Bae SY, Jung C, Park HJ, et al. Anti-tumor activity of yuanhuacine by regulating AMPK/mTOR signaling pathway and actin cytoskeleton organization in non-small cell lung cancer cells. *PLoS ONE.* (2015) 10:e0144368. doi: 10.1371/journal.pone.0144368
6. Song Y, Ye M, Zhou J, Wang ZW, Zhu X. Restoring E-cadherin expression by natural compounds for anticancer therapies in genital and urinary cancers. *Mol Ther Oncolytics.* (2019) 14:130–8. doi: 10.1016/j.omto.2019.04.005
7. Zhang CF, Zhang SL, He X, Yang XL, Wu HT, Lin BQ, et al. Antioxidant effects of Genkwa flos flavonoids on Freunds adjuvant-induced rheumatoid arthritis in rats. *J Ethnopharmacol.* (2014) 153:793–800. doi: 10.1016/j.jep.2014.03.046
8. Chen CY, Yang SC, Lee KH, Yang X, Wei LY, Chow LP, et al. The antitumor agent PBT-1 directly targets HSP90 and hnRNP A2/B1 and inhibits lung adenocarcinoma growth and metastasis. *J Med Chem.* (2014) 57:677–85. doi: 10.1021/jm401686b
9. Subramanian A, Tamayo P, Mootha VK, Mukherjee S, Ebert BL, Gillette MA, et al. Gene set enrichment analysis: a knowledge-based approach for interpreting genome-wide expression profiles. *Proc Natl Acad Sci USA.* (2005) 102:15545–50. doi: 10.1073/pnas.0506580102
10. Wang TH, Chan CW, Fang JY, Shih YM, Liu YW, Wang TV, et al. 2-O-Methylmagnolol upregulates the long non-coding RNA, GAS5, and enhances apoptosis in skin cancer cells. *Cell Death Dis.* (2017) 8:e2638. doi: 10.1038/cddis.2017.66
11. Mortazavi A, Williams BA, McCue K, Schaeffer L, Wold B. Mapping and quantifying mammalian transcriptomes by RNA-Seq. *Nat Methods.* (2008) 5:621–8. doi: 10.1038/nmeth.1226
12. Plesca D, Mazumder S, Almasan A. DNA damage response and apoptosis. *Methods Enzymol.* (2008) 446:107–22. doi: 10.1016/S0076-6879(08)01606-6
13. Kitazumi I, Tsukahara M. Regulation of DNA fragmentation: the role of caspases and phosphorylation. *FEBS J.* (2011) 278:427–41. doi: 10.1111/j.1742-4658.2010.07975.x
14. Lu W, Kang Y. Epithelial-mesenchymal plasticity in cancer progression and metastasis. *Dev Cell.* (2019) 49:361–74. doi: 10.1016/j.devcel.2019.04.010
15. Butler MS. The role of natural product chemistry in drug discovery. *J Nat Prod.* (2004) 67:2141–53. doi: 10.1021/np040106y
16. Chuang CY, Chang CP, Lee YJ, Lin WL, Chang WW, Wu JS, et al. PRMT1 expression is elevated in head and neck cancer and inhibition of protein arginine methylation by adenosine dialdehyde or PRMT1 knockdown downregulates proliferation and migration of oral cancer cells. *Oncol Rep.* (2017) 38:1115–23. doi: 10.3892/or.2017.5737

17. Han Y, Gao S, Muegge K, Zhang W, Zhou B. Advanced applications of RNA sequencing and challenges. *Bioinform Biol Insights*. (2015) 9(Suppl. 1):29–46. doi: 10.4137/BBI.S28991
18. Sherr CJ, Roberts JM. CDK inhibitors: positive and negative regulators of G1-phase progression. *Genes Dev*. (1999) 13:1501–12. doi: 10.1101/gad.13.12.1501
19. Elmore S. Apoptosis: a review of programmed cell death. *Toxicol Pathol*. (2007) 35:495–516. doi: 10.1080/01926230701320337
20. Sharma A, Singh K, Almasan A. Histone H2AX phosphorylation: a marker for DNA damage. *Methods Mol Biol*. (2012) 920:613–26. doi: 10.1007/978-1-61779-998-3_40
21. Fragkos M, Jurvansuu J, Beard P. H2AX is required for cell cycle arrest via the p53/p21 pathway. *Mol Cell Biol*. (2009) 29:2828–40. doi: 10.1128/MCB.01830-08
22. Nijkamp MM, Span PN, Hoogsteen IJ, van der Kogel AJ, Kaanders JH, Bussink J. Expression of E-cadherin and vimentin correlates with metastasis formation in head and neck squamous cell carcinoma patients. *Radiother Oncol*. (2011) 99:344–8. doi: 10.1016/j.radonc.2011.05.066

9

Functional Landscape of Dysregulated MicroRNAs in Oral Squamous Cell Carcinoma: Clinical Implications

Ruma Dey Ghosh [1], Arun Pattatheyil [2] and Susanta Roychoudhury [3]*

[1] Tata Translational Cancer Research Center, Tata Medical Center, Kolkata, India, [2] Department of Head and Neck Surgical Oncology, Tata Medical Center, Kolkata, India, [3] Saroj Gupta Cancer Centre and Research Institute, Kolkata, India

***Correspondence:**
Ruma Dey Ghosh
deyrumai@yahoo.co.in;
ruma.deyghosh@tmckolkata.com

MicroRNA (miRNA) dysregulation is associated with the pathogenesis of oral squamous cell carcinoma (OSCC), and its elucidation could potentially provide information on patient outcome. A growing body of translational research on miRNA biology is focusing on precision oncology, aiming to decode the miRNA regulatory network in the development and progression of cancer. Tissue-specific expression and stable presence in all body fluids are unique features of miRNAs, which could be potentially exploited in the clinical setting. Recent understanding of miRNA properties has led them to be useful, attractive, and potential tools either as biomarkers (distinct miRNA expression signature) for diagnosis and prognostic outcomes or as targets for novel therapeutic entities, enabling personalized treatment for OSCC. In this review, we discuss recent research on different aspects of alterations in miRNA profiles along with their clinical significance and strive to identify probable potential miRNA biomarkers for diagnosis and prognosis of OSCC. We also discuss the current understanding and scope of development of miRNA-based therapeutics against OSCC.

Keywords: dysregulated miRNA, miRNA biomarker, non-invasive biomarker, miRNA-based therapy, oral squamous cell carcinoma

INTRODUCTION

Oral squamous cell carcinoma (OSCC) is the second most common cancer reported in India. According to recent Globacon-2018 data, ~120,000 new cases of OSCC are detected every year in India (1, 2). It is the leading cause of cancer-associated death in the Indian male population. Annually, more than 72,000 deaths are attributed to this disease in this country (3). OSCC originates in mucosal epithelial cells of the oral cavity (4, 5). Tobacco (smoking/smokeless) and alcohol are the primary risk factors for OSCC. Chewing of areca nut, betel leaf, poor oral health hygiene, and human papillomavirus (HPV) infection are also important risk factors for OSCC. Treatment in the early stages of the disease offers the best chance of cure (4, 5). Surgery is the first line of treatment, whereas radiotherapy and chemotherapy are used as adjuvant therapies (6, 7). Treatment strategies mainly depend on the location of the primary tumor, identification of high-risk features by histopathology, stage of tumor, and comorbidities. The 5-year survival rate of patients with oral cancer is around 50%. Poor outcomes are attributed to disease recurrence (both second primaries and locoregional recurrence) and distant metastasis. Despite availability of risk information from histopathology, the pattern and timing of relapse and metastasis are difficult to predict. About 86% of the recurrence occurs within 24 months after primary treatment (7). Prognostic information is mainly derived from anatomic location; tumor stage; tumor thickness; and histological characteristics like cellular heterogeneity, degree of differentiation, depth of invasion, presence of nodal metastases, margin status, neural invasion, and pattern of invasion (6).

Biomarkers are quantifiable indicators associated with the specific disease conditions that facilitate decision-making by clinicians with respect to the most effective clinical interventions. In conventional practice, extra nodal extension (ENE), perineural invasion (PNI), and lymphovascular invasion (LVI) are considered histopathological biomarkers associated with poor disease prognosis (6, 7). Given that the genetics of OSCC is highly heterogeneous and complex, so far, no known molecular biomarker (except HPV positivity) has been used to subclassify OSCC accurately. Currently, only one epidermal growth factor receptor (EGFR)-specific targeted-immunotherapy with cetuximab antibody is available for the management of this cancer. Therefore, in the current scenario, early detection of the disease with identification of distinct prognostic subgroups to facilitate advanced treatment strategies is required for effective management of OSCC. Genomic, epigenomic, proteomic, and metabolomic high-throughput approaches have recently been used to discover and validate tumor biomarkers individually and/or in panels (8–13). Since microRNAs (miRNAs) are highly stable in tissues as well as in circulation, they are considered potential biomarkers for cancer detection and prognostication (14–18). Here, we review potential candidate miRNAs for their possible use as molecular biomarkers to improve the diagnosis and prognostication of OSCC and to stratify such patients into distinct prognostic subgroups. In this review, we have voyaged through various dysregulated miRNAs reported to be responsible for the pathogenesis, progression, and specific outcomes of OSCC. Their functional associations with overall therapeutic management, responsiveness, recurrence, and metastasis of OSCC are also elaborated upon.

BASICS OF MicroRNAs: ALTERED miRNA FUNCTION CAN FINE-TUNE CELL-FATE DECISION VIA ALTERED GENE AND PROTEIN EXPRESSION

Mature miRNAs are endogenous, single-stranded, evolutionarily conserved, non-coding RNAs ~19–26 nucleotides long; discovered by Lee et al. (19). miRNAs preferentially interact with complementary seed sequences in the 3′ untranslated regions (UTRs) of their target mRNAs. miRNA binding sites may also be present in the 5′ UTRs and coding sequences of target mRNAs (20). miRNA-mediated gene silencing is a fundamental biological process for cellular homeostasis, executed through translational inhibition followed by mRNA deadenylation and decay (21–23). Circulating cell-free miRNAs also play an important role in intracellular/intercellular communication through miRNA-mediated gene silencing (17, 24). As a result, miRNA expression profiles in tissues and circulation are associated with several pathophysiological conditions, including cancers (17, 25). Dysregulation in miRNA expression profile was first reported in leukemia (26). Therefore, a distinct miRNA expression signature that distinguishes normal tissues from cancer tissues could be a new "hallmark of cancer," which regulates almost all other cancer hallmarks defined earlier (18, 27, 28).

Functional dysregulation of mature miRNAs is associated with various kinds of pathological conditions. Dysregulation of miRNA expression and function may be due to one or more of the following: (1) altered miRNA biogenesis process: (a) epigenetic (methylation and histone modifications) alterations of miRNA genes, (b) altered activities of transcription factors, and (c) altered expression of miRNA-processing enzymes (Drosha, Dicer, etc.); (2) chromosomal instability, genomic instability, and presence of mutations in miRNA genes; (3) single-nucleotide polymorphisms (SNPs), deletions, and duplications in miRNA genes (pri-, pre-, and mature miRNA regions) as well as in the binding sequences on target mRNAs; (4) loss of miRNA-binding sites on target mRNAs; and (5) redirecting of the miRNA-induced silencing complex (miRISC) to multiple competitive miRNA-binding sites present in competing endogenous RNAs (ceRNAs), which act as miRNA sponges and inhibit their functions (17, 23, 28–30). All ceRNAs are naturally occurring, endogenous regulatory molecules, like long non-coding RNAs (lncRNAs), circular RNAs, pseudogenes, and some protein-coding mRNAs (29, 30). Notably, in miRNA-mediated regulatory networks, one miRNA can regulate many genes and a single gene can be regulated by many miRNAs (23).

The above-described processes ultimately lead to activation of some oncogenic genes/proteins and, at the same time, deactivation of some tumor suppressor genes/proteins. They also direct cellular signaling cascades toward making the cell fate verdict (23, 28). Eventually, these distinct alterations in miRNA expression profile drive a normal cell to transform into a cancer cell and dictate its progression, metastasis, stemness, and responsiveness to therapy (radiotherapy/chemotherapy) (17, 18).

DISTINCT MicroRNA SIGNATURES AS HALLMARKS OF ORAL SQUAMOUS CELL CARCINOMA

The utility of miRNAs as diagnostic and prognostic biomarkers of OSCC has not been convincingly established. Previous studies on miRNA expression profiling mainly focused on differential expression of miRNAs in normal and tumor tissues and body fluids (blood, saliva, serum, or plasma) from OSCC patients (10, 12). These studies have yielded a plethora of dysregulated (upregulated/downregulated) miRNAs in OSCC. Here, we used the miRCancer database, PubMed, and Google to search for relevant data and reevaluate miRNAs as potential biomarkers for the diagnosis, prognosis, and therapeutics of OSCC. miRCancer is an online, up-to-date database (last updated on August 27, 2019) that provides a comprehensive collection of miRNA expression profiles in various human cancers extracted from published literature available in PubMed (31).

MicroRNA PROFILING IN ORAL SQUAMOUS CELL CARCINOMA

Dysregulated miRNA Expression in Tumor Tissues

Tran et al. (32) performed the first high-throughput miRNA profiling in OSCC using nine OSCC cell lines. Subsequently, several investigators have studied miRNA profiles as prognostic biomarkers using primary tumor and paired control tissues from patients with head and neck squamous cell carcinoma (HNSCC) (33–35). The differential expression analysis revealed sets of mature miRNAs that were either upregulated or downregulated in the tumor tissues. Childs et al. (35) showed that miR-21, miR-155, miR-191, and miR-221 were upregulated, whereas miR-1, miR-133a, miR-205, and let-7d were downregulated in primary tumors at diagnosis (35, 36). Another retrospective study on 51 formalin-fixed HNSCC tumor samples revealed consistent expression of mature miRNAs in malignant tissues; miR-21, miR-155, let-7i, miR-142-3p, miR-423, miR-106b, miR-20a, and miR-16 were overexpressed, whereas miR-125b, miR-375, and miR-10a were underexpressed) (37). Lu et al. (38) showed that miR-10b, miR-196a, miR-196b, miR-582-5p, miR-15b, miR-301, miR-148b, and miR-128a were upregulated, whereas miR-503 and miR-31 were downregulated in six oral cancer cell lines compared with those in normal keratinocytes. Specific miRNAs related to the clinicopathological features of site-specific OSCC were investigated, which demonstrated a significant difference in let-7a, miR-200c, miR-34a levels between oropharyngeal and laryngeal cancers (39). In addition, miR-21, miR-200c, and miR-34a were upregulated, and miR-375 was downregulated in tumor tissues of all subsites when compared with those in paired control tissues (39). Studies also suggested that genes associated with the phosphoinositide 3-kinase (PI3K)/AKT and p53 signaling pathways, which are involved in the OSCC carcinogenesis process, were regulated through a set of dysregulated miRNAs, such as let-7a, let-7d, let-7f, miR-16, miR-29b, miR-142-3p, miR-144, miR-203, and miR-223 (40). Lamperska et al. (41) suggested that miR-21 and miR-205 could be used to analyze the clarity of surgical margins, but they failed to find a correlation between miRNA expression and clinical outcome and the course of illness. Here, we considered only those studies that reported targeted or genome-wide miRNA profiling either in cell lines or in tumor samples.

These studies make it obvious that malignant OSCC tumors have distinct miRNA expression profiles. Subsequently, the regulatory network composed of these distinct miRNAs in the malignant cell causes key downstream molecular alteration, which ultimately leads to a distinct patient outcome (17, 28, 42). It is evident from the above studies that the results are not always consistent. The source of the problem could be found within and among the studies. Variations are observed in study design, end point objective, selection of cell lines, use of appropriate controls (in most of the cases, adjacent normal tissues were used which could harbor genomic alterations), methodology, protocol or treatment strategies, and localized patient pools in these studies. Further, purity and availability of tumor tissue, stromal cell contamination, and small sample size may impact study results. In most of the studies, intra/inter tumor heterogeneity, variable etiopathogenesis, and heterogenous genetic constitution of each patient are important factors that lead to variations in results. Despite these limitations, the results of individual studies demonstrate that miRNAs may be useful as potential biomarkers to predict OSCC outcome. The present quantum of knowledge lays the groundwork for logical implementation and execution of large-scale studies with improved, standardized study protocols in the future.

miRNA Expression Signatures Associated With Risk Factors of OSCC

One miRNA profiling study comparing smoker and non-smoker patients reported high miR-155 expression in 58% of OSCC cases and 83% of dysplasia cases and subsequently suggested miR-155 as a driver of oral tumorigenesis in non-smokers (43).

The association of OSCC with betel quid was also analyzed in OSCC specimens by another investigator who discovered 84 betel quid-associated mature miRNAs, of which 19 were located on chromosome 14q32.2 (44). In this context, Hou et al. (45) established that specific polymorphisms in miR-499a are associated with OSCC progression. They discovered that the T/C+C/C genotypes of miR-499a increased the risk of betel quid-associated oral submucosal fibrosis (OSF) but decreased the risk of OSCC. Further, miR-499a T>C (rs3746444) influences the expression of miR-499-5p during OSCC carcinogenesis (45).

Several investigators have also conducted miRNA expression profiling to compare HPV-positive and -negative OSCC tumors and revealed that miR-127-3p, miR-363, miR-20a, miR-34a, let-7c-5p, and miR-9 could effectively distinguish between the two groups (39, 46–49). Different etiological factors causing distinct patterns of miRNA expression have also been well-established by several investigators. Most of the work has been done on HPV-associated OSCC. The studies reveal little effect of tobacco and betel quid on miRNA expression in OSCC compared with that in HPV-associated OSCC.

Dysregulated miRNAs in Tumor Cells Collected Through Non-invasive Brush Biopsy

Recently, the more advanced brush biopsy or other related scraper-based methods have offered non-invasive ways to identify OSCC-specific miRNA biomarkers for diagnosis and prognostication of the disease. Gissi et al., using brush biopsy samples from OSCCs and from regenerative areas after surgical resection and from their respective normal distant mucosa, revealed that miR-146a and miR-191 were significantly altered in the regenerative areas after OSCC resection (50). Studies also claim that brush biopsy samples may be superior to surgically dissected samples (51, 52). In brush biopsy, sampling sites within lesions that are not ulcerated and are non-necrotic and minimally friable make the samples homogeneous, with viable epithelial cells. It must be noted, however, that in case of smaller tumors (T1, T2), there is a chance of normal epithelial cell contamination in brush biopsy samples (51, 52). For high-throughput technology (next-generation sequencing), obtaining high quality and quantity of total RNA (or enriched miRNA) from brush biopsy samples is the main challenge (51). Quantitative real-time PCR (qRT-PCT) is a reliable method in this case. miRNA profiles in individual brush biopsy OSCC samples show ~50% overlap with miRNAs enriched in surgically obtained tumor tissue profiles (51). The non-invasive rapid brush biopsy methods are useful in obtaining homogeneous tumor cells. Over the years, given all the limitations, the accuracy in predicting OSCC-associated miRNA expression signature is still to be improved for clinical applications.

CELL-FREE MicroRNA PROFILING: POTENTIAL BIOMARKERS FOR LIQUID BIOPSY

The most fascinating aspect of miRNA biology is the stable presence of cell-free miRNAs in all biological fluids. Previous studies have demonstrated that the stability of circulating cell-free miRNA results from either internalization of miRNAs into exosomes or other microvesicles or formation of complexes between circulating miRNAs and specific proteins and lipids (14–16, 53). These cell-free miRNAs are probably released by cancer cells, necrotic cells, and/or apoptotic cells along with their associated proteins or lipids, such as the RNA-binding protein NPM1 (nucleophosmin), AGO proteins (argonaute 1/2), and high-density lipoprotein (HDL), to avoid RNase degradation in blood circulation (15, 16, 54). Further, the spectrum of these cell-free miRNAs is altered by various pathophysiological conditions, including cancer (42, 54–57). In OSCC, saliva is one of the important sources to identify reliable biomarkers for predicting diagnosis and prognosis. Blood (serum and plasma) is another important sampling source. The sources of these cell-free miRNAs are thought to be directly associated with tumor pathogenesis and/or other related systemic physiological (immune system/metabolic system) conditions (54–56).

Dysregulated Cell-Free miRNAs in Biological Fluids of OSCC Patients

Saliva

Studies using human saliva samples have shown that salivary cell-free miRNAs could be potential diagnostic biomarkers in OSCC patients compared with those in healthy individuals (58–60). Genome-wide expression patterns of miRNAs have revealed that miRNA expression is significantly altered in the saliva of OSCC patients compared with that in healthy controls. miR-125a, miR-136, miR-147, miR-1250, miR-148a, miR-200a, miR-632, miR-646, miR-668, miR-877, miR-503, miR-220a, and miR-323-5p were downregulated, and miR-24 and miR-27b were found to be upregulated. The studies revealed that miR-27b was significantly upregulated in OSCC patients compared with that in healthy controls, patients with OSCC in remission, and patients with oral lichen planus and served as a biomarker to detect OSCC. Finally, the studies concluded that miR-27b could be a valuable cell-free biomarker in saliva for distinguishing OSCC patients (60).

Plasma

A study using plasma samples obtained at different time points showed that plasma miR-146a levels were significantly higher in OSCC patients (sensitivity: >0.72) than in healthy controls, and these levels decreased drastically after tumor resection in these patients (61). Similarly, higher plasma miR-187-3p level was found to be another potential marker of OSCC diagnosis, and the plasma levels of miR-187-3p were significantly reduced after tumor resection in patients who had better prognosis (62). Studies have also suggested that circulating miR-196a, miR-196b, and miR-200b-3p levels in plasma might serve as a panel of plasma biomarkers for the early detection of oral cancer (63–65). In a separate study, three plasma miRNAs—miR-222-3p, miR-150-5p, and miR-423-5p—were identified for early detection of malignant OSCC (66). miR-222-3p and miR-423-5p negatively correlated with T stage, lymph node metastasis status, and clinical stage. A high diagnostic accuracy (area under curve = 0.88) was demonstrated for discriminating oral leukoplakia from OSCC (66).

Serum

A miRNA microarray experiment using serum samples from OSCC patients vs. healthy controls revealed 16 miRNAs were significantly upregulated and 10 were significantly downregulated in the patients. miR-483-5p expression was significantly correlated (sensitivity = 0.853, specificity = 0.746) with lymph node metastasis and shorter survival, suggesting increased miR-483-5p expression in OSCC and suggesting its potential as a novel diagnostic and prognostic biomarker for OSCC (67). Further, low serum miR-9 level correlated with poor prognosis of OSCC (68). Recently, another study compared the circulating miRNA profile with the respective tumor-specific dysregulated miRNA profile and suggested that hsa-miR-32-5p in serum is a potential non-invasive biomarker for OSCC (69).

Whole Blood

Circulating miR-21 level and *PTEN* expression observed in whole blood samples could be possible biomarkers for detection of OSCC (70). Ries et al. (71–73) suggested that whole-blood sample is more reliable than only one specific blood component (serum/plasma/circulating cells) for identifying miRNA biomarkers for OSCC using a minimally invasive method. Microarray-based miRNA expression profiling was performed on 20 whole-blood samples (in a PAXgene blood RNA tube) from OSCC patients and healthy volunteers, and the results were validated through qRT-PCR using another 57 OSCC patient samples and 33 healthy control samples. This study showed that miR-186 was downregulated and miR-3651 and miR-494 were upregulated significantly in OSCC (71). In further studies, the authors evaluated these circulating miRNA biomarkers with diagnostic and prognostic significance in different patient cohorts (72). They also showed that the circulating miRNA expression signature (from whole-blood sample) was different from the miRNA expression in OSCC tissues (73). This is probably because the changes in miRNA expression in circulation occur as a consequence of pathogenic reactions upon immune-pathogenic interactions in response to cancer.

On the basis of all these studies, we can suggest that liquid biopsy would be a reliable, consistent, rapid, easy, cheap, and minimally invasive method to determine miRNA expression signatures to predict OSCC diagnosis and prognosis (57, 74). Evident challenges persist in terms of quality and quantity (for high-throughput techniques) of RNA and usage of proper endogenous controls for data normalization (75–77). To overcome these issues, recently advanced instruments (Qubit, concentrator, droplet digital PCR) and advanced modified assay protocols (inclusion of exogenous spike-in-control and newly identified endogenous cell-free control miRNA) have been introduced to obtain reliable, potential predictive biomarkers for OSCC (75, 77, 78). We prepared a list of dysregulated miRNAs, in which each miRNA is representative of a particular miRNA expression signature in tumor tissues/cell lines and/or in circulation/other body fluids (**Supplementary Table 1**). Individual studies on the effect of one/two miRNAs with clinical significance were also included in this table. Each miRNA is accountable either for sole or cumulative functions related to OSCC pathogenesis, progression, differential tumor behavior, aggressiveness, invasion, and metastasis, resulting in distinct outcome for each patient with OSCC.

CLINICAL SIGNIFICANCE OF DYSREGULATED MicroRNAs IN THE DIAGNOSIS AND PROGNOSIS OF OSCC

miRNA Signature for Susceptibility to OSCC

A major goal of precision medicine is to assess disease risk based on the genetic makeup of an individual. SNPs in various miRNAs have also been shown to be associated with different cancers. Dysregulation due to distinct polymorphisms in mature miRNAs, particularly miR-196a2 rs11614913 C>T, miR-146a rs2910164 G>C, miR-149 rs2292832 C>T, and miR-499 rs3746444 A>G, are associated with the risk of OSCC (45, 63, 79). In addition, polymorphisms in miR-146a [genotype: CC vs. GG + CG; odds ratio (OR) $= 0.874, p = 0.041$] and miR-196a2 (genotype: TT vs. TC + CC; OR $< 1, p < 0.05$) increase the risk of OSCC, whereas the miR-499 polymorphisms (G allele and the GG genotype; OR $> 1, p < 0.05$) exert protective effects against OSCC risk. In this context, study results on miR-149 polymorphisms are not significant. They are associated with both increased risk of nodal metastasis and poor survival in OSCC, although another research group disclosed that they appeared to have no significant relationship with the risk of OSCC (80, 81).

miRNAs as Early Biomarkers for OSCC Diagnosis

Early detection of OSCC allows clinicians to provide proper administration of curative treatment long before it metastasizes and progresses to the advanced stages. The identification of biomarkers for early detection and prognostication of OSCC through minimally invasive or non-invasive methods acquires major emphasis in current investigative drives. A targeted miRNA expression profiling study (using 22 oral leukoplakia tissue samples with different grades of dysplasia, 17 OSCC samples, and six normal oral mucosa samples) demonstrated the prognostic values of miR-21, miR-181b, and miR-345 in oral leukoplakia with severe dysplasia. Although dysplasia grading is not a very reliable predictor, advanced aggressive dysplasia progresses to OSCC (82). Other studies using tumor tissues revealed that miR-137 and miR-29a/b/c could be potential biomarkers for early diagnosis of OSCC. miR-29s (miR-29a/b/c) were significantly downregulated in OSCC patients (83). Consecutively, circulating miR-223 and miR-10b in plasma were proposed to be potential biomarkers for early detection of oral cancer (38, 84). Further, miR-146a, miR-187-3p, miR-196a, miR-196b, miR-200b-3p, miR-222-3p, miR-223, miR-150-5p, and miR-423-5p levels in plasma could also be potential diagnostic markers for early detection of OSCC (61–66). A separate study described serum miR-32-5p as a potential biomarker for OSCC (69).

miRNAs as Biomarkers for OSCC Prognostication

Lymph Node Invasion and Distant Metastasis in OSCC

Epithelial–mesenchymal transition (EMT) of cancer cells is directly associated with cellular migration/invasion leading to cancer metastasis. In OSCC, ample dysregulated miRNAs have been found to be involved in EMT, invasion, and metastasis, which are primarily responsible for lymph node metastasis and distant metastasis.

In preclinical OSCC cell lines, miR-130b, miR-134, miR-149, miR-181d, miR-146b, miR-491, and miR-27a-3p are associated with EMT and cellular migration through targeting BMI1, MMP9, E-cadherin, and the YAP1-OCT4-Sox2 signaling axis (85, 86). High levels of miR-1275 and low levels of miR-222-3p and miR-423-5p are correlated with induced regional lymph node invasion in OSCC (40). Similarly, other studies have suggested that upregulation of miR-187, miR-196b, miR-372, miR-373, and miR-483 could be potential biomarkers for nodal metastasis in HNSCC (38, 62, 67, 87–90). ZEB1, Twist, and Snail (EMT-related transcription factors) are directly regulated by miR-429 and miR-101 and inversely by let-7d and mediate tumor growth and metastasis in OSCC (35, 91–93). Downregulation of miR-300 is another requirement for EMT initiation and maintenance, mediated through modulation of Twist expression and the transforming growth factor (TGF)β signaling pathway in OSCC (94). Bufalino et al. (95) demonstrated that lymph node metastasis resulted from downregulation of the miR-143/miR-145 cluster and consequent induction of activin-A, which contributed to poor prognosis through induced EMT. Similarly, RUNX2 is directly regulated by miR-376c-3p, which was found to be downregulated and to promote lymph node metastasis in OSCC (96). Other studies also demonstrated that the miR-23b/27b cluster regulates the MET oncogene, whereas miR-29a/b/c regulates the expression of *MMP2*, *LAMC2*, and

ITGA6, responsible for disease invasion and metastasis in OSCC (83, 97, 98). Further, miR-218 is directly correlated with increased invasion and cellular migration mediated through *LAMB3* and *RICTOR* and the focal adhesion and mTOR-Akt signaling pathways (99, 100). *EGFR*, *c-MET*, and *KRAS* are direct targets of miR-1 and miR-206. Both these miRNAs, particularly miR-206, are significantly associated with advanced tumor node metastasis (node positivity in the Tumor Node Metastasis staging system) and shorter overall survival in OSCC (101, 102). Moreover, high expression of miR-196a and miR-149 polymorphisms is associated with increased risk of nodal metastasis (63, 80).

Biomarkers for Locoregional Recurrence in OSCC

The evolution of second primary or locoregional recurrence is unpredictable. In most cases, relapses are detected in late stages, which significantly reduce survival and worsen morbidity. Salvage surgery can cure recurrent tumors effectively if detected early.

Low miR-422a expression in stage III–IV tumors promotes local recurrence *via* targeting oncogenic *CD73* when compared with that in oropharynx stage III–IV tumors, without relapse or with locoregional relapse within 2 years of posttreatment (103). Other studies have shown that miR-196a, miR-205, and miR-675 are significantly associated with locoregional recurrence at diagnosis and treatment in OSCC (35, 80, 103, 104). miR-451 was found to be significantly overexpressed (4.7-fold) in non-relapsed vs. relapsed patients (37). Furthermore, locoregional recurrence in OSCC is also significantly affected by polymorphisms in miR-196a (63). All these indicators could be building blocks for developing meaningful biomarkers for early disease prognostication, recurrence, and/or metastasis in the clinical setting.

Dysregulated miRNAs Associated With Response to Chemoradiation Therapy in OSCC

Until date, cetuximab is the only clinically applied targeted drug used to treat patients with OSCC. However, the occurrence of therapeutic resistance or non-responsiveness has been found during chemotherapy/radiotherapy treatment in patients with OSCC. Several studies identified miRNAs as potential biomarkers to predict the sensitivity/resistance of tumors to chemotherapy or a particular drug used in chemotherapy and radiotherapy for OSCC.

Henson et al. (105) showed that the amplification of chromosomal band 11q13, loss of distal 11q, and downregulation of miR-125b and miR-100 are associated with radioresistance and disease progression (105, 106). In our previous study, we identified six cisplatin resistance-specific signature miRNAs—miR-130b, miR-134, miR-149, miR-181d, miR-146b, and miR-491. These miRNAs function in OSCC mainly through modulating the expression of proteins related to cancer stem cells (augmentation of CD44, c-Myc, and Oct-4), drug resistance (upregulation of P-gp and MRP1), and EMT (increase in BMI1 and MMP9 expression and loss of E-cadherin) (85). Low miR-29a level is reported to be associated with induced drug resistance and invasion (97). High miR-196a and miR-21 levels enhance radioresistance through inhibiting annexin A1 and signal transducer and activator of transcription 3 (STAT3), respectively (107, 108). Moreover, low Dicer expression is associated with resistance to 5-fluorouracil-based chemoradiotherapy and shorter overall survival in patients with OSCC (109). In brief, upregulation of the let-7 family, miR-203, miR-23a, miR-214, miR-518c, and miR-608 and downregulation of miR-21 and miR-342 have been shown to be connected with the manifestation of chemosensitivity/chemoresistance in OSCC (91, 110, 111). Moreover, therapeutic resistance is mediated through EGFR and c-MET, which are further alleviated by low levels of miR-1 and miR-206 in OSCC (102). However, determination of the exact range (single/panel) of these miRNA biomarkers as well as the spectrum of their expression level needs to be extremely accurate, sensitive, and specific in order to predict optimum therapy response in OSCC.

Biomarkers for Prediction of Patient Survival in OSCC

The relation between disease-free survival and overall survival of OSCC patients and aberrant miRNA expression has been studied by several investigators. Early detection and prompt treatment using suitable multidisciplinary protocols could improve survival in OSCC. Earlier evidence has shown that irrespective of tumor size, poor patient survival is significantly correlated with lower expression levels of miR-9, miR-149, miR-150-5p, miR-200b, miR-205, miR-375, miR-483-5p, miR-542-3p, and let-7d (35, 62, 68, 103, 104, 112–118). Concurrently, it was also found that overexpression of miR-1246 and miR-675 and downregulation of miR-187 and miR-134 in plasma are associated with better patient survival in OSCC (35, 62, 67, 68, 103, 104, 112–118). Moreover, other studies discovered that decreased levels of Dicer and miR-206 correlate significantly with lower overall survival in OSCC (101, 109).

ADVANCED THERAPEUTICS BASED ON MicroRNA EXPRESSION IN ORAL SQUAMOUS CELL CARCINOMA

As described above, a variety of tumor-specific dysregulated miRNAs have been identified in OSCC, with either tumor suppressor or oncogenic functions. However, the challenges that remain for therapeutic application of miRNAs in OSCC are as follows: (a) miRNA selection, (b) complex regulatory mechanisms, (c) delivery, (d) pharmacokinetics, and (e) toxicity. Nevertheless, being endogenous molecules, miRNAs exhibit low toxicity in humans. Further, owing to their small size, miRNAs can be introduced into the system through different delivery methods.

In this context, so far, miRNA sponging, locked nucleic acid-mediated suppression of oncogenic miRNAs, and replacement of tumor-suppressive miRNAs using respective mimics/viral vectors/small compounds have already been used for different cancers (17, 119). To this end, the efficacy and accuracy of the miRNA delivery system are very important. Two main miRNA delivery approaches have been described: local (intra-tumor) and systemic. Systemic approaches would be suitable for metastatic or late-stage advanced cancers. The miRNA could be conjugated with a folate ligand, such as vitamin B9, for selective delivery to treat the cancer (17, 119). In addition, exosome/microvesicle/liposome-mediated delivery of miRNAs could also be used as novel tools for miRNA-based cancer therapy (53). Interestingly, therapeutic delivery of miRNA may be possible just through oral intake of vegetables, since it has been found that humans and animals can acquire plant miRNAs in their sera or body fluids through food intake (120). The first miRNA-based therapy specifically for cancer is MRX34, wherein a synthetic miR-34a mimic is loaded into liposomal nanoparticles (121). Quantification of MRX34 in non-human primates has established a satisfactory 7.7 h half-life in whole blood (122). Currently, only two observational miRNA-based therapies, miR-29b and miR-29, have progressed to clinical trials (Trial ref No.: NCT02009852 and NCT01927354, respectively) for OSCC. Further studies on miRNA-based diagnostics and therapies need to be evaluated extensively for OSCC treatment.

CONCLUSION

This review highlighted the functional landscape of dysregulated miRNAs in OSCC from a clinical perspective. We identified 17 miRNAs (let-7d, miR-1, miR-125b-5p, miR-138-5p, miR-142, miR-145, miR-155, miR-16, miR-196a, miR-196b, miR-200c, miR-20a-5p, miR-21-5p, miR-218, miR-31-5p, miR-34a, and miR-375) commonly dysregulated in OSCC and that have been found to have clinical significance in three or more extensive studies. We also found 22 miRNAs (let-7d, miR-125b-5p, miR-145, miR-146a, miR-150, miR-16, miR-184, miR-191, miR-196a, miR-196b, miR-21-5p, miR-223, miR-24, miR-26a, miR-27b, miR-29a, miR-31-5p, miR-32-5p, miR-375, miR-451, miR-9 and miR-99b-3p) to be significantly dysregulated in two or more clinical sample types (tumor tissues/epithelial cells and one or more circulating body fluid) collected from OSCC patients. These miRNAs could have the potential for clinical application for disease diagnosis, patient stratification, and therapy in OSCC. Six miRNAs (miR-146a, miR-148a, miR-24, miR-438-5p, miR-9, and miR-99b-3p) which are common to different types of biological fluid samples (blood/plasma/serum/saliva) from OSCC patients could be potential biomarkers through minimally invasive or non-invasive methods to predict OSCC more accurately. Logical selection, validation, and confirmation of these potential miRNA biomarkers (single/panel) are very important for augmenting their specific clinical applications in OSCC.

The number of human miRNAs (>2,600) in miRbase significantly increases in every successive version of the database (recent is v22.1) due to continuous inclusion of novel miRNAs (123). In most of the cases, the newer studies came up with new sets of dysregulated miRNA signatures for OSCC detection and prognostication. Therefore, large differences are frequently found in the results of similar older studies and current large-scale data sets. The ethnicity of the recruited patient population is also an important issue in this situation. In the current review, importantly, we summarized the recent progress on elucidating the clinical significance of miRNAs (tumor-associated or circulating), especially with respect to possible ways to develop miRNA-based detection and prognostication methods in conjunction with available techniques. Recent evidence increasingly demonstrates that cell-free miRNAs are evolving as consistent and reliable biomarkers for early detection, disease monitoring, and patient stratification, as well as guides to optimum treatment protocols for patients with OSCC.

In conclusion, a wide variety of dysregulated miRNAs contribute to the OSCC phenotype and differential patient outcomes, including tumor progression, therapy response, recurrence, metastasis, and survival. Moreover, miRNA-mediated regulatory mechanisms are complex and tangled with numerous interconnected physiological events. Here, one of the biggest challenges is to identify the tailor-made potentially relevant key miRNA candidates (single or in spectrum) along with or without their key targets for detection of disease and stratification of each patient with OSCC. Therefore, on the basis of our previous knowledge, careful, logical selection, and functional characterization of signature miRNAs (mentioned above) are very important. Standardized validation studies must be undertaken to ensure the sensitivity, specificity, and robustness of the signature miRNAs for individual patient conditions. Thus, well-designed, multicentered, prospective trials with large patient cohorts would be necessary to mitigate external variations in data sets. This will provide useful information for molecular diagnostics and determination of prognostic information for improved management of OSCC.

AUTHOR CONTRIBUTIONS

RG conceived the idea, collected all data, and designed and wrote the manuscript. SR and AP supervised and contributed with their expert comments and views in the logical presentation of manuscript and checked and edited the manuscript. All authors approved the final manuscript.

REFERENCES

1. Bray F, Ferlay J, Soerjomataram I, Siegel RL, Torre LA, Jemal A. Global cancer statistics 2018: GLOBOCAN estimates of incidence and mortality worldwide for 36 cancers in 185 countries. *CA Cancer J Clin.* (2018) 68:394–424. doi: 10.3322/caac.21492
2. Ferlay J, Colombet M, Soerjomataram I, Mathers C, Parkin DM, Pineros M, et al. Estimating the global cancer incidence and mortality in 2018: GLOBOCAN sources and methods. *Int J Cancer.* (2019) 144:1941–53. doi: 10.1002/ijc.31937
3. International Agency for Research on Cancer W. *India, Source: Globacon 2018.* The Global Cancer Observatory (2019). Available online at: https://gco.iarc.fr/today/data/factsheets/populations/356-india-fact-sheets.pdf
4. Leemans CR, Braakhuis BJ, Brakenhoff RH. The molecular biology of head and neck cancer. *Nat Rev Cancer.* (2011) 11:9–22. doi: 10.1038/nrc2982
5. Rischin D, Ferris RL, Le QT. Overview of advances in head and neck cancer. *J Clin Oncol.* (2015) 33:3225–6. doi: 10.1200/JCO.2015.63.6761
6. Chinn SB, Myers JN. Oral cavity carcinoma: current management, controversies, and future directions. *J Clin Oncol.* (2015) 33:3269–76. doi: 10.1200/JCO.2015.61.2929
7. Koyfman SA, Ismaila N, Crook D, D'Cruz AL. Management of the neck in squamous cell carcinoma of the oral cavity and oropharynx: ASCO Clinical Practice Guideline. *J Clin Oncol.* (2019) 37:1753–74. doi: 10.1200/JCO.18.01921
8. Wang Z, Jiang L, Huang C, Li Z, Chen L, Gou L, et al. Comparative proteomics approach to screening of potential diagnostic and therapeutic targets for oral squamous cell carcinoma. *Mol Cell Proteomics.* (2008) 7:1639–50. doi: 10.1074/mcp.M700520-MCP200
9. Schaaij-Visser TB, Brakenhoff RH, Leemans CR, Heck AJ, Slijper M. Protein biomarker discovery for head and neck cancer. *J Proteomics.* (2010) 73:1790–803. doi: 10.1016/j.jprot.2010.01.013
10. Kang H, Kiess A, Chung CH. Emerging biomarkers in head and neck cancer in the era of genomics. *Nat Rev Clin Oncol.* (2014) 12:11–26. doi: 10.1038/nrclinonc.2014.192
11. Wang Y, Springer S, Mulvey CL, Silliman N, Schaefer J, Sausen M, et al. Detection of somatic mutations and HPV in the saliva and plasma of patients with head and neck squamous cell carcinomas. *Sci Transl Med.* (2015) 7:293ra104. doi: 10.1126/scitranslmed.aaa8507
12. Cohen JD, Javed AA, Thoburn C, Wong F, Tie J, Gibbs P, et al. Combined circulating tumor DNA and protein biomarker-based liquid biopsy for the earlier detection of pancreatic cancers. *Proc Natl Acad Sci USA.* (2017) 114:10202–7. doi: 10.1073/pnas.1704961114
13. Cohen JD, Li L, Wang Y, Thoburn C, Afsari B, Danilova L, et al. Detection and localization of surgically resectable cancers with a multi-analyte blood test. *Science.* (2018) 359:926–30. doi: 10.1126/science.aar3247
14. Wang K, Zhang S, Weber J, Baxter D, Galas DJ. Export of microRNAs and microRNA-protective protein by mammalian cells. *Nucleic Acids Res.* (2010) 38:7248–59. doi: 10.1093/nar/gkq601
15. Arroyo JD, Chevillet JR, Kroh EM, Ruf IK, Pritchard CC, Gibson DF, et al. Argonaute2 complexes carry a population of circulating microRNAs independent of vesicles in human plasma. *Proc Natl Acad Sci USA.* (2011) 108:5003–8. doi: 10.1073/pnas.1019055108
16. Vickers KC, Palmisano BT, Shoucri BM, Shamburek RD, Remaley AT. MicroRNAs are transported in plasma and delivered to recipient cells by high-density lipoproteins. *Nat Cell Biol.* (2011) 13:423–33. doi: 10.1038/ncb2210
17. Iorio MV, Croce CM. MicroRNA dysregulation in cancer: diagnostics, monitoring and therapeutics. A comprehensive review. *EMBO Mol Med.* (2012) 4:143–59. doi: 10.1002/emmm.201100209
18. Dhawan A, Scott JG, Harris AL, Buffa FM. Pan-cancer characterisation of microRNA across cancer hallmarks reveals microRNA-mediated downregulation of tumour suppressors. *Nat Commun.* (2018) 9:5228. doi: 10.1038/s41467-018-07657-1
19. Lee RC, Feinbaum RL, Ambros V. The C. elegans heterochronic gene lin-4 encodes small RNAs with antisense complementarity to lin-14. *Cell.* (1993) 75:843–54. doi: 10.1016/0092-8674(93)90529-Y
20. Ebert MS, Sharp PA. Roles for microRNAs in conferring robustness to biological processes. *Cell.* (2012) 149:515–24. doi: 10.1016/j.cell.2012.04.005
21. Krol J, Loedige I, Filipowicz W. The widespread regulation of microRNA biogenesis, function and decay. *Nat Rev Genet.* (2010) 11:597–610. doi: 10.1038/nrg2843
22. Djuranovic S, Nahvi A, Green R. miRNA-mediated gene silencing by translational repression followed by mRNA deadenylation and decay. *Science.* (2012) 336:237–40. doi: 10.1126/science.1215691
23. Jonas S, Izaurralde E. Towards a molecular understanding of microRNA-mediated gene silencing. *Nat Rev Genet.* (2015) 16:421–33. doi: 10.1038/nrg3965
24. Redis RS, Calin S, Yang Y, You MJ, Calin GA. Cell-to-cell miRNA transfer: from body homeostasis to therapy. *Pharmacol Ther.* (2012) 136:169–74. doi: 10.1016/j.pharmthera.2012.08.003
25. Fang C, Li Y. Prospective applications of microRNAs in oral cancer. *Oncol Lett.* (2019) 18:3974–84. doi: 10.3892/ol.2019.10751
26. Calin GA, Dumitru CD, Shimizu M, Bichi R, Zupo S, Noch E, et al. Frequent deletions and down-regulation of micro- RNA genes miR15 and miR16 at 13q14 in chronic lymphocytic leukemia. *Proc Natl Acad Sci USA.* (2002) 99:15524–9. doi: 10.1073/pnas.242606799
27. Hanahan D, Weinberg RA. Hallmarks of cancer: the next generation. *Cell.* (2011) 144:646–74. doi: 10.1016/j.cell.2011.02.013
28. Bracken CP, Scott HS, Goodall GJ. A network-biology perspective of microRNA function and dysfunction in cancer. *Nat Rev Genet.* (2016) 17:719–32. doi: 10.1038/nrg.2016.134
29. Anastasiadou E, Jacob LS, Slack FJ. Non-coding RNA networks in cancer. *Nat Rev Cancer.* (2018) 18:5–18. doi: 10.1038/nrc.2017.99
30. Cai Y, Wan J. Competing endogenous RNA regulations in neurodegenerative disorders: current challenges and emerging insights. *Front Mol Neurosci.* (2018) 11:370. doi: 10.3389/fnmol.2018.00370
31. Xie B, Ding Q, Han H, Wu D. miRCancer: a microRNA-cancer association database constructed by text mining on literature. *Bioinformatics.* (2013) 29:638–44. doi: 10.1093/bioinformatics/btt014
32. Tran N, Mclean T, Zhang X, Zhao CJ, Thomson JM, O'brien C, et al. MicroRNA expression profiles in head and neck cancer cell lines. *Biochem Biophys Res Commun.* (2007) 358:12–7. doi: 10.1016/j.bbrc.2007.03.201
33. Chang SS, Jiang WW, Smith I, Poeta LM, Begum S, Glazer C, et al. MicroRNA alterations in head and neck squamous cell carcinoma. *Int J Cancer.* (2008) 123:2791–7. doi: 10.1002/ijc.23831
34. Wong TS, Liu XB, Wong BY, Ng RW, Yuen AP, Wei WI. Mature miR-184 as potential oncogenic microRNA of squamous cell carcinoma of tongue. *Clin Cancer Res.* (2008) 14:2588–92. doi: 10.1158/1078-0432.CCR-07-0666
35. Childs G, Fazzari M, Kung G, Kawachi N, Brandwein-Gensler M, Mclemore M, et al. Low-level expression of microRNAs let-7d and miR-205 are prognostic markers of head and neck squamous cell carcinoma. *Am J Pathol.* (2009) 174:736–45. doi: 10.2353/ajpath.2009.080731
36. Gombos K, Horvath R, Szele E, Juhasz K, Gocze K, Somlai K, et al. miRNA expression profiles of oral squamous cell carcinomas. *Anticancer Res.* (2013) 33:1511–7. Available online at: http://ar.iiarjournals.org/content/33/4/1511.full.pdf
37. Hui AB, Lenarduzzi M, Krushel T, Waldron L, Pintilie M, Shi W, et al. Comprehensive MicroRNA profiling for head and neck squamous cell carcinomas. *Clin Cancer Res.* (2010) 16:1129–39. doi: 10.1158/1078-0432.CCR-09-2166
38. Lu YC, Chen YJ, Wang HM, Tsai CY, Chen WH, Huang YC, et al. Oncogenic function and early detection potential of miRNA-10b in oral cancer as identified by microRNA profiling. *Cancer Prev Res.* (2012) 5:665–74. doi: 10.1158/1940-6207.CAPR-11-0358
39. Kalfert D, Pesta M, Kulda V, Topolcan O, Ryska A, Celakovsky P, et al. MicroRNA profile in site-specific head and neck squamous cell cancer. *Anticancer Res.* (2015) 35:2455–63. Available online at: http://ar.iiarjournals.org/content/35/4/2455.full.pdf
40. Manikandan M, Deva Magendhra Rao AK, Arunkumar G, Manickavasagam M, Rajkumar KS, Rajaraman R, et al. Oral squamous cell carcinoma: microRNA expression profiling and integrative analyses for elucidation of tumourigenesis mechanism. *Mol Cancer.* (2016) 15:28. doi: 10.1186/s12943-016-0512-8
41. Lamperska KM, Kozlowski P, Kolenda T, Teresiak A, Blizniak R, Przybyla W, et al. Unpredictable changes of selected miRNA in expression

profile of HNSCC. *Cancer Biomark.* (2016) 16:55–64. doi: 10.3233/CBM-150540

42. Zeljic K, Jovanovic I, Jovanovic J, Magic Z, Stankovic A, Supic G. MicroRNA meta-signature of oral cancer: evidence from a meta-analysis. *Ups J Med Sci.* (2018) 123:43–9. doi: 10.1080/03009734.2018.1439551
43. Towle R, Gorenchtein M, Garnis C, Dickman C, Zhu Y, Poh CF. Dysregulation of microRNAs across oral squamous cell carcinoma fields in non-smokers. *J Interdiscipl Med Dent Sci.* (2014) 2:131. doi: 10.4172/2376-032X.1000131
44. Shiah SG, Hsiao JR, Chang WM, Chen YW, Jin YT, Wong TY, et al. Downregulated miR329 and miR410 promote the proliferation and invasion of oral squamous cell carcinoma by targeting Wnt-7b. *Cancer Res.* (2014) 74:7560–72. doi: 10.1158/0008-5472.CAN-14-0978
45. Hou YY, Lee JH, Chen HC, Yang CM, Huang SJ, Liou HH, et al. The association between miR-499a polymorphism and oral squamous cell carcinoma progression. *Oral Dis.* (2015) 21:195–206. doi: 10.1111/odi.12241
46. Lajer CB, Garnaes E, Friis-Hansen L, Norrild B, Therkildsen MH, Glud M, et al. The role of miRNAs in human papilloma virus (HPV)-associated cancers: bridging between HPV-related head and neck cancer and cervical cancer. *Br J Cancer.* (2012) 106:1526–34. doi: 10.1038/bjc.2012.109
47. Network TCGA. Comprehensive genomic characterization of head and neck squamous cell carcinomas. *Nature.* (2015) 517:576–82. doi: 10.1038/nature14129
48. Hu J, Ge W, Xu J. HPV 16 E7 inhibits OSCC cell proliferation, invasion, and metastasis by upregulating the expression of miR-20a. *Tumour Biol.* (2016) 37:9433–40. doi: 10.1007/s13277-016-4817-4
49. Bozinovic K, Sabol I, Dediol E, Milutin Gasperov N, Manojlovic S, Vojtechova Z, et al. Genome-wide miRNA profiling reinforces the importance of miR-9 in human papillomavirus associated oral and oropharyngeal head and neck cancer. *Sci Rep.* (2019) 9:2306. doi: 10.1038/s41598-019-38797-z
50. Gissi DB, Morandi L, Gabusi A, Tarsitano A, Marchetti C, Cura F, et al. A noninvasive test for microRNA expression in oral squamous cell carcinoma. *Int J Mol Sci.* (2018) 19:1789. doi: 10.3390/ijms19061789
51. Adami GR, Tang JL, Markiewicz MR. Improving accuracy of RNA-based diagnosis and prognosis of oral cancer by using noninvasive methods. *Oral Oncol.* (2017) 69:62–7. doi: 10.1016/j.oraloncology.2017.04.001
52. Zhou Y, Kolokythas A, Schwartz JL, Epstein JB, Adami GR. microRNA from brush biopsy to characterize oral squamous cell carcinoma epithelium. *Cancer Med.* (2017) 6:67–78. doi: 10.1002/cam4.951
53. Kamerkar S, Lebleu VS, Sugimoto H, Yang S, Ruivo CF, Melo SA, et al. Exosomes facilitate therapeutic targeting of oncogenic KRAS in pancreatic cancer. *Nature.* (2017) 546:498–503. doi: 10.1038/nature22341
54. Redova M, Sana J, Slaby O. Circulating miRNAs as new blood-based biomarkers for solid cancers. *Future Oncol.* (2013) 9:387–402. doi: 10.2217/fon.12.192
55. Mitchell PS, Parkin RK, Kroh EM, Fritz BR, Wyman SK, Pogosova-Agadjanyan EL, et al. Circulating microRNAs as stable blood-based markers for cancer detection. *Proc Natl Acad Sci USA.* (2008) 105:10513–8. doi: 10.1073/pnas.0804549105
56. Turchinovich A, Weiz L, Langheinz A, Burwinkel B. Characterization of extracellular circulating microRNA. *Nucleic Acids Res.* (2011) 39:7223–33. doi: 10.1093/nar/gkr254
57. Rapado-Gonzalez O, Lopez-Lopez R, Lopez-Cedrun JL, Triana-Martinez G, Muinelo-Romay L, Suarez-Cunqueiro MM. Cell-free microRNAs as potential oral cancer biomarkers: from diagnosis to therapy. *Cells.* (2019) 8:1653. doi: 10.3390/cells8121653
58. Park NJ, Zhou H, Elashoff D, Henson BS, Kastratovic DA, Abemayor E, et al. Salivary microRNA: discovery, characterization, and clinical utility for oral cancer detection. *Clin Cancer Res.* (2009) 15:5473–7. doi: 10.1158/1078-0432.CCR-09-0736
59. Yang Y, Li YX, Yang X, Jiang L, Zhou ZJ, Zhu YQ. Progress risk assessment of oral premalignant lesions with saliva miRNA analysis. *BMC Cancer.* (2013) 13:129. doi: 10.1186/1471-2407-13-129
60. Momen-Heravi F, Trachtenberg AJ, Kuo WP, Cheng YS. Genomewide study of salivary microRNAs for detection of oral cancer. *J Dent Res.* (2014) 93:86S–93S. doi: 10.1177/0022034514531018
61. Hung PS, Liu CJ, Chou CS, Kao SY, Yang CC, Chang KW, et al. miR-146a enhances the oncogenicity of oral carcinoma by concomitant targeting of the IRAK1, TRAF6 and NUMB genes. *PLoS ONE.* (2013) 8:e79926. doi: 10.1371/journal.pone.0079926
62. Liu CJ, Lin JS, Cheng HW, Hsu YH, Cheng CY, Lin SC. Plasma miR-187* is a potential biomarker for oral carcinoma. *Clin Oral Investig.* (2016) 21:1131–8. doi: 10.1007/s00784-016-1887-z
63. Liu CJ, Tsai MM, Tu HF, Lui MT, Cheng HW, Lin SC. miR-196a overexpression and miR-196a2 gene polymorphism are prognostic predictors of oral carcinomas. *Ann Surg Oncol.* (2013) 20(Suppl 3):S406–14. doi: 10.1245/s10434-012-2618-6
64. Lu YC, Chang JT, Huang YC, Huang CC, Chen WH, Lee LY, et al. Combined determination of circulating miR-196a and miR-196b levels produces high sensitivity and specificity for early detection of oral cancer. *Clin Biochem.* (2015) 48:115–21. doi: 10.1016/j.clinbiochem.2014.11.020
65. Sun G, Cao Y, Wang P, Song H, Bie T, Li M, et al. miR-200b-3p in plasma is a potential diagnostic biomarker in oral squamous cell carcinoma. *Biomarkers.* (2018) 23:137–41. doi: 10.1080/1354750X.2017.1289241
66. Chang YA, Weng SL, Yang SF, Chou CH, Huang WC, Tu SJ, et al. A three-microRNA signature as a potential biomarker for the early detection of oral cancer. *Int J Mol Sci.* (2018) 19:758. doi: 10.3390/ijms19030758
67. Xu H, Yang Y, Zhao H, Yang X, Luo Y, Ren Y, et al. Serum miR-483-5p: a novel diagnostic and prognostic biomarker for patients with oral squamous cell carcinoma. *Tumour Biol.* (2016) 37:447–53. doi: 10.1007/s13277-015-3514-z
68. Sun L, Liu L, Fu H, Wang Q, Shi Y. Association of decreased expression of serum miR-9 with poor prognosis of oral squamous cell carcinoma patients. *Med Sci Monit.* (2016) 22:289–94. doi: 10.12659/MSM.895683
69. Schneider A, Victoria B, Lopez YN, Suchorska W, Barczak W, Sobecka A, et al. Tissue and serum microRNA profile of oral squamous cell carcinoma patients. *Sci Rep.* (2018) 8:675. doi: 10.1038/s41598-017-18945-z
70. Ren W, Qiang C, Gao L, Li SM, Zhang LM, Wang XL, et al. Circulating microRNA-21 (MIR-21) and phosphatase and tensin homolog (PTEN) are promising novel biomarkers for detection of oral squamous cell carcinoma. *Biomarkers.* (2014) 19:590–6. doi: 10.3109/1354750X.2014.955059
71. Ries J, Vairaktaris E, Agaimy A, Kintopp R, Baran C, Neukam FW, et al. miR-186, miR-3651 and miR-494: potential biomarkers for oral squamous cell carcinoma extracted from whole blood. *Oncol Rep.* (2014) 31:1429–36. doi: 10.3892/or.2014.2983
72. Ries J, Baran C, Wehrhan F, Weber M, Neukam FW, Krautheim-Zenk A, et al. Prognostic significance of altered miRNA expression in whole blood of OSCC patients. *Oncol Rep.* (2017) 37:3467–74. doi: 10.3892/or.2017.5639
73. Ries J, Baran C, Wehrhan F, Weber M, Motel C, Kesting M, et al. The altered expression levels of miR-186, miR-494 and miR-3651 in OSCC tissue vary from those of the whole blood of OSCC patients. *Cancer Biomark.* (2019) 24:19–30. doi: 10.3233/CBM-180032
74. Mazumder S, Datta S, Ray JG, Chaudhuri K, Chatterjee R. Liquid biopsy: miRNA as a potential biomarker in oral cancer. *Cancer Epidemiol.* (2019) 58:137–45. doi: 10.1016/j.canep.2018.12.008
75. Blondal T, Jensby Nielsen S, Baker A, Andreasen D, Mouritzen P, Wrang Teilum M, et al. Assessing sample and miRNA profile quality in serum and plasma or other biofluids. *Methods.* (2013) 59:S1–6. doi: 10.1016/j.ymeth.2012.09.015
76. Buschmann D, Haberberger A, Kirchner B, Spornraft M, Riedmaier I, Schelling G, et al. Toward reliable biomarker signatures in the age of liquid biopsies - how to standardize the small RNA-Seq workflow. *Nucleic Acids Res.* (2016) 44:5995–6018. doi: 10.1093/nar/gkw545
77. Garcia-Elias A, Alloza L, Puigdecanet E, Nonell L, Tajes M, Curado J, et al. Defining quantification methods and optimizing protocols for microarray hybridization of circulating microRNAs. *Sci Rep.* (2017) 7:7725. doi: 10.1038/s41598-017-08134-3
78. Gevaert AB, Witvrouwen I, Vrints CJ, Heidbuchel H, Van Craenenbroeck EM, Van Laere SJ, et al. MicroRNA profiling in plasma samples using qPCR arrays: recommendations for correct analysis and interpretation. *PLoS ONE.* (2018) 13:e0193173. doi: 10.1371/journal.pone.0193173
79. Orsos Z, Szanyi I, Csejtei A, Gerlinger I, Ember I, Kiss I. Association of pre-miR-146a rs2910164 polymorphism with the risk of head and neck cancer.

Anticancer Res. (2013) 33:341–6. Available online at: http://ar.iiarjournals.org/content/33/1/341.full.pdf

80. Tu HF, Liu CJ, Chang CL, Wang PW, Kao SY, Yang CC, et al. The association between genetic polymorphism and the processing efficiency of miR-149 affects the prognosis of patients with head and neck squamous cell carcinoma. *PLoS ONE.* (2012) 7:e51606. doi: 10.1371/journal.pone.0051606
81. Niu YM, Du XY, Lu MY, Xu QL, Luo J, Shen M. Significant association between functional microRNA polymorphisms and head and neck cancer susceptibility: a comprehensive meta-analysis. *Sci Rep.* (2015) 5:12972. doi: 10.1038/srep17149
82. Brito JA, Gomes CC, Guimaraes AL, Campos K, Gomez RS. Relationship between microRNA expression levels and histopathological features of dysplasia in oral leukoplakia. *J Oral Pathol Med.* (2014) 43:211–6. doi: 10.1111/jop.12112
83. Kinoshita T, Nohata N, Hanazawa T, Kikkawa N, Yamamoto N, Yoshino H, et al. Tumour-suppressive microRNA-29s inhibit cancer cell migration and invasion by targeting laminin-integrin signalling in head and neck squamous cell carcinoma. *Br J Cancer.* (2013) 109:2636–45. doi: 10.1038/bjc.2013.607
84. Tachibana H, Sho R, Takeda Y, Zhang X, Yoshida Y, Narimatsu H, et al. Circulating miR-223 in oral cancer: its potential as a novel diagnostic biomarker and therapeutic target. *PLoS ONE.* (2016) 11:e0159693. doi: 10.1371/journal.pone.0159693
85. Ghosh RD, Ghuwalewala S, Das P, Mandloi S, Alam SK, Chakraborty J, et al. MicroRNA profiling of cisplatin-resistant oral squamous cell carcinoma cell lines enriched with cancer-stem-cell-like and epithelial-mesenchymal transition-type features. *Sci Rep.* (2016) 6:23932. doi: 10.1038/srep23932
86. Zeng G, Xun W, Wei K, Yang Y, Shen H. MicroRNA-27a-3p regulates epithelial to mesenchymal transition via targeting YAP1 in oral squamous cell carcinoma cells. *Oncol Rep.* (2016) 36:1475–82. doi: 10.3892/or.2016.4916
87. Lu YC, Chang JT, Liao CT, Kang CJ, Huang SF, Chen IH, et al. OncomiR-196 promotes an invasive phenotype in oral cancer through the NME4-JNK-TIMP1-MMP signaling pathway. *Mol Cancer.* (2014) 13:218. doi: 10.1186/1476-4598-13-218
88. Tu HF, Chang KW, Cheng HW, Liu CJ. Upregulation of miR-372 and−373 associates with lymph node metastasis and poor prognosis of oral carcinomas. *Laryngoscope.* (2015) 125:E365–70. doi: 10.1002/lary.25464
89. Hou YY, You JJ, Yang CM, Pan HW, Chen HC, Lee JH, et al. Aberrant DNA hypomethylation of miR-196b contributes to migration and invasion of oral cancer. *Oncol Lett.* (2016) 11:4013–21. doi: 10.3892/ol.2016.4491
90. Lin SC, Kao SY, Chang JC, Liu YC, Yu EH, Tseng SH, et al. Up-regulation of miR-187 modulates the advances of oral carcinoma by targeting BARX2 tumor suppressor. *Oncotarget.* (2016) 7:61355–65. doi: 10.18632/oncotarget.11349
91. Chang CJ, Hsu CC, Chang CH, Tsai LL, Chang YC, Lu SW, et al. Let-7d functions as novel regulator of epithelial-mesenchymal transition and chemoresistant property in oral cancer. *Oncol Rep.* (2011) 26:1003–10. doi: 10.3892/or.2011.1360
92. Lei W, Liu YE, Zheng Y, Qu L. MiR-429 inhibits oral squamous cell carcinoma growth by targeting ZEB1. *Med Sci Monit.* (2015) 21:383–9. doi: 10.12659/MSM.893412
93. Wu B, Lei D, Wang L, Yang X, Jia S, Yang Z, et al. MiRNA-101 inhibits oral squamous-cell carcinoma growth and metastasis by targeting zinc finger E-box binding homeobox 1. *Am J Cancer Res.* (2016) 6:1396–407. Available online at: http://www.ajcr.us/files/ajcr0026756.pdf
94. Yu J, Xie F, Bao X, Chen W, Xu Q. miR-300 inhibits epithelial to mesenchymal transition and metastasis by targeting Twist in human epithelial cancer. *Mol Cancer.* (2014) 13:121. doi: 10.1186/1476-4598-13-121
95. Bufalino A, Cervigne NK, De Oliveira CE, Fonseca FP, Rodrigues PC, Macedo CC, et al. Low miR-143/miR-145 cluster levels induce activin a overexpression in oral squamous cell carcinomas, which contributes to poor prognosis. *PLoS ONE.* (2015) 10:e0136599. doi: 10.1371/journal.pone.0136599
96. Chang WM, Lin YF, Su CY, Peng HY, Chang YC, Lai TC, et al. Dysregulation of RUNX2/activin-A axis upon miR-376c downregulation promotes lymph node metastasis in head and neck squamous cell carcinoma. *Cancer Res.* (2016) 76:7140–50. doi: 10.1158/0008-5472.CAN-16-1188
97. Lu L, Xue X, Lan J, Gao Y, Xiong Z, Zhang H, et al. MicroRNA-29a upregulates MMP2 in oral squamous cell carcinoma to promote cancer invasion and anti-apoptosis. *Biomed Pharmacother.* (2014) 68:13–9. doi: 10.1016/j.biopha.2013.10.005
98. Fukumoto I, Koshizuka K, Hanazawa T, Kikkawa N, Matsushita R, Kurozumi A, et al. The tumor-suppressive microRNA-23b/27b cluster regulates the MET oncogene in oral squamous cell carcinoma. *Int J Oncol.* (2016) 49:1119–29. doi: 10.3892/ijo.2016.3602
99. Uesugi A, Kozaki K, Tsuruta T, Furuta M, Morita K, Imoto I, et al. The tumor suppressive microRNA miR-218 targets the mTOR component Rictor and inhibits AKT phosphorylation in oral cancer. *Cancer Res.* (2011) 71:5765–78. doi: 10.1158/0008-5472.CAN-11-0368
100. Kinoshita T, Hanazawa T, Nohata N, Kikkawa N, Enokida H, Yoshino H, et al. Tumor suppressive microRNA-218 inhibits cancer cell migration and invasion through targeting laminin-332 in head and neck squamous cell carcinoma. *Oncotarget.* (2012) 3:1386–400. doi: 10.18632/oncotarget.709
101. Lin F, Yao L, Xiao J, Liu D, Ni Z. MiR-206 functions as a tumor suppressor and directly targets K-Ras in human oral squamous cell carcinoma. *Onco Targets Ther.* (2014) 7:1583–91. doi: 10.2147/OTT.S67624
102. Koshizuka K, Hanazawa T, Fukumoto I, Kikkawa N, Matsushita R, Mataki H, et al. Dual-receptor (EGFR and c-MET) inhibition by tumor-suppressive miR-1 and miR-206 in head and neck squamous cell carcinoma. *J Hum Genet.* (2017). 62:113–21. doi: 10.1038/jhg.2016.47
103. Bonnin N, Armandy E, Carras J, Ferrandon S, Battiston-Montagne P, Aubry M, et al. MiR-422a promotes loco-regional recurrence by targeting NT5E/CD73 in head and neck squamous cell carcinoma. *Oncotarget.* (2016) 7:44023–38. doi: 10.18632/oncotarget.9829
104. Liu CJ, Shen WG, Peng SY, Cheng HW, Kao SY, Lin SC, et al. miR-134 induces oncogenicity and metastasis in head and neck carcinoma through targeting WWOX gene. *Int J Cancer.* (2014) 134:811–21. doi: 10.1002/ijc.28358
105. Henson BJ, Bhattacharjee S, O'dee DM, Feingold E, Gollin SM. Decreased expression of miR-125b and miR-100 in oral cancer cells contributes to malignancy. *Genes Chromosomes Cancer.* (2009) 48:569–82. doi: 10.1002/gcc.20666
106. Shiiba M, Shinozuka K, Saito K, Fushimi K, Kasamatsu A, Ogawara K, et al. MicroRNA-125b regulates proliferation and radioresistance of oral squamous cell carcinoma. *Br J Cancer.* (2013) 108:1817–21. doi: 10.1038/bjc.2013.175
107. Zhou X, Ren Y, Liu A, Jin R, Jiang Q, Huang Y, et al. WP1066 sensitizes oral squamous cell carcinoma cells to cisplatin by targeting STAT3/miR-21 axis. *Sci Rep.* (2014) 4:7461. doi: 10.1038/srep07461
108. Suh YE, Raulf N, Gaken J, Lawler K, Urbano TG, Bullenkamp J, et al. MicroRNA-196a promotes an oncogenic effect in head and neck cancer cells by suppressing annexin A1 and enhancing radioresistance. *Int J Cancer.* (2015) 137:1021–34. doi: 10.1002/ijc.29397
109. Kawahara K, Nakayama H, Nagata M, Yoshida R, Hirosue A, Tanaka T, et al. A low Dicer expression is associated with resistance to 5-FU-based chemoradiotherapy and a shorter overall survival in patients with oral squamous cell carcinoma. *J Oral Pathol Med.* (2014) 43:350–6. doi: 10.1111/jop.12140
110. Yu ZW, Zhong LP, Ji T, Zhang P, Chen WT, Zhang CP. MicroRNAs contribute to the chemoresistance of cisplatin in tongue squamous cell carcinoma lines. *Oral Oncol.* (2010) 46:317–22. doi: 10.1016/j.oraloncology.2010.02.002
111. Lin J, Lin Y, Fan L, Kuang W, Zheng L, Wu J, et al. miR-203 inhibits cell proliferation and promotes cisplatin induced cell death in tongue squamous cancer. *Biochem Biophys Res Commun.* (2016) 473:382–7. doi: 10.1016/j.bbrc.2016.02.105
112. Sun L, Yao Y, Liu B, Lin Z, Lin L, Yang M, et al. MiR-200b and miR-15b regulate chemotherapy-induced epithelial-mesenchymal transition in human tongue cancer cells by targeting BMI1. *Oncogene.* (2012) 31:432–45. doi: 10.1038/onc.2011.263
113. Liao L, Wang J, Ouyang S, Zhang P, Wang J, Zhang M. Expression and clinical significance of microRNA-1246 in human oral squamous cell carcinoma. *Med Sci Monit.* (2015) 21:776–81. doi: 10.12659/MSM.892508

114. Guan GF, Zhang DJ, Wen LJ, Xin D, Liu Y, Yu DJ, et al. Overexpression of lncRNA H19/miR-675 promotes tumorigenesis in head and neck squamous cell carcinoma. *Int J Med Sci.* (2016) 13:914–22. doi: 10.7150/ijms.16571
115. Xu P, Li Y, Zhang H, Li M, Zhu H. MicroRNA-340 mediates metabolic shift in oral squamous cell carcinoma by targeting glucose transporter-1. *J Oral Maxillofac Surg.* (2016) 74:844–50. doi: 10.1016/j.joms.2015.09.038
116. Qiao B, Cai JH, King-Yin Lam A, He BX. MicroRNA-542-3p inhibits oral squamous cell carcinoma progression by inhibiting ILK/TGF-beta1/Smad2/3 signaling. *Oncotarget.* (2017) 8:70761–76. doi: 10.18632/oncotarget.19986
117. Zhang B, Li Y, Hou D, Shi Q, Yang S, Li Q. MicroRNA-375 inhibits growth and enhances radiosensitivity in oral squamous cell carcinoma by targeting insulin like growth factor 1 receptor. *Cell Physiol Biochem.* (2017) 42:2105–17. doi: 10.1159/000479913
118. Koshizuka K, Hanazawa T, Kikkawa N, Katada K, Okato A, Arai T, et al. Antitumor miR-150-5p and miR-150-3p inhibit cancer cell aggressiveness by targeting SPOCK1 in head and neck squamous cell carcinoma. *Auris Nasus Larynx.* (2018) 45:854–65. doi: 10.1016/j.anl.2017.11.019
119. Rupaimoole R, Slack FJ. MicroRNA therapeutics: towards a new era for the management of cancer and other diseases. *Nat Rev Drug Discov.* (2017) 16:203–22. doi: 10.1038/nrd.2016.246
120. Zhang L, Hou D, Chen X, Li D, Zhu L, Zhang Y, et al. Exogenous plant MIR168a specifically targets mammalian LDLRAP1: evidence of cross-kingdom regulation by microRNA. *Cell Res.* (2012) 22:107–26. doi: 10.1038/cr.2011.158
121. Bouchie A. First microRNA mimic enters clinic. *Nat Biotechnol.* (2013) 31:577. doi: 10.1038/nbt0713-577
122. Kelnar K, Peltier HJ, Leatherbury N, Stoudemire J, Bader AG. Quantification of therapeutic miRNA mimics in whole blood from nonhuman primates. *Anal Chem.* (2014) 86:1534–42. doi: 10.1021/ac403044t
123. Griffiths-Jones S, Saini HK, Van Dongen S, Enright AJ. miRBase: tools for microRNA genomics. *Nucleic Acids Res.* (2008) 36:D154–8. doi: 10.1093/nar/gkm952

10

miR-22 and miR-205 Drive Tumor Aggressiveness of Mucoepidermoid Carcinomas of Salivary Glands

Erika Naakka[1,2], Mateus Camargo Barros-Filho[3], Shady Adnan-Awad[2,4], Ahmed Al-Samadi[1,2], Fábio Albuquerque Marchi[3], Hellen Kuasne[3], Katja Korelin[1,2], Ilida Suleymanova[1,2], Amy Louise Brown[5], Cristovam Scapulatempo-Neto[6], Silvia Vanessa Lourenço[7,8], Rogério Moraes Castilho[9], Luiz Paulo Kowalski[10,11], Antti Mäkitie[12,13,14], Vera Cavalcanti Araújo[5], Ilmo Leivo[15], Silvia Regina Rogatto[16,17], Tuula Salo[1,2,18,19,20] and Fabricio Passador-Santos[5]*

[1] Department of Oral and Maxillofacial Diseases, University of Helsinki, Helsinki, Finland, [2] Translational Immunology Research Program (TRIMM), University of Helsinki, Helsinki, Finland, [3] Centro Internacional de Pesquisa (CIPE) – A.C.Camargo Cancer Center, São Paulo, Brazil, [4] Hematology Research Unit, Department of Clinical Chemistry and Hematology, University of Helsinki, Helsinki University Hospital Comprehensive Cancer Center, Helsinki, Finland, [5] Department of Oral Pathology, Faculdade São Leopoldo Mandic, Campinas, Brazil, [6] Molecular Oncology Research Center, Barretos, and Diagnósticos da América (DASA), Barueri, Brazil, [7] Department of Pathology, A.C.Camargo Cancer Center, São Paulo, Brazil, [8] Department of General Pathology, Dental School, University of São Paulo, São Paulo, Brazil, [9] Department of Periodontics and Oral Medicine, University of Michigan School of Dentistry, Ann Arbor, MI, United States, [10] Department of Head and Neck Surgery and Otorhinolaryngology, A.C.Camargo Cancer Center, São Paulo, Brazil, [11] Department of Head and Neck Surgery, University of Sao Paulo Medical School, São Paulo, Brazil, [12] Department of Otorhinolaryngology – Head and Neck Surgery, University of Helsinki and Helsinki University Hospital, Helsinki, Finland, [13] Research Program in Systems Oncology, Faculty of Medicine, University of Helsinki, Helsinki, Finland, [14] Division of Ear, Nose and Throat Diseases, Department of Clinical Sciences, Intervention and Technology, Karolinska Institute and Karolinska Hospital, Stockholm, Sweden, [15] Institute of Biomedicine, Pathology, University of Turku and Turku University Hospital, Turku, Finland, [16] Department of Clinical Genetics, University Hospital of Southern Denmark, Vejle, Denmark, [17] Institute of Regional Health Research, University of Southern Denmark, Odense, Denmark, [18] Department of Pathology, Helsinki University Hospital, Helsinki, Finland, [19] Cancer and Translational Medicine Research Unit, University of Oulu, Oulu, Finland, [20] Medical Research Center, Oulu University Hospital, Oulu, Finland

Correspondence:
Fabricio Passador-Santos
fabricio.passador@slmandic.edu.br

Objectives: To integrate mRNA and miRNA expression profiles of mucoepidermoid carcinomas (MECs) and normal salivary gland (NSGs) tissue samples and identify potential drivers.

Material and Methods: Gene and miRNA expression arrays were performed in 35 MECs and six NSGs.

Results: We found 46 differentially expressed (DE) miRNAs and 3,162 DE mRNAs. Supervised hierarchical clustering analysis of the DE transcripts revealed two clusters in both miRNA and mRNA profiles, which distinguished MEC from NSG samples. The integrative miRNA-mRNA analysis revealed a network comprising 696 negatively correlated interactions (44 miRNAs and 444 mRNAs) involving cell signaling, cell cycle, and cancer-related pathways. Increased expression levels of miR-205-5p and miR-224-5p and decreased expression levels of miR-139-3p, miR-145-3p, miR-148a-3p, miR-186-5p, miR-338-3p, miR-363-3p, and miR-4324 were significantly related to worse overall survival in MEC patients. Two overexpressed miRNAs in MEC (miR-22 and miR-205) were selected for inhibition by the CRISPR-Cas9 method. Cell viability, migration, and invasion assays were performed using an intermediate grade MEC cell line. Knockout of miR-205 reduced cell viability and enhanced *ZEB2* expression, while miR-22 knockout reduced cell migration and invasion and enhanced *ESR1* expression. Our results indicate a distinct transcriptomic profile of MEC compared to NSG, and the integrative analysis highlighted miRNA-mRNA interactions involving cancer-related pathways, including PTEN and PI3K/AKT.

Conclusion: The *in vitro* functional studies revealed that miR-22 and miR-205 deficiencies reduced the viability, migration, and invasion of the MEC cells suggesting they are potential oncogenic drivers in MEC.

Keywords: mucoepidermoid carcinoma, salivary gland tumor, head and neck cancer, oral cancer, transcriptomic analysis, miR22, miR205, microRNA

INTRODUCTION

Mucoepidermoid carcinoma (MEC) is the most common salivary gland malignancy in major and minor glands, and the most common salivary gland cancer affecting pediatric patients (1). The clinical behavior is variable, ranging from indolent locally infiltrative lesions to highly aggressive and metastatic lesions (2, 3). The widely used histological grade system stratifies MECs into low, intermediate, or high-grade (I, II, or III, respectively) according to histologic characteristics (1, 4–6). Histologic grade and TNM status are commonly used parameters for treatment planning. Treatment of low- and intermediate-grade tumors is based on complete surgical removal of the tumor, while there is no consensus regarding the guidelines for intermediate histologic grade (2, 7–10). In high-grade MEC, the treatment is generally surgery, followed by postoperative radiotherapy. The survival rates for low-grade MEC is over 90% at 10 years, while 70% of intermediate-grade and only 25% of high-grade MEC patients are alive after 10 years (1).

The recurrent chromosome translocation t(11;19) with the resulting *CRTC1-MAML2* fusion oncogene has been described in 60-90% of MECs (10–17). The fusion transcript has been found specific for MECs when comparing with other types of salivary gland tumors (17). *CRTC1-MAML2* has also been considered a prognostic marker (18–20), although its use in prognostication has been questioned (12, 21).

The gene expression profile of MECs has been reported in two studies in which the authors investigated a few MEC cases and compared the differentially expressed (DE) mRNA transcripts with other salivary gland tumors (22, 23).

miRNA expression studies were performed on a few MEC samples focusing on specific gene/miRNA pathways, such as angiogenesis, mast cell activation, and apoptosis (24, 25). In six MEC and three normal salivary gland samples, Binmadi et al. reported 68 DE miRNAs (26) [25]. Among them, miR-302a was the most upregulated and miR-885-5p the most downregulated miRNA (26).

Here, we investigated mRNA and miRNA expression profiles of 35 fresh-frozen MECs and six normal salivary gland tissue samples, followed by an integrative miRNA-mRNA analysis to select potential drivers. In an intermediate grade MEC cell line (UM-HMC-2), we used the CRISPR/Cas9 method to knock down two miRNAs (miR-22 and miR-205) overexpressed in MEC tissues, with the aim of analyzing their role as oncogenic drivers in MEC.

MATERIAL AND METHODS

Patients and Tissue Specimens

We selected 35 MEC samples from patients treated at the A.C.Camargo Cancer Center and Barretos Cancer Hospital, Barretos, São Paulo, Brazil. Two experienced pathologists (FPS and VCA) in salivary gland tumors reviewed the diagnosis of all tumor cases and graded according to Auclair et al., 1992 (4). Demographic, clinical, pathological, therapeutic, and follow-up data were obtained from the patients' medical records (**Table 1**). A reference RNA (Human Universal Reference Total RNA, Clontech, Mountain View, California, USA) was used and hybridized with both tumor RNA and normal salivary gland RNA. Six surrounding normal salivary glands (NSG/control) tissues were removed during surgical procedures of six MEC patients, and they were hybridized with reference RNA to further compare their mRNA and miRNA expressions with MEC's (tumor) mRNA and miRNA expressions. All samples were collected from treatment-naive patients. Written informed consent was obtained from all patients before the sample collection. The National Human Research Ethics Committee approved the study (Protocol #1.380.762/2015).

miRNA Expression Analysis

miRNA expression analyses were performed in 25 out of the 35 fresh-frozen MEC samples and six NSG; no tissue or total RNA was available for analyses in the remaining 10 samples (**Table 1**). Hybridizations were performed using a one-color SurePrint 8X60K Human miRNA platform (G4870A, Agilent Technologies, Santa Clara, CA, USA), as recommended by the supplier. Background correction, quantile normalization, log2

TABLE 1 | Demographic, clinical histopathological, therapeutic and follow-up findings of 35 mucoepidermoid carcinomas patients evaluated by mRNA and miRNA expression analyses.

Characteristics	Number of patients	
	miRNA analysis	**mRNA analysis**
Age (mean ± SD)	48.7 ± 19.7	47.7 ± 19.8
Gender		
Female	12	20
Male	13	14
Race		
Caucasian	17	26
Asian	1	1
NA	7	7
Anatomical site		
Parotid gland	13	16
Intra oral minor salivary gland and others*	7	8
Hard/soft palate	2	4
Tongue	2	4
Submandibular gland	1	2
cT stage		
T1-T2	8	10
T3-T4	10	14
NA	7	10
cN stage		
N0	13	18
N1	1	2
N2	4	4
N3	0	0
NA	7	10
cM stage		
M0	17	21
M1	1	3
NA	7	10
Tumor Grade		
Low	14	19
Intermediate	6	7
High	5	8
Vital status		
Alive	15	21
Deceased (cause of death MEC)	8	10
NA or dead of other causes#	2	3
Local recurrence		
Yes	6	6
No	18	27
NA	1	1
Treatment		
Surgery	8	13
Surgery and Radiotherapy	15	19
None	2, one received palliative RT	2, one received palliative RT
Distant Metastasis		
Yes	3	5
No	21	28
NA	1	1
Follow-up: median months (IQ range)	49.0 (62.0)	49.5 (59.8)

*NA, Information not available; SD, standard deviation; IQ, Interquartile. *gingiva, maxillary sinus, eye, nasal fossa, nasal septum.*

transformation, and statistical tests were conducted using BRB ArrayTools software v. 4.4.0 (Biometric Research Branch, National Cancer Institute, Bethesda, MD, USA - https://brb.nci.nih.gov/BRB-ArrayTools/index.html). Sequences with more than 10% of MEC and NSG samples presenting undetectable expression (below background signal) were removed. The mean of the probes representing the same miRNA was used in the subsequent steps. miRNAs DE between MEC and NSG groups were identified with a p-value <0.05 (random variance t-test), false discovery rate (FDR) <0.05, and fold change (FC) ≥ 2 and ≤ -2. Supervised hierarchical clustering analysis was performed using 1-minus correlation distance and complete linkage (BRB array tools). Robustness of hierarchical clustering analyses was confirmed using pvclust package (R program) (**Supplementary Figure S1**). Data were deposited in the Gene Expression Omnibus (GEO) database with the accession number GSE199692.

Gene Expression Analysis

Array-based gene expression analysis was performed in 34 out of the 35 fresh-frozen MEC samples and five NSG; one MEC and one NGS sample were excluded based on inferior RNA quality (**Table 1**). Hybridizations were performed using Two-color SurePrint G3 Human Gene Expression Microarray 8x60K (G4851B, Agilent) platform, as previously described (27). Data processing and analyses were carried out using similar parameters described for miRNA profiling (BRB array tools). Identification of DE mRNAs (p-value < 0.001, FDR < 0.05, FC ≥ 2 and ≤ -2) and supervised hierarchical clustering analysis were performed as described above. Pvclust package (R program) was used to confirm the robustness of hierarchical clustering analyses (**Supplementary Figure S1**). The data were deposited in the GEO database (accession number GSE169754).

miRNA-mRNA Integrative Analysis

Target transcripts from the disrupted miRNAs were predicted using the miRWalk 2.0 tool (http://www.umm.uni-heidelberg.de/apps/zmf/mirwalk/), considering only the interactions predicted by at least three of four different bioinformatic algorithms (miRWalk, miRanda, RNAhybrid, and Targetscan). miRNA and mRNA expression data from 24 MEC samples tested by both procedures were integrated based on a significant negative correlation (Pearson correlation, p-value < 0.05) between predicted miRNA-mRNA interactions. Experimentally validated interactions were additionally obtained from the miRTarBase database (28).

Pathway Enrichment Analysis

Pathway enrichment analysis was performed with KOBAS 3.0 (http://kobas.cbi.pku.edu.cn) and pathDIP (http://ophid.utoronto.ca/pathDIP) tools, comprising PANTHER, Reactome, and KEGG databases. Default parameters were adopted in KOBAS 3.0, and only experimentally detected protein-protein interactions were considered in PathDIP. The threshold used in both *in silico* tools was defined as p-value < 0.001 (hypergeometric test) and adjuscted p-value < 0.05 (Benjamini and Hochberg method).

Cell Line Culture

Human Mucoepidermoid Carcinoma (UM-HMC-2) cells were isolated from the intermediate grade (stage IVb) parotid gland

MEC of a 59-year-old Caucasian female and cultured according to Warner et al. (29).

CRISPR/Cas9-Mediated Knockout of miRNA-22 and miR-205

miRNA-22 and miR-205 expression in UM-HMC-2 was confirmed using qRT-PCR (data not shown). Then, UM-HMC-2 cells were transfected with pSpCas9(BB)-2A-GF (PX458 expression vector, Addgene plasmid # 48138) expressing CRISPR-Cas9 and sgRNA targeting either miR-22 or miR-205 using Fugene HD transfection reagent (Promega, Madison, WI, USA). This resulted in transient expression of Cas9-sgRNA. Cells transfected with an empty plasmid were used as a control. After 72 hours, cells were sorted for GFP (Green fluorescent protein) positive population using a Sony SH800 cell sorter (Sony Biotechnology, San Jose, CA, USA), and were cloned as single cells per well in a flat bottom 96-well plate. Successfully expanded clones were then screened by capillary sequencing to detect nonhomologous end-joining CRISPR-Cas9 induced gene editing. Clones with predicted out of frame insertions and deletions (indels) were selected and expanded. The predicted effect of the CRISPR editing on miRNAs was assessed using the TIDE tool (30). Details of all sgRNAs and primers used in the experiments, as well as the CRISPR knockout efficiency, are summarized in the supplementary information (**Supplementary Figure S2A** and **Supplementary Table S1**).

qRT-PCR for miRNA

In addition to sequencing, CRISPR knockout of miR-22 and miR-205 was confirmed using qRT-PCR. The miRNA was extracted with miRNeasy Tissue/Cell Advanced Mini Kit (Qiagen, Hilden, Germany) and transcripted to cDNA using miScript II RT Kit (Qiagen) following manufacturer's instructions. The miScript universal primer and miRNA-specific primers for Hsa-miR-22-3p (MS00003220) and hsa-miR-205-5p (MS00003780) were purchased from Qiagen. The relative quantitative expressions were normalized to the endogenous control human RNU-6 (MS00033740) purchased also from Qiagen. Quantitative real-time PCR was performed on Applied Biosystems QuantStudio 5 Real-Time PCR System. qRT-PCR results are summarized in the supplementary information (**Supplementary Figure S2B**).

qRT-PCR for mRNA

In order to study the effect of miR-knockouts, 11 genes were selected and evaluated by qRT-PCR: *PTEN, LAMC1, CADM1, HER3, MYCBP, SNAI1, YAP1, CD147, SMAD4, ESR1* (*ESR1*) and *ZEB2*. One thousand ng of the total RNA was used for cDNA synthesis. Synthesis was done using iScript cDNA Synthesis Kit (Bio-Rad Laboratories, Hercules, CA, USA) according to the manufacturer's instructions. Two nanograms of cDNA was used for performing qRT-PCR with the Fast SYBR Green Master Mix (Thermo Fisher Scientific) as per the manufacturer's instructions. The relative quantitative expression was normalized to the endogenous control *GAPDH*. The primers were purchased from Metabion (Planegg, Germany) and the sequences are summarized in the supplementary information (**Supplementary Table S1**). Quantitative real-time PCR was performed on Applied Biosystems QuantStudio 5 Real-Time PCR System.

Cell Viability Assay

A CellTiter-Glo (CTG) 2.0 Luminescent Cell Viability Assay (Promega, Madison, WI, USA) was used to determine the effect of miR-22 and miR-205 on the cells' viability. Briefly, 100 µL of cell suspension was dispensed in the Perkin Elmer ViewPlate-96 microplate with a clear flat bottom and black well walls (Perkin Elmer Inc., Waltham, MA, USA) for a final concentration of 1000 cells per well. After 72 hours, 100 µL of the CellTiter-Glo reagent was dispensed into the wells, and the luminescence reads were measured using a PHERAstar plate reader (BMG Labtech, Ortenberg, Germany).

Scratch Wound Cell Migration and Invasion Assays

IncuCyte 96-well ImageLock Microplate wells (Sartorius, Göttingen, Germany) were coated with 300 µg/mL Myogel for migration and invasion assays (31). The cells were seeded at a density of 25,000 cells per well in 100 µL of complete medium for both assays. After 24 hours at 37°C, a 96-pin IncuCyte WoundMaker Tool (Sartorius) was used to make uniform wounds on the confluent monolayer of the cell. The wells were washed two times with media, and 100 µL of complete medium was added. For the invasion plate, 50 µL of Myogel-collagen gel (2.4 mg/mL Myogel, 0.8 mg/mL type I rat tail collagen) (Corning Incorporated, Corning, NY, USA) was added on top of the cells. After the gel was solidified, 50 µL of media was added, and the plates were transferred to an incubator. The wound closing was monitored automatically every 2 hours for two days using IncuCyte S3 Live-Cell Imaging System (Sartorius). Analysis of wound closing (width of the wound) was performed using Matlab. Mathematical function decorrelation was used to make the cells' intensity substantially higher than the background.

Spheroid Invasion Assay

The spheroid invasion assay was done according to Naakka et al. (32). The UM-HMC-2 cells were seeded at a concentration of 1000 cells per well in 50 µL of the complete medium using a U-shaped ultra-low attachment 96-well plate (Corning, New York, USA) and incubated for four days. Next, the spheroids were embedded in 50 µL Myogel-fibrin gel containing 0.5 mg/mL Myogel, 0.3 U/mL thrombin (Sigma-Aldrich), 33.3 mg/mL aprotinin (Sigma-Aldrich), and 0.5 mg/mL fibrinogen (Merck). After the Myogel-fibrin matrix (30 min) solidification, 100 µL of complete medium was added to the wells.

Images of the spheroids were captured daily using Nikon Eclipse TS100 Inverted Microscope (Nikon, Minato, Tokyo, Japan) at 4x magnification. Analysis of the spheroid invasion area and length of the longest branch was performed using ilastik (freeware) and Fiji ImageJ 1.51 software (33).

Statistical Analysis

All *in vitro* assays were repeated at least three times, each performed at least in triplicate. Statistical analyses were carried out with SPSS v.25.0 (IBM Corporation, Chicago, IL, USA) and the GraphPad Prism software (v. 6.0; GraphPad Software Inc., La Jolla, CA, USA). Student's T-test or One-way ANOVA followed by Bonferroni correction was used in posthoc analysis. A p-value < 0.05 was considered as statistically significant. Figures were created with Origin 2018b graphing software (OriginLab Corporation, Northampton, MA, USA).

Overall survival analysis was performed using the Kaplan-Meier estimator with the log-rank test in IBM SPSS Statistics for Windows, Version 25.0 (IBM Corp. Armonk, NY, USA). The miRNA expression values were dichotomized below and above the median (p-value < 0.05). A random variance t-test using BRB ArrayTools software (v. 4.4.0) was applied to investigate differences in the miRNA expression in relation to the histological grade, lymph node, and distant metastasis (p-value < 0.05, FDR < 0.05).

RESULTS

The mean age of whole patient group was 46.9 ± 20.2 years (range 12 to 82 years old). Female patients were more frequently affected by MEC than males (ratio 1.4:1). Parotid was the most common anatomical site, followed by minor salivary glands of the palate and other sites. Twenty cases presented with low histologic grade, seven with intermediate-grade, and nine with high-grade at diagnosis. T3-T4 tumors at diagnosis were found in 14 cases. Six patients presented lymph node involvement at diagnosis and three patients presented distant metastases at diagnosis. Twenty patients were treated with surgery and radiotherapy, while 14 received surgery only. Follow-up time ranged from 4 to 188 months (median 49,5 months). Demographic, clinical, histopathological, therapeutic and follow-up features are detailed in **Table 1**. The study design, methodologies, and the foremost results are presented in **Figure 1**.

miRNA and mRNA Expression Profile of MEC

After excluding uniformly low expressed miRNAs in MEC and NSG samples, 530 miRNAs and 19,911 mRNAs were considered for further analysis. We found 46 DE miRNAs (18 overexpressed

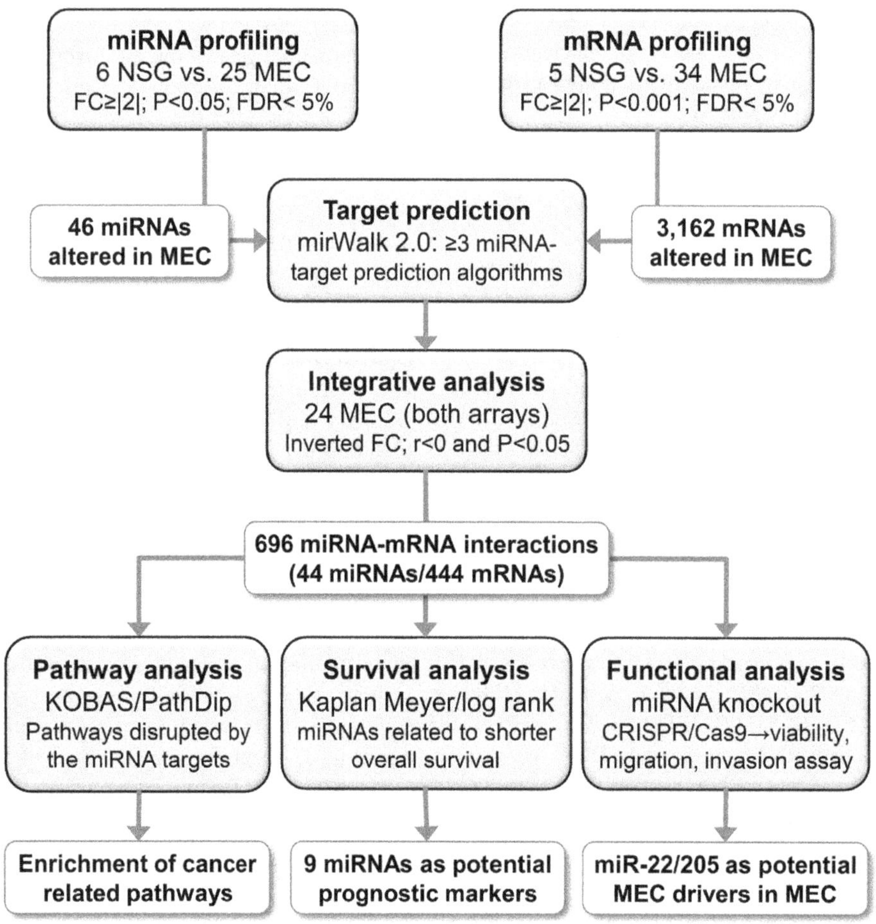

FIGURE 1 | Study design and main results obtained from the miRNA and mRNA expression analyses. First, a miRNA and mRNA global expression analyses revealed 46 miRNAs and 3,162 mRNAs differentially expressed in MEC compared to SNG. An integrative analysis was carried out using predicted miRNA-mRNA interactions, generating a network containing 44 miRNAs and 444 mRNAs (696 interactions). The target genes were associated with cancer-related pathways, and nine miRNAs were associated with shorter overall survival. A knockout assay was performed for miR-22 and miR-205 (CRISPR/Cas9), resulting in viability, migration, and invasion reduction, which indicate their role as putative cancer drivers in MEC.

and 28 underexpressed) in MEC (**Supplementary Table S2**). The most significant (P adjusted ≤ 0.005) overexpressed miRNAs included miR-21-5p (FC=10.2), miR-22-3p (FC=2.0), miR-181a-5p (FC=2.9), miR-205-3p (FC=14.7), and miR-224-3p (FC=5.3). The miR-363-3p (FC =-16.3), miR-625-5p (FC =-18.5), miR-885-5p (FC =-10.7), miR-892b (FC =-2.7), and miR-1288-3p (FC =-2.7) were significantly underexpressed (**Figure 2**). A similar approach used for mRNAs unveiled 3,162 mRNAs differentially expressed in MEC (1,488 overexpressed and 1,674 underexpressed (**Supplementary Table S3**).

Supervised hierarchical clustering analysis based on the DE transcripts revealed two clusters in both miRNA (**Figure 3A**) and mRNA (**Figure 3B**). Although these two main clusters completely separated MEC from NSG samples, no association was observed when comparing the clinical-pathological parameters (histological grade, lymph node involvement, and distant metastasis) with the clusters generated by both miRNA and mRNA analysis.

The miRNA-target prediction analysis resulted in 20,816 miRNA-mRNA putative interactions. The integrative analysis revealed a miRNA-mRNA network comprising 696 negatively correlated interactions and inverted FCs (44 miRNAs and 444 mRNAs) (**Supplementary Table S4**). The main biological pathways uncovered by miRNA targets corroborated by the integrative analysis were cell signaling, cell cycle, and cancer-related pathways (**Table 2**).

Lower expression levels of miR-582-5p, miR-3125, and miR-4324 were found in high-grade MEC compared to low and intermediate grades (**Supplementary Figure S3**). Increased expression levels of miR-205-5p and miR-224-5p (both overexpressed in MEC) and decreased expression levels of miR-139-3p, miR-145-3p, miR-148a-3p, miR-186-5p, miR-338-3p, miR-363-3p and miR-4324 were significantly related to worse overall survival in MEC patients (**Figure 4**).

Among the list of differentially expressed miRNAs, we selected miR-22 and miR-205 for functional assays for the following reasons: they were significantly overexpressed (adjuscted p-value <0.005) (**Figure 2**), presented high interactivity in the integrative analysis (>10 underexpressed mRNA predicted targets negatively correlated with the miRNA expression) (**Supplementary Table S4**), and showed clinical association with worse prognosis (increased miR-205 expression was associated with shorter overall survival) (**Figure 4**).

Knockout of miR-205 Decreases MEC Cell Viability While the Knockout of miR-22 Reduces MEC Cell Migration and Invasion

We explored the use of the CRISPR-Cas9-based method to knockout miR-22 and miR-205 in MEC. Cell viability, migration, and invasion assays were performed in the MEC cell line UM-HMC-2. The cell viability was the lowest in the miR-205 knockout, followed by miR-22-knockout cells, but with no statistical significance (**Figure 5A**).

The scratch wound migration assay showed that miR-22 and miR-205 knockouts reduced cell migration. The effect was the same in both knockout cell lines compared to the empty vector, but miR-22-knockout cells migrated significantly slower than the control cells (**Figures 5B–D** and **Supplementary Figure S4A**). The cell lines showed different invasion speeds, and the knockouts invaded slower in both scratch wound invasion (**Figures 5E–F** and **Supplementary Figure S4A**) and spheroid invasion assays (**Figures 5G–K** and **Supplementary Figure S4B**). Both miR-22 and miR-205 knockout cell lines invaded slower than the cell line with empty gRNA vectors. However, the effect was statistically significant only when miR-22-knockout cells were compared to the empty vector in the spheroid invasion assay.

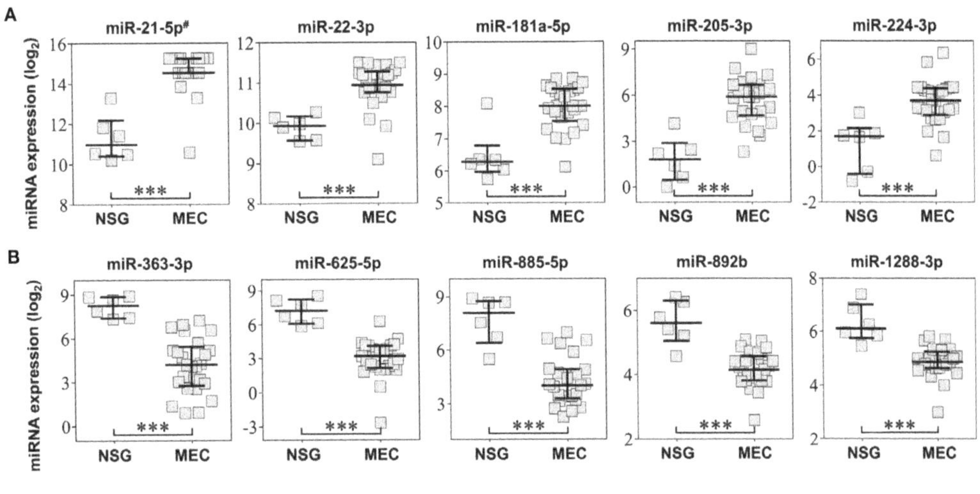

FIGURE 2 | Top five most significant overexpressed **(A)** and underexpressed **(B)** miRNAs obtained in the microarray analysis. The error bars and middle line represent the interquartile range and median, respectively. NSG: surrounding normal salivary gland tissues; MEC: mucoepidermoid carcinoma tissues. #miR-21-3p was omitted (both mature sequence from miR-21 precursor were highly significant). ***P < 0.001 (t test).

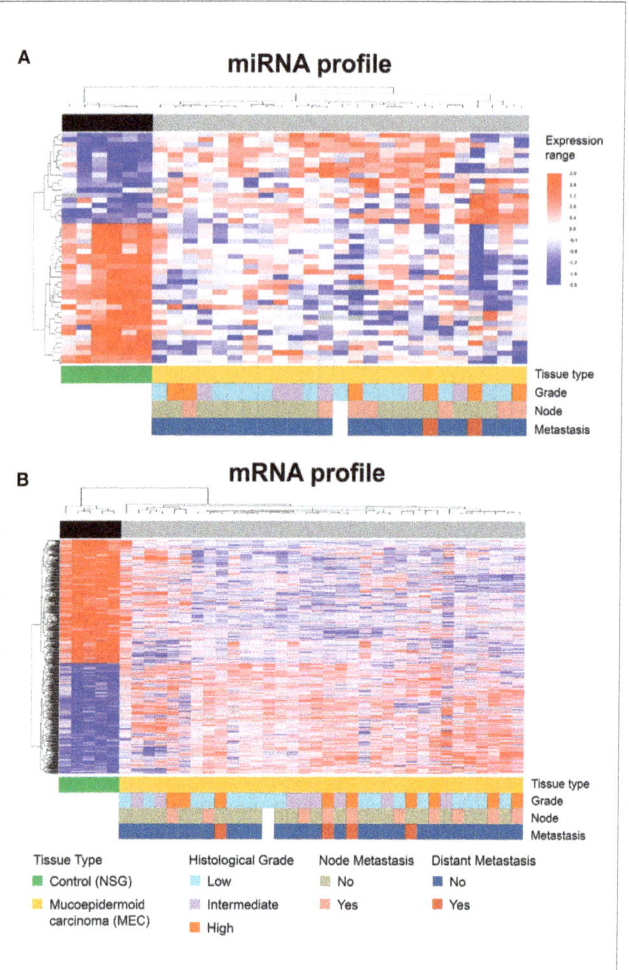

FIGURE 3 | Supervised hierarchical clustering analysis considering the miRNA **(A)** and mRNA **(B)** expression profiles. The dendrograms show a complete separation between MEC and NSG samples according to the 47 miRNAs **(A)** and 3,162 mRNA differentially expressed **(B)**. The samples are represented in columns and miRNAs/genes in rows.

Knockout of miR-22 Induces ESR1 and Knockout of miR-205 Induces ZEB2 Expression

In order to understand the mechanism behind the effect of miR-22 and miR-205 knockout on MEC cell behaviour, we studied the expression of specific molecules: *PTEN, LAMC1, CADM1, HER3, MYCBP, SNAI1, YAP1, CD147, SMAD4, ESR1* and *ZEB2* which, based on the literature, are known to be targets either for miR-22 or miR-205. We reported significant differences in two of the targets: estrogen receptor alpha (*ESR1*) for miR-22 and zinc finger E-box-binding homeobox 2 (*ZEB2*) and miR-205 (**Figure 6**). These molecules influence cell proliferation, migration and invasion (34–36). As expected, miR-22 knockout cells have significantly higher expression of *ESR1*, and miR-205 knockout cells have significantly higher expression of *ZEB2* compared with the empty vector.

DISCUSSION

Varied clinical behavior and multiple histologic grading systems have challenged pathologists in prognostication of MEC and clinicians in making an appropriate treatment decision for the patients (37). Moreover, the differential diagnosis between a salivary gland MEC and other lesions, such as salivary duct cyst, cystadenoma, or glandular odontogenic cyst may be difficult in some situations. In particular, small incisional biopsies are often problematic in the diagnostic workup. The presence of the *CRTC1-MAML2* fusion gene can be helpful for the diagnosis of MEC, but it is not found in all cases of MEC, and there is contradiction about some benign conditions (38–40). Mucoepidermoid carcinomas of the salivary gland are poorly explored at the molecular level. Therefore, genetic studies can unravel diagnostic, prognostic, and predictive markers, as reported in several tumor types.

TABLE 2 | Biological pathways enriched (P value < 0.001 and P adjusted < 0.05) by the genes detected in the miRNA-mRNA integrative analysis (KOBAS 3.0 and Pathdip *in silico* pathway tools).

Biological Pathways	Database	KOBAS 3.0		Pathdip*	
		P value	P adj	P value	P adj
Signal Transduction	Reactome	4E-12	4E-09	6E-05	8E-03
Post-translational protein modification	Reactome	1E-08	4E-06	2E-04	1E-02
Membrane Trafficking	Reactome	2E-07	2E-05	5E-04	2E-02
Diseases of signal transduction	Reactome	3E-06	2E-04	9E-05	8E-03
Signaling by Rho GTPases	Reactome	8E-06	4E-04	1E-04	1E-02
EPH-Ephrin signaling	Reactome	2E-05	8E-04	9E-05	8E-03
Cell Cycle	Reactome	2E-05	9E-04	4E-05	9E-03
RHO GTPase Effectors	Reactome	3E-05	1E-03	8E-06	3E-03
Proteoglycans in cancer	KEGG	2E-04	4E-03	5E-05	8E-03
Cell Cycle, Mitotic	Reactome	2E-04	4E-03	2E-04	1E-02
DNA Double-Strand Break Repair	Reactome	2E-04	5E-03	1E-03	3E-02
EPH-ephrin mediated repulsion of cells	Reactome	4E-04	8E-03	6E-04	2E-02
MicroRNAs in cancer	KEGG	9E-04	1E-02	6E-05	7E-03

*KEGG, Kyoto Encyclopedia of Genes and Genomes; *Experimentally detected protein-protein interactions.*

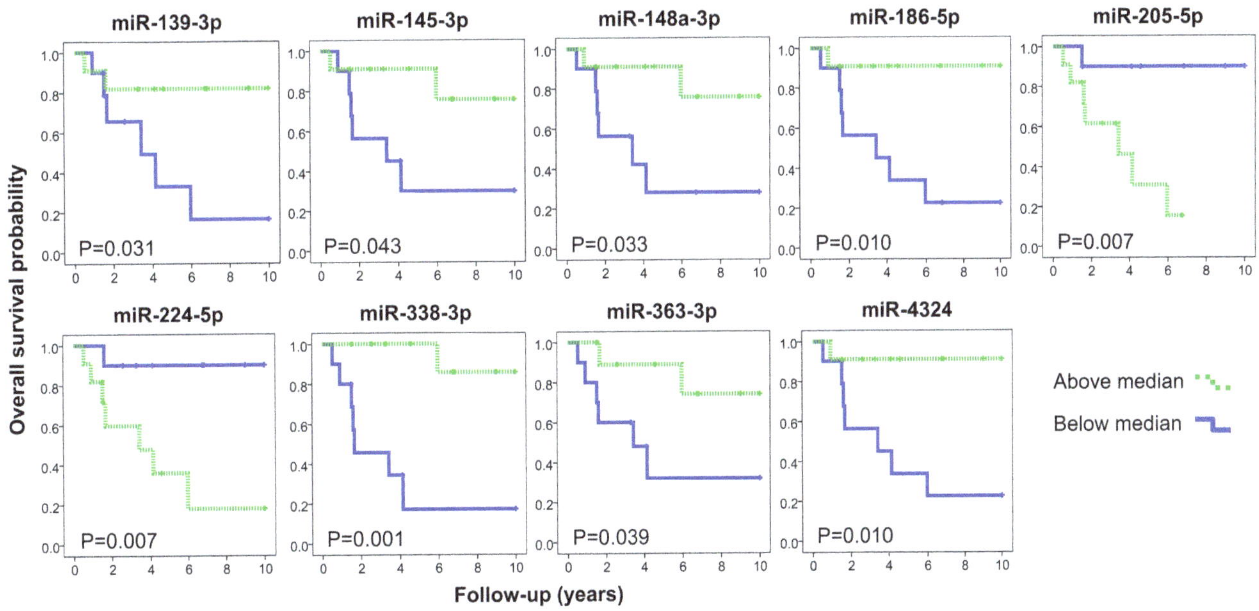

FIGURE 4 | Kaplan-Meier representation of overall survival according to the expression levels of nine miRNAs (log rank test P<0.05). The quantifications obtained by the microarray analysis were stratified in below (blue) and above (green) the median values. Note: miR-224-3p was omitted (both mature sequences from mir-224 precursor were associated with overall survival).

In the present study using large-scale expression analyses, we found 46 miRNAs and 3,162 mRNAs differentially expressed compared to normal salivary glands. In agreement with our present miRNA findings, a previous MEC study reported that miRNA-205 and miRNA-22 were amongst the highest overexpressed miRNAs in MEC, while miRNA-885-5p and miRNA-375 were downregulated (26).

Two earlier studies have investigated global gene expression in MEC (22, 23), but none of the genes reported were found in our analysis. A possible explanation for this discordance may be the small number of MEC cases (2 and 6) investigated in the earlier studies and/or the different methodological strategies. For instance, Leivo et al. (22) focused on comparing different histological types of salivary gland malignancies, which might explain the disparities compared with our findings.

Although we could not investigate the *CRTC1-MAML2* status in our sample set due to a lack of sample material, we observed a decreased *CRTC1* expression level. In MEC, the *CRTC1-MAML2* gene fusion activates *CREB/Cyclic* AMP related genes and possibly the Notch pathway (11, 41–45). Recently, Chen et al. (2021) (46) suggested that deregulated *p16-CDK4/6-RB* signaling is a cooperating event in the progression of MEC with the *CRTC1-MAML2* fusion. The authors also suggested that *EGFR* and *CDK4/6* inhibitors are potentially useful to treat MEC patients.

An integrative analysis was conducted to elucidate the role of miRNAs and their mRNA targets and the core genes and pathways involved in MEC. We found 669 miRNA-mRNA interactions (44 miRNAs and 444 mRNAs) involving cancer-related pathways such as miRNAs in cancer, cell cycle and signal transduction, ERK/MAPK signaling, EIF2 signaling, PI3K/AKT, among others. These findings provide supportive evidence for the detection of drivers involved in MEC pathogenesis. A set of these transcripts was associated with poor prognostic features, such as high histological grade. For instance, a decreased expression of miR-582-5p in MEC was related to high-grade tumors. Previously, miRNA-582-5p downregulation was described in salivary gland tumors (47, 48), and its induction inhibited invasion and migration in salivary adenoid cystic carcinoma (AdCC) (48). We found that the target of this miRNA, *EZH2*, was overexpressed and related to high-grade MEC (**Supplementary Table S4** and **Supplementary Figure S3**). *EZH2* is a member of the polycomb group of proteins involved with transcription regulation through chromatin remodeling (49). Increased EZH2 protein expression has been reported in MEC, myoepithelial carcinoma of salivary glands, and AdCC (50–52). In AdCC, increased EZH2 expression was associated with a worse prognosis.

Significantly decreased miR-4324 expression was detected in our high-grade MEC compared to low/intermediate-grade tumors, and it was also associated with shorter overall survival. miR-4324 has been shown to be underexpressed in a subset of *PTEN* deficient breast cancer patients with exceedingly poor prognoses (53). *PIK3CA* and *PTEN* inactivating mutations are frequent events in high-grade MEC (54). Interestingly, a highly predicted interaction between miR-205-3p and *PLAC8* from the PI3K pathway was observed in our integrative analysis. A recent study demonstrated that *PLAC8* contributes to cell proliferation and suppresses cell apoptosis in breast cancer by activating the PI3K/AKT/NF-κB pathway (55).

Based on established criteria, including increased expression levels, high interactivity in the integrative analysis, and

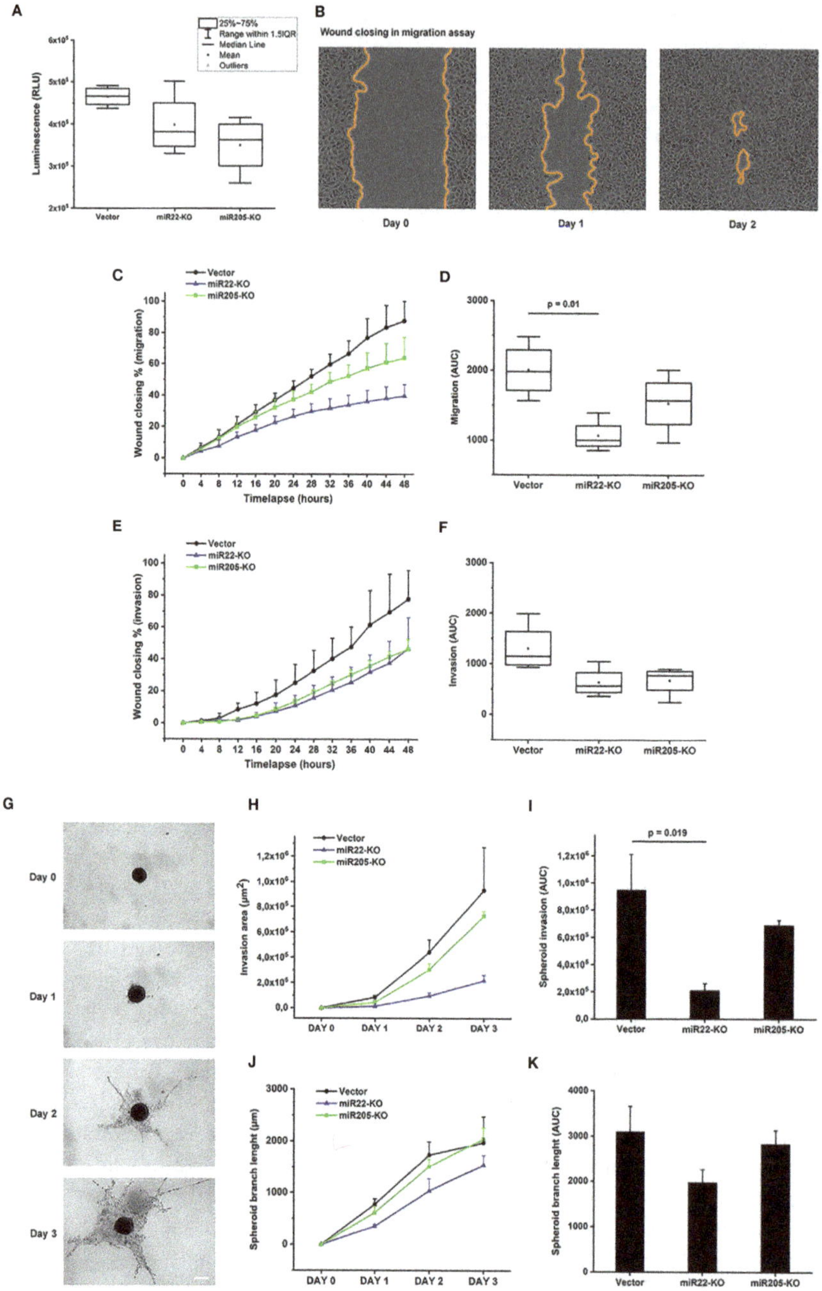

FIGURE 5 | Cell viability, migration and invasion assays performed using the UM-HMC-2 cell line. **(A)** UM-HMC-2 cells were cultured for three days and the cell viability was measured using luminescent cell viability assay. Although not statistically significant, the cell viability was decreased in both miR22- and miR205-knockout cell lines compared to the cell line transfected with an empty plasmid vector. **(B–D)** UM-HMC-2 cells were cultured on Myogel matrix and cell migration was evaluated using scratch wound cell migration assay. **(B)** Representative image of migration distance at 0, 24, and 48 hours after wounding. **(C, D)** Quantification of cell migration in scratch wound assay. miR22- and miR205-knockout cell lines migrated slower than the vector cell line. Statistically significant difference was denoted between vector and miR22-KO cell lines. **(E, F)** UM-HMC-2 cell invasion through Myogel-collagen in scratch wound cell invasion assay. UM-HMC-2 cells were cultured in Myogel-collagen matrix, and cell invasion was evaluated using scratch wound cell invasion assay. miR22- and miR205-knockout cell lines invaded slower than vector cell line (p-value > 0.05). **(G–K)** UM-HMC-2 cell invasion through Myogel-fibrin in spheroid invasion assay. Cells were cultured in U-shaped ultra-low attachment 96-well plate wells and embedded in Myogel-fibrin matrix. Spheroids were observed under a light microscope and the invasion area and the spheroid branch length were analyzed using ilastik and ImageJ software. **(G)** Representative images of spheroid invasion at different time points. Scale bar = 200 μm (Original magnification X4). **(H, I)** Quantification of cell invasion in 3D spheroid invasion assay. Knockout of miR22 and miR205 reduced tumor cell invasion. Difference between vector and miR22-KO cell lines reached statistical significance. **(J, K)** Quantification of spheroid branch length revealed that miR22- and miR205-knockout cell line spheroids did not extend as far as vector cell line (p-value > 0.05). Data are presented as means ± SD of 3-4 independent experiments, each at least in triplicate. $p < 0.05$ is considered as significantly different compared to vector control.

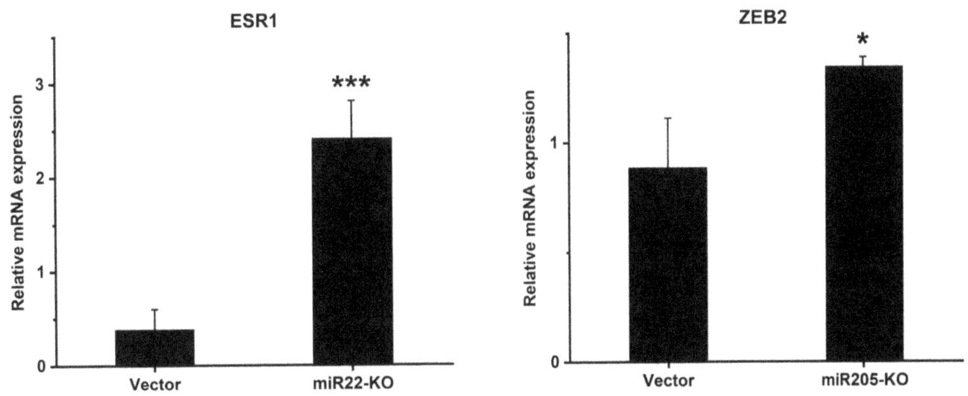

FIGURE 6 | mRNA expression levels of selected genes after miR-knockout. Expression levels of *ESR1* in miR22-KO and *ZEB2* in miR205-KO cell lines were analysed using qRT-PCR. The relative mRNA levels are shown after normalization to GAPDH. *ESR1*, Estrogen receptor alpha; *ZEB2*, Zinc finger E-box binding homeobox 2. Data are presented as means ± SD. $^*p \leq 0.05$, $^{***} \leq 0.001$.

association with clinical parameters, we selected two miRNAs, miR-205 and miR-22, for functional assays. These two miRNAs were among the highest overexpressed miRNAs in previously described MEC cases (26). miR-205 was one of the most significantly overexpressed miRNAs, and it was associated with shorter overall survival in our MEC cases. Overexpression of this miRNA has been reported in several cancers, including AdCC and head and neck squamous cell carcinomas (56–58). A previous study suggested that miR-205-5p targets *PTEN* to regulate the epithelial mesenchymal transition through the PI3K/AKT pathway (58).

Since miR-22 was one of the highest overexpressed miRNAs in MEC, it was selected for knockdown and functional experiments. Dysregulation of this miRNA has been reported in several tumor types (59) and implicated in the regulation of cell growth, cell cycle, apoptosis, and invasion (60, 61). *MYC* and *PI3K/AKT* can induce miR-22 gene expression, which in turn targets *PTEN* (62). Since PTEN is a repressor of AKT, miR-22 could act as a key element in a positive feedback of the *PI3K/AKT* pathway to cause downregulation of *PTEN* (59). As previously described in MEC (13), this miRNA also induces chromosomal instability (63). Knockdown of miR-22 showed a consistent reduction of viability, migration, and invasion of MEC cells. However, the effect on migration and invasion was stronger and seems not to be as a result of reduced viability which was only mild and not significant.

Previous studies have reported that miR-22 represses *ESR1* expression in breast cancer and lead to a reduction in estrogen signaling (34). In line with that, we showed that the miRNA-22 knockout increased *ESR1* expression levels. *ZEB2* was reported to negatively correlate with miR-205 levels in esophageal squamous cell carcinoma cells (35) and silencing of *ZEB2* lead to suppressed cell viability, migration, and invasion in laryngeal squamous cell carcinoma cells (36). Our data showed an upregulation of *ZEB2* in miR-205-knockout cells which is in line with the reports above. Additionally, *ZEB2* has been shown to directly bind to the E-cadherin promoter and repress its transcription (64). Loss of E-cadherin is one of the main initiation events of epithelial to mesenchymal transition (EMT) and thus plays an important role in cancer progression. The biological mechanism behind these actions remains to be elucidated in future studies.

CONCLUSION

Although we investigated a limited number of cases, we described a transcriptomic profile distinguishing MEC from normal salivary glands. The integrative analysis highlighted miRNA-mRNA interactions, and cancer-related pathways were described. Comparison with other studies using similar strategies was limited due to the absence of available miRNA-mRNAs expression data in public databases. However, our list of differentially expressed miRNAs-mRNAs revealed that PTEN and PI3K/AKT pathways were altered in MEC. Our *in vitro* functional assays indicate that miR-22 and miR-205 deficiencies reduce cell viability, migration, and invasion in a MEC cell line by enhancing the expression of *ZEB2* and *ESR1* mRNAs. Taken together, our findings suggest that these dysregulated miRNAs have a pathogenic role in MEC.

ETHICS STATEMENT

The studies involving human participants were reviewed and approved by The National Human Research Ethics Committee (Protocol #1.380.762/2015). Written informed consent to participate in this study was provided by the participants' legal guardian/next of kin.

AUTHOR CONTRIBUTIONS

Study concept and design: FP-S, TS, and SR. Data Acquisition:

EN, MB-F, HK, KT, and AB. Quality control and data algorithms: MB-F, SA, FM, IS, and SL. Data analysis and interpretation: FP-S, EN, MB-F, and FM. Statistical analysis: MB-F, SA, FM, and IS. Manuscript preparation: FP-S and EN. Manuscript editing: EN, FP-S, TS, and SR. Manuscript review: CS-N, RC, LK, AM, VA, IL, TS, SR, and AA-S. All authors contributed to the article and approved the submitted version.

ACKNOWLEDGMENTS

The authors would like to acknowledge Barretos Cancer Hospital and A.C.Camargo Cancer Center, SP, Brazil, for providing human specimens. The authors acknowledge the FIMM Sequencing Unit, Institute for Molecular Medicine Finland and DDCB core facility (FIMM High Throughput Biomedicine Unit), University of Helsinki, for technical support and Biostatistics Unit, University of Helsinki, for their biostatistical assistance. We would like to thank Annamari Arpalahti and Tapio Flinck for their technical assistance, and Dr. Clovis Antonio Lopes Pinto and Dr. Claudia Malheiros Coutinho Camillo for their help with sample collection.

SUPPLEMENTARY MATERIAL

Supplementary Figure S1 | Bootstrap analysis to estimate the cluster stability. B = 1000 bootstraps conducted with pvclust package (R program).

Supplementary Figure S2 | (A) CRISPR knockout efficiency and indel spectrum. The predicted effect of the CRISPR-editing on miRNAs was assessed using TIDE online tool by The Netherlands Cancer Institute, Amsterdam, Netherlands (https://tide.nki.nl/).

qRT-PCR assay reveals down-regulation of miR-22-3p ($p < 0.008$) and miR-205-5p ($p < 0.004$) expression in knockout cells compared to vector control.

Supplementary Figure S3 | Differentially expressed miRNAs according to the histological grade. miR-582-5p (FC= -5.1; P=0.0001; FDR =0.0066), miR-4324 (FC= -3.7, P=0.0019, FDR=0.0305) and miR-3125 (FC=-2.1, P=0.0031, FDR=0.0305) were all underexpressed in high-grade mucoepidermoid salivary gland carcinoma compared to low/intermediate grade. ***P < 0.001, **P < 0.01 (t test).

Supplementary Figure S4 | UM-HMC-2 cell migration and invasion assays. **(B)** Representative images of UM-HMC-2 cell migration and invasion distance at 0, 24, and 48 hours in wound scratch wound assay. **(B)** Representative images of UM-HMC-2 cell invasion through Myogel-fibrin in spheroid invasion assay at different time points. Scale bar = 200 µm (original magnification X4).

Supplementary Table S1 | Primers used in this study. Oligonucleotide pairs for construction of gRNA expression plasmids, primer sequences used to amplify the target site before the Sanger sequencing and primers for target gene qRT-PCR (F, forward; R, reverse).

Supplementary Table S2 | Differentially expressed miRNA in salivary gland **(A)** Mucoepidermoid carcinoma (MEC) compared to normal salivary gland (NSG) tissues.

Supplementary Table S3 | Differentially expressed mRNAs in MEC compared to non-neoplastic salivary gland tissues (excel file).

Supplementary Table S4 | MicroRNA and target-mRNA interactions retrieved from the integrative analysis, comprising the transcripts differentially expressed in MEC (excel file).

REFERENCES

1. Brandwein-Gensler M, Bell D, Inagaki H, Katabi N, Leivo I, Seethala R, et al. "Mucoepidemoid Carcinoma". In: AK El-Naggar, JKC Chan, J Grandis, T Takata, PJ Slootweg, editors. *WHO Classification of Head and Neck Tumors.* (2017) Lyon: IARC Press. p. 163–4.
2. Aro K, Leivo I, Mäkitie AA. Management and Outcome of Patients With Mucoepidermoid Carcinoma of Major Salivary Gland Origin: A Single Institution's 30-Year Experience. *Laryngoscope* (2008) 118:258–62. doi: 10.1097/MLG.0b013e31815a6b0b
3. Nance MA, Seethala RR, Wang Y, Chiosea SI, Myers EN, Johnson JT, et al. Treatment and Survival Outcomes Based on Histologic Grading in Patients With Head and Neck Mucoepidermoid Carcinoma. *Cancer* (2008) 113:2082–9. doi: 10.1002/cncr.23825
4. Auclair PL, Goode RK, Ellis GL. Mucoepidermoid Carcinoma of Intraoral Salivary Glands Evaluation and Application of Grading Criteria in 143 Cases. *Cancer* (1992) 69:2021–30. doi: 10.1002/1097-0142(19920415)69:8<2021::AID-CNCR2820690803>3.0.CO;2-7
5. Seethala RR. An Update on Grading of Salivary Gland Carcinomas. *Head Neck Pathol* (2009) 3:69–77. doi: 10.1007/s12105-009-0102-9
6. Brandwein MS, Ivanov K, Wallace DI, Hille JJ, Wang B, Fahmy A, et al. Mucoepidermoid Carcinoma: A Clinicopathologic Study of 80 Patients With Special Reference to Histological Grading. *Am J Surg Pathol* (2001) 25:835–45. doi: 10.1097/00000478-200107000-00001
7. Lau VH, Aoaud R, Farwell G, Donald PJ, Chen AM. Patterns of Nodal Involvement for Clinically N0 Saliavry Gland Carcinoma: Refining the Role of Elective Neck Irradiation. *Head Neck* (2014) 36:1435–9. doi: 10.1002/HED.23467
8. Moss WJ, Coffey CS, Brumund KT, Weisman RA. What is the Role of Elective Neck Dissection in Low-, Intermediate-, and High-Grade Mucoepidermoid Carcinoma? *Laryngoscope* (2016) 126:11–3. doi: 10.1002/lary.25588
9. Nobis CP, Rohleder NH, Wolff KD, Wagenpfeil S, Scherer EQ, Kesting MR. Head and Neck Salivary Gland Carcinomas - Elective Neck Dissection, Yes or No? *J Oral Maxillofac Surg* (2014) 72:205–10. doi: 10.1016/j.joms.2013.05.024
10. Shafique K, Zhang PJ, Montone KT, Song S, Livolsi VA, Baloch Z. Pathologic Grading of Mucoepidermoid Carcinomas of the Salivary Gland and Its Effect on Clinicopathologic Follow-Up: An Institutional Experience. *Hum Pathol* (2020) 98:89–97. doi: 10.1016/j.humpath.2020.02.001
11. Tonon G, Modi S, Wu L, Kubo A, Coxon AB, Komiya T, et al. T(11;19)(Q21; P13) Translocation in Mucoepidermoid Carcinoma Creates a Novel Fusion Product That Disrupts a Notch Signaling Pathway. *Nat Genet* (2003) 33:208–13. doi: 10.1038/ng1083
12. Tirado Y, Williams MD, Hanna EY, Kaye FJ, Batsakis JG, El-Naggar AK. CRTC1/MAML2 Fusion Transcript in High Grade Mucoepidermoid Carcinomas of Salivary and Thyroid Glands and Warthin's Tumors: Implications for Histogenesis and Biologic Behavior. *Genes Chromosomes Cancer* (2007) 46:708–15. doi: 10.1002/gcc.20458
13. Jee KJ, Persson M, Heikinheimo K, Passador-Santos F, Aro K, Knuutila S, et al. Genomic Profiles and CRTC1-MAML2 Fusion Distinguish Different Subtypes of Mucoepidermoid Carcinoma. *Mod Pathol* (2013) 26:213–22. doi: 10.1038/modpathol.2012.154
14. Saade RE, Bell D, Garcia J, Roberts D, Weber R. Role of CRTC1/MAML2 Translocation in the Prognosis and Clinical Outcomes of Mucoepidermoid Carcinoma. *JAMA Otolaryngol Head Neck Surg* (2016) 142:234–40. doi: 10.1001/jamaoto.2015.3270
15. Luk PP, Wykes J, Selinger CI, Ekmejian R, Tay J, Gao K, et al. Diagnostic and Prognostic Utility of Mastermind-Like 2 (MAML2) Gene Rearrangement Detection by Fluorescent *In Situ* Hybridization (FISH) in Mucoepidermoid Carcinoma of the Salivary Glands. *Oral Surg Oral Med Oral Pathol Oral Radiol* (2016) 121:530–41. doi: 10.1016/j.oooo.2016.01.003

16. Verdorfer I, Fehr A, Bullerdiek J, Scholz N, Brunner A, Krugman J, et al. Chromosomal Imbalances, 11q21 Rearrangement and MECT1-MAML2 Fusion Transcript in Mucoepidermoid Carcinomas of the Salivary Gland. *Oncol Rep* (2009) 22:305–11. doi: 10.3892/or_00000438
17. Seethala RR, Dacic S, Cieply K, Kelly LM, Nikiforova MN. A Reappraisal of the MECT1/MAML2 Translocation in Salivary Mucoepidermoid Carcinomas. *Am J Surg Pathol* (2010) 34:1106–21. doi: 10.1097/PAS.0b013e3181de3021
18. Behboudi A, Enlund F, Winnes M, Andrén Y, Nordkvist A, Leivo I, et al. Molecular Classification of Mucoepidermoid Carcinomas-Prognostic Significance of the MECT1-MAML2 Fusion Oncogene. *Genes Chromosomes Cancer* (2006) 45:470–81. doi: 10.1002/gcc.20306
19. Okabe M, Miyabe S, Nagatsuka H, Terada A, Hanai N, Yokoi M, et al. MECT1-MAML2 Fusion Transcript Defines a Favorable Subset of Mucoepidermoid Carcinoma. *Clin Cancer Res* (2006) 12:3902–7. doi: 10.1158/1078-0432.CCR-05-2376
20. Okumura Y, Nakano S, Murase T, Ueda K, Kawakita D, Nagao T, et al. Prognostic Impact of CRTC1/3-MAML2 Fusions in Salivary Gland Mucoepidermoid Carcinoma: A Multiinstitutional Retrospective Study. *Cancer Sci* (2020) 111:4195–204. doi: 10.1111/cas.14632
21. Seethala RR, Chiosea SI. MAML2 Status in Mucoepidermoid Carcinoma Can No Longer Be Considered a Prognostic Marker. *Am J Surg Pathol* (2016) 40:1151–3. doi: 10.1097/PAS.0000000000000676
22. Leivo I, Jee KJ, Heikinheimo K, Laine M, Ollila J, Nagy B, et al. Characterization of Gene Expression in Major Types of Salivary Gland Carcinomas With Epithelial Differentiation. *Cancer Genet Cytogenet* (2005) 156:104–13. doi: 10.1016/j.cancergencyto.2004.04.016
23. Francioso F, Carinci F, Tosi L, Scapoli L, Pezzetti F, Passerella E, et al. Identification of Differentially Expressed Genes in Human Salivary Gland Tumors by DNA Microarrays. *Mol Cancer Ther* (2002) 1:533–8.
24. Flores B de CT de CP, Lourenço SV, Damascena AS, Kowaslki LP, Soares FA, Coutinho-Camillo CM. Altered Expression of Apoptosis-Regulating miRNAs in Salivary Gland Tumors Suggests Their Involvement in Salivary Gland Tumorigenesis. *Virchows Arch* (2017) 470:291–9. doi: 10.1007/s00428-016-2049-z
25. Santos PRB, Coutinho-Camillo CM, Soares FA, Freitas VS, Vilas-Bôas DS, Xavier FCA, et al. MicroRNAs Expression Pattern Related to Mast Cell Activation and Angiogenesis in Paraffin-Embedded Salivary Gland Tumors. *Pathol Res Pract* (2017) 213:1470–6. doi: 10.1016/j.prp.2017.10.012
26. Binmadi N, Basile J, Perez P, Gallo A, Tandon M, Elias W, et al. miRNA Expression Profile of Mucoepidermoid Carcinoma. *Oral Dis* (2018) 24:537–43. doi: 10.1111/odi.12800
27. Lapa RML, Barros-Filho MC, Marchi FA, Domingues MAC, de Carvalho GB, Drigo SA, et al. Integrated miRNA and mRNA Expression Analysis Uncovers Drug Targets in Laryngeal Squamous Cell Carcinoma Patients. *Oral Oncol* (2019) 93:76–84. doi: 10.1016/j.oraloncology.2019.04.018
28. Huang HY, Lin YCD, Li J, Huang KY, Shrestha S, Hong HC, et al. MiRTarBase 2020: Updates to the Experimentally Validated microRNA-Target Interaction Database. *Nucleic Acids Res* (2020) 48:D148–54. doi: 10.1093/nar/gkz896
29. Warner KA, Adams A, Bernardi L, Nor C, Finkel KA, Zhang Z, et al. Characterization of Tumorigenic Cell Lines From the Recurrence and Lymph Node Metastasis of a Human Salivary Mucoepidermoid Carcinoma. *Oral Oncol* (2013) 49:1059–66. doi: 10.1016/j.oraloncology.2013.08.004
30. Ran AF, Hsu PD, Wright J, Agarwala V, Scott DA, Zhang F. Genome Engineering Using CRISPR-Cas9 System. *Nat Protoc* (2013) 8:2281–308. doi: 10.1038/nprot.2013.143
31. Salo T, Sutinen M, Hoque Apu E, Sundquist E, Cervigne NK, de Oliveira CE, et al. A Novel Human Leiomyoma Tissue Derived Matrix for Cell Culture Studies. *BMC Cancer* (2015) 15:1. doi: 10.1186/s12885-015-1944-z
32. Naakka E, Tuomainen K, Wistrand H, Palkama M, Suleymanova I, Al-Samadi A, et al. Fully Human Tumor-Based Matrix in Three-Dimensional Spheroid Invasion Assay. *J Vis Exp* (2019) 2019:1–7. doi: 10.3791/59567
33. Schindelin J, Arganda-Carrera I, Frise E, Verena K, Mark L, Tobias P, et al. Fiji - An Open Platform for Biological Image Analysis. *Nat Methods* (2012) 9:676–82. doi: 10.1038/nmeth.2019.Fiji
34. Pandey DP, Picard D. miR-22 Inhibits Estrogen Signaling by Directly Targeting the Estrogen Receptor α mRNA. *Mol Cell Biol* (2009) 29:3783–90. doi: 10.1128/MCB.01875-08
35. Matsushima K, Isomoto H, Yamaguchi N, Inoue N, Machida H, Nakayama T, et al. MiRNA-205 Modulates Cellular Invasion and Migration *via* Regulating Zinc Finger E-Box Binding Homeobox 2 Expression in Esophageal Squamous Cell Carcinoma Cells. *J Transl Med* (2011) 9:30. doi: 10.1186/1479-5876-9-30
36. Li Q, Ma L, Wu Z, Wang G, Huang Q, Shen Z, et al. Zinc Finger E–box Binding Homeobox 2 Functions as an Oncogene in Human Laryngeal Squamous Cell Carcinoma. *Mol Med Rep* (2019) 6:4545–52. doi: 10.3892/mmr.2019.10126
37. Cipriani NA, Lusardi JJ, Mcelherne J, Pearson AT, Olivas AD, Fitzpatrick C, et al. Mucoepidermoid Carcinoma: A Comparison of Histologic Grading Systems and Relationship to MAML2 Rearrangement and Prognosis. *Am J Surg Pathol* (2019) 43:885–97. doi: 10.1097/PAS.0000000000001252
38. Reddy R, Islam MN, Bhattacharyya I, Cohen DM, Fitzpatrick SG, Ganatra S. The Reliability of MAML2 Gene Rearrangement in Discriminating Between Histologically Similar Glandular Odontogenic Cysts and Intraosseous Mucoepidermoid Carcinomas. *Oral Surg Oral Med Oral Pathol Oral Radiol* (2019) 127:e136–47. doi: 10.1016/j.oooo.2018.12.003
39. Bishop JA, Yonescu R, Batista D, Warnock GR, Westra WH. Glandular Odontogenic Cysts (GOCs) Lack MAML2 Rearrangements: A Finding to Discredit the Putative Nature of GOC as a Precursor to Central Mucoepidermoid Carcinoma. *Head Neck Pathol* (2014) 8:287–90. doi: 10.1007/s12105-014-0534-8
40. Argyris PP, Wehrs RN, García JJ, Koutlas IG. Fluorescence *in-Situ* Hybridization Identifies Mastermind-Like 2 (MAML2) Rearrangement in Odontogenic Cysts With Mucous Prosoplasia: A Pilot Study. *Histopathology* (2015) 66:791–7. doi: 10.1111/his.12526
41. Conkright MD, Canettieri G, Screaton R, Guzman E, Miraglia L, Hogenesch JB, et al. TORCs: Transducers of Regulated CREB Activity. *Mol Cell* (2003) 12:413–23. doi: 10.1016/j.molcel.2003.08.013
42. Coxon A, Rozenblum E, Park YS, Joshi N, Tsurutani J, Dennis PA, et al. Mect1-Maml2 Fusion Oncogene Linked to the Aberrant Activation of Cyclic AMP/CREB Regulated Genes. *Cancer Res* (2005) 65:7137–44. doi: 10.1158/0008-5472.CAN-05-1125
43. Enlund F, Behboudi A, Andrén Y, Öberg C, Lendahl U, Mark J, et al. Altered Notch Signaling Resulting From Expression of a WAMTP1-MAML2 Gene Fusion in Mucoepidermoid Carcinomas and Benign Warthin's Tumors. *Exp Cell Res* (2004) 292:21–8. doi: 10.1016/j.yexcr.2003.09.007
44. Wu L, Liu J, Gao P, Nakamura M, Cao Y, Shen H, et al. Transforming Activity of MECT1-MAML2 Fusion Oncoprotein Is Mediated by Constitutive CREB Activation. *EMBO J* (2005) 24:2391–402. doi: 10.1038/sj.emboj.7600719
45. Chen J, Li JL, Chen Z, Griffin JD, Wu L. Gene Expression Profiling Analysis of CRTC1-MAML2 Fusion Oncogene-Induced Transcriptional Program in Human Mucoepidermoid Carcinoma Cells. *BMC Cancer* (2015) 15:1–13. doi: 10.1186/s12885-015-1827-3
46. Chen Z, Ni W, Li JL, Lin S, Zhou X, Sun Y, et al. The CRTC1-MAML2 Fusion Is the Major Oncogenic Driver in Mucoepidermoid Carcinoma. *JCI Insight* (2021) 6:1-18. doi: 10.1172/jci.insight.139497
47. Denaro M, Navari E, Ugolini C, Seccia V, Donati V, Casani AP, et al. A microRNA Signature for the Differential Diagnosis of Salivary Gland Tumors. *PLoS One* (2019) 14:1–16. doi: 10.1371/journal.pone.0210968
48. Wang WW, Chen B, Lei CB, Liu GX, Wang YG, Yi C, et al. miR-582-5p Inhibits Invasion and Migration of Salivary Adenoid Cystic Carcinoma Cells by Targeting FOXC1. *Jpn J Clin Oncol* (2017) 47:690–8. doi: 10.1093/jjco/hyx073
49. Kerppola TK. Polycomb Group Complexes - Many Combinations, Many Functions. *Trends Cell Biol* (2009) 19:692–704. doi: 10.1016/j.tcb.2009.10.001
50. Vékony H, Röser K, Löning T, Raaphorst FM, Leemans CR, van der Waal I, et al. Deregulated Expression of P16ink4a and P53 Pathway Members in Benign and Malignant Myoepithelial Tumours of the Salivary Glands. *Histopathology* (2008) 53:658–66. doi: 10.1111/j.1365-2559.2008.03184.x
51. Vékony H, Raaphorst FM, Otte AP, Van Lohuizen M, Leemans CR, van der Waal I, et al. High Expression of Polycomb Group Protein EZH2 Predicts Poor Survival in Salivary Gland Adenoid Cystic Carcinoma. *J Clin Pathol* (2008) 61:744–9. doi: 10.1136/jcp.2007.054262

52. Hajósi-Kalcakosz S, Vincze E, Dezso K, Paku S, Rókusz A, Sápi Z, et al. EZH2 Is a Sensitive Marker of Malignancy in Salivary Gland Tumors. *Diagn Pathol* (2015) 10:1–5. doi: 10.1186/s13000-015-0392-z
53. Wang DY, Gendoo DMA, Ben-David Y, Woodgett JR, Zacksenhaus E. A Subgroup of microRNAs Defines PTEN-Deficient, Triple-Negative Breast Cancer Patients With Poorest Prognosis and Alterations in RB1, MYC, and Wnt Signaling. *Breast Cancer Res* (2019) 21:1–13. doi: 10.1186/s13058-019-1098-z
54. Wang K, McDermott JD, Schrock AB, Elvin JA, Gay L, Karam SD, et al. Comprehensive Genomic Profiling of Salivary Mucoepidermoid Carcinomas Reveals Frequent BAP1, PIK3CA, and Other Actionable Genomic Alterations. *Ann Oncol* (2017) 28:748–53. doi: 10.1093/annonc/mdw689
55. Mao M, Chen Y, Jia Y, Yang J, Wei Q, Li Z, et al. PLCA8 Suppresses Breast Cancer Apoptosis by Activating the PI3k/AKT/NF-κb Pathway. *J Cell Mol Med* (2019) 23:6930–41. doi: 10.1111/jcmm.14578
56. Feng X, Matsuo K, Zhang T, Hu Y, Mays AC, Browne JD, et al. MicroRNA Profiling and Target Genes Related to Metastasis of Salivary Adenoid Cystic Carcinoma. *Anticancer Res* (2017) 37:3473–81. doi: 10.21873/anticanreS.11715
57. de Carvalho AC, Scapulatempo-Neto C, Maia DCC, Evangelista AF, Morini MA, Carvalho AL, et al. Accuracy of microRNAs as Markers for the Detection of Neck Lymph Node Metastases in Patients With Head and Neck Squamous Cell Carcinoma. *BMC Med* (2015) 13:1–14. doi: 10.1186/s12916-015-0350-3
58. Zhang P, Lu X, Shi Z, Li X, Zhang Y, Zhao S, et al. miR-205-5p Regulates Epithelial-Mesenchymal Transition by Targeting PTEN *via* PI3K/AKT Signaling Pathway in Cisplatin-Resistant Nasopharyngeal Carcinoma Cells. *Gene* (2019) 710:103–13. doi: 10.1016/j.gene.2019.05.058
59. Budd WT, Seashols-Williams SJ, Clark GC, Weaver D, Calvert V, Petricoin E, et al. Dual Action of miR-125b as a Tumor Suppressor and OncomiR-22 Promotes Prostate Cancer Tumorigenesis. *PLoS One* (2015) 10:1–21. doi: 10.1371/journal.pone.0142373
60. Tsuchiya N, Izumiya M, Ogata-Kawata H, Okamoto K, Fujiwara Y, Nakai M, et al. Tumor Suppressor miR-22 Determines P53-Dependent Cellular Fate Through Post-Transcriptional Regulation of P21. *Cancer Res* (2011) 71:4628–39. doi: 10.1158/0008-5472.CAN-10-2475
61. Xu D, Takeshita F, Hino Y, Fukunaga S, Kudo Y, Tamaki A, et al. miR-22 Represses Cancer Progression by Inducing Cellular Senescence. *J Cell Biol* (2011) 193:409–24. doi: 10.1083/jcb.201010100
62. Song SJ, Pandolfi PP. MiR-22 in Tumorigenesis. *Cell Cycle* (2014) 13:11–2. doi: 10.4161/cc.27027
63. Lee JH, Park SJ, Kim SW, Hariharasudhan G, Jung SM, Jun S, et al. C-Fos-Dependent miR-22 Targets MDC1 and Regulates DNA Repair in Terminally Differentiated Cells. *Oncotarget* (2017) 8:48204–21. doi: 10.18632/oncotarget.18389
64. Gregory PA, Bracken CP, Bert AG, Goodall GJ. MicroRNAs as Regulators of Epithelial-Mesenchymal Transition. *Cell Cycle* (2008) 7:3112–8. doi: 10.4161/cc.7.20.6851

11

Oncologic Outcomes of Patients with Sarcomatoid Carcinoma of the Hypopharynx

Liyuan Dai[1], *Qigen Fang*[1*†], *Peng Li*[1], *Fei Liu*[2] *and Xu Zhang*[1]

[1] *Department of Head Neck and Thyroid, Affiliated Cancer Hospital of Zhengzhou University, Henan Cancer Hospital, Zhengzhou, China,* [2] *Department of Oral Medicine, The First Affiliated Hospital of Zhengzhou University, Henan Cancer Hospital, Zhengzhou, China*

***Correspondence:**
Qigen Fang
qigenfang@126.com

†Present address:
Qigen Fang, Department of Head Neck and Thyroid, Affiliated Cancer Hospital of Zhengzhou University, Henan Cancer Hospital, Zhengzhou, China

Objectives: Sarcomatoid carcinoma (SaCa) of the hypopharynx is rare, and its clinical pathologic characteristics and prognosis remain unknown. Therefore, the study aimed to analyze the oncologic outcomes of patients with SaCa of the hypopharynx.

Methods: Patients with SaCa of the hypopharynx who were surgically treated in the period from January 1985 to December 2018 were enrolled from two clinical centers. A matched pair study was also performed, and each patient with SaCa of the hypopharynx was matched with one patient with squamous cell carcinoma (SCC) of the hypopharynx. The main study endpoint was disease-specific survival (DSS).

Results: A total of 62 patients (all male) were enrolled. Compared to patients with traditional SCC of the hypopharynx, patients with SaCa of the hypopharynx were older and had higher rates of perineural invasion, lymphovascular invasion and cancer cachexia. The 5-year DSS rate was 20% in patients with SaCa compared to 34% in patients in the matched group, and the difference was significant ($p = 0.016$). According to the univariate analysis, tumor stage, lymph node stage, disease stage, and cachexia were associated with DSS. According to the Cox model, neck lymph node metastasis and disease stage were independent predictors for worse DSS.

Conclusion: The prognosis of patients with SaCa of the hypopharynx is dismal, and this type of SaCa is associated with more aggressive biological behavior than traditional SCC of the hypopharynx; neck lymph neck node metastasis and disease stage were the most important predictors of DSS.

Keywords: sarcomatoid carcinoma, cancer of the hypopharynx, spindle cell carcinoma, head and neck spindle cell carcinoma, prognosis

INTRODUCTION

Since it was first reported by Virchow et al. (1) in 1864, sarcomatoid carcinoma (SaCa), a rare variant of squamous cell carcinoma (SCC), has been shown to be biphasic (2) and usually consists of both a conventional epithelial squamous cell component and a sarcomatous spindle cell component. Conventional SCC and sarcomatoid components have now been proven to arise monoclonally from a single stem cell (3–7). The disease is characterized by local recurrence and invasive growth, and is associated with poor prognosis. The tumor shows morphologic epithelial changes, where areas of squamous and spindle cell differentiation are observed (2–10).

The larynx is the most commonly involved site in SaCa of the head and neck region, followed by the oral cavity and hypopharynx (3). Cases of SaCa of the hypopharynx have only been described by a few authors (2, 3, 5–8, 11, 12); owing to the rarity of the disease, <50 cases have been reported, and detailed information regarding prognosis as well as prognostic factors for SaCa of the hypopharynx remain scarce. Therefore, we aimed to analyze the oncologic outcomes in SaCa of the hypopharynx by looking at outcomes occurring over a period of 30 years.

MATERIALS AND METHODS

The Zhengzhou University institutional research committee approved our study, all participants signed an informed consent agreement for medical research before initial treatment, and all experiments were performed in accordance with relevant guidelines and regulations.

The medical records of patients with primary spindle cell carcinoma or SaCa of the hypopharynx who were surgically treated from January 1985 to December 2018 were reviewed from two hospitals: Affiliated Cancer Hospital and The First Affiliated Hospital of Zhengzhou University. The two clinical centers had the same treatment principle for hypopharynx malignancies. Information regarding age, sex, operation record, treatment, pathologic report, and follow-up was collected and analyzed. Patients were restaged by the 7th edition AJCC classification. Cancer cachexia was defined as an unintentional weight loss of at least 5% of the premorbid weight occurring over 3–6 months (13). All the pathologic sections were re-evaluated by at least two head and neck pathologists for the accurate diagnosis of SaCa of the hypopharynx (**Figure 1**). Perineural invasion was considered to be present if tumor cells were identified within the perineural space and/or nerve bundle, and lymphovascular infiltration was positive if a tumor was noted within the lymphovascular channels (14). Drinkers were defined as those who consumed at least one alcoholic drink per day for at least 1 year, and smokers were defined as those who smoked on a daily basis or who had quit smoking for <5 years (15).

To compare the survival rates between patients with SaCa of the hypopharynx and those with SCC of the hypopharynx, patients with SCC of the hypopharynx were also reviewed during the same study period in the two hospitals. Each patient with SaCa of the hypopharynx was matched with one patient with SCC of the hypopharynx, and the matching process was performed according to age, sex, perineural invasion, lymphovascular invasion, and disease stage (15).

The propensity score matching was used to perform the pair matching process. A Pearson chi-square test or Fisher's exact test was used to compare the clinical pathologic variables between the two groups. Disease-specific survival (DSS) was the main study endpoint, and it was calculated by the Kaplan-Meier method. The factors that were significant in the univariable analysis were then analyzed in the Cox model to determine the independent risk factors. All statistical analyses were performed using SPSS 20.0. A p-value of <0.05 was considered significant.

RESULTS

There were 62 (all male) patients with SaCa of the hypopharynx enrolled in total: 25 (40.3%) patients from the Affiliated Cancer Hospital and 37 (59.7%) patients from the First Affiliated Hospital. The mean age was 65.3 years old, with a range from 51 to 76, and smoking and drinking were noted in 41 (66.1%) and 29 (46.8%) patients, respectively. Cachexia was noted in 37 (59.7%) patients. Tumor stages were distinguished as T1 in 10 (16.1%) patients, T2 in 20 (32.2%) patients, T3 in 16 (25.8%) patients, and T4 in 16 (25.8%) patients. A total of 45 (72.6%) patients underwent partial pharyngolaryngectomy, and 17 (27.4%) patients underwent total pharyngolaryngectomy. Thirty-seven (59.7%) patients underwent primary closure, 15 patients

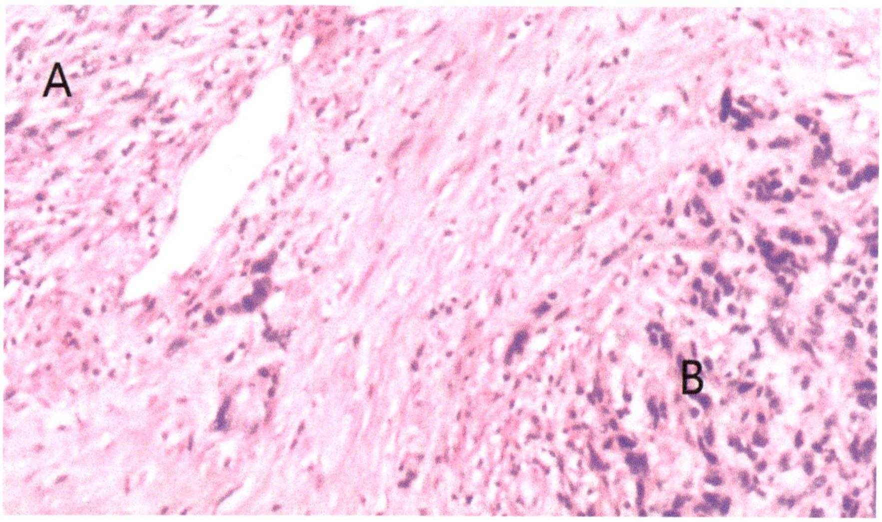

FIGURE 1 | Accurate diagnosis of sarcomatoid carcinoma (SaCa) of the hypopharynx showing morphologic epithelial changes, where areas of spindle cell **(A)** and squamous **(B)** differentiation are demonstrated (hematoxylin and eosin stain × 20).

(24.2%) underwent submental island flap reconstruction, and 10 patients (16.1%) underwent radial forearm flap reconstruction.

All patients underwent neck dissection, and a total of 59 selective neck dissections, 14 modified neck dissections, and five radical neck dissections were performed. Neck node metastasis was noted in 32 (51.6%) patients: N1 in 6 (18.8%, 6/32) patients, N2a in 10 (31.3%, 10/32) patients, N2b in 10 (31.3%, 10/32) patients, N2c in 3 (9.4%, 3/32) patients, and N3 in 3 (9.4%, 3/32) patients. The disease stages observed in patients were distinguished as I in 5 (8.1%) patients, II in 10 (16.1%) patients, III in 17 (27.4%) patients, and IV in 30 (48.4%) patients. Perineural invasion was reported in 23 (37.1%) patients, and lymphatic invasion was reported in 22 (35.5%) patients. A positive margin was demonstrated in 6 (9.7%) patients. Extracapsular extension of the node was reported in 17 (27.4%) patients. A total of 50 (80.6%) patients underwent postoperative radiotherapy, and 19 (30.6%) patients also received postoperative chemotherapy.

During the same period, there were 1,632 patients with traditional SCC of the hypopharynx. As described in **Table 1**, compared to traditional SCC of the hypopharynx, SaCa of the hypopharynx mainly affected male, older patients and was associated with a higher rate of perineural invasion; moreover, cancer cachexia was more common in patients with SaCa (all $p < 0.05$). No significant difference regarding tumor stage, neck lymph node stage, disease stage, lymphovascular invasion, or treatment was noted (all $p > 0.05$).

During our follow-up period with a mean time of 40.1 (range: 5–136) months, recurrence was noted in 49 (79.0%) patients: 22 (44.9%, 22/49) were cases of local recurrence, 14 (28.6%, 14/49) were cases of regional recurrence, 7 (14.3%, 7/49) were cases of loco-regional recurrence, and 6 (12.2%, 6/49) were cases of distant recurrence. Fifteen (30.6%, 15/49) patients experienced recurrence that was successfully salvaged by surgical treatment: 8 (53.3%, 8/15) patients underwent radical neck dissection, 5 (33.3%, 5/15) patients underwent total pharyngolaryngectomy, and 2 (13.3%, 2/15) patients underwent both radical neck dissection and total pharyngolaryngectomy. Forty-four (71.0%) patients died of the disease, and the 5- and 10-year DSS rates were 20 and 8%, respectively. After being matched, the two groups had no significant difference regarding age, sex, tumor stage, neck lymph node stage, disease stage, perineural invasion, lymphovascular invasion, or treatment (**Table 2**, all $p > 0.05$). In matched patients, the 5- and 10-year DSS rates were 34 and 28%, respectively, and the difference was significant ($p = 0.016$) (**Figure 2**).

With regard to the survival analysis in patients with SaCa, tumor stage, neck lymph node stage, disease stage, cachexia, and extracapsular extension were associated with the DSS rate according to the univariable analysis, and further Cox model analysis described that neck node stage and disease stage were the independent predictors for DSS rate (**Table 3**).

TABLE 1 | Comparison of clinical pathologic variables between patients with sarcomatoid carcinoma (SaCa) and patients with traditional hypopharynx squamous cell carcinoma (SCC).

	SaCa (n = 62)	SCC (n = 1,632)	p
Age			
≥65	47 (75.8%)	1,002 (61.4%)	
<65	15 (24.2%)	630 (38.6%)	0.022
Sex			
Male	62 (100%)	1,248 (76.5%)	
Female	0	384 (23.5%)	<0.001
Smokers			
Yes	41 (66.1%)	956 (58.6%)	
No	21 (33.9%)	676 (41.4%)	0.236
Drinkers			
Yes	29 (46.8%)	589 (36.1%)	
No	33 (53.2%)	1,043 (63.9%)	0.086
Cachexia			
Yes	37 (59.7%)	745 (45.6%)	
No	25 (40.3%)	887 (54.4%)	0.030
Tumor stage			
T1 + T2	30 (48.4%)	749 (45.9%)	
T3 + T4	32 (51.6%)	883 (54.1%)	0.699
Neck node stage			
N0	30 (48.4%)	715 (43.8%)	
N+	32 (51.6%)	917 (56.2%)	0.476
Disease stage			
I + II	15 (24.2%)	519 (31.8%)	
III + IV	47 (75.8%)	1113 (68.2%)	0.206
Perineural invasion#			
Yes	23 (37.1%)	287 (24.0%)	
No	39 (62.9%)	908 (76.0%)	0.020
Lymphovascular invasion*			
Yes	22 (35.5%)	248 (20.3%)	
No	40 (64.5%)	971 (79.7%)	0.004
Extracapsular spread&			
Yes	17 (27.4%)	333 (24.9%)	
No	45 (72.6%)	1004 (75.1%)	0.655
Treatment			
Surgery	12 (19.4%)	245 (15.0%)	
Surgery + radiotherapy	31 (50.0%)	822 (50.4%)	
Surgery + radiotherapy + chemotherapy	19 (30.6%)	565 (34.6%)	0.601

#Status of perineural invasion in 437 patients with traditional SCC was unknown.
**Status of lymphovascular invasion in 413 patients with traditional SCC was unknown.*
&Status of extracapsular spread in 295 patients with traditional SCC was unknown.
Gray value indicates significant variables.

DISCUSSION

Since SaCa was first reported in 1864 (1), a few studies have described its clinical and pathologic characteristics in the throat, the parotid gland and other subsites of the head and neck region (2–12). However, due to the rarity of the disease, <50 cases of SaCa of the hypopharynx have been previously reported (2–12), and the prognosis and prognostic factors remain unknown in SaCa of the hypopharynx; the current study was the first to present the clinical results of SaCa of the hypopharynx. SCC is the most common pathologic type found in head and neck cancer (16). Previous evidence has shown an evolution from

TABLE 2 | Comparison of clinical pathologic variables between patients with sarcomatoid carcinoma (SaCa) and matched patients with traditional hypopharynx squamous cell carcinoma (SCC).

	SaCa (*n* = 62)	SCC (*n* = 62)	$p^{\#}$
Age			
≥65	47 (75.8%)	47 (75.8%)	
<65	15 (24.2%)	15 (24.2%)	NS
Sex			
Male	62 (100%)	62 (100%)	
Female	0	0	NS
Smokers			
Yes	41 (66.1%)	37 (59.7%)	
No	21 (33.9%)	25 (40.3%)	NS
Drinkers			
Yes	29 (46.8%)	33 (53.2%)	
No	33 (53.2%)	29 (46.8%)	NS
Cachexia			
Yes	37 (59.7%)	37 (59.7%)	
No	25 (40.3%)	25 (40.3%)	NS
Tumor stage			
T1 + T2	30 (48.4%)	27 (43.5%)	
T3 + T4	32 (51.6%)	35 (56.5%)	NS
Neck lymph node stage			
N0	30 (48.4%)	34 (54.8%)	
N+	32 (51.6%)	28 (45.2%)	NS
Disease stage			
I + II	15 (24.2%)	15 (24.2%)	
III + IV	47 (75.8%)	47 (75.8%)	NS
Perineural invasion			
Yes	23 (37.1%)	23 (37.1%)	
No	39 (62.9%)	39 (62.9%)	NS
Lymphovascular invasion			
Yes	22 (35.5%)	22 (35.5%)	
No	40 (64.5%)	40 (64.5%)	NS
Extracapsular spread			
Yes	17 (27.4%)	14 (22.6%)	
No	45 (72.6%)	48 (77.4%)	NS
Treatment			
Surgery	12 (19.4%)	11 (17.7%)	
Surgery + radiotherapy	31 (50.0%)	33 (53.2%)	
Surgery + radiotherapy + chemotherapy	19 (30.6%)	18 (29.0%)	NS

#NS, not significant.

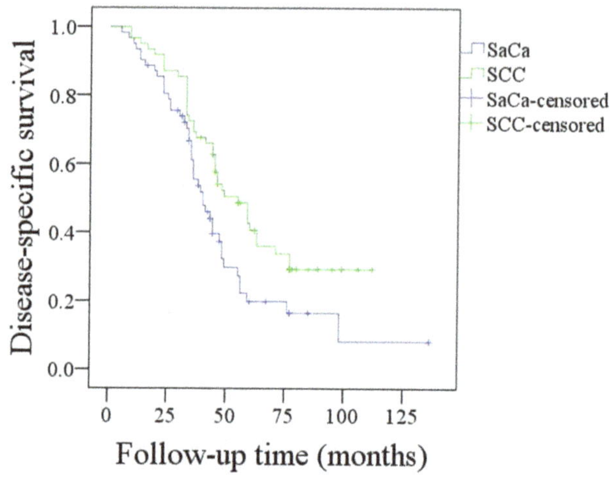

FIGURE 2 | Comparison of disease-specific survival between patients with sarcomatoid carcinoma (SaCa) of the hypopharynx and patients matched for squamous cell carcinoma (SCC) (*p* = 0.016).

TABLE 3 | Univariable and cox model analysis of predictors for the disease-specific survival in patients with hypopharynx sarcomatoid carcinoma.

Variables	Univariable	Cox model	
	p	*p*	Exp(B) (95% CI)
Age (<65 vs. ≥65)	0.185		
Smoke	0.385		
Alcohol	0.560		
Tumor stage (T1 + T2 vs. T3 + T4)	0.040	0.277	1.680 (0.402–7.011)
Node stage (N0 vs. N+)	<0.001	0.048	1.339 (1.011–4.697)
Disease stage (I+ II vs. III + IV)	0.013	0.002	2.090 (1.231–6.913)
Perineural invasion	0.175		
Lymphovascular invasion	0.403		
Cachexia	0.035	0.611	0.821 (0.287–4.341)
Extracapsular extension	0.021	0.058	1.339 (0.968–2.998)
Radiotherapy	0.689		
Chemotherapy	0.738		
Margin status	0.366		

Gray value indicates significant variables.

conventional epithelial cancer to SaCa as well as a malignant nature of the sarcomatoid component (7). There might be variations in survival between SaCa and conventional SCC. Our matched analysis supports the hypothesis that a significantly lower DSS rate is noted in patients with SaCa than in patients with SCC, and a similar finding was also reported by Chang et al. (8) in SaCa of the head and neck. However, it is prudent to conclude that the prognosis of SaCa of the hypopharynx is poorer than that of SCC of the hypopharynx: first, both studies had a limited sample size (62 cases and 18 cases), and second, even if the matching process had taken several confounding factors into consideration, the different radiation techniques and margin statuses were not analyzed between the two groups, owing to the long time span; these factors are typically independent negative prognostic predictors in head and neck cancer (17).

The detailed clinical pathologic characteristics of SaCa of the hypopharynx remain unclear. Gamez et al. (4) reported that the majority of patients with SaCa of the larynx were elderly males who presented with early-stage disease. Berthelet et al. (3) also reported a male prevalence and a low risk of lymph node metastasis in SaCa of the head and neck. Our findings partially supported these viewpoints: all patients were male, and compared to patients with traditional SCC, patients with SaCa were older. However, hoarseness was apparent even in every patient with early-stage SCC of the larynx; however, there are typically no obvious symptoms that appear until advanced-stage cancer of the hypopharynx occurs, which might explain why most of our patients presented with advanced-stage disease. Cancer cachexia is a common concomitant phenomenon in SCC of the head and neck, and approximately one-third of patients have cachexia at diagnosis (18, 19). This finding is partially reflected by the degree of tumor malignancy (20); data demonstrate a higher degree of tumor malignancy in patients with SaCa than in our patients with traditional SCC of the hypopharynx and in previous reports (18, 19). Additionally, perineural invasion and lymphovascular invasion are two of the most important prognostic factors in SCC of the head and neck, and it has been noted that there are higher rates of perineural invasion and lymphovascular invasion in patients with SaCa. These findings suggest that the biological behavior of SaCa is more aggressive and might result in poorer survival than that of SCC.

The prognosis of patients with SaCa of the head and neck is typically dismal. In a report by Berthelet et al. (3), a total of 17 patients were enrolled for analysis, and the authors described that the median survival time was 32 months, with an actual survival of 72 and 42% at 2 and 5 years, respectively. In another paper focusing on outcomes in SaCa of the larynx, the authors reported that the 5-year overall survival, progression-free survival, and local control rates were 63, 46, and 72%, respectively (4). This finding apparently conflicts with our findings. The 5-year DSS rate was found to be only 20% in the current study; the first possible explanation for this finding is that advanced stage disease predominated in the current study, unlike in the abovementioned studies. Similarly, in a report published by Chang et al. (8), of the 78 included patients, 64% (50) were classified as having T3 or T4 tumors at the time of diagnosis, and the 5-year survival rate was 14%. Second, all the cases of disease in the current study involved localization in the hypopharynx, and cancer of the hypopharynx is usually associated with a poorer prognosis than cancers in other subsites of the head and neck (21).

Overall lymph node metastasis is typically uncommon in SaCa of the head and neck. Gamez et al. (4) reported that positive neck disease represented only 5% of the cases of SaCa of the larynx, and Niu et al. (10) reported that 5 (20%) patients had pathologic node metastasis out of the 15 patients undergoing neck dissection. However, in the current study, it was noted that 32 (51.6%) patients had neck metastatic disease, and this striking difference might be associated with the anatomic characteristics of the hypopharynx. There are abundant lymphatic vessels in the hypopharynx, and movements related to swallowing and speech can promote the occurrence of metastasis. Moreover, routine neck dissection was included in the primary treatment strategy in the two cancer centers, but in the abovementioned studies, elective neck dissection was more commonly performed, and this discrepancy might mask the true incidence of metastasis.

Prognostic factors have been evaluated for SaCa of the head and neck. Chang et al. (8) found that in a surgical intervention group, only a history of previous SCC produced good outcomes. The practice of neck dissection, the use of adjuvant therapies, or cancer stage did not affect the overall survival rate. Niu et al. described that in SaCa of the parotid gland, perineural nerve invasion was the only independent predictor for DSS (10). In the current study, neck lymph node metastasis was significantly associated with the DSS rate in SaCa of the hypopharynx. A higher neck lymph node metastasis stage and disease stage were associated with a higher risk of death, and a similar finding was also noted in SCC of the head and neck (22, 23).

The effectiveness of radiotherapy and chemotherapy for increasing local-regional and distant control in SCC of the head and neck has been widely accepted, but there is little evidence in the literature on the role of such adjuvant treatments for the treatment of SaCa. In a report by Chang et al. (8), 41 (64.1%) of the patients received radiotherapy, and the author found that no apparent survival benefit was associated with radiotherapy. In another paper focusing on SaCa of the larynx (24), the authors reported that compared to a 57.1% DSS rate with nonsurgical treatment, surgery led to a 5-year DSS rate of 84.1%, and adjuvant radiotherapy was not advised. Similarly, we also failed to note that postoperative adjuvant treatment could improve DSS. However, owing to the difference in the lymph node metastasis rate and pattern between cancer of the larynx and hypopharynx, the application of adjuvant radiotherapy cannot be easily excluded, and more studies are needed to clarify this question.

In summary, the prognosis of patients with SaCa of the hypopharynx is dismal, and SaCa of the hypopharynx is associated with more aggressive biological behavior than traditional SCC of the hypopharynx; neck lymph node stage and disease stage were the most important predictors for DSS.

ETHICS STATEMENT

The Zhengzhou University institutional research committee approved our study and all participants signed an informed consent agreement for medical research before initial treatment. And all the related procedures were consistent with Ethics Committee regulations.

AUTHOR CONTRIBUTIONS

All authors contributed to data analysis, drafting, and revising the article, gave final approval of the version to be published, and agree to be accountable for all aspects of the work.

REFERENCES

1. Virchow R. *Die Krankhaften Geschwulste*. Berlin: Hirschwald (1864–1865).
2. Viswanathan S, Rahman K, Pallavi S, Sachin J, Patil A, Chaturvedi P, et al. Sarcomatoid (spindle cell) carcinoma of the head and neck mucosal region: a clinicopathologic review of 103 cases from a tertiary referral cancer centre. *Head Neck Pathol*. (2010) 4:265–75. doi: 10.1007/s12105-010-0204-4
3. Berthelet E, Shenouda G, Black MJ, Picariello M, Rochon L. Sarcomatoid carcinoma of the head and neck. *Am J Surg*. (1994) 168:455–8. doi: 10.1016/S0002-9610(05)80098-4
4. Gamez ME, Jeans E, Hinni ML, Moore E, Young G, Ma D, et al. Outcomes and patterns of failure of sarcomatoid carcinoma of the larynx: the Mayo Clinic experience. *Laryngoscope*. (2018) 128:373–7. doi: 10.1002/lary.26725
5. Rosko AJ, Birkeland AC, Wilson KF, Muenz DG, Bellile E, Bradford CR, et al. Tumor biomarkers in spindle cell variant squamous cell carcinoma of the head and neck. *Otolaryngol Head Neck Surg*. (2016) 155:106–12. doi: 10.1177/0194599816636612
6. Batsakis JG, Suarez P. Sarcomatoid carcinomas of the upper aerodigestive tracts. *Adv Anat Pathol*. (2000) 7:282–93. doi: 10.1097/00125480-200007050-00002
7. Choi HR, Sturgis EM, Rosenthal DI, Luna MA, Batsakis JG, El-Naggar AK. Sarcomatoid carcinoma of the head and neck: molecular evidence for evolution and progression from conventional squamous cell carcinomas. *Am J Surg Pathol*. (2003) 27:1216–20. doi: 10.1097/00000478-200309000-00004
8. Chang NJ, Kao DS, Lee LY, Chang JW, Hou MM, Lam WL, et al. Sarcomatoid carcinoma in head and neck: a review of 30 years of experience–clinical outcomes and reconstructive results. *Ann Plast Surg*. (2013) 71(Suppl. 1):S1–7. doi: 10.1097/SAP.0000000000000069
9. Huang SF, Chen IH, Liao CT, Chen TM, Lee KF. Sarcomatoid carcinoma of the parotid gland with apparent metastasis of epidermoid elements to cervical lymph nodes. *Acta Otolaryngol*. (2006) 126:667–71. doi: 10.1080/00016480500469560
10. Niu X. Sarcomatoid carcinoma in the parotid gland: a review of 30 years of experience. *Laryngoscope*. (2019) 129:1137–40. doi: 10.1002/lary.27474
11. Spencer MG, Elliott RIK, Wadsworth PV, Deutsch GP. Pseudosarcoma of the pharynx and larynx. *J Laryngol Otol*. (1983) 97:85–91. doi: 10.1017/S0022215100093853
12. Ampil FL. The controversial role of radiotherapy in spindle cell carcinoma (pseudosarcoma) of the head and neck. *Radiat Med*. (1985) 3:225–9.
13. Richey LM, George JR, Couch ME, Kanapkey BK, Yin X, Cannon T, et al. Defining cancer cachexia in head and neck squamous cell carcinoma. *Clin Cancer Res*. (2007) 13:6561–7. doi: 10.1158/1078-0432.CCR-07-0116
14. Fang Q, Li P, Qi J, Luo R, Chen D, Zhang X. Value of lingual lymph node metastasis in patients with squamous cell carcinoma of the tongue. *Laryngoscope*. (2019). doi: 10.1002/lary.27927. [Epub ahead of print].
15. Fang QG, Shi S, Liu FY, Sun CF. Squamous cell carcinoma of the oral cavity in ever smokers: a matched-pair analysis of survival. *J Craniofac Surg*. (2014)25:934–7. doi: 10.1097/SCS.0000000000000710
16. Liu F, Cheng GY, Fang QG, Sun Q. Natural history of untreated squamous cell carcinoma of the head and neck. *Clin Otolaryngol*. (2019) 44:200–3. doi: 10.1111/coa.13260
17. van der Veen J, Nuyts S. Can intensity-modulated-radiotherapy reduce toxicity in head and neck squamous cell carcinoma? *Cancers (Basel)*. (2017) 9:E135. doi: 10.3390/cancers9100135
18. Orell-Kotikangas H, Österlund P, Mäkitie O, Saarilahti K, Ravasco P, Schwab U, et al. Cachexia at diagnosis is associated with poor survival in head and neck cancer patients. *Acta Otolaryngol*. (2017) 137:778–85. doi: 10.1080/00016489.2016.1277263
19. Kwon M, Kim RB, Roh JL, Lee SW, Kim SB, Choi SH, et al. Prevalence and clinical significance of cancer cachexia based on time from treatment in advanced-stage head and neck squamous cell carcinoma. *Head Neck*. (2017) 39:716–23. doi: 10.1002/hed.24672
20. Gallagher IJ, Jacobi C, Tardif N, Rooyackers O, Fearon K. Omics/systems biology and cancer cachexia. *Semin Cell Dev Biol*. (2016) 54:92–103. doi: 10.1016/j.semcdb.2015.12.022
21. Sim F, Leidner R, Bell RB. Immunotherapy for head and neck cancer. *Oral Maxillofac Surg Clin North Am*. (2019) 31:85–100. doi: 10.1016/j.coms.2018.09.002
22. Fang QG, Shi S, Liu FY, Sun CF. Tongue squamous cell carcinoma as a possible distinct entity in patients under 40 years old. *Oncol Lett*. (2014) 7:2099–102. doi: 10.3892/ol.2014.2054
23. Fang QG, Shi S, Li ZN, Zhang X, Liua FY, Xu ZF, et al. Squamous cell carcinoma of the buccal mucosa: analysis of clinical presentation, outcome and prognostic factors. *Mol Clin Oncol*. (2013) 1:531–4. doi: 10.3892/mco.2013.86
24. Dubal PM, Marchiano E, Kam D, Dutta R, Kalyoussef E, Baredes S, et al. Laryngeal spindle cell carcinoma: a population-based analysis of incidence and survival. *Laryngoscope*. (2015) 125:2709–14. doi: 10.1002/lary.25383

12

Complete Response to Nivolumab in Recurrent/Metastatic HPV-Positive Head and Neck Squamous Cell Carcinoma Patient After Progressive Multifocal Leukoencephalopathy

Laura Deborah Locati[1†], Mara Serena Serafini[2†], Andrea Carenzo[2], Silvana Canevari[3], Federica Perrone[4], Ester Orlandi[5], Serena Delbue[6], Stefano Cavalieri[1], Giulia Berzeri[7], Anna Pichiecchio[7,8], Lisa Francesca Licitra[1,9], Enrico Marchioni[10†] and Loris De Cecco[2†]*

[1] Head and Neck Cancer Medical Oncology Unit, Fondazione Istituto di Ricovero e Cura a Carattere Scientifico (IRCCS) Istituto Nazionale dei Tumori, Milan, Italy, [2] Integrated Biology Platform, Department of Applied Research and Technology Development, Fondazione Istituto di Ricovero e Cura a Carattere Scientifico (IRCCS) Istituto Nazionale dei Tumori, Milan, Italy, [3] Fondazione Istituto di Ricovero e Cura a Carattere Scientifico (IRCCS) Istituto Nazionale dei Tumori, Milan, Italy, [4] Pathology Department, Fondazione Istituto di Ricovero e Cura a Carattere Scientifico (IRCCS) Istituto Nazionale dei Tumori, Milan, Italy, [5] Radiation Oncology Clinical Department, National Center of Oncological Hadrontherapy, Pavia, Italy, [6] Department of Biomedical, Surgical and Dental Sciences, University of Milan, Milan, Italy, [7] Department of Brain and Behavioral Sciences, University of Pavia, Pavia, Italy, [8] Advanced Imaging and Radiomics Center, Neuroradiology Department, Istituto di Ricovero e Cura a Carattere Scientifico (IRCCS) Mondino Foundation, Pavia, Italy, [9] Department of Hematology and Oncology, University of Milan, Milan, Italy, [10] Neuroncology Unit, Istituto di Ricovero e Cura a Carattere Scientifico (IRCCS) Mondino Foundation, Pavia, Italy

***Correspondence:**
Loris De Cecco
loris.dececco@istitutotumori.mi.it

†These authors have contributed equally to this work

In an immune-competent context nivolumab showed long-term benefit in overall survival in recurrent/metastatic head and neck squamous cell carcinoma (HNSCC); however, in special cancer population such as these patients with immunodeficiency and viral infections, data on checkpoint inhibitors (ICI) activity are scant. Herein, we report a patient with a Human papilloma virus (HPV)-related oropharyngeal cancer (OPC) and CD4 lymphocytopenia. After a first-line treatment complete remission, the patient experienced Human Polyomavirus (JCV) infection in the brain. Consequently, to the recovery from progressive multifocal leukoencephalopathy (PML) the patient metastasized and was enrolled in a single-arm trial with nivolumab (EudraCT number: 2017-000562-30). A complete and durable response (more 3 years) was observed after 10 nivolumab injections Q2wks, interrupted for persistent drug related G2 diarrhea and a syndrome of inappropriate antidiuretic hormone secretion. We describe the circulating immune profile (before-, during-, and after nivolumab), consistent with the clinical history. Moreover, during nivolumab treatment, brain MRI evidenced the presence of small punctuate areas of contrast enhancement, reflecting a mild immune response in perivascular spaces. By cytofluorimetry, we observed that during JCV infection the CD4/CD8 ratio of the patient was under the normal values. After JCV infection recovery and before nivolumab treatment, CD4/CD8 ratio reached the normality threshold, even if the $CD4^+$ T cell count remained largely under the normal values. During ICI, gene expression xCell analyses of circulating immune cells of the patient, showed a progressive normalization of the total immune profile, with significant boost in $CD4^+$ and $CD8^+$ T cells and a reduction in NK T, comparable to the circulating immune profile of reference tumor-free HNSCC patients. The present case supports the activity of ICI in a population of special cancer patients; whether JCV and HPV infections (alone or together) might have a possible role as immune booster(s), require further investigations.

Keywords: immunotherapy, HNSCC, oropharynx, HPV, case report, PML

INTRODUCTION

Head and neck squamous cell carcinoma (HNSCC) is the eighth most frequent cancer in the world (1). For patients with recurrent/metastatic (R/M) HNSCC the overall survival has been recently improved due to available new treatment options, especially immune checkpoint inhibitors (ICI, i.e., nivolumab, pembrolizumab). Nivolumab is a human immunoglobulin G4 (IgG4) antibody targeting programmed death-1 (PD-1), an inhibitory receptor on activated T cells. This antibody blocks the interaction with PD-1 receptor and its ligands, PD-L1 and PD-L2, leading to the inhibition of the patient immune response against cancer cells. Nivolumab was approved by the FDA for platinum-refractory R/M HNSCC patients and, as reported in the randomized trial CheckMate-141, showed benefit as compared to standard of care and, once response is obtained, it may be prolonged (2). However, despite those encouraging results, in this set of patients response is still limited (about 15%), and to our knowledge predictive biomarkers, such as PD-L1 expression, are still under investigation (3). At our knowledge, data on the activity of nivolumab in challenging populations (such as immunocompromised patients or those with HIV and viral hepatitis infections) are scant, mainly due to their under representation in clinical trials (4, 5). The present unique case report represents a remarkable portrait of peripheral blood immune profile before, during, and post nivolumab treatment in a platinum-refractory R/M HNSCC patient, with two concomitant viral infections, experiencing a long-term response.

CASE PRESENTATION

A 62-year-old man, an active smoker (>10 packs/year), was referred to our center (IRCCS Istituto Nazionale dei Tumori, Milan, Italy) in March 2017 due to a large lesion of the right infratemporal fossa (55 × 30 × 52 mm). His medical history was unremarkable apart from previous episodes of paroxysmal atrial fibrillation. A graphical representation of the case history is shown in **Figure 1**. Contrast head and neck magnetic resonance imaging (MRI) revealed a large mass with infiltration of the medial pterigoid muscles and the deep parotid lobe, until the lateral nasopharyngeal wall; posterior, the lesion infiltrated the prevertebral muscles, enclosing the right internal carotid together with multiple enlarged nodes in the ipsilateral neck (**Figure 2A**). Fine needle aspiration biopsy of the largest neck node (25 mm) demonstrated a poorly differentiated carcinoma, p16 immuno-histochemistry (IHC) positive in formalin-fixed, paraffin-embedded (FFPE) sections (6) and HPV viral infection confirmed by *in situ* hybridization (ISH). The patient was classified as cT4 N1 p16 positive, stage III according to the AJCC VIII classification. IHC analysis for PD-L1 expression was performed using IHC 22C3 pharmDx kit (Dako, Carpinteria, CA) on FFPE tissue. PD-L1 expression was evaluated both in tumor cells and in inflammatory cells and a combined proportion score (CPS) was determined and tumor infiltrating lymphocytes (TILs) were assessed on hematoxilin & eosin (H&E) slides (7). The analysis showed high PD-L1 expression both in tumor cells (40%) and infiltrating cells (20%) with a CPS = 55. In addition, we observed an enrichment (80%) of TILs. No residual FFPE tissue was available for additional deepen analysis.

FIRST-LINE ONCOLOGIC TREATMENT AND NEUROLOGICAL HISTORY

From June to August 2017 the patient received intensity-modulated radiation therapy (IMRT, 69.96 Gy in 33 fractions) concomitant to 2 courses of carboplatin (AUC 6), due to the previous paroxysmal atrial fibrillation, serum creatinine value at the upper level and tumor related weight loss. The patient obtained a complete clinical remission at the end of the treatment, despite an expected CRT myelotoxicity (**Figure 2B**). In November 2017, due to a subacute progressive gait ataxia and aphasia, a contrast brain head and neck MRI was performed (data not shown). The image confirmed the complete oncologic remission and in addition showed multiple T2 hyperintense alterations in the supra- and infratentorial white matter, not correlated with the oncological clinical history. From November till December 2017 the patient was treated with steroids (oral cortisone acetate; 62.5 mg daily), but no improvements of neurological symptoms were observed, and the patient was hospitalized at the Fondazione Istituto Neurologico Mondino (Pavia, Italy). Neurological examination revealed moderate cognitive impairment, severe mixed aphasia, mild right

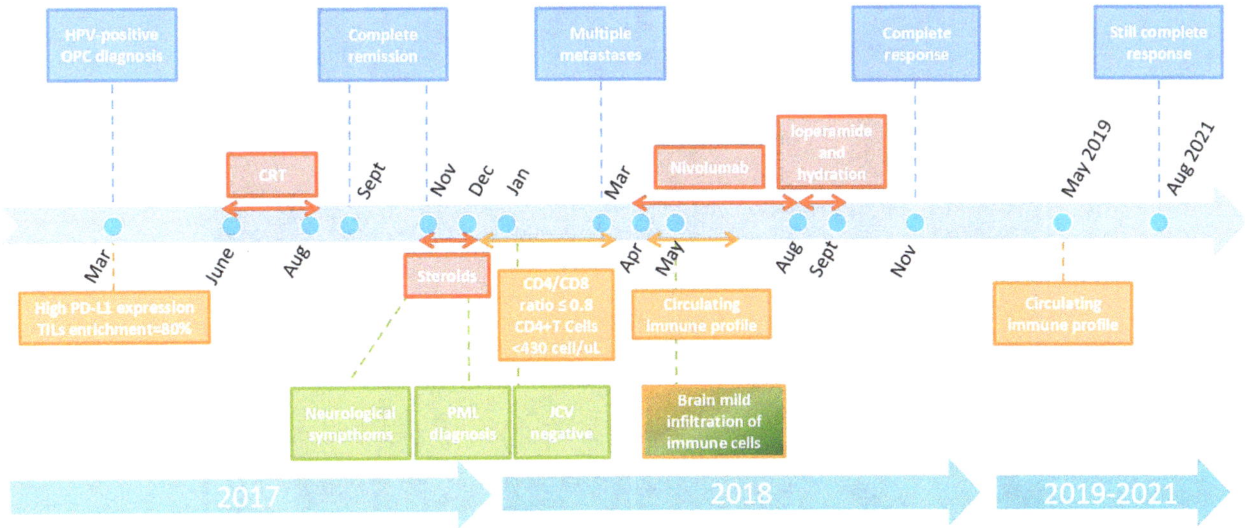

FIGURE 1 | Graphical timeline of case report with key oncologic, neurologic, and immunologic analyses and treatments. Color code for boxes: blue: oncologic history; red: treatments; light green: neurologic history; orange: immunologic analyses results. Every arrow indicates the duration of each treatment/immunologic situation. Dots represent specific key months. The scale is not strictly proportioned to dates.

hemiparesis, and cerebellar ataxia. The patient needed support for most daily life activities (modified Rankin scale—mRS—equal to 3) (8). Cerebrospinal fluid (CSF) analysis showed no inflammatory findings and no oligoclonal banding; Human Polyomavirus JC (JCV) DNA was isolated from 150 ml of CSF, using the commercial kit Nucleospin RNA virus (Macherey Nagel, Germany) and Real Time PCR, targeting the JCV Large- Antigen gene (9). Active JCV replication (4,700 copies/ml) was observed, and a brain MRI performed in December (**Figures 3A–D**), identified a large lesion in the left fronto-parietal white matter, characterized by hyperintensity on T2/FLAIR images, mild mass effect, and no contrast enhancement after gadolinium administration; b1000 images showed small areas of increased signal in a star-like («milky way») distribution pattern, though with incomplete correspondence hyposignal in the ADC map, which is a typical finding in "definite progressive multifocal leukoencephalopathy (PML)", reflecting diffusion restriction due to active demyelination. Steroid was withdrawn and over the following weeks, the patient experienced a gradual neurological improvement. Since January 2018, JCV viral load became undetectable in the CSF. In March 2018, aphasia and cognitive deficits were substantially improved and he was able to walk independently (mRS 2). Blood tests of lymphoid components, through cytofluorimetric analysis, were performed from December 2017 to March 2018. In December, during steroid treatment, CD4/CD8 ratio was inverted (CD8 >CD4; CD4/CD8 = 0.6, normal threshold >0.8), and the number circulating $CD4^+$ T cells were below the normal threshold (between 430 and 1,600 cells/μl) with an impaired count of 73 $CD4^+$ cells/μl. In January 2018, with the withdrawal of steroid, a slight improvement in $CD4^+$ T cell count was observed (161 cells/μl) and CD4/CD8 ratio was restored (CD4 >CD8, CD4/CD8 = 1.4). In March 2018, CD4/CD8 ratio was in the normal threshold (CD4/CD8 = 08), and $CD4^+$ T cell count was slightly increasing 165 cell/μl. However, $CD4^+$ T cells remained largely under the normal threshold.

MULTIPLE DISTANT METASTASIS AND SECOND-LINE TREATMENT

In March 2018, multiple distant metastases in skin, soft tissues, and bilateral lungs have been found at the follow-up 18FDG-PET scan (**Figures 2C, D**). In April 2018, the patient was enrolled in the study "A Single-Arm, Open-Label, Multicenter, Trial with Nivolumab in Subjects with Recurrent or Metastatic Platinum-refractory Squamous Cell Carcinoma of the Head and Neck" (EudraCT number: 2017-000562-30). During the following six months, the patient received 10 well-tolerated nivolumab infusions, each one of 240 mg every two weeks. A brain MRI, performed after the 4th nivolumab infusion (**Figures 3E–H**), showed a reduction in the extension of the left fronto-parietal lesion that no longer displayed mass effect, as evident on FLAIR images; b1000 images now showed an extensive area of hyposignal with correspondent hypersignal on ADC, reflecting extensive white matter destructuration without signs of ongoing active demyelination; areas of slight increased b1000 signal were still evident more anteriorly. T1 images after gadolinium injection showed the appearance of small punctuate areas of contrast enhancement, reflecting a mild immune response in perivascular spaces. Only a mild aphasia and apraxia without further deficits were present and JC viral load in the CSF continued

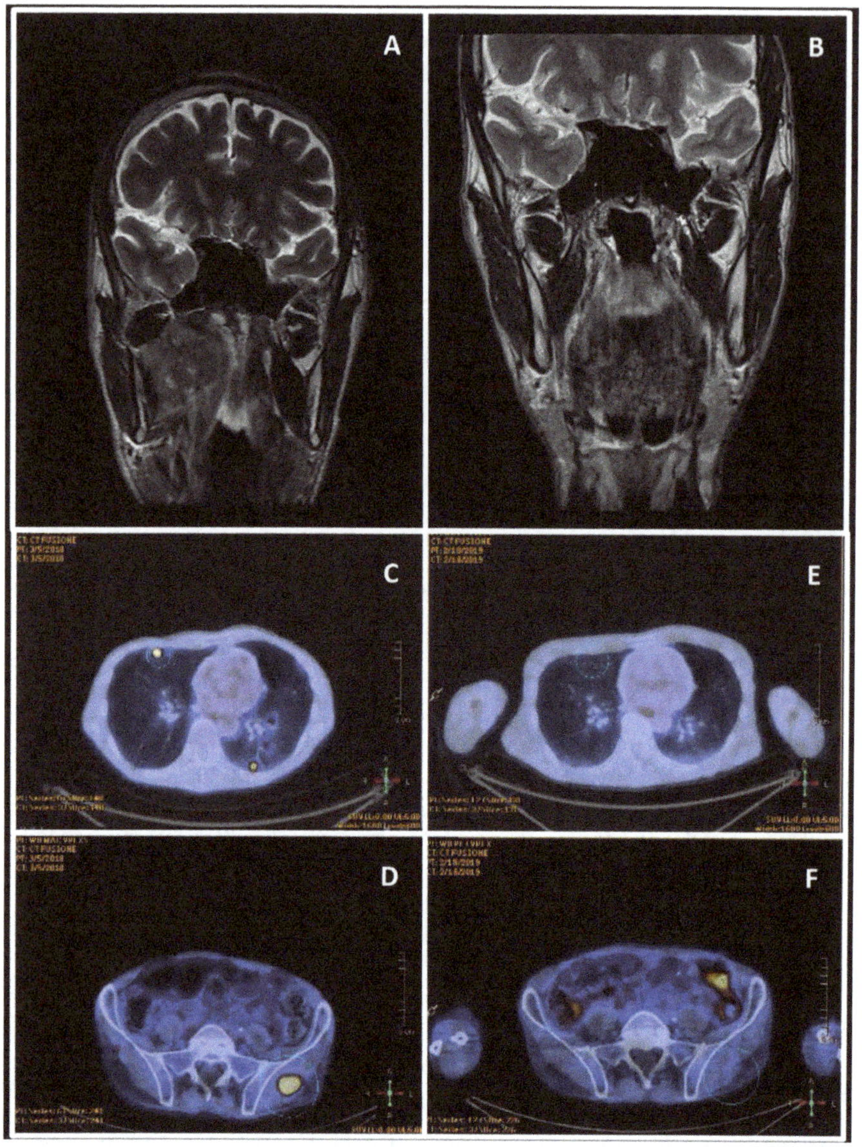

FIGURE 2 | Radiological assessments. **(A)** March 2017 Head and neck contrast-enhanced magnetic resonance imaging—before the primary treatment. **(B)** November 2017 Head and neck contrast-enhanced magnetic resonance imaging of complete remission after chemoradiation. **(C, D)** March 2018 Whole body FDG PET—at diagnosis of metastatic disease. **(E, F)** November 2018 Whole body FDG PET of complete response after nivolumab.

to be undetectable. Blood tests, through cytofluorimetric analysis, at the 5th cycle of nivolumab detected a CD4/CD8 ratio in the normal threshold (CD4/CD8 = 08), while $CD4^+$ T cell count remained largely under the normal values (160 cells/µl). In June 2018 a partial response according to the RECIST 1.1 criteria (5) was evident at the CT scan. In September 2018, nivolumab was withdrawn after 10 infusions, due to a G2 diarrhea (probably drug-related), persistent despite symptomatic treatment, and a syndrome of inappropriate antidiuretic hormone secretion (SIADH). Diagnosis of immune-mediated colitis was not endoscopically confirmed. Side effects were managed with loperamide and hydration, without using steroid or immunosuppressive therapy because of the risk of JC reactivation. In January 2019 a contrast brain MRI (**Figures 3I–L**) confirmed a substantial stability of imaging findings, disappearing of diffusivity abnormalities, but further evolution of cortical atrophy, even more evident at later follow-up evaluations. T1 images after gadolinium showed the disappearance of the small punctuate areas of enhancement that were previously evident during nivolumab treatment. In November 2019, a complete remission was confirmed by a CT scan total body (**Figures 2E, F**). At date, October 2021, the patient is still in complete remission for the HPV-related OPC and the JC infection.

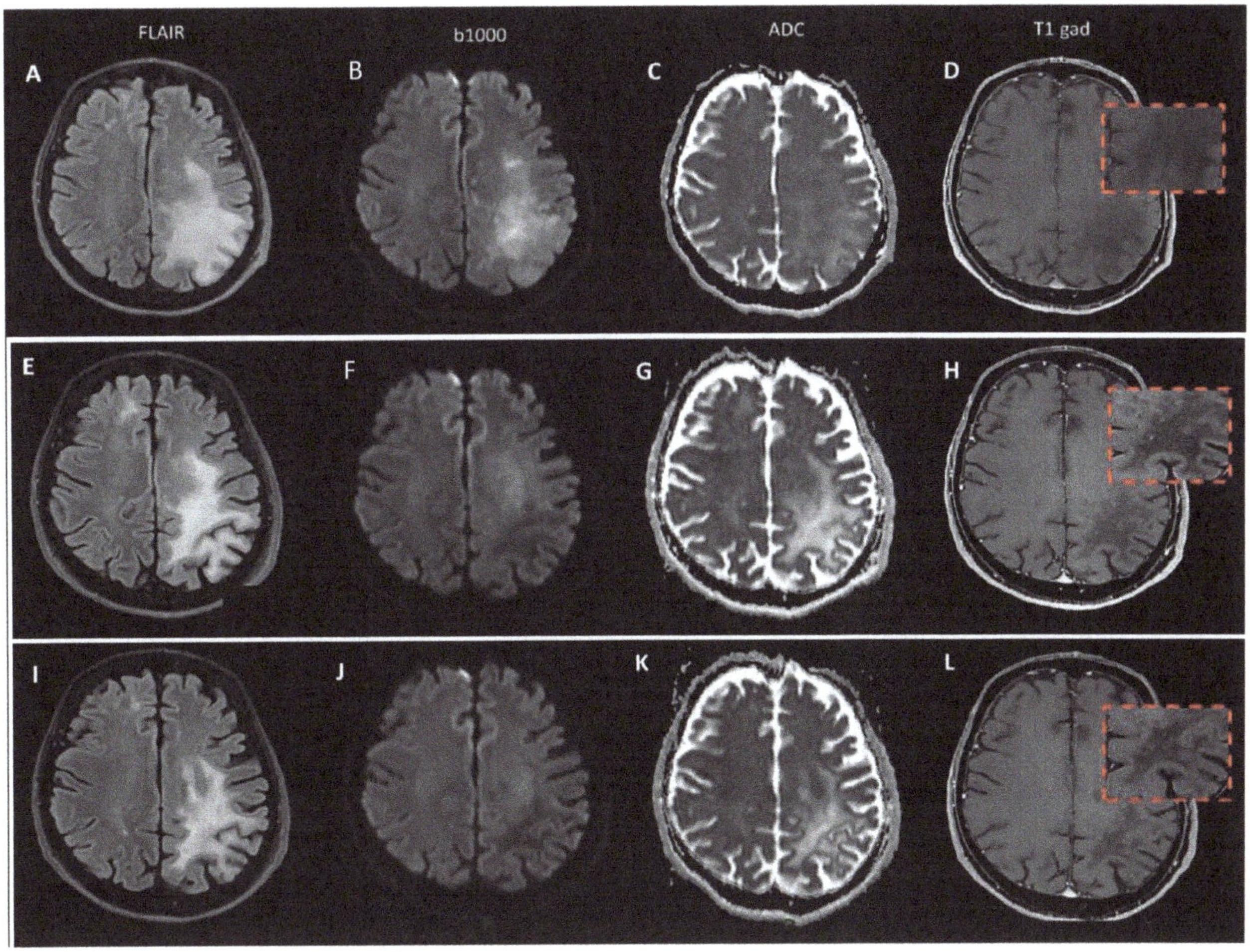

FIGURE 3 | Brain MRI. **(A–D)** December 2017 brain MRI at PML diagnosis. **(E–H)** May 2018 brain MRI during ICI treatment. **(I–L)** January 2019 brain MRI after ICI treatment.

CIRCULATING IMMUNE-PROFILE RESULTS

Recognizing the importance of profiling the immunological characteristics of the patient, blood samples collected before, during and after the single agent nivolumab treatment were employed to investigate, through a de-convolution gene expression method, the immune cells populations present in the peripheral blood. As reference, blood samples were also collected from 5 different HNSCC patients tumor-free after radical treatment. The reference patients were in the same age range and of the same gender (but one) of our patient, while they are heterogeneous in smoking history (3 heavy ex-smokers, 2 never smokers), site of the primary disease (two were p16 positive OPCs, 3 oral cavity cancer). Blood collection was made after signed informed consent from each patient. To perform the analysis, RNA was extracted from frozen blood buffycoat using RNeasy Lipid Tissue Mini Kit (Qiagen). Quality/quantity RNA had been assessed by 2200TapeStation system (Agilent), and Qubit 2.0 Fluorimetric Assay (Thermo Fisher Scientific), respectively. Gene expression experiments were performed using GeneChip WT Pico standard protocols (Affymetrix, ThermoFisher) on human Clariom-S chips. Probes were hybridized on GeneChip, that after washing and staining, through the Fluidics Station, were scanned with Affymetrix Gene Chip Scanner 3000 7G. Microarray data were compliant to MIAME (Minimum Information about a Microarray Experiment) and two gene expression matrices (5 different temporal samples from case report; 5 samples from reference patients) were deposited on GEO (accession number GSE161785). Bioinformatic analysis were performed on two different expression matrices, by the xCell approach (10).

Lymphoid cells with evident changes during and after nivolumab are reported in **Figure 4** (see **Supplementary Table** for all the xCell results and related statistics). At the beginning of April 2018 ("before-nivolumab"), all the considered lymphoid cells, with exclusion of NKT and $CD8^+$ Tem, exhibited a lower or absent expression compared to controls. In May and June 2018

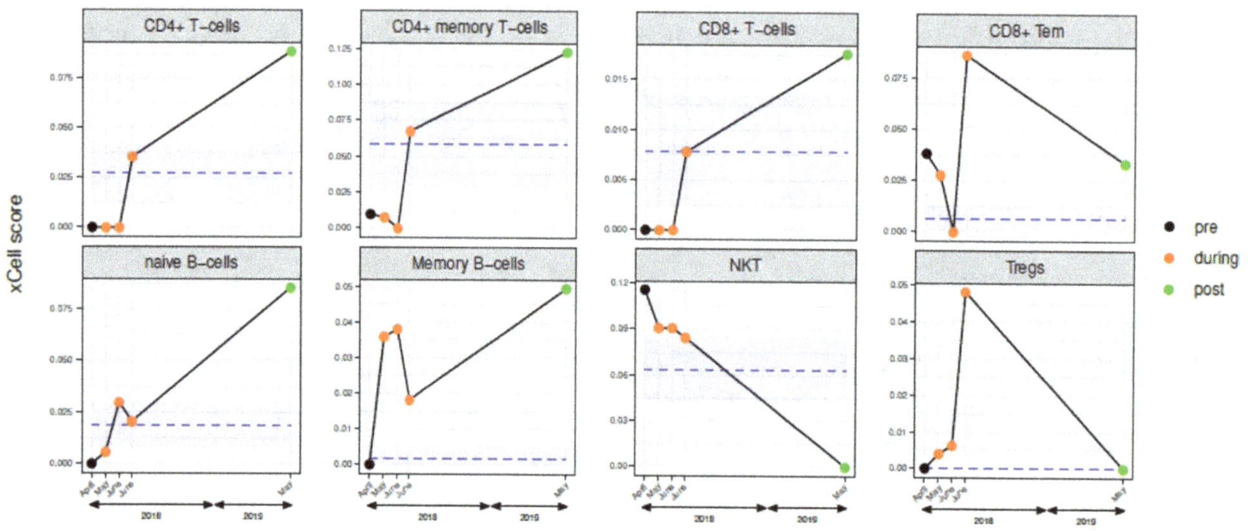

FIGURE 4 | Circulating immune cells characterization before, during, and after nivolumab treatment. Scores of selected lymphoid cells determined by xCell analysis of gene expression data of blood samples from: five samples case report patient (one pre-nivolumab: black dot; three during-nivolumab: orange dots; one post-nivolumab: green dot); mean and standard deviation of the five-reference xCell scores of tumor-free patients are represented by blue lines and light blue area, respectively. See **Table S1** for xCell data for the complete xCell scores ("lymphocytes" and "non-lymphocytes").

in two different blood samples ("during-nivolumab"), no relevant differences were observed for $CD4^+$ T cells, $CD4^+$ memory T cells, $CD8^+$ T cells, naïve B cells, and Tregs, compared to the baseline expression. On the contrary, a decrease for $CD8^+$ Tem and NKT and an increase for memory B cells were recorded. In comparison with the references' range of expression, the major immunological profile changes were recorded in the 3rd sample (7th nivolumab infusion): $CD4^+$ T cells, $CD4^+$ memory T cells, $CD8^+$ T cells, naïve B cells, NKT entered in the range, while $CD8^+$ Tem, memory B cells, and Tregs overtook the reference range. Interestingly, the immunological boost observed during the last sample "during-nivolumab", overtaking the controls, has been maintained one year later in May 2019.

DISCUSSION

We describe here the complete clinical and radiological remission of a metastatic, platinum-refractory, HPV-related OPC with ICI favorable markers (tumor PD-L1 and TILs IHC data) (3) in a patient who, after a partial recovery from CRT myelotoxicity and a complete recovery from a JC viral infection, received nivolumab. To our knowledge this is the first report of a complete durable response after ICI in a cancer patient with two viral infections (HPV in the tumor and JC in the cerebral system). Immunotherapy has been clinically used for the treatment of PML in patients with hematological malignancies, HIV-infection, or primary immune deficiencies, with erratic and conflicting results. In fact, while most patients show a decrease of PD1 expression on T-$CD4^+$ and $CD8^+$ lymphocytes as a result of PD1 blockade, only a proportion of them shows a consensual improvement of PML and even negative effects in transplant-receiver patients (11). In our case, PML was challenging and lately diagnosed since the patient had no personal history suggesting a primary immune deficiency and nivolumab was administrated after a transient immune suppression and PML remission. In the PML patients treated with ICI (12, 13), T cell profile seems the major determinant in eliciting a clinical and radiological response, being patients with higher amounts of terminally exhausted T cells less likely to respond to PD1 blockade (11, 14). Similar observations have been reported in patients receiving ICI for cancer treatment (15) and specifically in HNSCC (16). For these reasons, we decided to analyze the circulating immune profile of the case report patient before, during and after nivolumab, using the gene expression of frozen buffy coat and, as reference, HNSCC patients tumor-free after first-line treatment. The choice was based on the available material according to the trial protocol and on the evidence that gene expression data are comparable to cytofluorimetric data (10). At baseline we observed an immunoprofile consistent with the clinical history of our patient, with low levels of effector T cells ($CD4^+$ and $CD8^+$), and higher levels of $CD8^+$ memory and NKT-cells, in contrast with those reported for HNSCC patients (13), where, in an immunocompetent context, the response to nivolumab at baseline was associated with higher levels of $CD8^+$ T cells and lower levels of PD-1^+ Tregs. Even if the baseline immune profile of our patient could be interpreted as a negative predictor of response, the significant increase in relative levels of total $CD4^+$ T and memory B cells during ICI, maintained after the end of nivolumab, was in agreement with ICI efficacy. In addition, if we consider the particular immune status of this patient and we compare our data with those of PML patients, the increase of $CD4^+$ T cells during treatment seems consistent with the observation that $CD4^+$ T cell counts increased during ICI in responding PML patients (15). Indeed, the brain MRI during ICI showed the appearance of small punctuate areas of contrast enhancement within PML lesions, not present at the time of PML diagnosis, which spontaneously resolved, after nivolumab discontinuation. These areas, similarly to literature reported cases of ICI treated PML (17), are described as immune cell infiltrates in perivascular spaces and might be due to a collateral nivolumab boosting of a JC-specific cellular immunity. Nonetheless, PML was already evolving favorably in our patient before the start of nivolumab, questioning the contribution of nivolumab in JC virus clearance. Overall, the immune profile changes during treatment and the clinical outcome suggested that the immunotherapy was effective despite a persistent $CD4^+$ lymphocytopenia. Although the immune system impairment, we decided to no deepening into the lymphopenia of our patient since it might be specifically attributed to chemo-radiation treatment and steoroid administration, frequently recorded in HNSCC patients after primary treatment (18).

We should acknowledge some limitations of our study. First, the lack amount of available tumor tissue precluded the comparison between circulating immune cells with tumor immune microenvironment. Second, in adherence to the study protocol, the use of the entire blood samples for RNA extraction precluded a deeper evaluation of the intriguing Tregs expression during treatment, and long-term maintenance of high levels of memory B cells in comparison with samples of references. Third, the comparison with the literature reports (17) is indirect because an absolute counts of immune cells by cytofluorimetry has been reported in the literature, while our immune-profile was inferred from gene expression data. In conclusion, nivolumab induced a durable and complete response in a metastatic HNSCC patient with CD4 lymphocytopenia, experiencing two consecutive viral infections such as HPV and JCV. Our findings support the use of ICI in immune compromised subjects but whether JCV alone or in association with HPV infection could act as immune booster(s) requires further investigations.

ETHICS STATEMENT

Ethical review and approval was not required for the study on human participants in accordance with the local legislation and institutional requirements. The patients/participants provided their written informed consent to participate in this study. Written informed consent was obtained from the individual(s) for the publication of any potentially identifiable images or data included in this article.

AUTHOR CONTRIBUTIONS

Conception and design: LDL, LDC, and SiC. Financial support: LDC. Provision of study material: LDL and FP. Collection and assembly of data: LDL, EO, SD, GB, AP, and EM. Experimental data generation: MSS and LDC. Data analysis and interpretation: MSS, LDC, AC, SiC, StC, EM, and LFL. Manuscript writing: SiC, LDL, MSS, StC, LDC, and EM. All authors contributed to the article and approved the submitted version.

ACKNOWLEDGMENTS

The authors thank BMS for drug supply and AIRC for funding the present research results. The authors also thank the patient and his family for the publication of the present case report.

REFERENCES

1. Bray F, Ferlay J, Soerjomataram I, Siegel RL, Torre LA, Jemal A. Global Cancer Statistics 2018: GLOBOCAN Estimates of Incidence and Mortality Worldwide for 36 Cancers in 185 Countries. *CA Cancer J Clin* (2018) 68 (6):394–424. doi: 10.3322/caac.21492
2. Ferris RL, Blumenschein G Jr, Fayette J, Guigay J, Colevas AD, Licitra L, et al. Nivolumab vs Investigator's Choice in Recurrent or Metastatic Squamous Cell Carcinoma of the Head and Neck: 2-Year Long-Term Survival Update of CheckMate 141 With Analyses by Tumor PD-L1 Expression. *Oral Oncol* (2018) 81:45–51. doi: 10.1016/j.oraloncology.2018.04.008
3. Gavrielatou N, Doumas S, Economopoulou P, Foukas PG, Psyrri A. Biomarkers for Immunotherapy Response in Head and Neck Cancer. *Cancer Treat Rev* (2020) 84:101977. doi: 10.1016/j.ctrv.2020.101977
4. Johnson DB, Sullivan RJ, Menzies AM. Immune Checkpoint Inhibitors in Challenging Populations. *Cancer* (2017) 123(11):1904–11. doi: 10.1002/cncr.30642
5. Florou V, Puri S, Garrido-Laguna I, Wilky BA. Considerations for Immunotherapy in Patients With Cancer and Comorbid Immune Dysfunction. *Ann Transl Med* (2021) 9(12):1035. doi: 10.21037/atm-20-5207
6. Amin MB, Greene FL, Edge SB, Compton CC, Gershenwald JE, Brookland RK, et al. The Eighth Edition AJCC Cancer Staging Manual: Continuing to Build a Bridge From a Population-Based to a More "Personalized" Approach to Cancer Staging. *CA Cancer J Clin* (2017) 67(2):93–9. doi: 10.3322/caac.21388
7. Alfieri S, Carenzo A, Platini F, Serafini MS, Perrone F, Galbiati D, et al. Tumor Biomarkers for the Prediction of Distant Metastasis in Head and Neck Squamous Cell Carcinoma. *Cancers (Basel)* (2020) 12(4):922. doi: 10.3390/cancers12040922
8. Banks JL, Marotta CA. Outcomes Validity and Reliability of the Modified Rankin Scale: Implications for Stroke Clinical Trials - A Literature Review and Synthesis. *Stroke* (2007) 38(3):1091–6. doi: 10.1161/01.STR.0000258355.23810.c6
9. Delbue S, Sotgiu G, Fumagalli D, Valli M, Borghi E, Mancuso R, et al. A Case of a Progressive Multifocal Leukoencephalopathy Patient With Four Different JC Virus Transcriptional Control Region Rearrangements in Cerebrospinal Fluid, Blood, Serum, and Urine. *J Neurovirol* (2005) 11(1):51–7. doi: 10.1080/13550280590900382

10. Aran D, Hu Z, Butte AJ. Xcell: Digitally Portraying the Tissue Cellular Heterogeneity Landscape. *Genome Biol* (2017) 18(1):220. doi: 10.1186/s13059-017-1349-1
11. Medrano C, Vergez F, Mengelle C, Faguer S, Kamar N, Del Bello A. Effectiveness of Immune Checkpoint Inhibitors in Transplant Recipients With Progressive Multifocal Leukoencephalopathy. *Emerg Infect Dis* (2019). doi: 10.3201/eid2511.190705
12. Cortese I, Muranski P, Enose-Akahata Y, Ha SK, Smith B, Monaco M, et al. Pembrolizumab Treatment for Progressive Multifocal Leukoencephalopathy. *N Engl J Med* (2019) 380(17):1597–605. doi: 10.1056/nejmoa1815039
13. Concha-Benavente F, Gillison ML, Blumenschein GR, Harrington K, Fayette J, Colevas AD, et al. Characterization of Potential Predictive Biomarkers of Response to Nivolumab in CheckMate 141 in Patients With Squamous Cell Carcinoma of the Head and Neck (SCCHN). *J Clin Oncol* (2017) 6050. doi: 10.1200/jco.2017.35.15_suppl.6050
14. Pawlitzki M, Schneider-Hohendorf T, Rolfes L, Meuth SG, Wiendl H, Schwab N, et al. Ineffective Treatment of PML With Pembrolizumab: Exhausted Memory T-Cell Subsets as a Clue? *Neurol Neuroimmunol Neuroinflamm* (2019) 6(6):e627. doi: 10.1212/NXI.0000000000000627
15. Miller BC, Sen DR, Al Abosy R, Bi K, Virkud YV, LaFleur MW, et al. Subsets of Exhausted CD8+ T Cells Differentially Mediate Tumor Control and Respond to Checkpoint Blockade. *Nat Immunol* (2019) 20(3):326–36. doi: 10.1038/s41590-019-0312-6
16. Feng B, Hess J. Immune-Related Mutational Landscape and Gene Signatures: Prognostic Value and Therapeutic Impact for Head and Neck Cancer. *Cancers* (2021) 13(5):1162. doi: 10.3390/cancers13051162
17. Walter O, Treiner E, Bonneville F, Mengelle C, Vergez F, Lerebours F, et al. Treatment of Progressive Multifocal Leukoencephalopathy With Nivolumab. *N Engl J Med* (2019) 380(17):1674–6. doi: 10.1056/nejmc1816198
18. Kuss I, Hathaway B, Ferris RL, Gooding W, Whiteside TL. Decreased Absolute Counts of T Lymphocyte Subsets and Their Relation to Disease in Squamous Cell Carcinoma of the Head and Neck. *Clin Cancer Res* (2004) 10 (11):3755–62. doi: 10.1158/1078-0432.CCR-04-0054

13

Enabling Precision Medicine for Rare Head and Neck Tumors: The Example of BRAF/MEK Targeting in Patients with Metastatic Ameloblastoma

Maxime Brunet [1], *Emmanuel Khalifa* [2] *and Antoine Italiano* [1,3,4*]

[1] Department of Medicine, Institut Bergonié, Bordeaux, France, [2] Department of Tumor Genetics, Institut Bergonié, Bordeaux, France, [3] Faculty of Médicine, University of Bordeaux, Bordeaux, France, [4] INSERM, ACTION U1218, Bordeaux, France

Correspondence:
Antoine Italiano
a.italiano@bordeaux.unicancer.fr

Background: Ameloblastoma is a rare head and neck tumor characterized by a high incidence of BRAF mutation providing a rationale for the use of BRAF inhibitors in patients with advanced disease.

Methods: We report the case of a 26-year old female presenting with metastatic ameloblastoma. A molecular screening of the tumor revealed a BRAF V600E mutation.

Results: The patient started treatment with dabrafenib and trametinib and experienced complete response which is still ongoing 30 weeks after treatment onset.

Conclusions: The complete response observed here illustrate the role of molecular profiling in complicate clinical situation of rare head and neck cancer and the potential benefit of BRAF-targeted therapy in ameloblastoma carrying *BRAF* V600E mutation.

Keywords: ameloblastoma, BRAF, targeted therapeutic drugs, rare tumor, precision oncology

INTRODUCTION

Precision oncology aims to tailor the therapeutic strategy based on tumor's molecular alterations. Previous studies have suggested the validity of such approach in rare and ultra-rare tumor subtypes, including rare head and neck cancers; with the identification of targetable alterations in up to 93% of cases (1). Ameloblastomas are rare tumors, which often have a benign course. Metastatic evolution is extremely rare and there is no standard of care for patients in this setting.

CASE REPORT

In November 2018, a 26-year old female was referred for hemoptysis and cough of several weeks' duration. Her past medical history was significant for the diagnosis, at the age of 13 years, of an ameloblastoma of the right mandible (tooth 48) treated by surgery with clear margins and no evidence of locoregional relapse since then. A CT scan was performed which showed numerous bilateral nodules. The patient underwent a CT-guided percutaneous lung biopsy of one of these nodules. Histological examination was in favor of lung metastasis of ameloblastoma.

The patient was enrolled in our molecular screening program after signature of informed consent (Bergonié Institut Profiling study, NCT02534649) and gave also written informed consent for the publication of this case report. Next-generation sequencing of the metastatic tumor sample was performed as previously described and revealed the presence of a *BRAF* gene V600E mutation [**Figure 1**; (2)]. Given the lack of validated standard treatment for advanced ameloblastoma, the molecular tumor board recommended initiation of a BRAF-targeted therapy. The patient started treatment with dabrafenib (150 mg BID) combined with trametinib (2 mg QD). The first TEP-CT

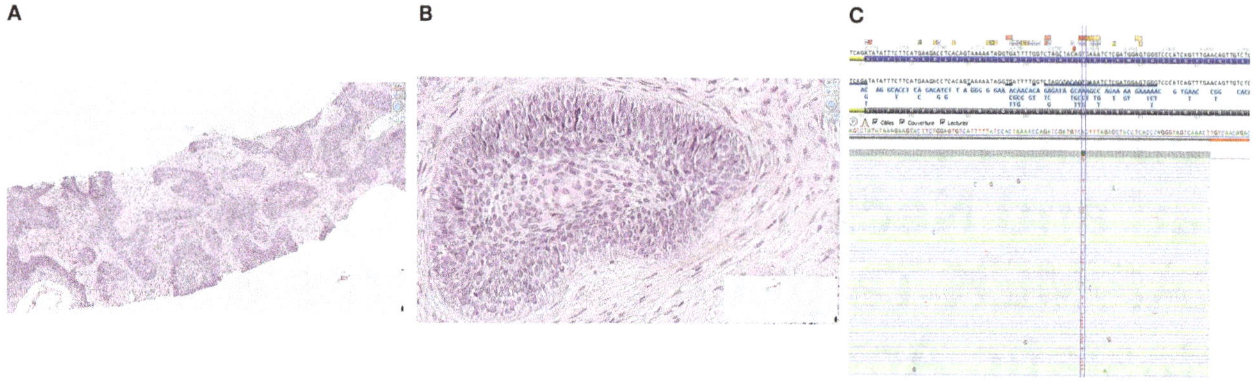

FIGURE 1 | Histological features of ameloblastoma (**A**: low magnification, **B**: high magnification) and BRAF V600E gene mutation assessed by next-generation sequencing **(C)**.

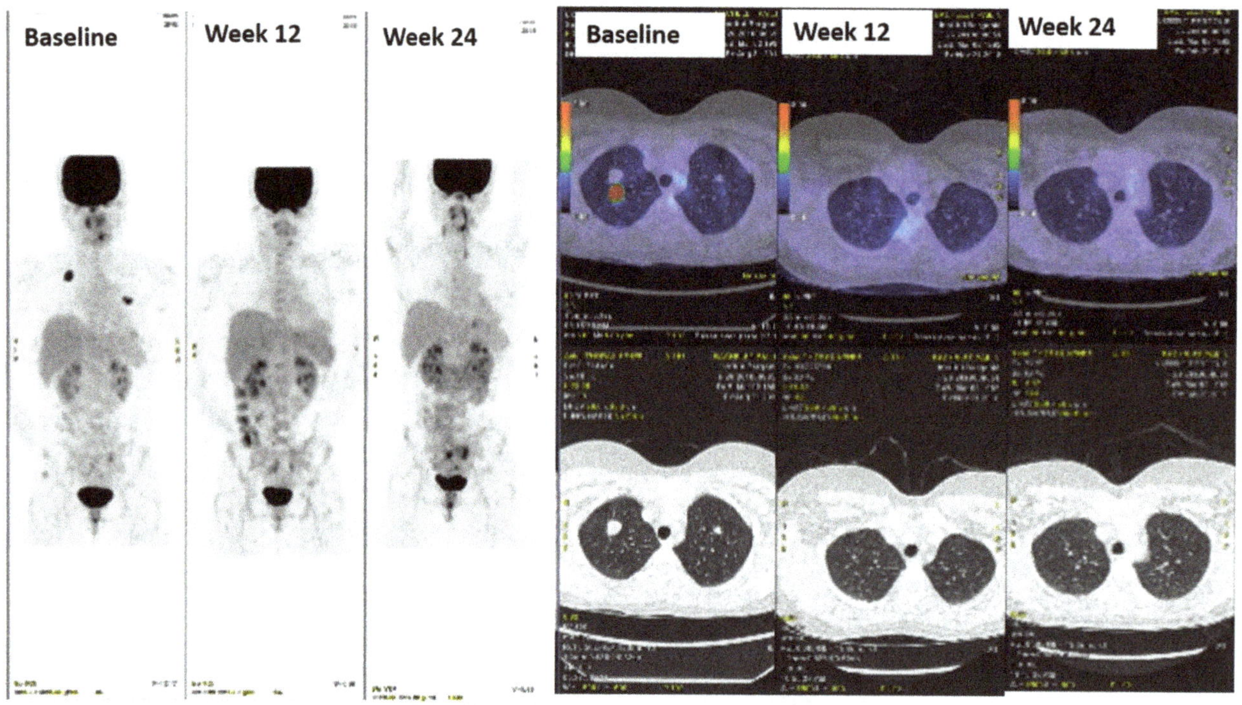

FIGURE 2 | Sustained complete response to dabrafenib + trametinib in a patient with ameloblastoma metastatic to the lungs.

scan performed 12 weeks after treatment onset showed competed response according to RECIST and PERCIST criteria (**Figure 2**). The patient is still doing well and in complete remission 30 weeks after treatment initiation.

DISCUSSION

The ameloblastoma is a histologically almost always benign odontogenic tumor of the jaw bones with a potential of locoregional recurrence (3). Distant metastases are extremely rare.

Anecdotal response has been reported with platinum salts agents but there is no standard of care in this setting (4). A seminal study investigating the molecular landscape of ameloblastomas revealed that ameloblastomas are characterized by the a frequent incidence of BRAF V600E mutations particularly in tumors located in the mandibular region while mutations of the SMO gene (39%) were predominant in maxillary tumors (82%) (5). This study and others provided a rationale to investigate BRAF targeting in patients with advance ameloblastoma. Previous case reports have suggested the clinical activity of BRAF inhibitor such as vemurafenib in patients with advanced ameloblastoma (**Table 1**). We opted here for the combination of a BRAF and MEK inhibitors. Indeed, several studies performed in melanomas, and other BRAF-driven malignancy, showed that acquired resistance to

TABLE 1 | Clinical reports of BRAF-targeting in advanced ameloblastoma.

References	Clinical setting	Tumor stage	Treatment	Outcome
Fernandes et al. (6)	29 years old female	Locally advanced	Vemurafenib	Partial response PFS not reached at 11 months after treatment onset
Tan et al. (7)	85 years old male	Locally advanced	Dabrafenib	Partial response
Faden and Algazi (8)	83 years old male	Locally advanced	Dabrafenib	Partial response PFS not reached at 12 months
Kaye et al. (9)	40 years old male	Metastatic	Dabrafenib + trametinib	Partial response Not reached at 5 months after treatment onset

BRAF inhibitors frequently develops through reactivation of the mitogen-activated protein kinase (MAPK) pathway, resulting in limited progression-free survival (10) In addition, the use of BRAF inhibitors as single agent may induce the development of secondary skin tumors, originating from a paradoxical activation of the MAPK pathway in cells without a *BRAF* mutation (10). In melanomas, combining a BRAF inhibitor with a MEK inhibitor addresses the limitations of single-agent BRAF inhibitors and results in a significant delay in the emergence of resistance, with a longer overall than with BRAF inhibitor alone, as well as a decreased incidence of BRAF-inhibitor–induced skin tumors (10). The toxicity of such a combination profile is generally good with the most common adverse events being rash, pyrexia, asthenia, headache, nausea, and arthralgia (11). The complete response observed here illustrate the role of molecular profiling in complicate clinical situation of rare head and neck cancer and the potential benefit of BRAF-targeted therapy in ameloblastoma carrying *BRAF* V600E mutation.

ETHICS STATEMENT

This study was approved by the institutional review board of Institut Bergonié.

AUTHOR CONTRIBUTIONS

AI: conception and design. EK and AI: collection and assembly of data. All authors: data analysis, interpretation, manuscript writing, and final approval of manuscript.

REFERENCES

1. Kato S, Kurasaki K, Ikeda S, Kurzrock R. Rare tumor clinic: the University of California San Diego Moores Cancer Center experience with a precision therapy approach. *Oncologist.* (2018) 23:171–8. doi: 10.1634/theoncologist.2017-0199
2. Cousin S, Grellety T, Toulmonde M, Auzanneau C, Khalifa E, Laizet Y, et al. Clinical impact of extensive molecular profiling in advanced cancer patients. *J Hematol Oncol.* (2017) 10:45. doi: 10.1186/s13045-017-0411-5
3. Sciubba J. Odontogenic tumors. In: Barnes L, Eveson J, Reichart P, Sidransky D, editors. *World Health Organization Classification of Tumors, Pathology and Genetics of Head and Neck Tumors.* Lyon: IARC Press (2005). p. 287–93.
4. McClary AC, West RB, McClary AC, Pollack JR, Fischbein NJ, Holsinger CF, et al. Ameloblastoma: a clinical review and trends in management. *Eur Arch Otorhinolaryngol.* (2016) 273:1649–61. doi: 10.1007/s00405-015-3631-8
5. Sweeney RT, McClary AC, Myers BR, Biscocho J, Neahring L, Kwei KA, et al. Identification of recurrent SMO and BRAF mutations in ameloblastomas. *Nat Genet.* (2014) 46:722–5. doi: 10.1038/ng.2986
6. Fernandes GS, Girardi DM, Bernardes JPG, Fonseca FP, Fregnani ER. Clinical benefit and radiological response with BRAF inhibitor in a patient with recurrent ameloblastoma harboring V600E mutation. *BMC Cancer.* (2018) 18:887. doi: 10.1186/s12885-018-4802-y
7. Tan S, Pollack JR, Kaplan MJ, Colevas AD, West RB. BRAF inhibitor treatment of primary BRAF-mutant ameloblastoma with pathologic assessment of response. *Oral Surg Oral Med Oral Pathol Oral Radiol.* (2016) 122:e5–7. doi: 10.1016/j.oooo.2015.12.016
8. Faden DL, Algazi A. Durable treatment of ameloblastoma with single agent BRAFi Re: Clinical and radiographic response with combined BRAF-targeted therapy in stage 4 ameloblastoma. *J Natl Cancer Inst.* (2016) 109:djw190. doi: 10.1093/jnci/djw190
9. Kaye FJ, Ivey AM, Drane WE, Mendenhall WM, Allan RW. Clinical and radiographic response with combined BRAF-targeted therapy in stage 4 ameloblastoma. *J Natl Cancer Inst.* (2014) 107:378. doi: 10.1093/jnci/dju378
10. Torres-Collado AX, Knott J, Jazirehi AR. Reversal of resistance in targeted therapy of metastatic melanoma: lessons learned from vemurafenib ($BRAF^{V600E}$-Specific Inhibitor). *Cancers.* (2018) 10:E157. doi: 10.3390/cancers10060157
11. Knispel S, Zimmer L, Kanaki T, Ugurel S, Schadendorf D, Livingstone E. The safety and efficacy of dabrafenib and trametinib for the treatment of melanoma. *Expert Opin Drug Saf.* (2018) 17:73–87. doi: 10.1080/14740338.2018.1390562

14

Exosomes in Head and Neck Squamous Cell Carcinoma

Cheng Xiao [1], *Fang Song* [2], *Yu Long Zheng* [1], *Jiong Lv* [3], *Qiang Feng Wang* [1] *and Nong Xu* [1*]

[1] *Department of Medical Oncology, College of Medicine, The First Affiliated Hospital, Zhejiang University, Hangzhou, China,*
[2] *Department of Anesthesiology, College of Medicine, The First Affiliated Hospital, Zhejiang University, Hangzhou, China,*
[3] *Department of Oral and Maxillofacial Surgery, College of Medicine, The First Affiliated Hospital, Zhejiang University, Hangzhou, China*

Correspondence:
Nong Xu
nongxu@zju.edu.cn

Exosomes are small membranous vesicles that contain proteins, lipids, genetic material, and metabolites with abundant information from parental cells. Exosomes carry and deliver bioactive contents that can reprogram the functions of recipient cells and modulate the tumor microenvironment to induce pathological events through cell-to-cell communication and signal transduction. Tumor-derived exosomes (TDEs) in head and neck squamous cell carcinoma (HNSCC) are involved in most aspects of cancer initiation, invasion, progression, immunoregulation, therapeutic applications, and treatment resistance. In addition, HNSCC-derived exosomes can be used to obtain information on diagnostic and therapeutic biomarkers in circulating blood and saliva. Currently, the biology, mechanisms, and applications of TDEs in HNSCC are still unclear, and further research is required. In this review, we discuss various aspects of exosome biology, including exosomal components, exosomal biomarkers, and molecular mechanisms involved in immunoregulation, cancer metastasis, and therapy resistance. We also describe recent applications to update our understanding of exosomes in HNSCC.

Keywords: exosomes, head and neck squamous cell carcinoma, tumor microenvironment, biomarkers, therapy resistance

INTRODUCTION

Head and neck cancer (HNC) is one of the most widespread malignancies worldwide. Although continual progress has been made in the treatment of HNC, the 5-year overall survival rate of advanced HNC remains low at approximately 50% (1, 2). HNC frequently develops from mucosal surfaces of the mouth, including the oral cavity (tongue, lip, buccal, gingiva, and palate), oropharynx, larynx, and perioral skin carcinoma (3). More than 90% of HNCs are head and neck squamous cell carcinoma (HNSCC). The exact etiology of HNSCC remains unclear; however, tobacco and alcohol consumption are major risk factors for HNSCC, as demonstrated in epidemiological studies. Mucosal human papilloma virus (HPV) is also related to a subset of HNSCCs; ~25.9% of HNSCCs are HPV positive, whereas the prevalence of HPV in oropharyngeal squamous cell carcinoma (SCC) is 34.1%, which is higher than that in oral SCC (4).

Exosomes, which were first discovered in 1983, are 30–150 nm mature double membrane multivesicular bodies (MVBs) originating from the endosomal pathway (5). Exosomes exist in the extracellular space and in liquids, such as blood, urine, and saliva (6). Exosomes are associated with many physiologic aspects of the disease via intercellular communication and signal transduction, indicating that exosomes have potential clinical applications as biomarkers and therapeutic targets. Tumor-derived exosomes (TDEs) contain a cytomembrane, proteins, nucleic acids, lipids, and other substances from parental tumor cells (7). Moreover, exosomes are known to be involved in nearly all stages of cancer (8–11). Growing evidence has demonstrated that TDEs participate in the development, progression, and treatment of cancer by mediating intercellular communication and signal transduction (12, 13). The bioactive components of HNSCC-derived exosomes, such as microRNAs, transcription factors, and oncogenic proteins, play key roles in mediating tumorigenesis, tumor microenvironment reprogramming, immune tolerance, promoting metastasis, and therapy resistance. For example, intracellular annexin 1 (ANXA1) regulates epidermal growth factor receptor (EGFR) activity and alter the release of EGFR-containing TDEs in HNCs (14). Exosomes produced by hypoxic oral SCC cells deliver viral *miR-21* to normoxic cells, inducing the epithelial-mesenchymal transition (EMT) to promote cell migration and invasion (15). Another study showed that exosomal nuclear factor-κB-activating kinase-associated protein 1 (NAP1) derived from oral cancer promotes the cytotoxicity of natural killer (NK) cells via activation of the interferon regulatory factor (IRF-3) signaling pathway in recipient cells (16). In addition, *miR-34a-5p* in cancer-associated fibroblast (CAF)-derived exosomes in oral SCC stimulates the proliferation and metastasis of oral cancer cells through the AKT/glycogen synthease kinase-3β/β-catenin/Snail signaling cascade (17). A recent study demonstrated that thrombospondin 1 derived from oral SCC exosomes is also involved in the polarization of macrophages to M1-like tumor-associated macrophages and promotes the invasion of cancer cells (18). HNSCC-derived exosomes containing EphrinB1 may manipulate the tumor microenvironment through induction of tumor innervation (19). Additionally, Sento demonstrated that oral SCC-derived exosomes promote tumor growth by activating the phosphatidylinositol 3-kiase (PI3K)/AKT, mitogen-activated protein kinase (MAPK)/extracellular signal-regulated kinase (ERK), and c-Jun N-terminal kinase-1/signal transducer and activator of transcription (STAT) 2 pathways (20). Emerging evidence has supported the vital role of TDEs in the development, progression, and treatment of HNSCC.

In this review, we summarize many aspects of exosome biology and functions in HNSCC.

BIOGENESIS, FEATURES, AND COMPONENTS OF EXOSOMES

Inward Budding and MVB Formation

Different types of vesicles, including extracellular vesicles (EVs), MVBs, and exosomes, have been described and often labeled interchangeably in many previous studies. Although these different types of vesicles share overlapping features, they have distinct morphologies, properties, biogenesis mechanisms, and functional roles. Plasma membrane components and enclosing cytosolic components are incorporated into the invaginating membrane, resulting in the formation of early endosomes (21). Exosomes typically originate from inward budding from the membrane and are then released into the extracellular space via activation of Ca^{2+}-dependent or Rab-GTPases (22). Briefly, exosomes are generated from early endosomes, mature into MVBs, and are then secreted into the extracellular space upon fusion with the plasma membrane. First, exosomes start as early endosomes, which are formed by endocytosis of the plasma membrane. The biogenesis of exosomes and sorting of functional cargo is precisely regulated by certain mechanisms involving multiple factors. The most commonly described pathway for exosomes biogenesis is the endosomal sorting complex required for transport (ESCRT) machinery. Four types of ESCRTs (ESCRT-0–III) are involved in regulating MVB formation, vesicle budding, and protein cargo sorting (23). The ESCRT mechanism is initiated and sequestrated by ubiquitinated proteins to domains of the endosomal membrane via ubiquitin binding subunits of ESCRT-0 in the endosomal membrane, then interacting with the ESCRT-I and ESCRT-II complexes inducing membrane deformation into buds. Finally, the ESCRT-III complex separates from the MVBs membrane (23–25). However, the machinery that drives the load of protein cargo into ESCRT-dependent exosomes is still unclear.

Cells also utilize ESCRT-independent pathways, involving insphingosine-1-phosphate, ceramide, tetraspanin-enriched microdomains, and sphingomyelinase, for exosome production and release (26–28). These ESCRT-independent mechanisms may participate in promoting domain-induced budding, sorting of bioactive molecules into exosomes, segregation of cargo within the endosomal membrane, and exosome formation.

The ESCRT-dependent and -independent mechanisms of exosome release are based on the cell origin. In addition, membrane proteins of lysosomes and late endosomes may be important for the biogenesis and secretion of exosomes (29).

Regulated Secretion and Intercellular Interactions

Exosome secretion is involved in various signaling pathways. For example, the key regulatory role of RAB family proteins in trafficking intracellular exosomes was demonstrated by Colombo et al. (30). Another report showed that the Wnt pathway is particularly important for the dysregulation of exosome release in cancer cells (31). Additionally, the secretion of exosomes is mediated through exocytosis-associated molecular motors and cytoskeletal proteins (32). Spontaneous secretion of exosomes usually occurs at the steady state; however, some conditions are known to stimulate exosomes. Indeed, cell intrinsic signals are known to enhance the release of high levels of TDEs from cancer cells via activation of oncogenic signaling pathways or regulation of membrane fusion machinery (33). In addition, evidence suggests that microenvironmental conditions enhance exosome release from cancer cells (15, 34). Exosomes are then released into the extracellular environment through exocytosis or degraded by fusing with lysosomes. As previously described, Rab GTPases are essential regulators of exosome secretion. Furthermore, several studies have shown that soluble N-ethylmaleimide-sensitive component attachment protein receptor complexes, which are involved in membrane fusion machinery, may affect the secretion of exosomes (35–37).

Ultimately, exosomes are internalized by recipient cells through receptor-mediated endocytosis, pinocytosis, phagocytosis, or fusion with the cell membrane, resulting in delivery of molecular and genetic components into the recipient cells (30). Exosomes target recipient cells after secretion into the extracellular space and then induce changes in downstream signaling pathways. The specificity of target recipient cells is dependent on the type of ligand/receptor pairs present on exosomes and recipient cells; and a study provides further insight that glycans are key players in the process of exosomes uptake (38). A schematic representation of exosome biogenesis and secretion pathways is shown in **Figure 1**.

FEATURES AND COMPONENTS OF EXOSOMES

Typical exosomes exhibit a particular biconcave or cup-like shape and are observed as spheroids under transmission electron microscopy (39). Exosome contents are rich in nucleic acids, cytosolic/endosome proteins, and cytoskeleton components, which have unique biological activities (40). The components of TDEs are distinct from those of exosomes released from healthy cells. TDEs deliver functional cargo, including oncogenes and oncogenic proteins that can exert biological activities. The functional cargoes, such as protein cargo, RNA cargo, and DNA cargo, of TDEs in the tumor microenvironment have an important role in promoting cancer progression and metastasis (**Figure 1**) (33). Protein cargoes, including different oncoproteins, immunomodulatory molecules, and growth factors, act as mediators of tumorigenesis. TDEs also contain abundant nucleic acids, such as microRNAs (miRNAs), mRNA, long noncoding RNAs, and DNAs, which deliver genetic information (41–43).

Many researchers have analyzed the functions of miRNAs in exosomes, and various specific miRNA cargoes and extracellular components have been detected in exosomes. These observations highlight the specificity of exosomal miRNAs, distinct miRNA signatures of exosomes, and various functions of exosomal miRNAs. A series of experiments have analyzed the function of the miRNAs in exosomes since their initial description (44). It has been reported that there was a selection of specific miRNA cargoes and extracellular exports in exosomes (30). These observations highlight the specificity of exosomal miRNAs, distinct miRNA signatures of exosomes, and various functions of exosomal miRNAs. Exosomal miRNAs are associated with a variety of pathological activities, including tumorigenesis, invasion, progression, angiogenesis, metastasis,

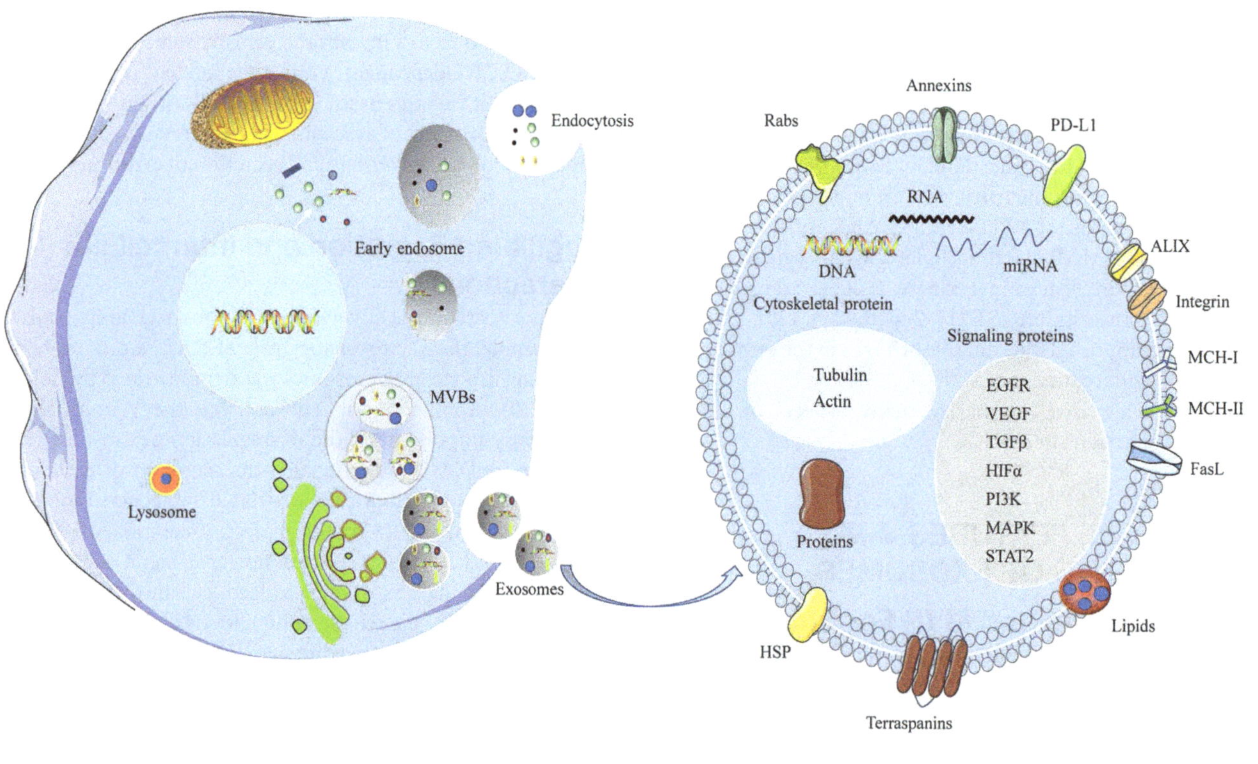

FIGURE 1 | A schematic representation of biogenesis and components of the HNSCC-derived exosomes. Invagination of the plasma membrane form early endosomes, followed by budding of payload into the endosomal membrane to form multivesicular endosomes (MVBs). Maturation of the late endosome through fusion with the plasma membrane and release of exosomes. Some of the late endosome fuse with lysosomes for lysosomal degradation. The HNSCC-derived exosomes contain various cellular ingredients, such as nucleic acids, lipid, and proteins, which act as key molecules of signaling transduction.

and chemoresistance. However, not all exosomal miRNAs are implicated in tumor-supportive mechanisms. miRNAs of exosomes are highly functional, with roles in intercellular communication and tumor microenvironment regulation, indicating that exosomal miRNAs play important roles in diagnostic and therapeutic applications.

In addition, exosomes contain ceramides, lipids, sphingolipids, cholesterol, and glycerophospholipids. Because exosomes originate from the fusion of endocytic compartments with the plasma membrane, the protein, lipid, and double lipid layer compositions can be used to identify exosomes. The most commonly identified markers are ALIX and tetraspanins, such as CD9, CD63, CD81, and CD82 (23).

FUNCTIONS OF EXOSOMES IN HNSCC

Exosomes have been identified as bioactive and informative nano-sized MVBs that influence many aspects of the development and progression of HNSCC. Here, we discuss recent findings of the mechanisms through which HNSCC-derived exosomes modulate the immune response, tumor microenvironment, cell-to-cell communication, and tumor invasion. We also describe exosomes as potential biomarkers and discuss their applications in cancer therapy and therapy resistance.

EXOSOMES AS POTENTIAL BIOMARKERS

In the clinical setting, some relevant biomarkers have been shown to influence treatments for patients with HNSCC. Several reports have shown that liquid biopsies, including biopsies of circulating tumor DNA, circulating tumor cells, and exosomal miRNAs, can have potential clinical applications in HNC (45). Moreover, HPV status is a prognostic factor in HNSCC; patients with HPV positivity have better responsiveness to chemotherapy and radiotherapy and are more susceptible to immune surveillance. In addition, miRNAs are independent prognostic markers for patients with HPV-negative HNSCC (46), and EGFR overexpression is associated with poorer prognosis and outcomes in HNSCC (47). However, further studies are needed to establish biomarkers for staging HNSCC and facilitating therapeutic decision-making.

Exosomes modulate various pathological activities to promote cancer cell growth, invasion, and distant metastasis. TDEs also carry valuable genomic and proteomic information and can provide information regarding alterations in genomic and proteomic profiles of exosomes from patients with cancer in response to anticancer therapies (48). Such proteomic and genetic components are well-protected within the lipid bilayer and can be preserved without significant loss of functional profiling. Therefore, exosomes may serve as promising markers for monitoring cancer progression and therapeutic responses (49).

TDEs can be obtained from blood or saliva of patients with HNSCC, indicating that TDEs may represent a real-time, non-invasive, clinically relevant biomarker of cancer progression, and treatment responses (45, 50–53). For example, the number of exosomes in the plasma has been shown to be a prognosis indicator for HNSCC. Gimzewski reported that elevated exosome numbers, exosome sizes, and interexosomes were detected in the saliva of patients with oral cancer (54). In addition, patients with HNSCC with advanced-stage disease and shorter overall survival usually exhibit elevated levels of exosomes in the plasma, indicating that plasma exosomes in HNSCC may have applications in monitoring tumor progression (52, 54). One previous study demonstrated that TDE signatures could serve as candidate biomarkers for early cancer diagnosis, monitoring, and surveillance in HPV-16-associated oropharyngeal (55). Moreover, a non-invasive method involving Fourier-transform infrared spectroscopy of salivary exosomes was shown to have high sensitivity and specificity in the diagnosis of oral cancer (56).

Non-coding RNAs from plasma exosomes have been extensively studied as potential biomarkers in HNSCC because they are derived from whole tumor cells and may therefore represent whole cellular RNAs (57, 58). Several studies have reported that cancer cells can selectively pack selected miRNAs into exosomes, and these selective exosomal miRNAs then act as tumor suppressors or oncogenes in HNSCC (59–61). Additionally, a hypoxic microenvironment can stimulate oral SCC to generate *miR-21*-rich exosomes, which are associated with lymph node metastasis (15). Serum exosomal *miR-21* and homeobox transcript antisense RNA (*HOTAIR*) are also significantly associated with the clinical characteristics of laryngeal SCC (59). In a previous study, elevated CAF-derived exosomal *miR-196a* levels were shown to be correlated with cisplatin resistance in HNSCC through targeting cyclin-dependent kinase (CDK) N1B and inhibitor of growth family member 5 (ING5), indicating that this miRNA may serve as a promising predictor of cisplatin resistance and poor survival in HNSCC (60). A study by Zhou and colleagues revealed that there were significant differences in expression between exosomal miRNAs and cellular miRNAs in laryngeal SCC (61). Furthermore, oral cancer-derived salivary exosomal *miR-512-3p* and *miR-412-3p* may serve as potential biomarkers (62). In another example, Inazawa and colleagues found that exosomal *miR-1246* induces cell motility and invasion through directly targeting differentially expressed in normal vs. neoplastic/MAPK-activating death domain-containing 2D in oral SCC (63). Collectively, these results suggested that exosomal miRNAs could serve as excellent diagnostic and prognostic biomarkers.

Analysis of exosomal proteins is a novel tool for developing exosomes as potential biomarkers for HNSCC. More than 80% of HNSCCs exhibit overexpression of EGFR in the membrane, and hyperactivity EGFR plays an important role in tumorigenesis development and drug-resistance mechanisms by activating various signaling pathways, including the PI3K/AKT, RAS/MEK/ERK, and Janus kinase (JAK)/STAT pathways, in HNSCC. A recent study showed that EGFR can be secreted from cells via the transport of exosomes and that these EGFR-containing exosomes have the ability to regulate autocrine VEGF production in endothelial cells (64). Exosomal EGFR mediates metastasis and tumor immunity in lung cancer (65). ANXA1, a tumor suppressor in HNSCC, regulates EGFR activity and exosomal phospho-EGFR release, revealing that exosomal EGFR and phospho-EGFR may be prognostic biomarkers in HNSCC (14). Additionally, the levels of exosomal EGFR and phospho-EGFR are reduced after cetuximab treatment, indicating that exosomes can serve as biomarkers to monitor cetuximab treatment (66).

Analysis of exosome protein profiles showed that the characteristics and functions of exosomes from HPV-positive/-negative HNC differed significantly. HPV-positive exosomes had low p53 levels and did not contain cyclin D1, but did harbor p16, E6/E7, and the T-cell inhibitory protein PTPN11 (67). A recent study revealed that proteome analysis of salivary extracellular vesicles may yield prognostic biomarkers for oral SCC (68).

The microenvironment of HNSCC is highly immunosuppressive, and the programmed cell death (PD)-1/PD-ligand 1 (PD-L1) pathway plays an important role in HNSCC. High levels of PD-L1 are associated with poor outcomes in various types of cancer, including HNSCC. PD-1 checkpoint inhibitors were found to be safe and effective in platinum-refractory recurrent or metastatic HNSCC (69, 70). Furthermore, a study by Whiteside and colleagues indicated that PD-L1$^+$ exosomes in the plasma were related to immune suppression and disease progression. Additionally, blocking PD-L1$^+$ exosome signaling to PD-1$^+$ T cells attenuated immune suppression in patients with HNSCC (71). In another study, Ferris reported that JAK2/STAT1 signaling was involved in EGFR-mediated immune evasion in HNSCC and that therapies targeting this signaling pathway may be beneficial for blocking PD-L1 upregulation in HNSCC (72). Moreover, elevated heat-shock protein 90 levels in TDEs have been reported to serve as potential biomarkers for clinical stage and prognosis in patients with oral cancer (73). A recent study showed that plasma-derived exosomes were associated with disease progression of HNSCC after separation into CD3$^+$ and CD3$^-$ fractions (74). Furthermore, HNSCC-derived exosomes have been shown to exhibit synergistic interactions with invadopodia, indicating that exosomes play key roles in promoting cancer invasion (35). TDEs inducing transcriptome reprogramming can cause cancer-associated pathologies in HNSCC, including angiogenesis, immunoregulation, and metastasis; these functional differences in HNSCC may serve as candidate markers (75).

A growing body of evidence has shown that the characteristics of TDEs and exosomal components (e.g., exosomal miRNAs, exosomal proteins) may serve as potential noninvasive biomarkers for the detection, monitoring, and treatment of HNSCC (**Figure 2**). However, methods for TDE isolation and separation are complicated and time-consuming, and additional studies of TDEs as non-invasive biomarkers are needed.

ROLES IN REGULATING THE TUMOR MICROENVIRONMENT

Immune Cells

The tumor microenvironment is formed by stromal cells and is associated with malignant progression (76). Moreover, TDEs play important roles in regulating the tumor microenvironment of HNC (77). The immunological activities of exosomes are related to many aspects of immune regulation, including antigen presentation, immune activation, immune surveillance, and immune suppression. Tumor-infiltrating myeloid-derived suppressor cells (MDSCs), tumor-associated macrophages (TAMs), and regulatory T cells (Tregs) are known mediators of the immunosuppressive microenvironment and limit the efficacy of immune therapy in HNC (78). Exosomes that contain immunosuppressive molecules can facilitate immunosuppression in cancer, which helps cancer cells escape from immune responses, thereby promoting tumorigenesis (79, 80). Additionally, exosome-associated bioactive proteins and RNAs have been shown to regulate the immune system (81, 82). Exosomes may mediate immune suppression through

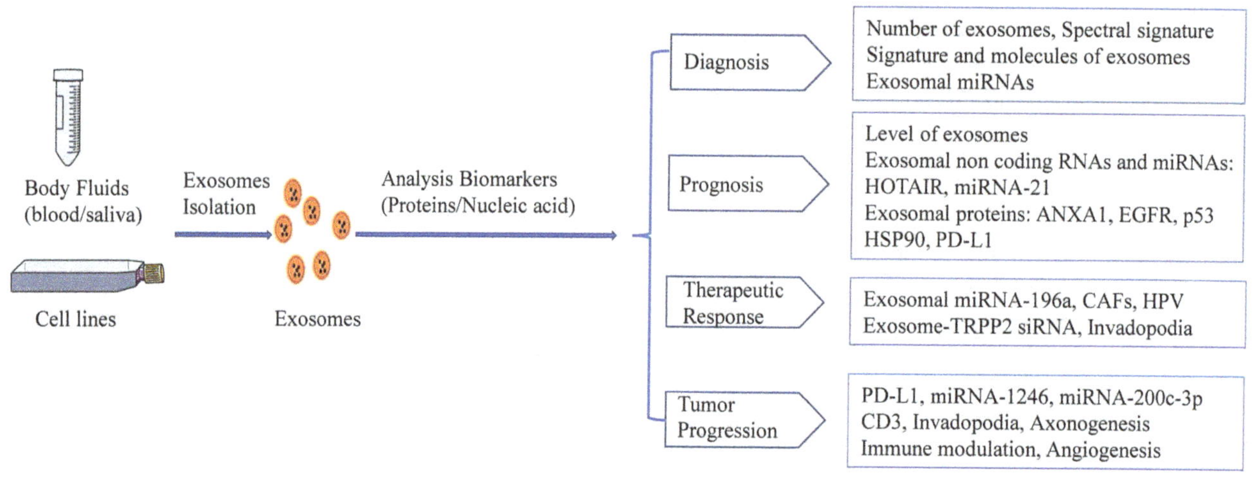

FIGURE 2 | HNSCC-derived exosomes act as biomarkers. Exosomal biomarkers screening of diagnostics, prognosis, or therapeutics in HNSCC.

directly/indirectly inhibiting the functions of T cells and NK cells and then altering the number or activity of immune suppressor cells, including MDSCs, Tregs, and HLA-DR cells (83). Exosomes are also involved in different soluble factors such as check-point receptor ligands (PD-L1), inhibitory cytokines (IL-10 and TGF-β1), death receptor ligands (FasL), ectoenzymes, and prostaglandin E2 responsible for antitumor immunity in the tumor microenvironment (84, 85). In lymphocytes and NK cells, exosomes are associated with disease stage and activity in patients with HNC, suggesting that plasma exosomes may be related to HNC progression (86). In cancer, exosome signaling may affect the immune system by inhibiting the maturity of antigen-presenting cells and TDEs that carry and transfer tumor antigens to antigen-presenting cells, thereby inducing T cell- or NK cell-dependent immune responses (87). In a similar study, TDEs containing FasL and tumor necrosis factor α were found to induce T-cell apoptosis, thereby establishing an immunosuppressive tumor microenvironment to support tumor progression (88). TDEs derived from multiple HNCC cell lines induce a suppressive phenotype in $CD8^+$ T cells through galectin-1, indicating that tumor-derived immunosuppressive exosomes may be potential therapeutic targets for preventing T-cell dysfunction and enhancing antitumor immune responses (89). As previously mentioned, the levels of oral SCC-derived $FasL^+$ microvesicles are correlated with tumor burden, and the $FasL^+$ microvesicles are involved in mediating apoptosis in activated T lymphocytes via receptor and mitochondrial pathways (51). A recent study showed that $CD4^+CD39^+$ Tregs produce adenosine by exposure to $CD39^+CD73^+$ exosomes from plasma in patients with HNSCC, thereby supporting tumor immune escape (90). Additionally, a recent study showed that oxygen pressure regulates the tumor microenvironment by altering exosomal miRNAs, which subsequently regulate the *miR-21*/phosphatase and tensin homolog (PTEN)/PD-L1 axis (91).

HPV-Positive and -Negative Exosomes

The molecular and functional profiles of exosomes from HPV-positive and -negative HNSCC are different. An early study demonstrated that HNSCC-derived exosomes have different effects on the immune system in HPV-positive and -negative HNSCC. However, there are no differences in suppressive $CD4^+$ and $CD8^+$ T cells between HPV-positive and -negative exosomes, although the responses of human monocyte-derived dendritic cells (DCs) and mature DCs to exosomes are different. HPV-positive exosomes promote DC maturation, whereas HPV-negative exosomes suppress DC maturation. HPV-negative exosomes suppress the expression of antigen processing machinery, whereas HPV-positive exosomes do not (67). HPV-positive exosomes that promote DC maturation may also stimulate antitumor immune responses, thereby improving clinical outcomes in patients with HPV-positive HNSCC (67). HPV has been shown to utilize host exosomes for cell-cell communication and to induce EGFR expression and AKT signaling in recipient cells. One study found that exosomal NAP1 derived from oral cancer cells can promote the activation of NK cells by increasing the expression and phosphorylation of IRF-3 (92).

Fibroblasts

CAFs are particularly important for regulating tumor progression. Mesenchymal stem cells reprogrammed by TDEs mediate pro-angiogenic activity and convert stromal cells into CAFs; these cells are a major component of the tumor microenvironment and play key roles in promoting tumor progression (93). HNC-derived CAFs are innately resistant to cisplatin. Indeed, a study by Zhang showed that exosomal *miR-196a* derived from HNC causes cisplatin resistance by targeting CDKN1B and ING5, highlighting the roles of CAF-derived exosomal *miR-196a* in promoting cell proliferation and inhibiting cell apoptosis in the HNC microenvironment (60). Moreover, high expression of microfibril associated protein 5 in CAF-derived exosomes may contribute to the proliferation and metastasis of oral SCC via activation of the MAPK and AKT signaling pathways (94). Additionally, TDEs have been shown to deliver caveolin-1 to the tumor microenvironment to mediate the EMT and CAFs in tongue SCC (95). In a similar study, CAF-derived exosomal *miR-34a-5p* was found to be associated with oral cancer cell proliferation and metastasis in oral SCC (17). Thus, TDEs are emerging as potent mediators of the tumor microenvironment in HNSCC (**Figure 3**).

ROLES OF TDES IN REGULATING CANCER PROGRESSION AND METASTASIS

Many studies have evaluated the roles of TDEs in cancer initiation and progression. Numerous molecules in TDEs have been implicated in the initiation and progression of cancer cells or the tumor microenvironment (96). Indeed, TDEs can transform epithelial cells into cancerous cells, thereby initiating tumorigenesis. Studies have shown that TDEs reprogram the functions of recipient cells and facilitate premetastatic niche transformation to promote metastasis through cell-cell communication or autocrine signals. Additionally, TDEs facilitate tumor progression by delivery of factors necessary for sustaining tumor growth via utilizing autocrine or juxtacrine signaling (97). Furthermore, many studies have shown that RNA from TDEs can promote metastasis (57). The shuttling of miRNA molecules may cause tumorigenesis, tumor progression, and mRNA entry into recipient cells, resulting in protein translation and metastasis (44). The EMT has been implicated in cancer cell progression and metastasis, and TDEs deliver functional complexes by membrane fusion with recipient cells and binding of the recipient cell membrane receptors to promote the EMT (98).

Exosomes derived from hypoxic oral SCC cells promote cell migration and invasion by delivering *miR-21* to normoxic cells in HNSCC (15). Nakashima conducted a study indicating that *miR-200c-3p* had invasive capacity in the human oral SCC microenvironment (99). Moreover, CAFs contribute to the proliferation and metastasis of oral cancer cells via

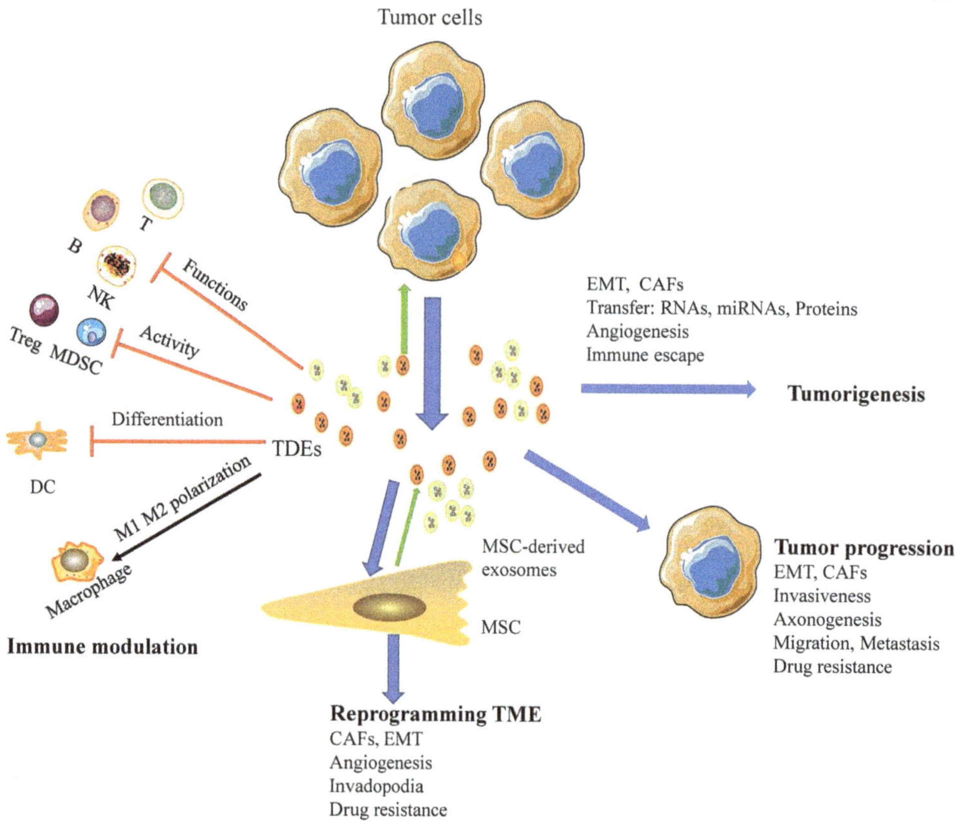

FIGURE 3 | A macroscopic view of the functions of HNSCC-derived exosomes in the tumor microenvironment. Exosomes reduce tumor immunosurveillance by interfering with the immune system: (a) inhibit the functions of immune cells; (b) suppress the activity of Tregs, MDSCs; (c) interference the differentiation of DC; (d) TAMs polarization. HNSCC-derived exosomes mediated metastasis via stimulating proliferation of endothelial cells, EMT, CAFs, and promote angiogenesis as well as re-programming of the stromal compartment. Also HNSCC-derived exosomes influence cancer progression, promoting cancer cell growth, and invasive behavior of cancer cells and development of therapy resistance.

exosome-mediated paracrine *miR-34a-5p* signaling (17). Several studies have reported the heterogeneity of transforming growth factor (TGF) β signaling in oral cavity SCC. TGFβ expressed on the surface of TDEs can differentiate fibroblasts into myofibroblasts, thereby promoting tumor progression and metastasis in oral cavity SCC (100). Additionally, exosomes target different organs via variations in integrin molecules expressed on the surface. Released exosomes can be delivered to distant organs to promote oncogenic activity by constructing a suitable premetastatic tumor microenvironment for tumor migration. Thus, TDEs contribute to the development of this premetastatic niche and induce metastatic potential in recipient cells. A recent study showed that exosomes can transport EGFR to the liver to remodel the liver microenvironment (101). TDEs can transfer oncogenic EGFR to endothelial cells, triggering upregulation of vascular endothelial growth factor (VEGF) and autocrine VEGF in endothelial cells exposed to cancer cell-related MVs (64). Moreover, oral cancer cell-derived MVs promote endothelial cell angiogenesis through the Shh/RhoA signaling pathway (102). Additional experiments have demonstrated that exosomal *miR-150* promotes tumorigenesis by upregulating VEGF, and another study showed that HNSCC-derived exosomes stimulate angiogenesis *in vitro* and *in vivo* through functional reprogramming of endothelial cells (103). These studies suggest that exosomal miRNA could affect the biology of endothelial cells; then the exosomal miRNA induces angiogenesis in HNC through different regulation pathways.

TDEs modulate the immune response in tumor microenvironment interactions implicated in cancer progression. Oral SCC-derived exosomes induced M1-like TAMs polarized and promoted tumor metastasis (18). And tumor released exosomes containing EphrinB1 potentiate induce axonogenesis will promote tumor innervation in HNSCC (19). And the delivery of miRNA-21-abundant exosomes promote EMT-mediated M2-like polarization of TAMs may promote tumor progression of HNSCC (104). Another study demonstrated that exosomes derived from irradiated HNSCC cells can modify cancer cell movement and promote migration of recipient cells through AKT-signaling (105). In an additional series of experiments, exosomes were recruited to the plasma membrane of invadopodia, and knockdown of Rab27a decreased exosome secretion and extracellular matrix digestion associated with maturing invadopodia (35). The mechanisms through which TDEs regulate cancer progression and metastasis are illustrated in **Figure 3**.

THERAPEUTIC APPLICATION

Exosomes are cell-derived nanoparticles that have unique properties, such as low immunogenicity, strong ability to cross physiological barriers, good biodistribution and bioavailability, and reduced immunogenicity. Thus, TDEs may have important roles as potential vehicles for anticancer drugs. In addition, exosomes can be remodeled through their parental cells or supplemented with desired biological activity (106). Exosomes have been designed as promising therapeutic agents in the treatment of various cancers (107–109). Because patients with metastatic HNSCC have a poor prognosis and do not typically respond well to traditional therapies, efficient targeted delivery of conventional chemotherapeutic drugs may be facilitated by innovative approaches to engineering drug delivery systems, such as exosomes.

Drug carrier exosomes have been isolated from various types of cells, including HEK-293 cells, immature DCs, macrophages, and cancer cells. Different therapeutic agents, including proteins, small interfering RNAs (siRNAs), miRNAs, and targeted drugs, can be incorporated into exosomes via electroporation, chemical-based transfection, modification of parental cells, or direct incubation, thereby increasing bioactivity and achieving targeted delivery in patients. The James Graham Brown Cancer Center initiated a phase I clinical trial to test the therapeutic effects of plant exosomes in HNC (NCT01668849). In various types of cancer, exosomes have been shown to shuttle miRNAs and soluble proteins as therapeutic molecules into recipient cells and tissues (107, 110). A hypoxic microenvironment promotes the generation of *miR-21*-rich exosomes by oral SCC in a hypoxia-inducible factor (HIF)-1a- and HIF-2a-dependent manner, and these *miR-21*-rich exosomes then mediate migration and invasion behaviors. Restoration of *miR-21* expression in HIF-1a- and HIF-2a-depleted exosomes rescues oral SCC migration and invasion (15). Moreover, hypoxic TDEs mediate MDSC function through the *miR-21*/PTEN/PD-L1 axis in oral SCC (91). These findings indicate the therapeutic value of exosome inhibition for oral SCC treatment.

Anti-EGFR nanobodies anchored on extracellular vesicles via glycosyl phosphatidylinositol may improve the targeting ability of extracellular vesicles, highlighting the potential applications of these extracellular vesicles as a drug delivery system and new tool in EGFR-expressing tumor cells (111). The blood-brain barrier restricts drugs from entering into the brain, which can reduce the therapeutic effects of brain cancer treatments. Brain endothelial cell-derived exosomes can deliver anticancer drugs across the blood-brain barrier for the treatment of brain cancer. Additionally, exosome-based drug carriers can mediate permeability across the blood-brain barrier, enabling the drug to target cancer cells (112).

The main rational approaches for inhibiting exosome-mediated tumor-promoting potential have focused on blocking exosome release and suppressing the communication of tumor cells with recipient cells. TDEs are known to be abundantly secreted from cancer cells, making them potential targets for anticancer therapy. Direct targeting of the exosome release process has also been studied for the treatment of cancer. Exosome-delivered transient receptor potential polycystic 2 (TRPP2) siRNA markedly suppresses TRPP2 expression and inhibits the EMT, suggesting that exosome-TRPP2 siRNA may be an effective RNA-based gene therapy in the treatment of HNC (113). Invadopodia also enhance exosome secretion; accordingly, silencing the expression of invadopodia may suppress TDE biogenesis and release (114). Another potential strategy for exosomal dysregulation is the inhibition of exosome uptake. Treatment with heparin blocks the uptake of exosomes by oral SCC cells, thereby attenuating exosome-induced cancer progression to inhibit the growth and progression of oral SCC cells (20). However, the use of these reagents for eliminating exosomes is currently limited to research use only because these reagents may also induce off-target effects. Further studies are needed to explore the translational implications of exosome-targeted reagents.

Owing to the potential presence of TDEs and the unique biomarkers associated with these vesicles, TDEs may also have applications as vaccine immunotherapies (115). Antigen-presenting exosomes from B lymphocytes and DCs containing MHCI/II complexes could stimulate $CD4^+$ and $CD8^+$ T cells as therapeutic HPV vaccines (116). Additionally, HPV oncogenes play vital roles in HPV-induced carcinogenesis, and silencing of endogenous HPV E6/E7 expression affects both the contents and levels of MVs released from HPV-positive cancer cells (117). These findings indicate that inhibition of endogenous HPV E6/E7 expression may have therapeutic applications. HPV vaccines based on endogenously engineered exosomes for HNC have been evaluated in several phase I clinical trials (118). However, additional studies are required to determine the feasibility and safety of TDEs as cancer vaccines. One of the major challenges in developing this approach is establishing scalable, reproducible methods for exosome production. MSCs may have uses in exosome production at a clinically applicable scale owing to their ability of produce large amounts of exosomes.

Collectively, these studies suggest that exosome-based strategies may have many benefits over conventional drug regimens; however, there are some limitations and challenges to the use of exosomes. First, because TDEs contain genetic components from cancer cells, cancer cells may not be suitable parental cells for exosome targeting in clinical applications. Additionally, efficient loading of exosomes without significant alterations to the structure and content of exosomal membranes may be difficult. Overall, these reports indicate that exosomes may function as exceptional gene delivery vectors that are safe, efficient, organ-/cell-specific, and nonimmunogenic. Nevertheless, significant efforts are required to before clinical applications are feasible.

ANTI-CANCER THERAPY RESISTANCE

Current therapy options for HNSCC include surgery, radiotherapy, chemotherapy, anti-EGFR-antibody treatment, and immunotherapy (119). However, drug resistance remains a major obstacle for achieving successful curative treatment of cancer. Drug resistance includes endogenous drug resistance, innate drug resistance, and acquired drug resistance. Acquired drug resistance is a process through which cancer cells exposed to chemotherapy, radiation, or targeted therapy show reprogramming of their genome to acquire resistance to the therapy. Cancer cells may mitigate the effects of radiation and chemotherapy through different mechanisms (120, 121).

Given the important roles of exosomes in cellular communication and the tumor microenvironment, many studies have indicated that exosomes are involved in anticancer therapy resistance. In one mechanism, exosomes sequester cytotoxic drugs in intracellular vesicles and subsequently negate the effects of drugs within the cells (122). Owing to the nature of exosomes as mediators of cell-cell communication in the tumor microenvironment, these exosomes play important roles in therapy resistance by transferring various contents, such as miRNAs, mRNAs, DNAs, and proteins, to induce extrinsic therapy resistance (123). Similarly, exosomes also promote therapy resistance by transferring mRNAs, miRNAs, and other components. In addition, TDEs mediate therapy resistance by different mechanism, including improved DNA repair, anti-apoptotic signaling, or delivery of transporters to treatment-sensitive cells. As mediators of mesenchymal stem cells and the EMT, exosomes also promote tumor microenvironment-associated treatment resistance (123).

Exosomes derived from drug-resistant cancer cells mediate drug resistance through direct shuttling of drugs out of the cells (124). The AKT pathway is a frequently mutated oncogenic pathway in HNSCC and functions as a key regulator of radiation resistance and a major driver of cellular movement and migration (125). Exosomes derived from irradiated HNSCC cells trigger the AKT pathway to promote migration and increase chemotaxis in recipient cancer cells (105). Radiation therapy may increase the invasive and metastatic properties of HNSCC via release of an abundance of exosomes in hypoxic cancer tissue after radiotherapy (126–128). In patients with melanoma receiving PD-1 blockade therapy, the level of circulating exosomal PD-L1 correlates with tumor burden and response to therapy (129). The PD-1/PD-L1 immune checkpoint signaling axis exhibits remarkable responses in platinum-refractory recurrent or metastatic HNSCC; PD-L1-containing TDEs, which transfer functional PD-L1 and inhibit immune responses, may be regulators and biomarkers of resistance to PD-1 blockade therapy. In addition, exosomes derived from cisplatin-resistant HNSCC cells deliver *miR-21* to parental cells and induce cisplatin resistance, suggesting that these exosomes may function primarily through gene regulation (130). TDEs have been implicated in contributing to drug resistance in HNSCC (**Figure 3**).

FUTURE IMPLICATIONS

TDEs contain numerous bioactive cellular molecules and genetic characteristics, enabling them to alter the functions of recipient cells and the tumor microenvironment. Accordingly, TDEs play important regulatory roles in cancer. Indeed, TDEs are involved in many aspects of intercellular substance transmission and signal transfer, contributing to the initiation, development, metastasis, treatment resistance, and immunosuppression of HNSCC. In HNSCC, TDEs may serve as potential clinical biomarkers of progression or responses to therapy owing to their various functional contents (proteins, genes) and elements of the parental cancer cells. Nevertheless, exosomes have not yet been applied in the treatment of HNSCC. Further studies are needed to elucidate the molecular mechanisms involved in the release of exosomes and to explore the clinical applications of these vesicles. Understanding how cancer cells utilize TDEs to promote cancer growth and progression may lead to the development of novel therapies for HNSCC. Therefore, much work is needed to establish exosome-based therapies for the treatment of HNSCC.

AUTHOR CONTRIBUTIONS

CX, FS, and NX: review concept, review design, interpretation, manuscript preparation, and manuscript review. YZ, JL, and QW: manuscript preparation and manuscript review.

REFERENCES

1. Bray F, Ferlay J, Soerjomataram I, Siegel RL, Torre LA, Jemal A. Global cancer statistics 2018: GLOBOCAN estimates of incidence and mortality worldwide for 36 cancers in 185 countries. *Cancer J Clin.* (2018) 68:394–424. doi: 10.3322/caac.21492
2. Ang KK, Harris J, Wheeler R, Weber R, Rosenthal DI, Nguyen-Tan PF, et al. Human papillomavirus and survival of patients with oropharyngeal cancer. *N Engl J Med.* (2010) 363:24–35. doi: 10.1056/NEJMoa0912217
3. Lydiatt WM, Patel SG, O'Sullivan B, Brandwein MS, Ridge JA, Migliacci JC, et al. Head and neck cancers-major changes in the American Joint Committee on cancer eighth edition cancer staging manual. *Cancer J Clin.* (2017) 67:122–37. doi: 10.3322/caac.21389
4. Kreimer AR, Clifford GM, Boyle P, Franceschi S. Human papillomavirus types in head and neck squamous cell carcinomas worldwide: a systematic review. *Cancer Epidemiol Biomark Prev.* (2005) 14:467–75. doi: 10.1158/1055-9965.EPI-04-0551
5. Pan BT, Johnstone RM. Fate of the transferrin receptor during maturation of sheep reticulocytes *in vitro*: selective externalization of the receptor. *Cell.* (1983) 33:967–78. doi: 10.1016/0092-8674(83)90040-5
6. Keller S, Ridinger J, Rupp AK, Janssen JW, Altevogt P. Body fluid derived exosomes as a novel template for clinical diagnostics. *J Transl Med.* (2011) 9:86. doi: 10.1186/1479-5876-9-86
7. Xin T, Greco V, Myung P. Hardwiring stem cell communication through tissue structure. *Cell.* (2016) 164:1212–25. doi: 10.1016/j.cell.2016.02.041
8. Steinbichler TB, Dudas J, Riechelmann H, Skvortsova, II. The role of exosomes in cancer metastasis. *Semin Cancer Biol.* (2017) 44:170–81. doi: 10.1016/j.semcancer.2017.02.006

9. Becker A, Thakur BK, Weiss JM, Kim HS, Peinado H, Lyden D. Extracellular vesicles in cancer: cell-to-cell mediators of metastasis. *Cancer Cell.* (2016) 30:836–48. doi: 10.1016/j.ccell.2016.10.009
10. Liu Y, Cao X. Organotropic metastasis: role of tumor exosomes. *Cell Res.* (2016) 26:149–50. doi: 10.1038/cr.2015.153
11. Zhang Y, Wang XF. A niche role for cancer exosomes in metastasis. *Nat Cell Biol.* (2015) 17:709–11. doi: 10.1038/ncb3181
12. Zhang HG, Grizzle WE. Exosomes: a novel pathway of local and distant intercellular communication that facilitates the growth and metastasis of neoplastic lesions. *Am J Pathol.* (2014) 184:28–41. doi: 10.1016/j.ajpath.2013.09.027
13. Wang Z, Chen JQ, Liu JL, Tian L. Exosomes in tumor microenvironment: novel transporters and biomarkers. *J Transl Med.* (2016) 14:297. doi: 10.1186/s12967-016-1056-9
14. Raulf N, Lucarelli P, Thavaraj S, Brown S, Vicencio JM, Sauter T, et al. Annexin A1 regulates EGFR activity and alters EGFR-containing tumour-derived exosomes in head and neck cancers. *Eur J Cancer.* (2018) 102:52–68. doi: 10.1016/j.ejca.2018.07.123
15. Li L, Li C, Wang S, Wang Z, Jiang J, Wang W, et al. Exosomes derived from hypoxic oral squamous cell carcinoma cells deliver miR-21 to normoxic cells to elicit a prometastatic phenotype. *Cancer Res.* (2016) 76:1770–80. doi: 10.1158/0008-5472.CAN-15-1625
16. Wang Y, Qin X, Zhu X, Chen W, Zhang J, Chen W. Oral cancer-derived exosomal NAP1 enhances cytotoxicity of natural killer cells via the IRF-3 pathway. *Oral Oncol.* (2018) 76:34–41. doi: 10.1016/j.oraloncology.2017.11.024
17. Li YY, Tao YW, Gao S, Li P, Zheng JM, Zhang SE, et al. Cancer-associated fibroblasts contribute to oral cancer cells proliferation and metastasis via exosome-mediated paracrine miR-34a-5p. *EBioMedicine.* (2018) 36:209–20. doi: 10.1016/j.ebiom.2018.09.006
18. Xiao M, Zhang J, Chen W, Chen W. M1-like tumor-associated macrophages activated by exosome-transferred THBS1 promote malignant migration in oral squamous cell carcinoma. *J Exp Clin Cancer Res.* (2018) 37:143. doi: 10.1186/s13046-018-0815-2
19. Madeo M, Colbert PL, Vermeer DW, Lucido CT, Cain JT, Vichaya EG, et al. Cancer exosomes induce tumor innervation. *Nat Commun.* (2018) 9:4284. doi: 10.1038/s41467-018-06640-0
20. Sento S, Sasabe E, Yamamoto T. Application of a persistent heparin treatment inhibits the malignant potential of oral squamous carcinoma cells induced by tumor cell-derived exosomes. *PLoS ONE.* (2016) 11:e0148454. doi: 10.1371/journal.pone.0148454
21. Abels ER, Breakefield XO. Introduction to extracellular vesicles: biogenesis, RNA cargo selection, content, release, and uptake. *Cell Mol Neurobiol.* (2016) 36:301–12. doi: 10.1007/s10571-016-0366-z
22. Blott EJ, Griffiths GM. Secretory lysosomes. *Nat Rev Mol Cell Biol.* (2002) 3:122–31. doi: 10.1038/nrm732
23. Colombo M, Moita C, van Niel G, Kowal J, Vigneron J, Benaroch P, et al. Analysis of ESCRT functions in exosome biogenesis, composition and secretion highlights the heterogeneity of extracellular vesicles. *J Cell Sci.* (2013) 126 (Pt 24):5553–65. doi: 10.1242/jcs.128868
24. Henne WM, Buchkovich NJ, Emr SD. The ESCRT pathway. *Dev Cell.* (2011) 21:77–91. doi: 10.1016/j.devcel.2011.05.015
25. Katzmann DJ, Babst M, Emr SD. Ubiquitin-dependent sorting into the multivesicular body pathway requires the function of a conserved endosomal protein sorting complex, ESCRT-I. *Cell.* (2001) 106:145–55. doi: 10.1016/S0092-8674(01)00434-2
26. Airola MV, Hannun YA. Sphingolipid metabolism and neutral sphingomyelinases. *Handb Exp Pharmacol.* (2013) 215:57–76. doi: 10.1007/978-3-7091-1368-4_3
27. Castro BM, Prieto M, Silva LC. Ceramide: a simple sphingolipid with unique biophysical properties. *Prog Lipid Res.* (2014) 54:53–67. doi: 10.1016/j.plipres.2014.01.004
28. Perez-Hernandez D, Gutierrez-Vazquez C, Jorge I, Lopez-Martin S, Ursa A, Sanchez-Madrid F, et al. The intracellular interactome of tetraspanin-enriched microdomains reveals their function as sorting machineries toward exosomes. *J Biol Chem.* (2013) 288:11649–61. doi: 10.1074/jbc.M112.445304
29. Zhu H, Guariglia S, Yu RY, Li W, Brancho D, Peinado H, et al. Mutation of SIMPLE in charcot-marie-tooth 1c alters production of exosomes. *Mol Biol Cell.* (2013) 24:1619–37, S1–3. doi: 10.1091/mbc.e12-07-0544
30. Colombo M, Raposo G, Thery C. Biogenesis, secretion, and intercellular interactions of exosomes and other extracellular vesicles. *Annu Rev Cell Dev Biol.* (2014) 30:255–89. doi: 10.1146/annurev-cellbio-101512-122326
31. Ekstrom EJ, Bergenfelz C, von Bulow V, Serifler F, Carlemalm E, Jonsson G, et al. WNT5A induces release of exosomes containing pro-angiogenic and immunosuppressive factors from malignant melanoma cells. *Mol Cancer.* (2014) 13:88. doi: 10.1186/1476-4598-13-88
32. Vlassov AV, Magdaleno S, Setterquist R, Conrad R. Exosomes: current knowledge of their composition, biological functions, and diagnostic and therapeutic potentials. *Biochim Biophys Acta.* (2012) 1820:940–8. doi: 10.1016/j.bbagen.2012.03.017
33. Bebelman MP, Smit MJ, Pegtel DM, Baglio SR. Biogenesis and function of extracellular vesicles in cancer. *Pharmacol Ther.* (2018) 188:1–11. doi: 10.1016/j.pharmthera.2018.02.013
34. Wang T, Gilkes DM, Takano N, Xiang L, Luo W, Bishop CJ, et al. Hypoxia-inducible factors and RAB22A mediate formation of microvesicles that stimulate breast cancer invasion and metastasis. *Proc Natl Acad Sci USA.* (2014) 111:E3234–42. doi: 10.1073/pnas.1410041111
35. Hoshino D, Kirkbride KC, Costello K, Clark ES, Sinha S, Grega-Larson N, et al. Exosome secretion is enhanced by invadopodia and drives invasive behavior. *Cell Rep.* (2013) 5:1159–68. doi: 10.1016/j.celrep.2013.10.050
36. Verweij FJ, Bebelman MP, Jimenez CR, Garcia-Vallejo JJ, Janssen H, Neefjes J, et al. Quantifying exosome secretion from single cells reveals a modulatory role for GPCR signaling. *J Cell Biol.* (2018) 217:1129–42. doi: 10.1083/jcb.201703206
37. Wei Y, Wang D, Jin F, Bian Z, Li L, Liang H, et al. Pyruvate kinase type M2 promotes tumour cell exosome release via phosphorylating synaptosome-associated protein 23. *Nat Commun.* (2017) 8:14041. doi: 10.1038/ncomms14041
38. Williams C, Pazos R, Royo F, Gonzalez E, Roura-Ferrer M, Martinez A, et al. Assessing the role of surface glycans of extracellular vesicles on cellular uptake. *Sci Rep.* (2019) 9:11920. doi: 10.1038/s41598-019-48499-1
39. Yellon DM, Davidson SM. Exosomes: nanoparticles involved in cardioprotection? *Circ Res.* (2014) 114:325–32. doi: 10.1161/CIRCRESAHA.113.300636
40. Thery C, Boussac M, Veron P, Ricciardi-Castagnoli P, Raposo G, Garin J, et al. Proteomic analysis of dendritic cell-derived exosomes: a secreted subcellular compartment distinct from apoptotic vesicles. *J Immunol.* (2001) 166:7309–18. doi: 10.4049/jimmunol.166.12.7309
41. Zhou W, Fong MY, Min Y, Somlo G, Liu L, Palomares MR, et al. Cancer-secreted miR-105 destroys vascular endothelial barriers to promote metastasis. *Cancer Cell.* (2014) 25:501–15. doi: 10.1016/j.ccr.2014.03.007
42. Melo SA, Sugimoto H, O'Connell JT, Kato N, Villanueva A, Vidal A, et al. Cancer exosomes perform cell-independent microRNA biogenesis and promote tumorigenesis. *Cancer Cell.* (2014) 26:707–21. doi: 10.1016/j.ccell.2014.09.005
43. Wilusz JE, Sunwoo H, Spector DL. Long noncoding RNAs: functional surprises from the RNA world. *Genes Dev.* (2009) 23:1494–504. doi: 10.1101/gad.1800909
44. Valadi H, Ekstrom K, Bossios A, Sjostrand M, Lee JJ, Lotvall JO. Exosome-mediated transfer of mRNAs and microRNAs is a novel mechanism of genetic exchange between cells. *Nat Cell Biol.* (2007) 9:654–9. doi: 10.1038/ncb1596
45. Nonaka T, Wong DTW. Liquid biopsy in head and neck cancer: promises and challenges. *J Dental Res.* (2018) 97:701–8. doi: 10.1177/0022034518762071
46. Hess J, Unger K, Maihoefer C, Schuttrumpf L, Wintergerst L, Heider T, et al. A five-microRNA signature predicts survival and disease control of patients with head and neck cancer negative for HPV infection. *Clin Cancer Res.* (2019) 25:1505–16. doi: 10.1158/1078-0432.CCR-18-0776
47. Xu MJ, Johnson DE, Grandis JR. EGFR-targeted therapies in the post-genomic era. *Cancer Metastasis Rev.* (2017) 36:463–73. doi: 10.1007/s10555-017-9687-8

48. Whiteside TL. The potential of tumor-derived exosomes for noninvasive cancer monitoring. *Expert Rev Mol Diagnos.* (2015) 15:1293–310. doi: 10.1586/14737159.2015.1071666
49. Wortzel I, Dror S, Kenific CM, Lyden D. Exosome-mediated metastasis: communication from a distance. *Dev Cell.* (2019) 49:347–60. doi: 10.1016/j.devcel.2019.04.011
50. Principe S, Hui AB, Bruce J, Sinha A, Liu FF, Kislinger T. Tumor-derived exosomes and microvesicles in head and neck cancer: implications for tumor biology and biomarker discovery. *Proteomics.* (2013) 13:1608–23. doi: 10.1002/pmic.201200533
51. Kim JW, Wieckowski E, Taylor DD, Reichert TE, Watkins S, Whiteside TL. Fas ligand-positive membranous vesicles isolated from sera of patients with oral cancer induce apoptosis of activated T lymphocytes. *Clin Cancer Res.* (2005) 11:1010–20.
52. Theodoraki MN, Hoffmann TK, Jackson EK, Whiteside TL. Exosomes in HNSCC plasma as surrogate markers of tumour progression and immune competence. *Clin Exp Immunol.* (2018) 194:67–78. doi: 10.1111/cei.13157
53. Zlotogorski-Hurvitz A, Dayan D, Chaushu G, Salo T, Vered M. Morphological and molecular features of oral fluid-derived exosomes: oral cancer patients versus healthy individuals. *J Cancer Res Clin Oncol.* (2016) 142:101–10. doi: 10.1007/s00432-015-2005-3
54. Sharma S, Gillespie BM, Palanisamy V, Gimzewski JK. Quantitative nanostructural and single-molecule force spectroscopy biomolecular analysis of human-saliva-derived exosomes. *Langmuir.* (2011) 27:14394–400. doi: 10.1021/la2038763
55. Kannan A, Hertweck KL, Philley JV, Wells RB, Dasgupta S. Genetic mutation and exosome signature of human papilloma virus associated oropharyngeal cancer. *Sci Rep.* (2017) 7:46102. doi: 10.1038/srep46102
56. Zlotogorski-Hurvitz A, Dekel BZ, Malonek D, Yahalom R, Vered M. FTIR-based spectrum of salivary exosomes coupled with computational-aided discriminating analysis in the diagnosis of oral cancer. *J Cancer Res Clin Oncol.* (2019) 145:685–94. doi: 10.1007/s00432-018-02827-6
57. Momen-Heravi F, Bala S. Emerging role of non-coding RNA in oral cancer. *Cell Signal.* (2018) 42:134–43. doi: 10.1016/j.cellsig.2017.10.009
58. Rabinowits G, Bowden M, Flores LM, Verselis S, Vergara V, Jo VY, et al. Comparative analysis of microRNA expression among benign and malignant tongue tissue and plasma of patients with tongue cancer. *Front Oncol.* (2017) 7:191. doi: 10.3389/fonc.2017.00191
59. Wang J, Zhou Y, Lu J, Sun Y, Xiao H, Liu M, et al. Combined detection of serum exosomal miR-21 and HOTAIR as diagnostic and prognostic biomarkers for laryngeal squamous cell carcinoma. *Med Oncol.* (2014) 31:148. doi: 10.1007/s12032-014-0148-8
60. Qin X, Guo H, Wang X, Zhu X, Yan M, Wang X, et al. Exosomal miR-196a derived from cancer-associated fibroblasts confers cisplatin resistance in head and neck cancer through targeting CDKN1B and ING5. *Genome Biol.* (2019) 20:12. doi: 10.1186/s13059-018-1604-0
61. Huang Q, Yang J, Zheng J, Hsueh C, Guo Y, Zhou L. Characterization of selective exosomal microRNA expression profile derived from laryngeal squamous cell carcinoma detected by next generation sequencing. *Oncol Rep.* (2018) 40:2584–94. doi: 10.3892/or.2018.6672
62. Gai C, Camussi F, Broccoletti R, Gambino A, Cabras M, Molinaro L, et al. Salivary extracellular vesicle-associated miRNAs as potential biomarkers in oral squamous cell carcinoma. *BMC Cancer.* (2018) 18:439. doi: 10.1186/s12885-018-4364-z
63. Sakha S, Muramatsu T, Ueda K, Inazawa J. Exosomal microRNA miR-1246 induces cell motility and invasion through the regulation of DENND2D in oral squamous cell carcinoma. *Sci Rep.* (2016) 6:38750. doi: 10.1038/srep38750
64. Al-Nedawi K, Meehan B, Kerbel RS, Allison AC, Rak J. Endothelial expression of autocrine VEGF upon the uptake of tumor-derived microvesicles containing oncogenic EGFR. *Proc Natl Acad Sci USA.* (2009) 106:3794–9. doi: 10.1073/pnas.0804543106
65. Huang SH, Li Y, Zhang J, Rong J, Ye S. Epidermal growth factor receptor-containing exosomes induce tumor-specific regulatory T cells. *Cancer Invest.* (2013) 31:330–5. doi: 10.3109/07357907.2013.789905
66. van Dommelen SM, van der Meel R, van Solinge WW, Coimbra M, Vader P, Schiffelers RM. Cetuximab treatment alters the content of extracellular vesicles released from tumor cells. *Nanomedicine.* (2016) 11:881–90. doi: 10.2217/nnm-2015-0009
67. Ludwig S, Sharma P, Theodoraki MN, Pietrowska M, Yerneni SS, Lang S, et al. Molecular and functional profiles of exosomes from HPV(+) and HPV(-) head and neck cancer cell lines. *Front Oncol.* (2018) 8:445. doi: 10.3389/fonc.2018.00445
68. Winck FV, Prado Ribeiro AC, Ramos Domingues R, Ling LY, Riano-Pachon DM, Rivera C, et al. Insights into immune responses in oral cancer through proteomic analysis of saliva and salivary extracellular vesicles. *Sci Rep.* (2015) 5:16305. doi: 10.1038/srep16305
69. Ferris RL, Blumenschein G Jr, Fayette J, Guigay J, Colevas AD, Licitra L, et al. Nivolumab for recurrent squamous-cell carcinoma of the head and neck. *N Engl J Med.* (2016) 375:1856–67. doi: 10.1056/NEJMoa1602252
70. Chow LQM, Haddad R, Gupta S, Mahipal A, Mehra R, Tahara M, et al. Antitumor activity of pembrolizumab in biomarker-unselected patients with recurrent and/or metastatic head and neck squamous cell carcinoma: results from the phase Ib KEYNOTE-012 expansion cohort. *J Clin Oncol.* (2016) 34:3838–45. doi: 10.1200/JCO.2016.68.1478
71. Theodoraki MN, Yerneni SS, Hoffmann TK, Gooding WE, Whiteside TL. Clinical significance of PD-L1(+) exosomes in plasma of head and neck cancer patients. *Clin Cancer Res.* (2018) 24:896–905. doi: 10.1158/1078-0432.CCR-17-2664
72. Concha-Benavente F, Srivastava RM, Trivedi S, Lei Y, Chandran U, Seethala RR, et al. Identification of the cell-intrinsic and -extrinsic pathways downstream of EGFR and IFNgamma that induce PD-L1 expression in head and neck cancer. *Cancer Res.* (2016) 76:1031–43. doi: 10.1158/0008-5472.CAN-15-2001
73. Ono K, Eguchi T, Sogawa C, Calderwood SK, Futagawa J, Kasai T, et al. HSP-enriched properties of extracellular vesicles involve survival of metastatic oral cancer cells. *J Cell Biochem.* (2018) 119:7350–62. doi: 10.1002/jcb.27039
74. Theodoraki MN, Hoffmann TK, Whiteside TL. Separation of plasma-derived exosomes into CD3((+)) and CD3((-)) fractions allows for association of immune cell and tumour cell markers with disease activity in HNSCC patients. *Clin Exp Immunol.* (2018) 192:271–83. doi: 10.1111/cei.13113
75. Qadir F, Aziz MA, Sari CP, Ma H, Dai H, Wang X, et al. Transcriptome reprogramming by cancer exosomes: identification of novel molecular targets in matrix and immune modulation. *Mol Cancer.* (2018) 17:97. doi: 10.1186/s12943-018-0846-5
76. Quail DF, Joyce JA. Microenvironmental regulation of tumor progression and metastasis. *Nat Med.* (2013) 19:1423–37. doi: 10.1038/nm.3394
77. Dayan D, Salo T, Salo S, Nyberg P, Nurmenniemi S, Costea DE, et al. Molecular crosstalk between cancer cells and tumor microenvironment components suggests potential targets for new therapeutic approaches in mobile tongue cancer. *Cancer Med.* (2012) 1:128–40. doi: 10.1002/cam4.24
78. Davis RJ, Van Waes C, Allen CT. Overcoming barriers to effective immunotherapy: MDSCs, TAMs, and Tregs as mediators of the immunosuppressive microenvironment in head and neck cancer. *Oral Oncol.* (2016) 58:59–70. doi: 10.1016/j.oraloncology.2016.05.002
79. Filipazzi P, Burdek M, Villa A, Rivoltini L, Huber V. Recent advances on the role of tumor exosomes in immunosuppression and disease progression. *Semin Cancer Biol.* (2012) 22:342–9. doi: 10.1016/j.semcancer.2012.02.005
80. Monypenny J, Milewicz H, Flores-Borja F, Weitsman G, Cheung A, Chowdhury R, et al. ALIX regulates tumor-mediated immunosuppression by controlling EGFR activity and PD-L1 presentation. *Cell Rep.* (2018) 24:630–41. doi: 10.1016/j.celrep.2018.06.066
81. van der Grein SG, Nolte-'t Hoen EN. "Small Talk" in the Innate immune system via RNA-containing extracellular vesicles. *Front Immunol.* (2014) 5:542. doi: 10.3389/fimmu.2014.00542
82. Aucher A, Rudnicka D, Davis DM. MicroRNAs transfer from human macrophages to hepato-carcinoma cells and inhibit proliferation. *J Immunol.* (2013) 191:6250–60. doi: 10.4049/jimmunol.1301728
83. Vincent-Schneider H, Stumptner-Cuvelette P, Lankar D, Pain S, Raposo G, Benaroch P, et al. Exosomes bearing HLA-DR1 molecules need dendritic cells to efficiently stimulate specific T cells. *Int Immunol.* (2002) 14:713–22. doi: 10.1093/intimm/dxf048
84. Whiteside TL. Exosomes and tumor-mediated immune suppression. *J Clin Invest.* (2016) 126:1216–23. doi: 10.1172/JCI81136

85. Shi L, Chen S, Yang L, Li Y. The role of PD-1 and PD-L1 in T-cell immune suppression in patients with hematological malignancies. *J Hematol Oncol.* (2013) 6:74. doi: 10.1186/1756-8722-6-74
86. Ludwig S, Floros T, Theodoraki MN, Hong CS, Jackson EK, Lang S, et al. Suppression of lymphocyte functions by plasma exosomes correlates with disease activity in patients with head and neck cancer. *Clin Cancer Res.* (2017) 23:4843–54. doi: 10.1158/1078-0432.CCR-16-2819
87. Wolfers J, Lozier A, Raposo G, Regnault A, Thery C, Masurier C, et al. Tumor-derived exosomes are a source of shared tumor rejection antigens for CTL cross-priming. *Nat Med.* (2001) 7:297–303. doi: 10.1038/85438
88. Zhang HG, Grizzle WE. Exosomes and cancer: a newly described pathway of immune suppression. *Clin Cancer Res.* (2011) 17:959–64. doi: 10.1158/1078-0432.CCR-10-1489
89. Maybruck BT, Pfannenstiel LW, Diaz-Montero M, Gastman BR. Tumor-derived exosomes induce CD8(+) T cell suppressors. *J Immunother Cancer.* (2017) 5:65. doi: 10.1186/s40425-017-0269-7
90. Schuler PJ, Saze Z, Hong CS, Muller L, Gillespie DG, Cheng D, et al. Human CD4+ CD39+ regulatory T cells produce adenosine upon co-expression of surface CD73 or contact with CD73+ exosomes or CD73+ cells. *Clin Exp Immunol.* (2014) 177:531–43. doi: 10.1111/cei.12354
91. Li L, Cao B, Liang X, Lu S, Luo H, Wang Z, et al. Microenvironmental oxygen pressure orchestrates an anti- and pro-tumoral gammadelta T cell equilibrium via tumor-derived exosomes. *Oncogene.* (2019) 38:2830–43. doi: 10.1038/s41388-018-0627-z
92. Zhou J, Li M, Lim WQ, Luo Z, Phua SZF, Huo R, et al. A transferrin-conjugated hollow nanoplatform for redox-controlled and targeted chemotherapy of tumor with reduced inflammatory reactions. *Theranostics.* (2018) 8:518–32. doi: 10.7150/thno.21194
93. Whiteside TL. Exosome and mesenchymal stem cell cross-talk in the tumor microenvironment. *Semin Immunol.* (2018) 35:69–79. doi: 10.1016/j.smim.2017.12.003
94. Principe S, Mejia-Guerrero S, Ignatchenko V, Sinha A, Ignatchenko A, Shi W, et al. Proteomic analysis of cancer-associated fibroblasts reveals a paracrine role for MFAP5 in human oral tongue squamous cell carcinoma. *J Proteome Res.* (2018) 17:2045–59. doi: 10.1021/acs.jproteome.7b00925
95. Vered M, Lehtonen M, Hotakainen L, Pirila E, Teppo S, Nyberg P, et al. Caveolin-1 accumulation in the tongue cancer tumor microenvironment is significantly associated with poor prognosis: an *in-vivo* and *in-vitro* study. *BMC Cancer.* (2015) 15:25. doi: 10.1186/s12885-015-1030-6
96. Milane L, Singh A, Mattheolabakis G, Suresh M, Amiji MM. Exosome mediated communication within the tumor microenvironment. *J Control Release.* (2015) 219:278–94. doi: 10.1016/j.jconrel.2015.06.029
97. Syn N, Wang L, Sethi G, Thiery JP, Goh BC. Exosome-mediated metastasis: from epithelial-mesenchymal transition to escape from immunosurveillance. *Trends Pharmacol Sci.* (2016) 37:606–17. doi: 10.1016/j.tips.2016.04.006
98. Blackwell RH, Foreman KE, Gupta GN. The role of cancer-derived exosomes in tumorigenicity & epithelial-to-mesenchymal transition. *Cancers.* (2017) 9:E105. doi: 10.3390/cancers9080105
99. Kawakubo-Yasukochi T, Morioka M, Hazekawa M, Yasukochi A, Nishinakagawa T, Ono K, et al. miR-200c-3p spreads invasive capacity in human oral squamous cell carcinoma microenvironment. *Mol Carcinogenesis.* (2018) 57:295–302. doi: 10.1002/mc.22744
100. Languino LR, Singh A, Prisco M, Inman GJ, Luginbuhl A, Curry JM, et al. Exosome-mediated transfer from the tumor microenvironment increases TGFbeta signaling in squamous cell carcinoma. *Am J Transl Res.* (2016) 8:2432–7.
101. Zhang H, Deng T, Liu R, Bai M, Zhou L, Wang X, et al. Exosome-delivered EGFR regulates liver microenvironment to promote gastric cancer liver metastasis. *Nat Commun.* (2017) 8:15016. doi: 10.1038/ncomms15016
102. Huaitong X, Yuanyong F, Yueqin T, Peng Z, Wei S, Kai S. Microvesicles releasing by oral cancer cells enhance endothelial cell angiogenesis via Shh/RhoA signaling pathway. *Cancer Biol Ther.* (2017) 18:783–91. doi: 10.1080/15384047.2017.1373213
103. Ludwig N, Yerneni SS, Razzo BM, Whiteside TL. Exosomes from HNSCC promote angiogenesis through reprogramming of endothelial cells. *Mol Cancer Res.* (2018) 16:1798–808. doi: 10.1158/1541-7786.MCR-18-0358
104. Hsieh CH, Tai SK, Yang MH. Snail-overexpressing cancer cells promote M2-like polarization of tumor-associated macrophages by delivering MiR-21-abundant exosomes. *Neoplasia.* (2018) 20:775–88. doi: 10.1016/j.neo.2018.06.004
105. Mutschelknaus L, Azimzadeh O, Heider T, Winkler K, Vetter M, Kell R, et al. Radiation alters the cargo of exosomes released from squamous head and neck cancer cells to promote migration of recipient cells. *Sci Rep.* (2017) 7:12423. doi: 10.1038/s41598-017-12403-6
106. Batrakova EV, Kim MS. Using exosomes, naturally-equipped nanocarriers, for drug delivery. *J Control Release.* (2015) 219:396–405. doi: 10.1016/j.jconrel.2015.07.030
107. Yim N, Ryu SW, Choi K, Lee KR, Lee S, Choi H, et al. Exosome engineering for efficient intracellular delivery of soluble proteins using optically reversible protein-protein interaction module. *Nat Commun.* (2016) 7:12277. doi: 10.1038/ncomms12277
108. Syn NL, Wang L, Chow EK, Lim CT, Goh BC. Exosomes in cancer nanomedicine and immunotherapy: prospects and challenges. *Trends Biotechnol.* (2017) 35:665–76. doi: 10.1016/j.tibtech.2017.03.004
109. Wu K, Xing F, Wu SY, Watabe K. Extracellular vesicles as emerging targets in cancer: recent development from bench to bedside. *Biochim Biophys Acta Rev Cancer.* (2017) 1868:538–63. doi: 10.1016/j.bbcan.2017.10.001
110. Li L, Piontek K, Ishida M, Fausther M, Dranoff JA, Fu R, et al. Extracellular vesicles carry microRNA-195 to intrahepatic cholangiocarcinoma and improve survival in a rat model. *Hepatology.* (2017) 65:501–14. doi: 10.1002/hep.28735
111. Kooijmans SA, Aleza CG, Roffler SR, van Solinge WW, Vader P, Schiffelers RM. Display of GPI-anchored anti-EGFR nanobodies on extracellular vesicles promotes tumour cell targeting. *J Extracell Vesicles.* (2016) 5:31053. doi: 10.3402/jev.v5.31053
112. Yang T, Martin P, Fogarty B, Brown A, Schurman K, Phipps R, et al. Exosome delivered anticancer drugs across the blood-brain barrier for brain cancer therapy in Danio rerio. *Pharm Res.* (2015) 32:2003–14. doi: 10.1007/s11095-014-1593-y
113. Wang C, Chen L, Huang Y, Li K, Jinye A, Fan T, et al. Exosome-delivered TRPP2 siRNA inhibits the epithelial-mesenchymal transition of FaDu cells. *Oncol Lett.* (2019) 17:1953–61. doi: 10.3892/ol.2018.9752
114. Murphy DA, Courtneidge SA. The 'ins' and 'outs' of podosomes and invadopodia: characteristics, formation and function. *Nat Rev Mol Cell Biol.* (2011) 12:413–26. doi: 10.1038/nrm3141
115. Sharma A, Khatun Z, Shiras A. Tumor exosomes: cellular postmen of cancer diagnosis and personalized therapy. *Nanomedicine.* (2016) 11:421–37. doi: 10.2217/nnm.15.210
116. Hao S, Bai O, Li F, Yuan J, Laferte S, Xiang J. Mature dendritic cells pulsed with exosomes stimulate efficient cytotoxic T-lymphocyte responses and antitumour immunity. *Immunology.* (2007) 120:90–102. doi: 10.1111/j.1365-2567.2006.02483.x
117. Honegger A, Leitz J, Bulkescher J, Hoppe-Seyler K, Hoppe-Seyler F. Silencing of human papillomavirus (HPV) E6/E7 oncogene expression affects both the contents and the amounts of extracellular microvesicles released from HPV-positive cancer cells. *Int J Cancer.* (2013) 133:1631–42. doi: 10.1002/ijc.28164
118. Di Bonito P, Accardi L, Galati L, Ferrantelli F, Federico M. Anti-cancer vaccine for HPV-associated neoplasms: focus on a therapeutic HPV vaccine based on a novel tumor antigen delivery method using endogenously engineered exosomes. *Cancers.* (2019) 11:E138. doi: 10.3390/cancers11020138
119. Cramer JD, Burtness B, Le QT, Ferris RL. The changing therapeutic landscape of head and neck cancer. *Nat Rev Clin Oncol.* (2019). doi: 10.1038/s41571-019-0227-z. [Epub ahead of print].
120. Meads MB, Gatenby RA, Dalton WS. Environment-mediated drug resistance: a major contributor to minimal residual disease. *Nat Rev Cancer.* (2009) 9:665–74. doi: 10.1038/nrc2714
121. Moitra K, Lou H, Dean M. Multidrug efflux pumps and cancer stem cells: insights into multidrug resistance and therapeutic development. *Clin Pharmacol Ther.* (2011) 89:491–502. doi: 10.1038/clpt.2011.14
122. Shedden K, Xie XT, Chandaroy P, Chang YT, Rosania GR. Expulsion of small molecules in vesicles shed by cancer cells: association with gene expression and chemosensitivity profiles. *Cancer Res.* (2003) 63:4331–7.

123. Steinbichler TB, Dudas J, Skvortsov S, Ganswindt U, Riechelmann H, Skvortsova II. Therapy resistance mediated by exosomes. *Mol Cancer.* (2019) 18:58. doi: 10.1186/s12943-019-0970-x
124. Namee NM, O'Driscoll L. Extracellular vesicles and anti-cancer drug resistance. *Biochim Biophys Acta Rev Cancer.* (2018) 1870:123–36. doi: 10.1016/j.bbcan.2018.07.003
125. Bussink J, van der Kogel AJ, Kaanders JH. Activation of the PI3-K/AKT pathway and implications for radioresistance mechanisms in head and neck cancer. *Lancet Oncol.* (2008) 9:288–96. doi: 10.1016/S1470-2045(08)70073-1
126. Pickhard AC, Margraf J, Knopf A, Stark T, Piontek G, Beck C, et al. Inhibition of radiation induced migration of human head and neck squamous cell carcinoma cells by blocking of EGF receptor pathways. *BMC Cancer.* (2011) 11:388. doi: 10.1186/1471-2407-11-388
127. Beck C, Piontek G, Haug A, Bas M, Knopf A, Stark T, et al. The kallikrein-kinin-system in head and neck squamous cell carcinoma (HNSCC) and its role in tumour survival, invasion, migration and response to radiotherapy. *Oral Oncol.* (2012) 48:1208–19. doi: 10.1016/j.oraloncology.2012.06.001
128. Mutschelknaus L, Peters C, Winkler K, Yentrapalli R, Heider T, Atkinson MJ, et al. Exosomes derived from squamous head and neck cancer promote cell survival after ionizing radiation. *PLoS ONE.* (2016) 11:e0152213. doi: 10.1371/journal.pone.0152213
129. Chen G, Huang AC, Zhang W, Zhang G, Wu M, Xu W, et al. Exosomal PD-L1 contributes to immunosuppression and is associated with anti-PD-1 response. *Nature.* (2018) 560:382–6. doi: 10.1038/s41586-018-0392-8
130. Liu T, Chen G, Sun D, Lei M, Li Y, Zhou C, et al. Exosomes containing miR-21 transfer the characteristic of cisplatin resistance by targeting PTEN and PDCD4 in oral squamous cell carcinoma. *Acta Biochim Biophys Sin.* (2017) 49:808–16. doi: 10.1093/abbs/gmx078

15

Leukoplakia: An Invasive Cancer Hidden within the Vocal Folds: A Multivariate Analysis of Risk Factors

Hanna Klimza[1†], Wioletta Pietruszewska[2†], Oskar Rosiak[3], Joanna Morawska[2], Piotr Nogal[1] and Małgorzata Wierzbicka[1]*

[1] Department of Otolaryngology and Laryngological Oncology, Poznań University of Medical Sciences, Poznań, Poland, [2] Department of Otolaryngology, Head and Neck Oncology, Medical University of Lodz, Lodz, Poland, [3] Balance Disorder Unit, Department of Otolaryngology, Medical University of Lodz, Lodz, Poland

***Correspondence:**
Hanna Klimza
hnogala@wp.pl

†These authors have contributed equally to this work

Introduction: Discerning the preoperative nature of vocal fold leukoplakia (VFL) with a substantial degree of certainty is fundamental, seeing that the histological diagnosis of VFL includes a wide spectrum of pathology and there is no consensus on an appropriate treatment strategy or frequency of surveillance. The goal of our study was to establish a clear schedule of the diagnostics and decision-making in which the timing and necessity of surgical intervention are crucial to not miss this cancer hidden underneath the white plaque.

Material and Methods: We define a schedule as a combination of procedures (white light and Narrow Band Imaging diagnostic tools), methods of evaluating the results (a combination of multiple image classifications in white light and Narrow Band Imaging), and taking into account patient-related risk factors, precise lesion location, and morphology. A total number of 259 patients with 296 vocal folds affected by leukoplakia were enrolled in the study. All patients were assessed for three classifications, in detail according to Ni 2019 and ELS 2015 for Narrow Band Imaging and according to Chen 2019 for white light. In 41 of the 296 folds (13.9%), the VFL specimens in the final histology revealed invasive cancer. We compared the results from the classifications to the final histology results.

Results: The results showed that the classifications and evaluations of the involvement of anterior commissure improve the clinical utility of these classifications and showed improved diagnostic performance. The AUC of this model was the highest (0.973) with the highest sensitivity, specificity, PPV, and NPV (90.2%, 89%, 56.9%, and 98.3%, respectively).

Conclusion: The schedule that combines white light and Narrow Band Imaging, with a combination of the two classifications, improves the specificity and predictive value, especially of anterior commissure involvement.

Keywords: vocal fold leukoplakia, narrow band imaging (NBI), glottic cancer, white light, anterior commissure (AC)

INTRODUCTION

Vocal fold leukoplakia (VFL) is a clinical term that describes a white patch or plaque resulting from epithelial parakeratosis, but does not specify what is hidden within the lesion. The histological diagnosis of VFL includes a wide spectrum of pathology, through stages of dysplasia to invasive cancer (1, 2). Additionally, there is no consensus on the threshold for surgical intervention, appropriate treatment strategy (wait and see policy, sampling, or excisional surgery), or the frequency of surveillance (3, 4). Therapeutic decisions balance high-quality voice preservation and oncological safety, thus caution is taken while referring a patient for surgical treatment and techniques are chosen to eliminate a superficial lesion while preserving the underlying vibratory mucosa. Some authors claim that a 'wait and see' approach is appropriate for smooth lesions, while some believe that more aggressive treatment should be performed (5, 6). In any event, the most popular treatment of VFL is surgery, even though in 50% of specimens, the final histology does not show dysplasia or cancer (7, 8). In aiming to resolve these discrepancies, diagnostic methods and recommendations such as the schedule for VFL management should be of utmost importance (9).

White light (WL) laryngoscopy is the first line and the most important diagnostic tool in the assessment of the pathologies of the larynx, including VFL (10, 11). However, it has limitations, especially in the assessment of underlying vascularization, which can be resolved by using additional light settings. Narrow Band Imaging (NBI) is a well-established bioendoscopic technique that uses filtered wavelengths to enhance the microvascular pattern and its alterations are associated with preneoplastic and neoplastic transformation of the upper aerodigestive tract mucosa (12–16). NBI using blue light (wavelength peak of 400 to 430 nm) and green light (wavelength peak of 515 to 555 nm), which correspond to the absorption peaks of hemoglobin (12), enhances the physicians' chances to detect and delineate the suspicious mucosal lesions in a non-invasive way, and is thus beneficial to the diagnosis of a variety of benign and malignant lesions (14). NBI proved to be a useful diagnostic tool for the assessment of laryngeal leukoplakia; however, there is no clear place or recommendations for using NBI in preoperative assessments of VFL (17, 18) or establishing this method as the guidance for management (19)

The researchers' hypothesis assumes the confirmation of a simple diagnostic schedule by using WL and NBI for patients with laryngeal leukoplakia in stratifying cancer risk to avoid false negative or false positive histological findings and vocal fold damage.

Therefore, the primary aim of this paper is to present the gathered and analyzed data to express which factors increase the risk of malignant transformation inside leukoplakia to avoid under- or overtreatment.

The second goal of our study was to confirm the usefulness of a clear diagnostic and decision-making schedule in which the timing and need for surgical intervention are crucial to not miss this cancer hidden underneath the white plaque.

MATERIAL AND METHODS

Study Population

A prospective study was conducted according to the guidelines of the Declaration of Helsinki and approved by the Ethics Committee of the Medical University of Lodz (RNN/225/19/KE, 9 April 2019) at the Poznan and Lodz Otolaryngology Tertiary Referral University Departments, between January 2015 and March 2020.

259 consecutive patients were enrolled – 212 men (81.85% of the cohort), 47 women (18.15%). The mean age was 62.08 years for males, and 61.2 years for females. VFL was diagnosed on 296 vocal folds.

The inclusion criteria were: a diagnosis of vocal fold leukoplakia confirmed by endoscopic evaluation under white light and NBI, no prior vocal fold-related medical intervention or procedures. Exclusion criteria were: other benign lesions (cysts, polyps, Reinke's edema, or papilloma) in endoscopic evaluation; a history of laryngeal surgery, trauma, or intubation; a history of radiotherapy and chemotherapy for head and neck, as well as a lack of written consent from the patient and the presence of changes in endoscopic evaluation suggestive of an advanced neoplasm.

Clinical Diagnostic Work-Up

All patients were assessed with a flexible transnasal video endoscope (Olympus Medical Systems Corporation, Tokyo, Japan) by means of WL and NBI. In the first step, the VFL in white light was observed regarding the texture, color, size, redness, symmetry, and thickness (according to the Chen 2019 classification). A fingertip control switch on the endoscope then changed the view to the NBI mode, and the vascular pattern was assessed, with close attention paid to the presence of intraepithelial papillary capillary loops (IPCLs) (according to the Ni 2019 (20) and European Laryngological Society (ELS) 2015 classifications).

Two independent physicians from each institution (JJ, HK, WP, JM), with at least 3 years of experience in the use of NBI, independently assessed each patient. For high-risk leukoplakia in the Chen classification, the cut-off point was 3 (elevated and rough leukoplakia); in the Ni classification, the cut-off point was 5 (IPCLs outside leukoplakia); and in the ELS classification, the cut-off point was 2 (perpendicular vessels).

Based on these classifications, the patients were qualified as at low or high risk of leukoplakia. The combination of these three classifications and cut-off points in the preoperative assessment of VFL was described by Pietruszewska et al. (2021) (9). Therefore, we used this scoring methodology for the leukoplakia image in WL and NBI.

In addition to the WL and NBI classification scores, additional variables were the patient's age, sex, smoking habits, uni- or bilateral lesions, anterior commissure (AC) involvement, and the uni- or multifocal nature of the lesions.

All patients underwent transoral microsurgery by cold instrumentation, and specimens were sent for final histology. A frozen section was not performed due to the very small size of the specimens, which encompassed only the epithelial layer.

Histopathological diagnosis was performed according to the WHO classification system to classify the resected tissue as low-risk or high-risk dysplasia (21). The main predictive variables taken into consideration were the vascular pattern according to the Ni classification (2019), the ELS classification (2015), and the morphological characteristics according to the Chen classification (2019), along with the final histological findings.

Statistical Methodology

Data were stored in a computer-based filing system and reported as absolute and relative frequencies. Statistical analysis was performed in STATISTICA 13.1 Software (Dell, USA). The cut-off values for classifications with more than two degrees were established based on the receiver operating characteristic (ROC) curve analysis, and the highest Youden's index in each classification determined the proposed cut-off value, as per Fluss et al. (22). To assess the diagnostic performance of the clinical classifications, the measures of occurrence (sensitivity, specificity, and accuracy) and the possibility of discriminating (positive and negative predictive values) for clinical classifications of WL and NBI endoscopy were calculated per the determined cut-off values. ROC curve comparisons for the analyzed classifications are presented in **Figure 1**. Odds Ratio's for particular types of non-dychotomized classification systems by Ni 2019 and Chen 2019 are provided as **Supplementary Material** (**Supplementary Figures 1, 2**).

Multivariate Analysis

Multivariate analysis was performed by means of logistic regression, the results of which are presented in a format suggested by Peng et al. (23) To perform logistic regression analysis on the probability of developing invasive cancer from leukoplakia, the following leukoplakia and epidemiological characteristics were analyzed in a univariate analysis: age, gender, leukoplakia localization, the focality of the leukoplakia, involvement of the anterior commissure, history of smoking, and the results of clinical classifications in WL and NBI. All variables were analyzed using the Likelihood Ratio (LR) test. The test was considered statistically significant if the p-value was < 0.05. The LR test results and the inclusion of variables for further multivariate analysis are summarised in **Table 1**.

The variables were checked for interactions and linearity of predictors using the LR test. No interactions between variables were detected. The linearity test result for age was $p = 0.59$; therefore, the variable was linear. A mixed effects logistic regression model was constructed to model a binary outcome of 0 (not developing invasive cancer) or 1 (developing invasive cancer under the leukoplakia). The equation to predict the probability of developing invasive cancer under the leukoplakia is presented below:

$$\text{Predicted logit} = (-7,753 + (1,628) \cdot \textit{Anterior Commisure Involvement} + (2,496) \cdot \textit{WL} + (3,742) \cdot \textit{ELS})$$

The model's predictive ability was validated using the V-fold cross-validation method with 10 subsets of data. The model's goodness of fit was evaluated with the Hosmer-Lemeshow test (p=0.623). The discrimination curves for the regression model and the V-fold cross-validation are depicted in **Figure 2**. The results of the multivariate analysis are summarised in **Table 2**. The predictive and diagnostic capabilities of the model were evaluated using ROC analysis, which is shown in **Table 3**.

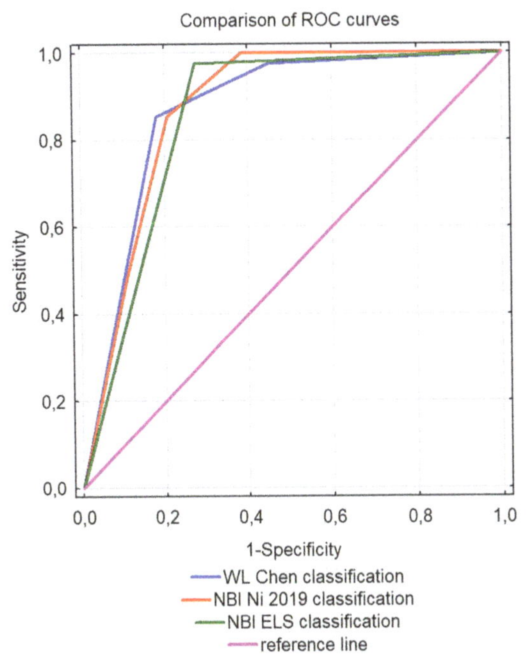

FIGURE 1 | The receiver operating characteristic (ROC) curves comparison for the analyzed clinical classifications.

RESULTS

Invasive cancer was confirmed in 41 (13.6%) out of the 296 VFL specimens in the final histology. Among this group, the mean age was 64.24, with 5 (12.2%) females and 36 (87.8%) males. 38 (92.7%) of the 41 patients were heavy smokers, and 23 (56.1%) were heavy drinkers. Taking into consideration the precise localization of the plaque carrying cancer, all 41 (100%) specimens were unilateral, but in 16 (39%), the lesions spread in the AC. Taking into account the number of VFL points, 24 (58.5%) presented unifocal and 17 (41.5%) multifocal. The complete characteristics of the study group divided by histopathological results Are available in the **Supplementary Material**.

Figure 3. Leukoplakia in WL (acc. to Chen type II) and NBI (acc. to Ni type V, acc. to ELS type II).

Using the Chen classification, out of the total number of 41 lesions only 1 (2.4%) was assessed as type 1 (flat and smooth), 5 (12.2%) as type 2 (elevated and smooth), and 35 (85.4%) as type 3 (rough).

TABLE 1 | Summary of univariate analysis conducted as the first step towards formulating a logistic regression model.

Variable	P (LR) Univariate analysis	Included in further analysis	OR (95%CI)
Age	0.068	No	1.033 (0.997;1.071)
Age categorized 0: below 60. 1: 60 and older	0.017	Yes	2.53 (1.124;5.708)
Gender 0: male 1: female	0.196	No	1.844 (0.069;4.933)
Leukoplakia localization 0: unilateral 1: bilateral	<0.001	Yes	0.03 (0; 0.42)[#]
Focality of leukoplakia 0: unifocal 1: multifocal	0.877	No	0.49 (0.486;1.852)
Anterior commissure involvement 0: not involved 1: involved	0.049	Yes	1.91 (1.03;3.802)
Smoking 0: non-smoker 1: current or former smoker	0.014	Yes	3.646 (1.085;12.25)
WL classification acc. to Chen's 2019 classification 0: stage I and II 1: stage III	<0.001	Yes	26.504 (10.531;66.705)
NBI ELS classification 0: longitudinal vessels 1: perpendicular vessels	<0.001	Yes	105.71 (14.259;783.725)
NBI Ni's 2019 classification 0: stage to IV 1: stage V and VI	<0.001	Yes	22.23 (8.884;55.641)

Haldane-Anscombe correction was applied to account for cells with 0 cases.

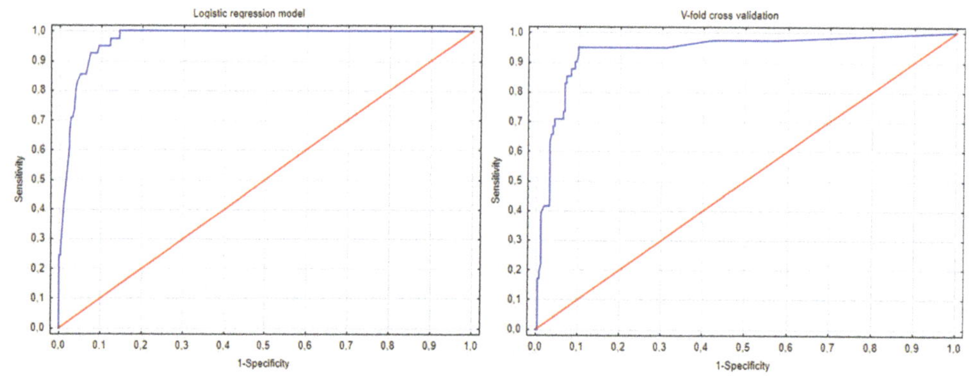

FIGURE 2 | The receiver operating characteristic (ROC) curves of the proposed logistic regression model and the v-fold cross validation of the model.

Using the Ni classification, 2 (4.9%) lesions were assessed as type 3 (IPCLs can be seen at the surface of the vocal fold mucosa surrounding the leukoplakia without clear boundaries), 4 (9.8%) as type 4 (IPCLs can be observed on the surface of the white plaque), 15 (36.6%) as type 5 (IPCLs can be seen on the vocal fold mucosa outside the leukoplakia with regular boundaries), and 20 (48.8%) as type 6 (IPCLs can be seen on the vocal fold mucosa outside the leukoplakia and on the surface of the plaque).

Using the ELS classification: 1 (0.4%) of the 41 had type 1 (longitudinal vascular pattern) and 40 (97.5%) had type 2 (perpendicular vascular pattern) leukoplakia.

Univariate Analysis

Univariate analysis revealed that bilateral vocal fold changes were 0.03 times less likely to present as invasive cancer ($p < 0.001$). However, this observation was not included in the regression model because there were no cases of invasive cancer present in bilateral VFL.

Considering age as a continuous variable, the LR test results were close to statistical significance (p=0.068). However, in order to include age in the multivariate analysis, age was dichotomized using the Weight of Effect (WOE), and similar WOE values were combined into two categories: patients up to 60 years and older

TABLE 2 | Summary of multivariate analysis using logistic regression, including the parameters for the regression model and goodness of fit test results.

Predictor	β	SEβ	Wald's χ^2	df	p	e^β (Odds Ratio) [95%CI]
Constant	-7.753	3.373	5.285	1	0.022	NA
Anterior commissure involvement	1.628	0.684	5.672	1	0.017	5.094 [1.334;19.452]
0: not involved						
1: involved						
WL Chen's 2019 classification	2.496	0.687	13.203	1	<0.001	12.134 (3.157;46.638)
0: stage I and II						
1: stage III						
NBI ELS classification	3.742	1.144	10.702	1	0.001	42.183 (4.482;397.015)
0: longitudinal vessels						
1: perpendicular vessels						

NA, not applicable.

TABLE 3 | Diagnostic performance of the analyzed endoscopic classifications and proposed cut-off values for determining the risk of cancer development under vocal fold leukoplakia.

Clinical classification	Youden's index	Proposed cut-off value	AUC	Sensitivity	Specificity	PPV	NPV
WL Chen's 2019 classification	0.67	3	0.867	85.4%	82%	43.2%	97.2%
Narrow Band Imaging ELS classification	0.7	1	0.851	97.6%	72.5%	36.4%	99.5%
NBI Ni's 2019 classification	0.65	5	0.823	85.4%	79.2%	39.8%	97.1%
Proposed logistic regression model			0.973	92.7%	92.9%	67.9%	98.8%

AUC, Area under curve; PPV, positive predictive value; NPV, negative predictive value; WL, white light; NBI, narrow band imaging

than 60. In this case, people over 60 were 2.53 times more likely to develop cancer under the leukoplakia (p=0.017). A history of smoking (present or former tobacco users) was associated with a 3.646 times increase in the probability of developing cancer. Neither gender nor the focality of the leukoplakia (multifocal or unifocal plaques on one vocal fold) was associated with statistically significant odds of malignant transformation under VFL.

Multivariate Analysis

In the multivariate analysis using a logistic regression model, VFL involving the anterior commissure was 5.094 times more likely to present with invasive cancer (p=0.017). The plaques that were rough and elevated (stage III in WL) were also associated with significantly higher odds of developing cancer (OR 12.124, p <0.001). The presence of a perpendicular blood vessel pattern surrounding the plaque (ELS grade 2) was associated with a 42.183 times higher risk of malignant transformation (p <0.001). The results of the multivariate analysis are presented in **Table 2**.

Diagnostic Performance

To evaluate the diagnostic performance of different clinical classifications regarding the risk of malignant transformation in clinical leukoplakia, we compared the AUC (Area Under Curve) values, sensitivity, specificity, and positive and negative predictive values. Among the clinical classifications proposed by different authors, the highest AUC of 0.867 in the ROC analysis was reported for WL evaluation according to Chen et al. (2019), with a sensitivity of 85.4% and specificity of 82%, and Negative Predictive Value (NPV) at 97.2%; however, Positive Predictive Value (PPV) was low at 43.2%.

The evaluation of leukoplakia with NBI utilizing the Ni 2019 classification did not significantly improve the diagnostic performance, with specificity being lower than WL (79.2% *vs.* 82%), sensitivity at the same level, similar to NPV of 97.1%, and an even lower PPV (39.8% *vs.* 43.2%).

Introducing the ELS classification to the NBI endoscopy shows better results than the Ni 2019 classification, with slightly higher AUC at 0.851, higher sensitivity (97.6% *vs.* 85.4%) but with lower specificity (72.5% *vs.* 79.2%).

The diagnostic algorithm derived from the logistic regression analysis, which included evaluation of a patient in NBI, WL, and evaluation of anterior commissure involvement, improves the clinical utility of these classifications and shows improved diagnostic performance. The AUC of this model was the highest (0.973), with the highest sensitivity, specificity, PPV, and NPV (90.2%, 89%, 56.9%, and 98.3%, respectively).

DISCUSSION

In the presented study, we have shown the tactics to resolve the clinical challenges that laryngologists face balancing therapeutic decisions in vocal fold leukoplakia. The philosophy of managing such patients is to consider both oncological efficacy and functional outcomes. Thus, our hypothesis assumed that a combination of procedures (WL and NBI), scoring systems (combining multiple image classifications in WL and NBI), patient-dependent variables, and the precise location of the plaque contribute to the ability to not miss the cancer.

Since its first introduction in the late 1990s, the use of NBI has considerably contributed to physicians' ability to non-invasively detect and delineate the suspicious mucosal lesions (19). Nowadays, NBI is a mainstay of diagnostics, although in VFL,

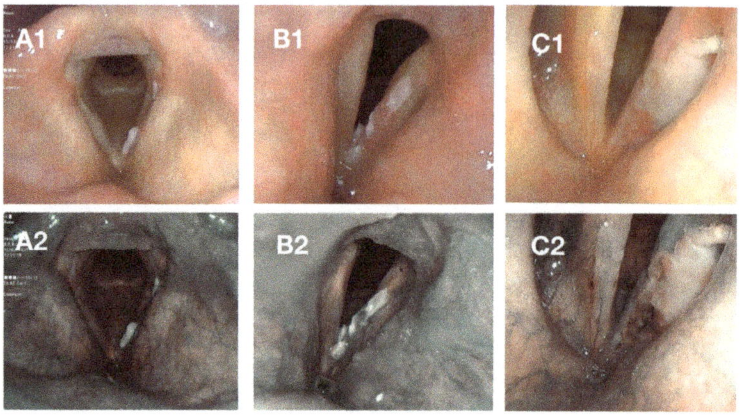

FIGURE 3 | Case A – elevated and smooth leukoplakia seen in white light [WL] **(A1)** and Narrow Band Imaging [NBI] **(A2)** with no evidence of neoplastic proliferation and only low-grade dysplasia in histopathological examination. Case B – elevated and rough leukoplakia in WL **(B1)** with pathologic vessels visible in the periphery of the plaque in NBI **(B2)**, high-grade dysplasia in histopathological examination. Case C – elevated and rough leukoplakia **(C1)** with pathologic vessels visible in the periphery of leukoplakia on the frontal part of the left vocal fold in NBI **(C2)** with invasive carcinoma in histopathological examination.

it has some limitations connected with the umbrella effect due to thick layers of keratin covering the vascular pattern. Nevertheless, in recent years, this impediment has been overcome through the assessment of the vascularization outside the plaque, and a number of studies have proved that NBI can be applied with success in VFL (24–26). But the problem remains in standardizing cut-off points and translating the NBI findings into firm indications for surgery or, on the contrary, to continue with watchful waiting.

Different classifications in recent decades (12, 16–19) were proposed. However, there is still the need for a common, unified schedule to be shared among clinicians to describe WL findings and NBI-enhanced vascular patterns to distinguish the nature of VFL.

In 2015, ELS introduced a simplified classification for vascular changes of the vocal folds divided between longitudinal and perpendicular vascular changes. The perpendicular changes present as intraepithelial papillary capillary loops (IPCLs) that are connected with laryngeal papillomatosis, precancerous, and cancerous lesions (27). Many authors confirmed the high accuracy of ELS classification in determining between benign and malignant lesions (28–30). In 2019, Ni et al. improved the classification from 2011, adding another six types that cover vocal fold leukoplakia. Both classifications are based on the morphological changes present in laryngeal IPCLs to distinguish them between benign and malignant lesions (31). In the new classification, the focality is on the presence of perpendicular vessels outside or on the surface of the plaque, which suggests a malignant lesion. The pathological vessels seen in NBI are visualized as brown dots of different sizes and are twisted, earthworm-like. The accuracy of this classification in the assessment of VFL was 90.8%, which is significantly better than that of conventional WL endoscopy (70%) (31, 32).

Our paper presented similar results. Using NBI in laryngeal leukoplakia diagnosis revealed high accuracy, especially when using the ELS classification. Specifically, the accuracy was 93.9%, according to ELS, and 85.1%, according to the NI 2019 classification. The combined use of contact endoscopy (CE) and NBI has already been suggested for visualizing specific vascular changes indicative of glottic neoplasia (33). However, inter-rater reliability and agreement in three classification systems proved to be the best for vascular changes by the ELS and was significantly higher than those by Ni et al. and Puxeddu et al. (33).

Other than NBI endoscopy, systems like the Storz Professional Image Enhancement System have also been increasingly used in patients with suspected lesions of the larynx and hypopharynx (34). Both methods are comparable in the detection and analysis of superficial neoangiogenesis, and both methods are efficient in observing epithelial and subepithelial microvascular irregularities and pathologies, but NBI has been more popularized (35). A conventional laryngoscope using white light plays the main role in the decision-making process concerning VFL in the majority of laryngology departments. In 2019, Chen et al. proposed a new WL classification for VFL connected with the morphological features of the lesions, and distinguished three types of plaque: flat and smooth, elevated and smooth, and rough. They showed a high correlation between the morphological features of the laryngeal leukoplakia and their final histology result (19).

Another issue is the precise location of the lesion in the glottis area. It is known that the anterior commissure raises oncological concern because it represents a weak point with regard to tumor spread (36, 37). There are different degrees of AC involvement (36), but this stratification is concerned with tumor infiltration and not with the location of the leukoplakia. The very small distance between anterior commissure mucosa and thyroid cartilage, and the lack of perichondrium or periosteum in the AC area promote the spread of cancer, even in early invasion (38, 39). This should not affect the risk of cancer in VFL, which affects the superficial epithelial layers. Nevertheless, the AC is a site susceptible to the influence of tobacco smoke carcinogens on the epithelium.

Thus, we wanted to check whether the plaque in the AC location should be treated more suspiciously. We confirmed that this area should receive greater attention because the odds of cancer developing under a leukoplakia plaque in lesions involving AC were 5.094 times higher than those not involving the anterior commissure.

In this paper, we stabilize the schedule to recognize cancer under VFL plaque on a large, multicenter group of patients. The flowchart used in this research followed the schedule published by Pietruszewska et al., but we add an additional variable, AC involvement, which in our opinion, is crucial for cancer prediction. The algorithm includes a scheme of action based on a physical examination: morphology of plaque in WL according to the Chen classification, the vascular pattern in NBI scored according to the ELS classification, and the precise localization of the plaque.

Our results showed a high correlation between both the ELS and Chen classifications and the pathological outcomes, which is comparable to the results of Lin et al. (40) and Lu et al. (41). Therefore, we believe that the combined classifications of ELS and Chen, and the addition of the focus on AC involvement play a basic role in the diagnosis of laryngeal leukoplakia, especially in determining and distinguishing between those that are benign and those that are malignant. These findings have clinical importance for initial VFL diagnosis, directing patients for surgery, and routine endoscopic surveillance.

This study has some strengths and limitations. The strong points of this study include the creation of a new schedule for VFL diagnostics based on WL and NBI with regard to AC location in one of the biggest clinical groups of VFL. The combination of methods applied according to the proposed schedule proved effective in distinguishing cancer underneath the leukoplakia and gives direct suggestions for treatment options. However, there are still several weaknesses in the study. The main issue concerns the prevalence of NBI in laryngology departments; this method is not as popular as white light endoscopy, and additionally, the learning curve of NBI is quite long.

CONCLUSIONS

The ability to detect invasive cancer under leukoplakia remains a diagnostic challenge. An algorithm that combines WL and NBI, and the combination of two classifications, improves the specificity and positive predictive value, especially in anterior commissure involvement.

ETHICS STATEMENT

The studies involving human participants were reviewed and approved by Komisja Bioetyczna przy Uniwersytecie Medycznym im. Karola Marcinkowskiego w Poznaniu/ Bioethics Committee of Poznań University of Medical Sciences/. Written informed consent for participation was not required for this study in accordance with the national legislation and the institutional requirements.

AUTHOR CONTRIBUTIONS

MW and WP contributed to conception and design of the study. HK, PN, OR, and JM organized the database. OR performed the statistical analysis. HK wrote the first draft of the manuscript. HK, OR, MW, and WP wrote sections of the manuscript. All authors contributed to manuscript revision, read, and approved the submitted version.

REFERENCES

1. Gale N, Poljak M, Zidar N. Update From the 4th Edition of the World Health Organization Classification of Head and Neck Tumours: What Is New in the 2017 WHO Blue Book for Tumours of the Hypopharynx, Larynx, Trachea and Parapharyngeal Space. *Head Neck Pathol* (2017) 11(1):23–32. doi: 10.1007/s12105-017-0788-z
2. Zhu H, Xu W, Li Y, Cheng L. Observation of Clinicopathological Characteristics of Vocal Fold Leukoplakia and Laryngopharyngeal Reflux. *Chin J Otorhinolaryngol Head NeckSurg* (2014) 49:368–73. doi: 10.3760/cma.j.issn.1673-0860.2014.05.004
3. Panwar A, Lindau R3rd, Wieland A. Management of Prema- Lignant Lesions of the Larynx. *Expert Rev Anticancer Ther* (2013) 13:1045–51. doi: 10.1586/14737140.2013.829643
4. Kim CM, Chhetri DK. Triological Best Practice: When Is Surgical Intervention Indicated for Vocal Fold Leukoplakia? *Laryngoscope* (2020) 130(6):1362–3. doi: 10.1002/lary.28527
5. Mehanna H, Paleri V, Robson A, Wight R, Helliwell T. Consensus Statement by Otorhinolaryngologists and Pathologists on the Diagnosis and Management of Laryngeal Dysplasia. *Clin Otolaryngol* (2010) 35:170–6. doi: 10.1111/j.1749-4486.2010.02119.x
6. Karatayli-Ozgursoy S, Pacheco-Lopez P, Hillel AT, Best SR, Bishop JA, Akst LM. Laryngeal Dysplasia, Demographics, and Treatment: A Single-Institution, 20-Year Review. *JAMA Otolaryngol Head Neck Surg* (2015) 141:313–8. doi: 10.1001/jamaoto.2014.3736
7. Isenberg JS, Crozier DL, Dailey SH. Institutional and Comprehensive Review of Laryngeal Leukoplakia. *Ann Otol Rhinol Laryngol* (2008) 117:74–9. doi: 10.1177/000348940811700114
8. Cui W, Xu W, Yang Q, Hu R. Clinicopathological Parameters Associated With Histological Background and Recurrence After Surgical Intervention of Vocal Cord Leukoplakia. *Med (Baltimore)* (2017) 96:e7033. doi: 10.1097/MD.0000000000007033
9. Pietruszewska W, Morawska J, Rosiak O, Leduchowska A, Klimza H, Wierzbicka M. Vocal Fold Leukoplakia: Which of the Classifications of

White Light and Narrow Band Imaging Most Accurately Predicts Laryngeal Cancer Transformation? Proposition for a Diagnostic Algorithm. *Cancers* (2021) 13:3273. doi: 10.3390/cancers13133273
10. Young C-K, Lin W-N, Lee L-Y, Lee LA, Hsin LJ, Liao CT, et al. Laryngoscopic Characteristics in Vocal Leukoplakia: Inter-Rater Reliability and Correlation With Histology Grading. *Laryngoscope* (2015) 125:E62–6. doi: 10.1002/lary.24884
11. Fang T-J, Lin W-N, Lee L-Y, et al. Classification of Vocal Fold Leukoplakia by Clinical Scoring. *Head Neck* (2016) 38(Suppl 1):E1998–2003. doi: 10.1002/hed.24368
12. Ni XG, He S, Xu ZG, Gao L, Lu N, Yuan Z, et al. Endoscopic Diagnosis of Laryngeal Cancer and Precancerous Lesions by Narrow Band Imaging. *J Laryngol Otol* (2011) 125:288–96. doi: 10.1017/S0022215110002033
13. Piazza C, Del Bon F, Peretti G, Nicolai P. Narrow Band Imaging in Endoscopic Evaluation of the Larynx. *CurrOpinOtolaryngol Head Neck Surg* (2012) 20:472–6. doi: 10.1097/MOO.0b013e32835908ac
14. Kraft M, Fostiropoulos K, Gürtler N, Arnoux A, Davaris N, Arens C. Value of Narrow Band Imaging in the Early Diagnosis of Laryngeal Cancer. *Head Neck* (2016) 38:15–20. doi: 10.1002/hed.23838
15. Lin YC, Wang WH, Lee KF, Tsai WC, Weng HH. Value of Narrow Band Imaging Endoscopy in Early Mucosal Head and Neck Cancer. *Head Neck* (2012) 34:1574–9. doi: 10.1002/hed.21964
16. Takano JH, Yakushiji T, Kamiyama I, Nomura T, Katakura A, Takano N, et al. Detecting Early Oral Cancer: Narrowband Imaging System Observation of the Oral Mucosa Microvasculature. *Int J Oral MaxillofacSurg* (2010) 39:208–13. doi: 10.1016/j.ijom.2010.01.007
17. Klimza H, Jackowska J, Tokarski M, Piersiala K, Wierzbicka M. Narrow-Band Imaging (NBI) for Improving the Assessment of Vocal Fold Leukoplakia and Overcoming the Umbrella Effect. *PloS One* (2017) 12:e0180590. doi: 10.1371/journal.pone.0180590
18. Stanikova L, Satankova J, Kucova H, Walderova R, Zelenik K, Kominek P. The Role of Narrow-Band Imaging (NBI) Endoscopy in Optical Biopsy of Vocal Cord Leukoplakia. *Eur Arch Otorhinolaryngol* (2017) 274:355–9. doi: 10.1007/s00405-016-4244-6
19. Chen M, Li C, Yang Y, Cheng L, Wu H. A Morphological Classification for Vocal Fold Leukoplakia. *Braz J Otorhinolaryngol* (2019) 85(5):588–96. doi: 10.1016/j.bjorl.2018.04.014
20. Ni XG, Zhu JQ, Zhang QQ, Zhang BG, Wang GQ. Diagnosis of Vocal Cord Leukoplakia: The Role of a Novel Narrow Band Imaging Endoscopic Classification. *Laryngoscope* (2019) 129(2):429–34. doi: 10.1002/lary.27346
21. Gale N, Hille J, Jordan RC, Nadal A, Williams MD. Precursor Lesions. Dysplasia. In: AK El-Naggar, JKC Chan, JR Grandis, T Takata, PJ Slootweg, editors. *WHO Classification of Head and Neck Tumours.* Lyon: IARC (2017). p. 91–3.
22. Fluss R, Faraggi D, Reiser B. Estimation of the Youden Index and its Associated Cutoff Point. *Biometrical J* (2005) 47:458–72. doi: 10.1002/bimj.200410135
23. Peng C-YJ, Lee KL, Ingersoll GM. An Introduction to Logistic Regression Analysis and Reporting. *J Educ Res* (2002) 96:1:3–14. doi: 10.1080/00220670209598786
24. Bertino G, Cacciola S, Fernandes WB Jr, Fernandes CM, Occhini A, Tinelli C, et al. Effectiveness of Narrow Band Imaging in the Detection of Premalignant and Malignant Lesions of the Larynx: Validation of a New Endoscopic Clinical Classification. *Head Neck* (2015) 37:215–22. doi: 10.1002/hed.23582
25. Stanikova L, Satankova J, Kucova H, Walderova R, Zelenik K, Kominek P. The Role of Narrow-Band Imaging (NBI) Endoscopy in Optical Biopsy of Vocal Cord Leukoplakia. *Eur Arch Otorhinolaryngol* (2017) 274(1):355–9. doi: 10.1007/s00405-016-4244-6
26. Klimza H, Jackowska J, Tokarski M, Piersiala K, Wierzbicka M. Narrow-Band Imaging (NBI) for Improving the Assessment of Vocal Fold Leukoplakia and Overcoming the Umbrella Effect. *PloS One* (2017) 12(6):e0180590. doi: 10.1371/journal.pone.0180590
27. Arens C, Piazza C, Andrea M, Dikkers FG, Tjon Pian Gi REA, Voigt-Zimmermann S, et al. Proposal for a Descriptive Guideline of Vascular Changes in Lesions of the Vocal Folds by the Committee on Endoscopic Laryngeal Imaging of the European Laryngological Society. *Eur Arch Otorhinolaryngol* (2016) 273:1207–14. doi: 10.1007/s00405-015-3851-y
28. Šifrer R, Šereg-Bahar M, Gale N, Hočevar-Boltežar I. The Diagnostic Value of Perpendicular Vascular Patterns of Vocal Cords Defined by Narrow-Band Imaging. *Eur Arch Otorhinolaryngol* (2020) 277(6):1715–23. doi: 10.1007/s00405-020-05864-5
29. Šifrer R, Rijken JA, Leemans CR, Eerenstein SEJ, van Weert S, Hendrickx JJ, et al. Evaluation of Vascular Features of Vocal Cords Proposed by the European Laryngological Society. *Eur Arch Otorhinolaryngol* (2018) 275(1):147–51. doi: 10.1007/s00405-017-4791-5
30. Missale F, Taboni S, Carobbio ALC, Mazzola F, Berretti G, Iandelli A, et al. Validation of the European Laryngological Society Classification of Glottic Vascular Changes as Seen by Narrow Band Imaging in the Optical Biopsy Setting. *Eur Arch Otorhinolaryngol* (2021) 278(7):2397–409. doi: 10.1007/s00405-021-06723-7
31. Ni X-G, Wang G-Q, Hu F-Y, Xu XM, Xu L, Liu XQ, et al. Clinical Utility and Effectiveness of a Training Programme in the Application of a New Classification of Narrow-Band Imaging for Vocal Cord Leukoplakia: A Multicentre Study. *Clin Otolaryngol* (2019) 00:1–7. doi: 10.1111/coa.13361
32. Campo F, Ralli M, Di Stadio A, Greco A, Pellini R, de Vincentiis M. Role of Narrow Band Imaging Endoscopy in Preoperative Evaluation of Laryngeal Leukoplakia: A Review of the Literature. *Ear Nose Throat J* (2020) 20:145561320973770. doi: 10.1177/0145561320973770
33. Mehlum CS, Døssing H, Davaris N, Giers A, Grøntved ÅM, Kjaergaard T, et al. Interrater Variation of Vascular Classifications Used in Enhanced Laryngeal Contact Endoscopy. *Eur Arch Otorhinolaryngol* (2020) 277(9):2485–92. doi: 10.1007/s00405-020-06000-z
34. Puxeddu R, Sionis S, Gerosa C, Carta F. Enhanced Contact Endoscopy for the Detection of Neoangiogenesis in Tumors of the Larynx and Hypopharynx. *Laryngoscope* (2015) 125(7):1600–6. doi: 10.1002/lary.25124
35. Staníková L, Walderová R, Jančatová D, Formánek M, Zeleník K, Komínek P. Comparison of Narrow Band Imaging and the Storz Professional Image Enhancement System for Detection of Laryngeal and Hypopharyngeal Pathologies. *Eur Arch Otorhinolaryngol* (2018) 275(7):1819–25. doi: 10.1007/s00405-018-4987-3
36. Rucci L, Gammarota L, Borghi Cirri MB. Carcinoma of the Anterior Commissure of the Larynx: I. Embryological and Anatomic Considerations. *Ann Otol Rhinol Laryngol* (1996) 105(4):303–8. doi: 10.1177/000348949610500412
37. Prades JM, Peoc'h M, Petcu C, Karkas A, Dumollard JM, Gavid M. The Anterior Commissure of the Human Larynx Revisited. *Surg Radiol Anat* (2017) 39(8):871–6. doi: 10.1007/s00276-017-1814-2
38. Krespi YP, Meltzer CJ. Laser Surgery for Vocal Cord Carcinoma Involving the Anterior Commissure. *Ann Otol Rhinol Laryngol* (1989) 98(2):105–9. doi: 10.1177/000348948909800204
39. Bagatella F, Bignardi L. Morphological Study of the Laryngeal Anterior Commissure With Regard to the Spread of Cancer. *Acta Otolaryngol* (1981) 92(1-2):167– 171. doi: 10.3109/00016488109133252
40. Lin C, Zhang S, Lu L, Wang M, Qian X. Diagnostic Value and Pathological Correlation of Narrow Band Imaging Classification in Laryngeal Lesions. *Ear Nose Throat J* (2020) 8:145561320925327. doi: 10.1177/0145561320925327
41. Lu G, Guo W, Zhang Q, Song X. Endoscopic Diagnosis Value of Narrow Band Imaging Ni Classification in Vocal Fold Leukoplakia and Early Glottic Cancer. *Am J Otolaryngol* (2021) 42(3):102904. doi: 10.1016/j.amjoto.2021.102904

16

Psorachromene Suppresses Oral Squamous Cell Carcinoma Progression by Inhibiting Long Non-Coding RNA GAS5 Mediated Epithelial-Mesenchymal Transition

Tong-Hong Wang[1,2,3†], *Yann-Lii Leu*[4,5,6†], *Chin-Chuan Chen*[1,4], *Tzong-Ming Shieh*[7], *Jang-Hau Lian*[8] *and Chi-Yuan Chen*[1,2*]

[1] Tissue Bank, Chang Gung Memorial Hospital, Tao-Yuan, Taiwan, [2] Research Center for Chinese Herbal Medicine, Graduate Institute of Health Industry Technology and Research Center for Food and Cosmetic Safety, College of Human Ecology, Chang Gung University of Science and Technology, Tao-Yuan, Taiwan, [3] Department of Hepato-Gastroenterology, Liver Research Center, Chang Gung Memorial Hospital, Tao-Yuan, Taiwan, [4] Graduate Institute of Natural Products, Chang Gung University, Tao-Yuan, Taiwan, [5] Chinese Herbal Medicine Research Team, Healthy Aging Research Center, Chang Gung University, Tao-Yuan, Taiwan, [6] Center for Traditional Chinese Medicine, Chang Gung Memorial Hospital, Tao-Yuan, Taiwan, [7] Department of Dental Hygiene, China Medical University, Taichung, Taiwan, [8] Genomic Medicine Core Laboratory, Chang Gung Memorial Hospital, Tao-Yuan, Taiwan

***Correspondence:**
Chi-Yuan Chen
d49417002@gmail.com

† These authors have contributed equally to this work

The extract of the seeds of *Psoralea corylifolia* Linn. (*P. corylifolia*) have been shown to display anti-tumor activity. However, the prospects of the active compounds from this plant in the treatment of oral squamous cell carcinoma (OSCC) remains unclear. In the present study, the antitumor effects of psorachromene, a flavonoid extracted from the seeds of *P. corylifolia*, were investigated using cells and animal models of OSCC; the downstream regulatory mechanisms were also elucidated. The results showed that psorachromene significantly repressed cell proliferation, migration, and invasiveness and increased the toxic effects of chemotherapeutic agents against OSCC cells. The repressive effects of psorachromene were attributable to the inhibition of EGFR-Slug signaling, and the induction of G2/M arrest and apoptosis in the OSCC cells. Additionally, we found that psorachromene induced the expression of tumor suppressor long non-coding ribonucleic acid (RNA) growth arrest-specific transcript 5 (GAS5) and the activation of its downstream anticancer mechanisms. Animal experiments also showed noticeable inhibition of tumor growth, without significant physiological toxicity. The findings indicate that psorachromene displays anti-tumor activity in OSCC, and warrants further investigation as a potential agent for clinical application.

Keywords: psorachromene, oral squamous cell carcinoma (OSCC), long non-coding RNA, growth arrest-specific transcript 5 (GAS5), epidermal growth factor receptor (EGFR)

INTRODUCTION

Oral cancer is the eleventh most common malignancy worldwide (1). In Taiwan, more than 4,700 people are diagnosed with oral cancer each year, and ~2,200 people die from it. Among all types of oral cancer, oral squamous cell carcinoma (OSCC) is the most common, with an incidence of ~90% (2). Smoking, drinking alcohol, and chewing tobacco or betel seeds are risk factors for OSCC (3–5).

Currently, the mainstay treatment for OSCC is surgical resection, with adjuvant chemotherapy or radiotherapy (6, 7). In addition, epidermal growth factor receptor (EGFR) and cyclooxygenase-2 (COX-2) inhibitors are also used in the treatment of OSCC (8, 9). However, the benefits of these therapies remain sub-optimal, and their side effects have a considerable impact on patients' quality of life. Therefore, oral cancer research continues to focus on the development of effective new treatment methods with minimal side effects.

Cancer-causing gene mutations are one of the major causes of OSCC (10–12). Previous studies have shown that over 75% of OSCC shows epidermal growth factor receptor (EGFR; also known as ErbB1 or HER1) overexpression; EGFR expression has shown a significantly positive association with the degree of malignancy (13–15). Therefore, inhibiting the growth of cancer cells by EGFR signaling inhibition is one of the current treatment strategies for OSCC (16, 17). Various EGFR inhibitors including anti-EGFR monoclonal antibodies (cetuximab and panitumumab) and small-molecule EGFR tyrosine kinase inhibitors (gefitinib, afatinib, and erlotinib) have been developed, and have demonstrated efficacy in OSCC (16, 18–20). However, only the monoclonal antibody cetuximab is currently approved for the treatment of OSCC; it has demonstrated significant inhibition of the progress of OSCC, with extension of survival (21, 22). Unfortunately, for reasons that are not fully clear, only $\sim$50% of patients respond to cetuximab (23, 24).

Traditional Chinese medicine (TCM) has long been used for the treatment of diseases in Asian countries (25, 26). Unlike Western medicine, TCM provides effective treatment options with relatively milder adverse effects (27–29). However, differences in the quality of TCM therapeutics and the levels of active ingredients usually result in variable therapeutic effects (30). In order to achieve more stable therapeutic effects, the active ingredients of many traditional Chinese medicinal materials have been purified and identified (31–33). The identified compounds can be used at lower doses with more specific therapeutic efficacy. Currently, many compounds extracted from TCM therapeutics, e.g., artemisinin, curcumin, resveratrol, and paclitaxel, which are used in the treatment of cancer have shown good efficacy (34–38). Among them, paclitaxel, camptothecin, and vinblastine, have also been approved for the treatment of various cancers, including lung cancer, liver cancer, and oral cancer (39).

Psoralea corylifolia L. is a TCM herb that is commonly used in Asian countries for the treatment of bacterial infections, inflammation, and cancer (40–44). *P. corylifolia* L. contains flavonoids such as bavachin, isobavachalcone, and neobavaisoflavone; polyphenols such as psoralidin, psoralen, and isopsoralen; and benzene ring compounds such as backuchiol; in addition, the herb has been found to have biological activity and various therapeutic effects (42). Psorachromene is an isoflavone component isolated from the fruit kernels of *P. corylifolia* L. (45). A few studies have investigated the mechanism of action of psorachromene. Recent reports indicate that psorachromene has anti-inflammatory effects that may inhibit inflammatory reactions caused by inducible NO synthase (iNOS) and cyclo-oxygenase (COX) expression induced by bacterial infection (46). However, there have been no studies on its anticancer effects. In this study, we investigated the anticancer activity of psorachromene in oral cancer, and studied its downstream regulatory mechanisms.

MATERIALS AND METHODS

Cell Lines and Culture Media

SAS is a human tongue squamous cell carcinoma cell line from the Japanese Collection of Research Bioresources (Tokyo, Japan) (47). OECM1 is a Taiwanese human gingival squamous carcinoma cell line; its derivation has been described in a previous study (47). Both cell lines were cultured in Dulbecco's modified Eagle's medium (DMEM) containing 10% fetal bovine serum (FBS), 1.2 g/L sodium bicarbonate, 0.5 mM sodium pyruvate, and 2.5 mM L-glutamine. The culture media, FBS, and chemical compounds were purchased from Life Technologies (Grand Island, NY, USA). The cells were cultured at 37°C in a humidified 5% CO_2 incubator.

Reagents and Antibodies

The crude materials of the *P. corylifolia* seed were purchased from Chuang Song Zong Pharmaceutical Co., Ltd (Kaohsiung, Taiwan). The dried seeds of *P. corylifolia* were infused in ethanol and were filtered to obtain the crude extract. The crude extract was partitioned in n-hexane/water (1:1). The n-hexane soluble extract was then fractionated by column chromatography on silica gel, eluting with n-hexane: ethylacetate to isolate psorachromene. The purity of psorachromene was determined by nuclear magnetic resonance analysis. Antibodies against vimentin, E-cadherin, slug, cleaved-PARP (cl-PARP, Asp214), and caspase 9 were obtained from Cell Signaling (Temecula, CA, USA). Antibodies against EGFR and β-actin were purchased from Santa Cruz Biotechnology (Santa Cruz, CA, USA). Prestained protein marker and TOOLSmart RNA extractor were purchased from BIOTOOLS (New Taipei City, Taiwan). The cisplatin and doxorubicin were purchased from Sigma-Aldrich (St. Louis, MO, USA), and the reagents for gel electrophoresis were purchased from Bio-Rad (Berkeley, CA, USA).

Cell Viability Assays

Cell viability was determined using the sulforhodamine B (SRB) assay by staining with trypan blue, as described previously (48, 49).

Terminal Deoxynucleotidyl Transferase dUTP Nick End Labeling (TUNEL) Assay

The apoptotic status of the treated cells was determined using a DeadEnd^{TM} Fluorometric TUNEL Assay Kit (Promega, Madison, WI) according to the manufacturers' protocol. In summary, the SAS cells were treated with psorachromene (50 μM) for 24 h and were then subjected to a terminal deoxynucleotidyl transferase dUTP nick end labeling (TUNEL) assay. The apoptotic cells (DAPI and TUNEL double stained cells) were enumerated using a fluorescence microscope (magnification, ×100). Cells in five different microscopic fields/dish were analyzed for each experiment.

Western Blotting

Cells were washed twice with phosphate-buffered saline (PBS), lysed in 200 μL of RIPA lysis buffer (Biotools Co. Ltd., Taiwan) containing protease inhibitors, and incubated on ice for 10 min. The samples were then centrifuged at 12,000 rpm for 30 min at 4°C, and the protein-containing supernatants were collected. The protein concentrations were determined using the Bio-Rad protein assay, and western blotting was performed as described previously (49).

Phenotypic Analysis for Clonogenic, Migration, and Invasion Ability

The clonogenic, migration, and invasion assays were performed as described previously (47).

Cell-Cycle Analysis

Cells were trypsinized, washed twice, and incubated in PBS containing 0.12% Triton X-100, 0.12 mmol/L EDTA, and 100 mg/mL ribonuclease A. Propidium iodide (50 μg/mL) was then added to each sample, and they were kept at 4°C for 20 min. Cell cycle distribution was then analyzed using flow cytometry (Beckman Coulter Epics Elite, Beckman, Inc.).

Whole-Transcriptome Sequencing

RNA extraction and whole-transcriptome sequencing was performed as described in a previous study (25).

Detection of lncRNA GAS5

RNA from the cells were isolated using a RNeasy mini kit (QIAGEN, Gaithersburg, MD, USA), according to the manufacturer's instructions. Two micrograms of RNA sample were subjected to reverse transcription (RT) using the reverse transcription kit (Applied Biosystems, Foster City, CA, USA). The expression of lncRNA GAS5 was detected by quantitative polymerase chain reaction (PCR) using the TaqMan gene expression assay (Applied Biosystems, Foster City, CA, USA), as described previously (50). Glyceraldehyde 3-phosphate dehydrogenase (GAPDH) was used as an internal control.

RNA Interference (RNAi)

Human lncRNA GAS5 were downregulated using a mixture of four small interfering RNAs (siRNAs) (ON-TARGETplus SMARTpool; Dharmacon, Lafayette, CO) as previously described (50). In summary, the four siRNAs targeting lncRNA GAS5 (GenBank accession no. NR_002578.2) covered the following: nucleotides 385-403 from the start codon (lncRNA GAS5-1: AGGCAGACCUGUUAUCCUA), nucleotides 248-266 (lncRNA GAS5-2: UGGAUGACUUGCUUGGGUA), nucleotides 567-585 (lncRNA GAS5-3: GAUGGAGUCUCAUGGCACA), and nucleotides 301-319 (lncRNA GAS5-4: AGGUAUGGAGAGUCGGCUU). Transfection was performed using the Dharmafect 1 transfection reagent (Dharmacon) according to the manufacturer's instructions.

In vivo Tumor Xenograft Study

The *in vivo* antitumor activity of psorachromene against SAS cells was studied using 6-week-old nude BALB/c nu/nu male mice. SAS cells (5×10^5) were subcutaneously implanted in the right flank of the mice on day 0. The mice were then randomized

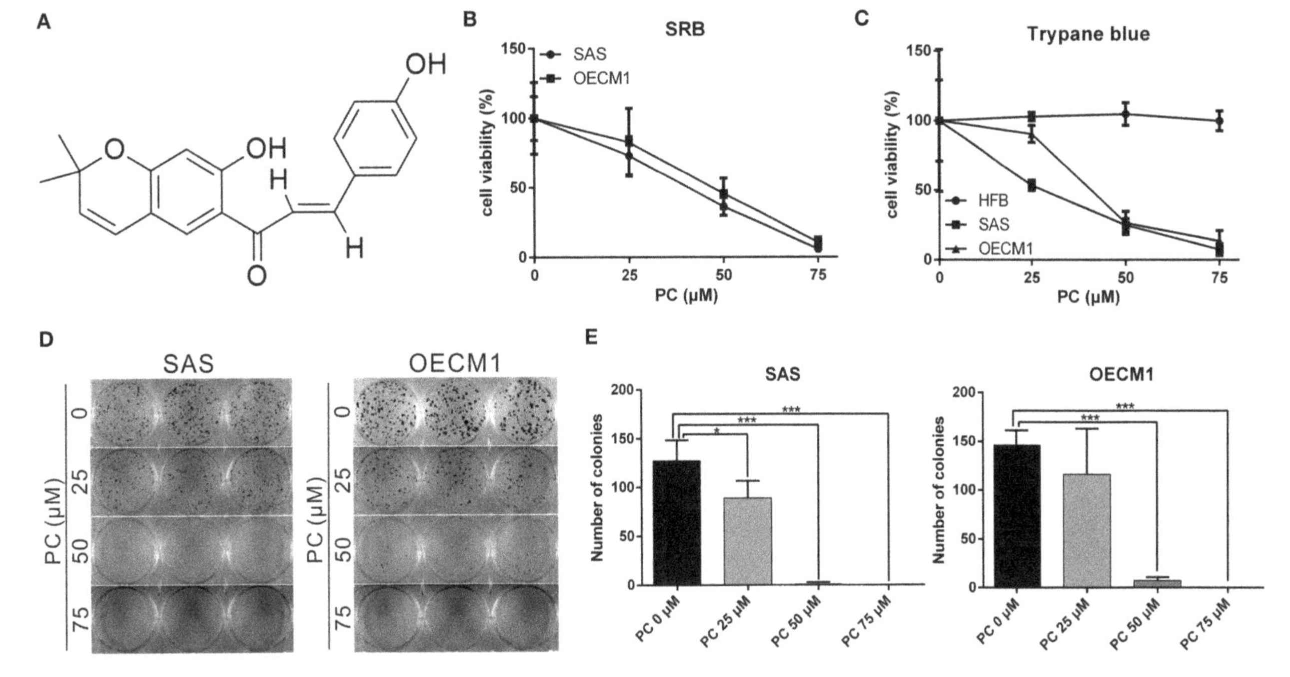

FIGURE 1 | Inhibition of the proliferation of OSCC cells by psorachromene. **(A)** Chemical structure of psorachromene. SAS and OECM1 cells were treated with different concentrations of psorachromene or vehicle (DMSO), and the cell proliferation status was analyzed using the SRB assay **(B)**, trypan blue staining assay **(C)**, and colony formation assay **(D,E)**. The results are the mean of three independent experiments. Significant differences vs. the control groups, *$p < 0.05$, ***$p < 0.001$.

on day 7 into vehicle control and treatment groups of six animals each. Psorachromene and cisplatin were administered intraperitoneally thrice weekly, with 100 μL of psorachromene (25 mg/kg of body weight), cisplatin (2 mg/kg), or an equal volume of dimethyl sulfoxide (DMSO), which served as a control. The tumor volume was evaluated every 2 days using calipers, based on the following formula: tumor volume = length × width^2/2. Their body weights and food consumption were also determined to evaluate apparent signs of toxicity. The tumor-bearing mice were weighed and sacrificed on day 22 for assaying the tumor biology. All animal experiments were performed in accordance with the guidelines for the Animal Care Ethics Commission of the Chang Gung Memorial Hospital, under an approved animal protocol (IACUC approval no. 2018031301).

Immunohistochemistry

The tumors were fixed in formalin and embedded in paraffin. Consecutive 2-μm-thick sections were obtained from the paraffin-embedded tissue blocks, and were floated onto glass slides. The slide-mounted tissue sections were subjected to immunohistochemical staining as described previously (51).

Statistics

All data have been presented as means ± standard deviations (SD). The Student's t-test was employed for comparison, and all analyses were performed using the Statistical Package for the Social Sciences version 12.0 (SPSS, Inc.). Differences between the variables were considered significant for p-values of > 0.05.

RESULTS

Psorachromene Inhibited the Growth of OSCC Cells and Promoted Their Apoptosis

Psorachromene is a flavonoid extracted from the seeds of *P. corylifolia* L. (**Figure 1A**). In this study, we treated OSCC cells and human fibroblast cell lines with different concentrations of psorachromene and analyzed the cell proliferation status using Sulforhodamine B (SRB) assay to determine whether psorachromene has inhibitory activity on OSCC. The results showed that psorachromene could significantly inhibit the growth of SAS and OECM1 cells starting from concentrations of 25 μM; the inhibitory effect became more significant with increasing psorachromene concentrations (**Figure 1B**). Similar results were obtained on the trypan blue staining assay.

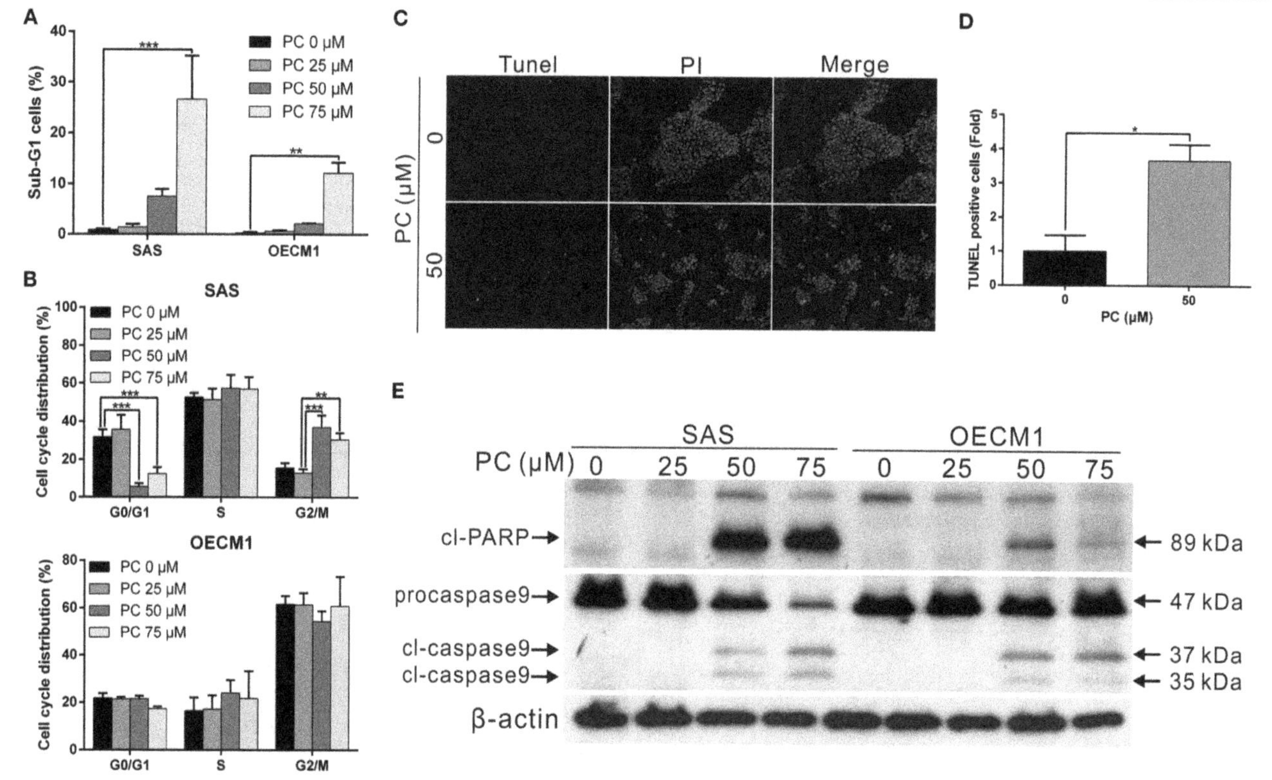

FIGURE 2 | Inhibition of cell cycle progression and promotion of apoptosis in OSCC cells by psorachromene. **(A,B)** Effect of psorachromene on cell cycle progression in SAS and OECM1 cells. The cells were treated with vehicles or different concentrations of psorachromene for 24 h. Cell cycle distribution was analyzed by flow cytometry. **(C)** SAS cells were treated with or without psorachromene, and cell apoptosis was determined using a terminal deoxynucleotidyl transferase dUTP nick end labeling (TUNEL) assay. Green punctate staining (white arrows) represents TUNEL-positive cells. Apoptotic cells were identified as DAPI and TUNEL double-stained cells. Magnification: 100×. Quantitative results seen in **(D)**. **(E)** Western blot analysis showing the effect on caspase 9 and PARP activity in OSCC cells after 48 h of psorachromene treatment. $^{*}p < 0.05$, $^{**}p < 0.01$, $^{***}p < 0.001$.

Psorachromene significantly inhibited the growth of SAS and OECM1 cells in a dose dependent manner. However, no inhibitory effect was observed on the growth of human fibroblast cell line HFB (**Figure 1C**). This indicated that psorachromene selectively inhibits the growth in OSCC cells without significant toxicity to normal cells. We also evaluated the impact of psorachromene on the colony forming ability of OSCC. The results showed significant inhibitory activity in a dose-dependent manner. At a concentration of 50 μM, psorachromene inhibited the colony forming ability of OSCC cells by more than 90% (**Figures 1D,E**), confirming its inhibitory activity on the growth of OSCC cells.

To determine the mechanism of inhibition of OSCC, we further compared the cell cycle progression between cells treated and not treated with psorachromene. Those treated with psorachromene were found to have been arrested in the G2 phase, their numbers in the sub-G1 phase were significantly higher compared to the control group (**Figures 2A,B**). These findings suggested that psorachromene inhibits cell cycle progression and promotes cell apoptosis. The results of the TUNEL assay also demonstrated that the number of apoptotic cells in the psorachromene treatment group were significantly higher compared with the control group (**Figures 2C,D**). Furthermore, the results of western blotting analysis confirmed the activation of caspase-9 and the cleavage of poly (ADP-ribose) polymerases (PARPs) by psorachromene, indicating that it promotes cell apoptosis by activating apoptosis-related proteins (**Figure 2E**).

Psorachromene Inhibits the Migration and Invasiveness of OSCC

Invasion and metastasis are the major contributors to the refractory nature of cancer. We conducted a wound-healing assay to evaluate whether psorachromene may affect cell migration; this was performed to further evaluate the potential of psorachromene in inhibiting metastasis and invasiveness in OSCC cells. The results showed that at a concentration of 25 μM, psorachromene significantly inhibited cell migration ability, and the inhibitory effects increased with the concentration of psorachromene. At a concentration of 75 μM, psorachromene inhibited the migration ability of SAS and OECM cells by 51.3 and 19.1%, respectively (**Figures 3A,B**). Furthermore, the invasion assay demonstrated that psorachromene may inhibit cell invasion by up to 83.7% at a concentration of 75 μM (**Figures 3C,D**).

Psorachromene Inhibits Epithelial-Mesenchymal Transition (EMT)

Epithelial-mesenchymal transition (EMT) is an important process in cancer cell metastasis, that weakens intercellular adhesions and facilitates metastasis. To determine whether

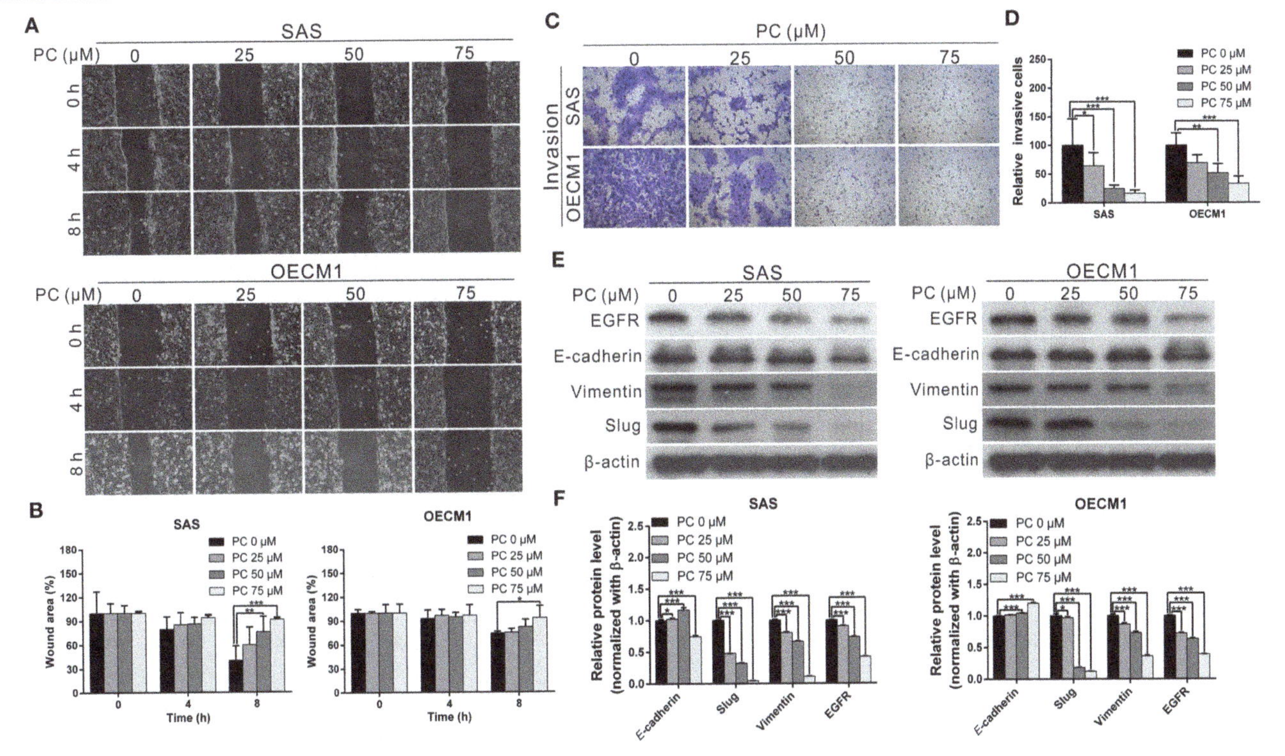

FIGURE 3 | Inhibition of cell metastasis ability in OSCC by psorachromene by inhibition of the progression of epithelial-mesenchymal transition. **(A)** The effect of psorachromene on the wound-healing ability of SAS and OECM1 cells. Quantitative results are seen in **(B)**. **(C,D)** The effect of psorachromene on the invasiveness of SAS and OECM1 cells. **(E)** Western blotting was used to examine the levels of EMT regulatory proteins in OSCC cells treated with psorachromene for 48 h. The quantified results are shown in **(F)**. $^{*}p < 0.05$, $^{**}p < 0.01$, $^{***}p < 0.001$.

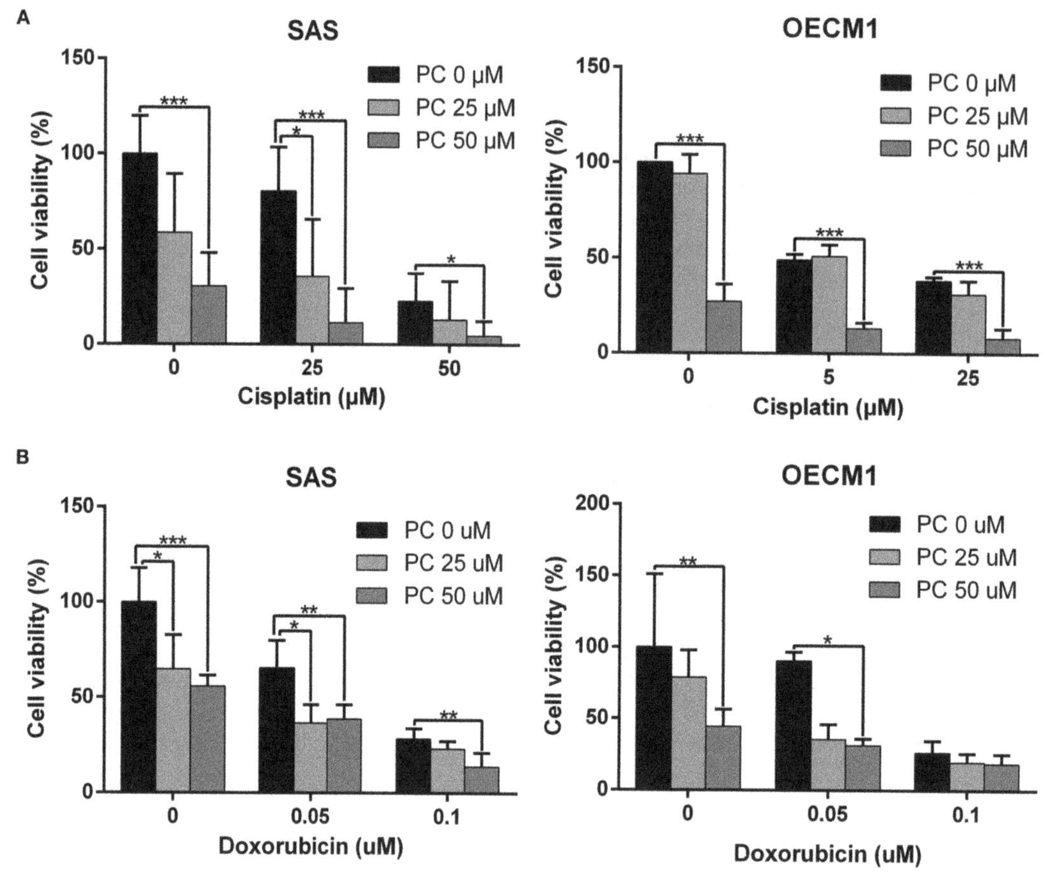

FIGURE 4 | Psorachromene combined with cisplatin and doxorubicin has additive effect. The effects of psorachromene combined with cisplatin and doxorubicin on proliferation of SAS **(A)** and OECM1 **(B)** cells. $^{*}p < 0.05$, $^{**}p < 0.01$, $^{***}p < 0.001$. All experiments were performed in triplicate.

psorachromene regulates EMT when inhibiting OSCC migration and invasion abilities, we performed western blotting to analyze the effects of psorachromene on EMT associated proteins. The results indicated that the expression of EMT-promoting proteins such as vimentin and slug was significantly lower in psorachromene-treated cells compared with the control group. However, the expression of E-cadherin did not change significantly (**Figures 3E,F**), suggesting that psorachromene may inhibit OSCC migration and invasion by inhibiting EMT.

Slug is a downstream gene regulated by the EGFR signaling pathway. We also evaluated whether psorachromene affects EGFR expression, and found its expression in psorachromene-treated cells to be significantly lower compared to the control group (**Figures 3E,F**). The results indicated that psorachromene may inhibit the expression of slug, and the progression of EMT by downregulating EGFR expression.

Psorachromene May Enhance the Therapeutic Effects of Cisplatin and Doxorubicin on OSCC

Cisplatin and doxorubicin are the commonly used chemotherapeutic drugs in the treatment of OSCC (52–54). In order to determine whether combining psorachromene with these drugs may improve their therapeutic effects on OSCC, we administered psorachromene, cisplatin, and doxorubicin alone, or in combination to the OSCC cells; we also evaluated its inhibitory effects on the growth of these cells. Cisplatin and doxorubicin alone had an inhibitory effect on OSCC; however, combination with psorachromene significantly enhanced the inhibition of OSCC. Compared to cisplatin or doxorubicin alone, the combination with psorachromene enhanced the toxicity on OSCC cells by up to 3.3-fold (**Figures 4A,B**). The combination index also demonstrated the additive effect of psorachromene in combination with cisplatin and doxorubicin (**Table 1**).

Psorachromene Inhibits Tumor Growth in Mice

The anticancer effects of psorachromene *in vivo* were verified using a mouse xenograft model; the effects of psorachromene on tumor growth in mice were similar to those of the cell experiments. The tumor growth rate was significantly reduced in mice treated with psorachromene. After 2 weeks of administering the drug, the tumor volume in the psorachromene-treated group was reduced by ~75.5% compared with the control group (**Figures 5A,B**), and the tumor inhibitory effect was equivalent to that of the cisplatin-treated group (84.6%).

In addition, there were no significant differences in body weight between the psorachromene-treated and control groups (**Figure 5C**), indicating that psorachromene may not have significant physiological toxicity.

In addition, we analyzed the expression of EGFR and EMT-related proteins including slug, vimentin, and E-cadherin in murine tumor tissues using immunohistochemical staining, and found that psorachromene may significantly inhibit the expression of EGFR and EMT-promoting proteins (**Figure 5D**). The results of this experiment were identical to those of cellular experiments, suggesting that psorachromene may inhibit EMT.

Psorachromene May Inhibit the Activation of Signaling Pathways Associated With Cell Growth and Extracellular Structure Organization

To understand its anticancer mechanisms of action, we treated SAS and OECM1 cell lines with psorachromene, and performed whole-transcriptome sequencing to identify the genes and signaling pathways that may be regulated by psorachromene. Heatmap analysis showed that after psorachromene treatment, gene expression was significantly altered compared with the control group (**Figure 6A**). We further performed ingenuity pathway analysis, and found that psorachromene mainly regulates the LKB1 and ErbB/EGFR signaling pathways (**Figure 6B**), affects the energy metabolism of cells, and the composition and generation of the extracellular matrix, thereby inhibiting their growth and metastasis.

Psorachromene Exerts Anticancer Effects by Inducing the Expression of Long Non-coding RNA GAS5

Previous studies have confirmed that long non-coding RNAs (lncRNAs) play an important role in cell physiological regulation, and drug responses. To understand the role of lncRNAs in the anti-OSCC mechanisms of action of psorachromene, we analyzed the previously-mentioned transcriptome sequencing data, and found that 12 lncRNAs demonstrated a higher than 2-fold change in expression after psorachromene treatment, compared to the control group (**Figure 6C**). Among these lncRNAs, growth arrest-specific transcript 5 (GAS5) has recently been discovered to suppress cancer. It has been shown to inhibit the growth and metastasis of OSCC by regulating the miR-21/PTEN axis. To confirm the regulatory relation between psorachromene and GAS5, we performed real-time reverse transcriptase-PCR to determine the expression of GAS5 in OSCC cells. The results indicated that the expression of GAS5 in SAS and OECM1 cells treated with psorachromene was significantly higher than that of the control group (**Figure 6D**); this indicates that psorachromene may inhibit the growth and metastasis of OSCC by inducing GAS5 mediated anticancer mechanisms.

We performed a rescue assay to further verify the mentioned conditions. The results showed that psorachromene significantly inhibited the growth and migration of OSCC cells. After silencing GAS5 expression, we found that the inhibitory effects of psorachromene on OSCC cells were attenuated (**Figures 7A–D**); this indicated that the anti-OSCC action of psorachromene is partly achieved by regulating the lncRNA-GAS5 anticancer pathway.

TABLE 1 | The combination index.

	PC (μM)	DOX (μM)	CI
SAS	25	0.05	0.68011
	25	0.1	0.50582
	50	0.05	1.04119
	50	0.1	0.84218
OECM1	25	0.05	0.79836
	25	0.1	1.18195
	50	0.05	1.51916
	50	0.1	1.84227
	PC (μM)	**CIS (μM)**	**CI**
SAS	25	25	0.99174
	25	50	0.63005
	50	25	0.96329
	50	50	0.75840
OECM1	25	5	1.93719
	25	25	0.84726
	50	5	0.84689
	50	25	0.76593

DISCUSSION

Psorachromene is a flavonoid component of *P. corylifolia* L., accounting for 0.0016% of the total extract from the seeds of *P. corylifolia* L (55). Current understanding on the biological functions of psorachromene is limited. Only a few studies have reported on its anti-inflammatory activity, which may inhibit inducible nitric oxide synthase (iNOS) and COX expression induced by lipopolysaccharide (LPS), thereby inhibiting inflammatory reaction (46). However, no studies have evaluated its anticancer effects. In this study, we investigated the inhibitory activity of psorachromene on OSCC, and found that it significantly inhibited the growth, migration, and invasiveness of OSCC cells, and suppressed EMT by inducing the expression of lncRNA-GAS5. The results of our animal experiments also showed that it may significantly inhibit the growth of tumor cells and the expression of EMT-associated proteins. To the best our knowledge, this is the first study to demonstrate that psorachromene regulates lncRNAs to exert its antitumor effects.

Previous studies have shown that ~80% of OSCC over-express EGFR; this leads to uncontrolled cell growth and enhances the metastatic ability of the cells (13, 56). It also enhances the resistance of OSCC to chemotherapeutic drugs including, cisplatin, 5-fluorouracil (5FU), and doxorubicin (57–59). Previous studies have also confirmed that the use of the EGFR inhibitor gefitinib in combination with cisplatin enhanced the therapeutic effects of the latter on

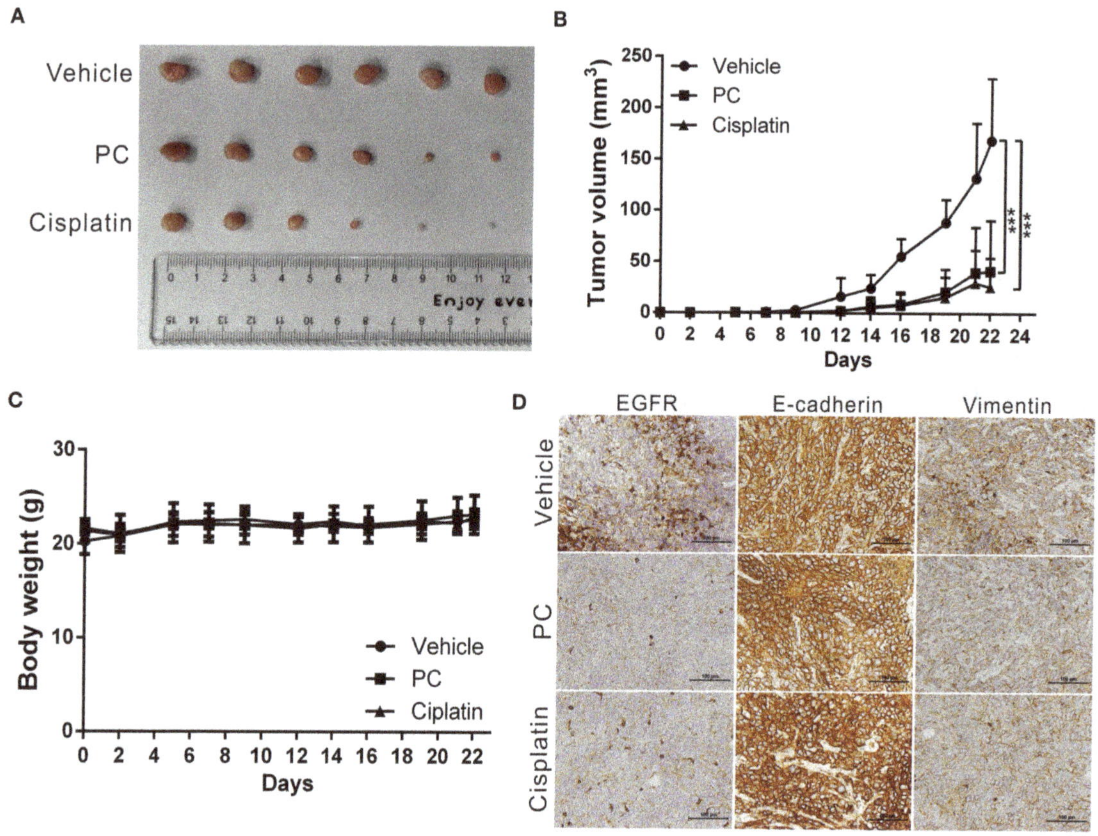

FIGURE 5 | Psorachromene inhibits tumor growth in mice. **(A)** A total of 5 × 10^6 SAS cells were inoculated into nude mice (n = 6). Representative images show the tumor xenografts at 3 weeks after implantation. Psorachromene significantly reduced tumor growth. **(B)** Tumor volumes were calculated every 3 days after injection. The volume of each tumor was calculated as follows: length × width^2 × 0.5. Bars indicate S.D. ***$p < 0.001$. **(C)** Body weights were calculated every 3 days after injection. **(D)** Immunohistochemical staining represents the effect of psorachromene on the expression of EGFR and EMT associated proteins in mice xenograft tumors. Magnification: 400×.

OSCC (20). This study demonstrated similar results. In addition to the inhibition of EGFR expression, psorachromene has synergistic activity with cisplatin and doxorubicin in the treatment of OSCC, with no significant physiological toxicities. Therefore, psorachromene has considerable potential for use as a therapeutic adjuvant in the treatment of OSCC.

To identify the genes and anticancer signaling pathways that may be regulated by psorachromene, we performed whole-transcriptome sequencing that examined the gene expression profiling of psorachromene in treated and untreated cells. The results showed that psorachromene mainly regulates the expression of genes associated with cell growth, extracellular matrix composition, and inflammation, among others, thereby inhibiting the growth and metastasis of OSCC cells; this was consistent with the results observed on cell functional assay. The inhibitory effect of psorachromene on the Erb-1 pathway indicates that it has considerable potential in the treatment of cancers that overexpress EGFR (including cancers of the breast and liver); it may also synergize with other anticancer drugs to enhance their therapeutic efficacy.

This study revealed that psorachromene induces lncRNA-GAS5 expression, which is a known anticancer lncRNA, and participates in the regulation of many important physiological processes, including cell growth, apoptosis, cell cycle progression, and EMT (60, 61). The low expression of GAS5 is closely related to the poor prognosis and chemoresistance of many cancers (62–65). Overexpression of GAS5 could enhance the inhibitory effect of Gefitinib on EGFR phosphorylation and its downstream signaling activation, while enhancing the sensitivity of lung cancer cells to EGFR-TKI (66). In addition, the chemotherapeutic drug, Lapatinib, can also enhance the response of breast cancer cells to trastuzumab by inducing GAS5 expression (67). Some studies have also suggested that GAS5 is significantly downregulated in OSCC cells, and that GAS5 expression may inhibit the growth and metastasis of OSCC by regulating the miR-21/PTEN axis (68). In this study, we found that psorachromene may induce GAS5 expression. It is speculated that the inhibitory effects of psorachromene on OSCC are partly attributable to GAS5-mediated anticancer mechanisms. Moreover, this result also shows the potential of psorachromene as a

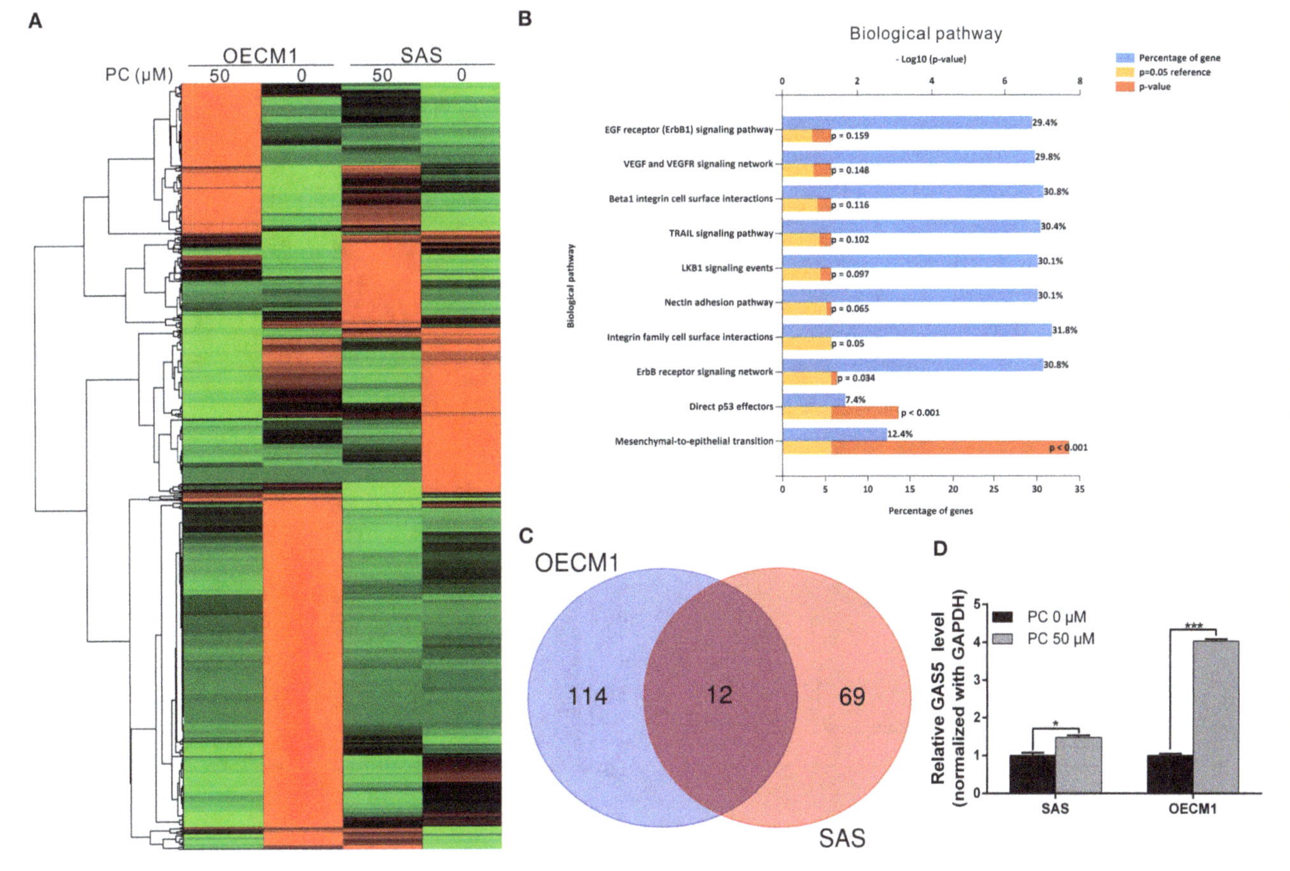

FIGURE 6 | Psorachromene-induced regulation of gene expression related to cell growth and extracellular structure organization. **(A)** Heatmap comparing significantly different expression of genes in SAS and OECM1 cells treated with or without psorachromene. The bar charts represent the enriched biological pathways **(B)** associated with the differentially expressed genes after psorachromene treatment. **(C)** The whole-transcriptome sequencing data shows that 12 lncRNAs manifested higher than a 2-fold change in expression after psorachromene treatment in both cell lines. **(D)** SAS and OECM1 cells were treated with psorachromene for 48 h, and GAS5 expression was analyzed using quantitative real-time RT-PCR. $^{*}p < 0.05$, $^{***}p < 0.001$.

therapeutic adjuvant that enhances the sensitivity of cancer cells to chemotherapeutic drugs by inducing the expression of GAS5.

Previous studies have demonstrated that long non-coding RNAs are involved in the regulation of a wide range of gene expression or protein stability. However, recent studies have shown that GAS5 does not regulate EGFR expression (66). We speculate that psorachromene regulates GAS5 and EGFR expression through two independent mechanisms; however, the detailed regulatory mechanism is yet to be delineated. In addition, the results of whole-transcriptome sequencing analysis showed that numerous lncRNAs are also regulated by psorachromene; the role of these lncRNAs in the anticancer mechanisms of psorachromene warrant further research.

In cell cycle analysis related to psorachromene treatment, the distribution of cell cycle between SAS and OECM1 cells is quite different. The inhibitory effect of psorachromene on SAS cells is better than that of OECM1. We speculated that the anti-OSCC effect of psorachromene may be induced by specific receptors. The genetic background difference between cells leads to the differences in receptor expression, which affect the anti-OSCC effect of psorachromene. However, the receptor that is targeted by psorachromene to achieve its anticancer mechanism and its detailed downstream regulation mechanism still need to be clarified to improve the clinical applicability of psorachromene.

The concentrations of psorachromene in *P. corylifolia* L. are not high; in addition, it has a simple structure. Therefore, psorachromene is mainly synthesized chemically for commercial formulations. Structural modifications may be introduced in the future to increase its anticancer activity and intracellular availability. In this study, we demonstrated the potential anticancer activity of psorachromene using cell and animal experiments; we also found that it affects certain relevant regulatory pathways. The small-molecule compounds that are commonly used in clinical practice only block specific carcinogenic pathways; in contrast, psorachromene has a wide range of targets. In addition, the animal experiments did not demonstrate significant differences in physiological toxicity compared to these molecules. In view of these findings, psorachromene holds

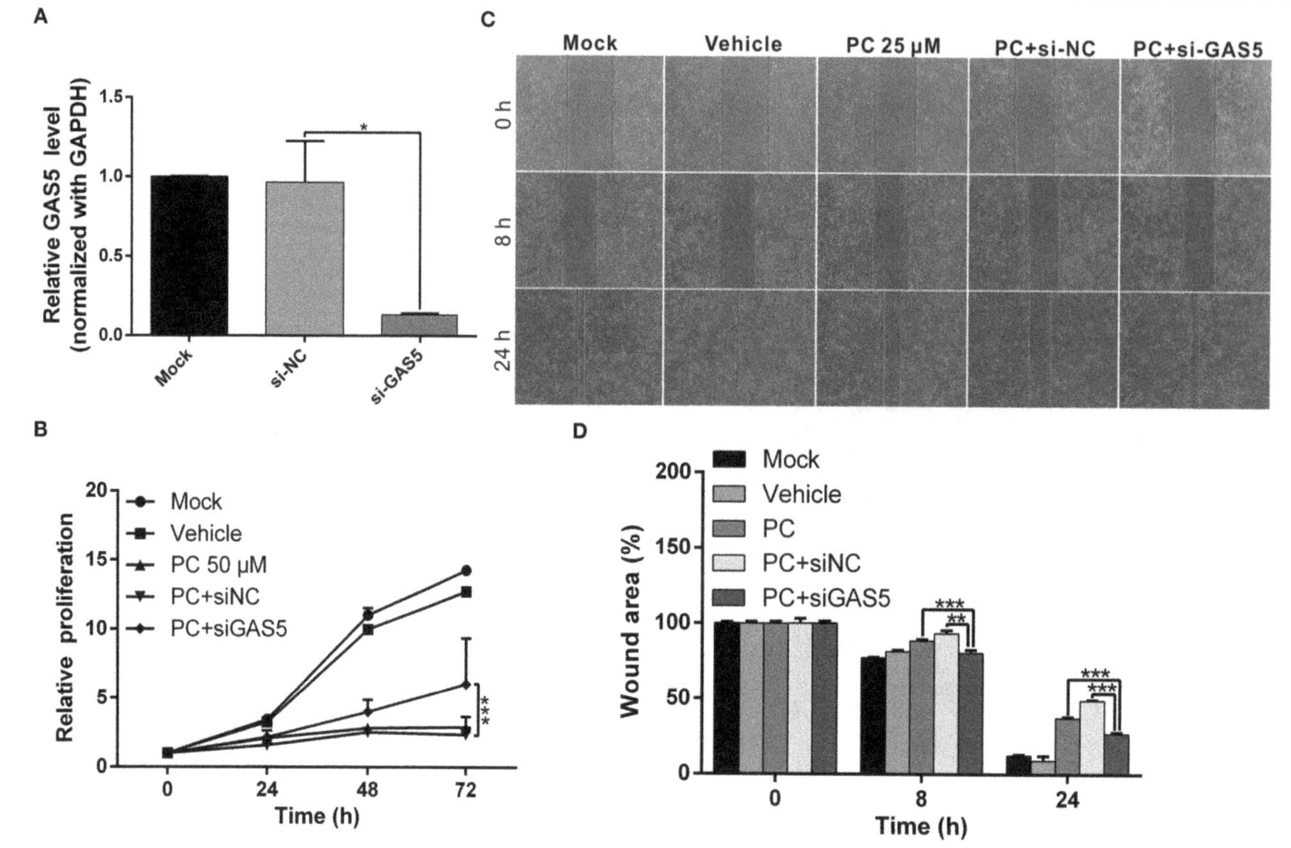

FIGURE 7 | The anticancer effect of psorachromene is exerted by inducing expression of lncRNA-GAS5. **(A)** Real-time PCR analysis shows the effect of siRNA treatments on the expression of GAS5 in OECM1 cells. GAPDH served as an internal control. **(B,C)** The inhibitory effects of psorachromene on cell proliferation and migration were significantly reversed by treatment with GAS5 siRNA (50 nM) in the OECM1 cells. The quantitative cell migration result was shown in **(D)**. $^{*}p < 0.05$, $^{**}p < 0.01$, $^{***}p < 0.001$.

promise as a new therapeutic agent for OSCC. Further studies with larger sample sizes are needed to validate our findings.

ETHICS STATEMENT

The animal study was reviewed and approved by Animal Care Ethics Commission of the Chang Gung Memorial Hospital (IACUC approval no. 2018031301).

AUTHOR CONTRIBUTIONS

C-YC, T-HW, and Y-LL contributed to the conception and design of the study. C-YC, T-HW, Y-LL, C-CC, T-MS, and J-HL performed the experiments and statistical analyses. T-HW and C-YC prepared the first draft of the manuscript. All authors contributed to manuscript revision and have read and approved the submitted version.

ACKNOWLEDGMENTS

The authors would like to thank the staff of the Tissue Bank and Genomic Medicine Core Laboratory at the Chang Gung Memorial Hospital, Lin-Kou, Taiwan for the excellent tissue processing and data analysis support.

REFERENCES

1. Ghantous Y, Abu Elnaaj I. Global incidence and risk factors of oral cancer. *Harefuah.* (2017) 156:645–9.
2. Bagan J, Sarrion G, Jimenez Y. Oral cancer: clinical features. *Oral Oncol.* (2010) 46:414–7. doi: 10.1016/j.oraloncology.2010.03.009
3. Nagler R, Dayan D. The dual role of saliva in oral carcinogenesis. *Oncology.* (2006) 71:10–7. doi: 10.1159/000100445
4. Chen YJ, Chang JT, Liao CT, Wang HM, Yen TC, Chiu CC, et al. Head and neck cancer in the betel quid chewing area: recent advances in molecular carcinogenesis. *Cancer Sci.* (2008) 99:1507–14. doi: 10.1111/j.1349-7006.2008.00863.x
5. Zygogianni AG, Kyrgias G, Karakitsos P, Psyrri A, Kouvaris J, Kelekis N, et al. Oral squamous cell cancer: early detection and the role of alcohol and smoking. *Head Neck Oncol.* (2011) 3:2. doi: 10.1186/1758-3284-3-2
6. Huang SH, O'sullivan B. Oral cancer: current role of radiotherapy and chemotherapy. *Med Oral Patol Oral Cir Bucal.* (2013) 18:e233–40. doi: 10.4317/medoral.18772
7. Gharat SA, Momin M, Bhavsar C. Oral squamous cell carcinoma: current treatment strategies and nanotechnology-based approaches for prevention and therapy. *Crit Rev Ther Drug Carrier Syst.* (2016) 33:363–400. doi: 10.1615/CritRevTherDrugCarrierSyst.2016016272
8. Hamakawa H, Nakashiro K, Sumida T, Shintani S, Myers JN, Takes RP, et al. Basic evidence of molecular targeted therapy for oral cancer and salivary gland cancer. *Head Neck.* (2008) 30:800–9. doi: 10.1002/hed.20830
9. Agnihotri NS, Astekar M. The role of novel prognostic markers PROX1 and FOXC2 in carcinogenesis of oral squamous cell carcinoma. *J Exp Ther Oncol.* (2018) 12:171–84.
10. Choi S, Myers JN. Molecular pathogenesis of oral squamous cell carcinoma: implications for therapy. *J Dent Res.* (2008) 87:14–32. doi: 10.1177/154405910808700104
11. Ramos-Garcia P, Ruiz-Avila I, Gil-Montoya JA, Ayen A, Gonzalez-Ruiz L, Navarro-Trivino FJ, et al. Relevance of chromosomal band 11q13 in oral carcinogenesis: an update of current knowledge. *Oral Oncol.* (2017) 72:7–16. doi: 10.1016/j.oraloncology.2017.04.016
12. Lindemann A, Takahashi H, Patel AA, Osman AA, Myers JN. Targeting the DNA damage response in OSCC with TP53 mutations. *J Dent Res.* (2018) 97:635–44. doi: 10.1177/0022034518759068
13. Kimura I, Kitahara H, Ooi K, Kato K, Noguchi N, Yoshizawa K, et al. Loss of epidermal growth factor receptor expression in oral squamous cell carcinoma is associated with invasiveness and epithelial-mesenchymal transition. *Oncol Lett.* (2016) 11:201–7. doi: 10.3892/ol.2015.3833
14. Xie X, Wang Z, Chen F, Yuan Y, Wang J, Liu R, et al. Roles of FGFR in oral carcinogenesis. *Cell Prolif.* (2016) 49:261–9. doi: 10.1111/cpr.12260
15. Huang SF, Chien HT, Cheng SD, Chuang WY, Liao CT, Wang HM. EGFR copy number alterations in primary tumors, metastatic lymph nodes, and recurrent and multiple primary tumors in oral cavity squamous cell carcinoma. *BMC Cancer.* (2017) 17:592. doi: 10.1186/s12885-017-3586-9
16. Soria JC, Felip E, Cobo M, Lu S, Syrigos K, Lee KH, et al. Afatinib versus erlotinib as second-line treatment of patients with advanced squamous cell carcinoma of the lung (LUX-Lung 8): an open-label randomised controlled phase 3 trial. *Lancet Oncol.* (2015) 16:897–907. doi: 10.1016/S1470-2045(15)00006-6
17. Fujiwara T, Eguchi T, Sogawa C, Ono K, Murakami J, Ibaragi S, et al. Carcinogenic epithelial-mesenchymal transition initiated by oral cancer exosomes is inhibited by anti-EGFR antibody cetuximab. *Oral Oncol.* (2018) 86:251–7. doi: 10.1016/j.oraloncology.2018.09.030
18. Cohen RB. Current challenges and clinical investigations of epidermal growth factor receptor (EGFR)- and ErbB family-targeted agents in the treatment of head and neck squamous cell carcinoma (HNSCC). *Cancer Treat Rev.* (2014) 40:567–77. doi: 10.1016/j.ctrv.2013.10.002
19. Brands RC, Muller-Richter UD, De Donno F, Seher A, Mutzbauer G, Linz C, et al. Co-treatment of wild-type EGFR head and neck cancer cell lines with afatinib and cisplatin. *Mol Med Rep.* (2016) 13:2338–44. doi: 10.3892/mmr.2016.4786
20. Khalil A, Jameson MJ. The EGFR inhibitor gefitinib enhanced the response of human oral squamous cell carcinoma to cisplatin *in vitro*. *Drugs R D.* (2017) 17:545–55. doi: 10.1007/s40268-017-0204-x
21. Rabinowits G, Haddad RI. Overcoming resistance to EGFR inhibitor in head and neck cancer: a review of the literature. *Oral Oncol.* (2012) 48:1085–9. doi: 10.1016/j.oraloncology.2012.06.016
22. Lopez-Verdin S, Lavalle-Carrasco J, Carreon-Burciaga RG, Serafin-Higuera N, Molina-Frechero N, Gonzalez-Gonzalez R, et al. Molecular markers of anticancer drug resistance in head and neck squamous cell carcinoma: a literature review. *Cancers.* (2018) 10:E376. doi: 10.3390/cancers10100376
23. Perri F, Longo F, Ionna F, Caponigro F. Recent results of cetuximab use in the treatment of squamous cell carcinoma of the head and neck. *Onco Targets Ther.* (2009) 2:243–50. doi: 10.2147/OTT.S6056
24. Naruse T, Yanamoto S, Matsushita Y, Sakamoto Y, Morishita K, Ohba S, et al. Cetuximab for the treatment of locally advanced and recurrent/metastatic oral cancer: an investigation of distant metastasis. *Mol Clin Oncol.* (2016) 5:246–52. doi: 10.3892/mco.2016.928
25. Chen CY, Chen CC, Shieh TM, Hsueh C, Wang SH, Leu YL, et al. Corylin suppresses hepatocellular carcinoma progression via the inhibition of epithelial-mesenchymal transition, mediated by long noncoding RNA GAS5. *Int J Mol Sci.* (2018) 19:E380. doi: 10.3390/ijms19020380
26. An W, Lai H, Zhang Y, Liu M, Lin X, Cao S. Apoptotic pathway as the therapeutic target for anticancer traditional chinese medicines. *Front Pharmacol.* (2019) 10:758. doi: 10.3389/fphar.2019.00758
27. He DY, Dai SM. Anti-inflammatory and immunomodulatory effects of paeonia lactiflora pall., a traditional chinese herbal medicine. *Front. Pharmacol.* (2011) 2:10. doi: 10.3389/fphar.2011.00010
28. Ji L, Tong X, Wang H, Tian H, Zhou H, Zhang L, et al. Efficacy and safety of traditional chinese medicine for diabetes: a double-blind, randomised, controlled trial. *PLoS ONE.* (2013) 8:e56703. doi: 10.1371/journal.pone.0056703
29. Jiao L, Dong C, Liu J, Chen Z, Zhang L, Xu J, et al. Effects of Chinese medicine as adjunct medication for adjuvant chemotherapy treatments of non-small cell lung cancer patients. *Sci Rep.* (2017) 7:46524. doi: 10.1038/srep46524
30. Zhang A, Sun H, Wang X. Potentiating therapeutic effects by enhancing synergism based on active constituents from traditional medicine. *Phytother Res.* (2014) 28:526–33. doi: 10.1002/ptr.5032
31. Xu L, Zhao W, Wang D, Ma X. Chinese medicine in the battle against obesity and metabolic diseases. *Front Physiol.* (2018) 9:850. doi: 10.3389/fphys.2018.00850
32. Jiang Z, Gao W, Huang L. Tanshinones, critical pharmacological components in *Salvia miltiorrhiza*. *Front Pharmacol.* (2019) 10:202. doi: 10.3389/fphar.2019.00202
33. Zhu H, Liu C, Hou J, Long H, Wang B, Guo D, et al. Gastrodia elata blume polysaccharides: a review of their acquisition, analysis, modification, and pharmacological activities. *Molecules.* (2019) 24:E2436. doi: 10.3390/molecules24132436
34. Ye MX, Li Y, Yin H, Zhang J. Curcumin: updated molecular mechanisms and intervention targets in human lung cancer. *Int J Mol Sci.* (2012) 13:3959–78. doi: 10.3390/ijms13033959
35. Terlikowska KM, Witkowska AM, Zujko ME, Dobrzycka B, Terlikowski SJ. Potential application of curcumin and its analogues in the treatment strategy of patients with primary epithelial ovarian cancer. *Int J Mol Sci.* (2014) 15:21703–22. doi: 10.3390/ijms151221703
36. Hong M, Tan HY, Li S, Cheung F, Wang N, Nagamatsu T, et al. Cancer stem cells: the potential targets of Chinese medicines and their active compounds. *Int J Mol Sci.* (2016) 17:E893. doi: 10.3390/ijms17060893
37. Houh YK, Kim KE, Park S, Hur DY, Kim S, Kim D, et al. The effects of artemisinin on the cytolytic activity of natural killer (NK) cells. *Int J Mol Sci.* (2017) 18:E1600. doi: 10.3390/ijms18071600
38. Slezakova S, Ruda-Kucerova J. Anticancer activity of artemisinin and its derivatives. *Anticancer Res.* (2017) 37:5995–6003. doi: 10.21873/anticanres.12046
39. Cragg GM, Pezzuto JM. Natural products as a vital source for the discovery of cancer chemotherapeutic and chemopreventive agents. *Med Princ Pract.* (2016) 25(Suppl 2):41–59. doi: 10.1159/000443404
40. Kim YJ, Lim HS, Lee J, Jeong SJ. Quantitative analysis of *Psoralea corylifolia* Linne and its neuroprotective and anti-neuroinflammatory effects in HT22 hippocampal cells and BV-2 microglia. *Molecules.* (2016) 21:E1076. doi: 10.3390/molecules21081076

41. Li CC, Wang TL, Zhang ZQ, Yang WQ, Wang YF, Chai X, et al. Phytochemical and pharmacological studies on the genus psoralea: a mini review. *Evid Based Complement Alternat Med.* (2016) 2016:8108643. doi: 10.1155/2016/8108643
42. Zhang X, Zhao W, Wang Y, Lu J, Chen X. The chemical constituents and bioactivities of *Psoralea corylifolia* Linn.: a review. *Am J Chin Med.* (2016) 44:35–60. doi: 10.1142/S0192415X16500038
43. Hung YL, Fang SH, Wang SC, Cheng WC, Liu PL, Su CC, et al. Corylin protects LPS-induced sepsis and attenuates LPS-induced inflammatory response. *Sci Rep.* (2017) 7:46299. doi: 10.1038/srep46299
44. Alam F, Khan GN, Asad M. *Psoralea corylifolia* L.: ethnobotanical, biological, and chemical aspects: a review. *Phytother Res.* (2018) 32:597–615. doi: 10.1002/ptr.6006
45. Choi YH, Yon GH, Hong KS, Yoo DS, Choi CW, Park WK, et al. *In vitro* BACE-1 inhibitory phenolic components from the seeds of *Psoralea corylifolia. Planta Med.* (2008) 74:1405–8. doi: 10.1055/s-2008-1081301
46. Kim DH, Li H, Han YE, Jeong JH, Lee HJ, Ryu JH. Modulation of inducible nitric oxide synthase expression in LPS-stimulated BV-2 microglia by prenylated chalcones from *Cullen corylifolium* (L.) medik. through Inhibition of I-kappaBalpha degradation. *Molecules.* (2018) 23:E109. doi: 10.3390/molecules23010109
47. Chen CY, Chiou SH, Huang CY, Jan CI, Lin SC, Hu WY, et al. Tid1 functions as a tumour suppressor in head and neck squamous cell carcinoma. *J Pathol.* (2009) 219:347–55. doi: 10.1002/path.2604
48. Chen CY, Yang SC, Lee KH, Yang X, Wei LY, Chow LP, et al. The antitumor agent PBT-1 directly targets HSP90 and hnRNP A2/B1 and inhibits lung adenocarcinoma growth and metastasis. *J Med Chem.* (2014) 57:677–85. doi: 10.1021/jm401686b
49. Chen CY, Jan CI, Pi WC, Wang WL, Yang PC, Wang TH, et al. Heterogeneous nuclear ribonucleoproteins A1 and A2 modulate expression of Tid1 isoforms and EGFR signaling in non-small cell lung cancer. *Oncotarget.* (2016) 7:16760–72. doi: 10.18632/oncotarget.7606
50. Wang TH, Chan CW, Fang JY, Shih YM, Liu YW, Wang TV, et al. 2-O-Methylmagnolol upregulates the long non-coding RNA, GAS5, and enhances apoptosis in skin cancer cells. *Cell Death Dis.* (2017) 8:e2638. doi: 10.1038/cddis.2017.66
51. Chen CC, Chen CY, Ueng SH, Hsueh C, Yeh CT, Ho JY, et al. Corylin increases the sensitivity of hepatocellular carcinoma cells to chemotherapy through long noncoding RNA RAD51-AS1-mediated inhibition of DNA repair. *Cell Death Dis.* (2018) 9:543. doi: 10.1038/s41419-018-0575-0
52. Chu Q, Amano O, Kanda Y, Kunii S, Wang Q, Sakagami H. Tumor-specific cytotoxicity and type of cell death induced by gefitinib in oral squamous cell carcinoma cell lines. *Anticancer Res.* (2009) 29:5023–31.
53. Sivanantham B, Sethuraman S, Krishnan UM. Combinatorial effects of curcumin with an anti-neoplastic agent on head and neck squamous cell carcinoma through the regulation of EGFR-ERK1/2 and apoptotic signaling pathways. *ACS Comb Sci.* (2016) 18:22–35. doi: 10.1021/acscombsci.5b00043
54. Iocca O, Farcomeni A, Di Rocco A, Di Maio P, Golusinski P, Pardinas Lopez S, et al. Locally advanced squamous cell carcinoma of the head and neck: a systematic review and Bayesian network meta-analysis of the currently available treatment options. *Oral Oncol.* (2018) 80:40–51. doi: 10.1016/j.oraloncology.2018.03.001
55. Khushboo PS, Jadhav VM, Kadam VJ, Sathe NS. *Psoralea corylifolia* Linn.-"Kushtanashini." *Pharmacogn Rev.* (2010) 4:69–76. doi: 10.4103/0973-7847.65331
56. Sarkis SA, Abdullah BH, Abdul Majeed BA, Talabani NG. Immunohistochemical expression of epidermal growth factor receptor (EGFR) in oral squamous cell carcinoma in relation to proliferation, apoptosis, angiogenesis and lymphangiogenesis. *Head Neck Oncol.* (2010) 2:13. doi: 10.1186/1758-3284-2-13
57. Yamano Y, Uzawa K, Saito K, Nakashima D, Kasamatsu A, Koike H, et al. Identification of cisplatin-resistance related genes in head and neck squamous cell carcinoma. *Int J Cancer.* (2010) 126:437–49. doi: 10.1002/ijc.24704
58. Celentano A, Mccullough M, Cirillo N. Glucocorticoids reduce chemotherapeutic effectiveness on OSCC cells via glucose-dependent mechanisms. *J Cell Physiol.* (2019) 234:2013–20. doi: 10.1002/jcp.27227
59. Maji S, Shriwas O, Samal SK, Priyadarshini M, Rath R, Panda S, et al. STAT3- and GSK3beta-mediated Mcl-1 regulation modulates TPF resistance in oral squamous cell carcinoma. *Carcinogenesis.* (2019) 40:173–83. doi: 10.1093/carcin/bgy135
60. Ma C, Shi X, Zhu Q, Li Q, Liu Y, Yao Y, et al. The growth arrest-specific transcript 5 (GAS5): a pivotal tumor suppressor long noncoding RNA in human cancers. *Tumour Biol.* (2016) 37:1437–44. doi: 10.1007/s13277-015-4521-9
61. Ghaforui-Fard S, Taheri M. Growth arrest specific transcript 5 in tumorigenesis process: an update on the expression pattern and genomic variants. *Biomed Pharmacother.* (2019) 112:108723. doi: 10.1016/j.biopha.2019.108723
62. Pickard MR, Williams GT. Regulation of apoptosis by long non-coding RNA GAS5 in breast cancer cells: implications for chemotherapy. *Breast Cancer Res Treat.* (2014) 145:359–70. doi: 10.1007/s10549-014-2974-y
63. Guo LJ, Zhang S, Gao B, Jiang Y, Zhang XH, Tian WG, et al. Low expression of long non-coding RNA GAS5 is associated with poor prognosis of patients with thyroid cancer. *Exp Mol Pathol.* (2017) 102:500–4. doi: 10.1016/j.yexmp.2017.05.008
64. Yang Y, Shen Z, Yan Y, Wang B, Zhang J, Shen C, et al. Long non-coding RNA GAS5 inhibits cell proliferation, induces G0/G1 arrest and apoptosis, and functions as a prognostic marker in colorectal cancer. *Oncol Lett.* (2017) 13:3151–8. doi: 10.3892/ol.2017.5841
65. Avgeris M, Tsilimantou A, Levis PK, Tokas T, Sideris DC, Stravodimos K, et al. Loss of GAS5 tumour suppressor lncRNA: an independent molecular cancer biomarker for short-term relapse and progression in bladder cancer patients. *Br J Cancer.* (2018) 119:1477–86. doi: 10.1038/s41416-018-0320-6
66. Dong S, Qu X, Li W, Zhong X, Li P, Yang S, et al. The long non-coding RNA, GAS5, enhances gefitinib-induced cell death in innate EGFR tyrosine kinase inhibitor-resistant lung adenocarcinoma cells with wide-type EGFR via downregulation of the IGF-1R expression. *J Hematol Oncol.* (2015) 8:43. doi: 10.1186/s13045-015-0140-6
67. Li W, Zhai L, Wang H, Liu C, Zhang J, Chen W, et al. Downregulation of LncRNA GAS5 causes trastuzumab resistance in breast cancer. *Oncotarget.* (2016) 7:27778–86. doi: 10.18632/oncotarget.8413
68. Zeng B, Li Y, Jiang F, Wei C, Chen G, Zhang W, et al. LncRNA GAS5 suppresses proliferation, migration, invasion, and epithelial-mesenchymal transition in oral squamous cell carcinoma by regulating the miR-21/PTEN axis. *Exp Cell Res.* (2019) 374:365–73. doi: 10.1016/j.yexcr.2018.12.014

17

Pembrolizumab in a Patient with a Metastatic CASTLE Tumor of the Parotid

Lisa Lorenz[1†], Joscha von Rappard[1†], Walter Arnold[2†], Nicole Mutter[3], Udo Schirp[4], Andreas Scherr[5] and Andreas Werner Jehle[1,6]*

[1] Department of Internal Medicine, Hirslanden Klinik St. Anna, Lucerne, Switzerland, [2] Department of Pathology, Cantonal Hospital Lucerne, Lucerne, Switzerland, [3] Department of Oncology, Hirslanden Klinik St. Anna, Lucerne, Switzerland, [4] Institute of Radiology and Nuclear Medicine, Hirslanden Klinik St. Anna, Lucerne, Switzerland, [5] Department of Pneumology, Hirslanden Klinik St. Anna, Lucerne, Switzerland, [6] Transplantation Immunology and Nephrology, University Hospital Basel, Basel, Switzerland

***Correspondence:**
Andreas Werner Jehle
andreas.jehle@hirslanden.ch;
andreas.jehle@unibas.ch

[†] These authors have contributed equally to this work

Carcinoma showing thymus-like elements (CASTLE) is a rare tumor, most commonly found in the thyroid gland. Here we report a case of CASTLE tumor localized to the parotid gland, recognized in retrospect after a late manifestation of symptomatic pleural carcinomatosis. The original tumor in the parotid gland was treated by surgery followed by radiotherapy. Ten years later, a metastatic disease with recurrent pleural effusions occurred. Pleural carcinomatosis was strongly positive for CD5, CD117, and p63 as was the original tumor of the parotid, which allowed the diagnosis of a CASTLE tumor. Additionally, the pleural tumor expressed high levels of programmed death ligand 1 (PD-L1), and the patient underwent treatment with the monoclonal PD-L1 inhibitor pembrolizumab achieving a partial remission. To the best of our knowledge, this is the first patient with a metastatic CASTLE tumor treated with a PD-L1 inhibitor.

Keywords: CASTLE, parotid, extrathyroidal, carcinoma, thymus-like, PD-L1, immunotherapy, checkpoint inhibitor

BACKGROUND

Carcinoma showing thymus-like differentiation (CASTLE) is a rare tumor usually of the thyroid gland or adjacent soft tissues of the neck (1). The entity was first described as an intrathyroidal epithelial thymoma by Miyauchi et al. (2) and later renamed as CASTLE by Chan and Rosai, who proposed that these tumors arise either from ectopic thymuses or from remnants of the branchial pouches that differentiate along the thymic line (3).

CASTLE tumors show not only structural similarity to thymic tissue but also express molecular markers of thymomas and thymic carcinomas (4, 5). In immunohistochemical staining, they are positive for CD5 in nearly all cases and positive for CD117 and p63, but negative for markers of thyroid carcinomas, such as thyroglobulin and calcitonin (5).

CASTLE tumors are indolent and slow-growing malignant neoplasms. In about 30–50% of cases, that describe the nodal status, lymph node involvement is reported and in 14–29% metastatic disease (6). Radical surgery is the treatment of choice for CASTLE, and radiotherapy is considered in patients with positive lymph node status. For advanced and metastatic disease, the standard treatment is chemotherapy (6). However, because of the rarity of CASTLE, data on the effectiveness of adjuvant radiotherapy and chemotherapy is missing.

Immunotherapy has become a cornerstone in the treatment of several malignancies in the past few years and involves the use of immune checkpoint inhibitors including antibodies against programmed cell death protein 1 (PD-1), and programmed death ligand 1 (PD-L1) (7). When PD-1, which is primarily expressed on activated T cells, binds PD-L1 on tumor cells, the cytotoxic T-cell response is reduced. PD-L1 expression is associated with a better response to anti-PD-1 treatment in non-small cell lung cancer (8, 9) as well as in thymic carcinoma (10). Herein, we report what we believe is the first case of a metastatic CASTLE tumor systemically treated with the PD-L1 inhibitor pembrolizumab.

CASE PRESENTATION

A 79-year old woman was hospitalized on April 25, 2018, at which time she had progressive dyspnea over the past 5 weeks, productive cough, poor appetite, and weight loss of 5 kg over the last 6 months currently weighing 81 kg. Her medical history included an invasive ductal breast cancer pT1cN0M0 G2 ER 90%, PR 20% 20 years ago treated with lumpectomy, radiotherapy, and tamoxifen until 2004, and an undifferentiated cancer of the right parotid pT1 (17 mm) pN2 (1/2 positive in level I, 1/11 positive in level II, no extranodal extensions) pM0 diagnosed 2008 and treated with a total parotidectomy achieving R0 margins and a selective neck dissection levels II-IV followed by radiotherapy.

On physical examination, the patient was in mild respiratory distress. The pulmonary exam revealed dullness to percussion, decreased fremitus, and decreased breathing sounds in up to two-thirds of the left lung field. Oxygen saturation was 92% with the patient breathing ambient air, and arterial blood gases showed partial respiratory insufficiency. A chest X-ray confirmed a left-sided pleural effusion, and thoracentesis removed 1.5 liters of turbid fluid. Biochemical analysis of the fluid established an exudative etiology. Atypical cells with immunocytochemical positivity for p40, cytokeratin 5, and p63 in the cytopathology specimen were primarily suggestive of a non-small cell lung cancer, and a CT scan of the thorax showed a mass (4.2 × 2.2 × 2.8 cm) in the right upper lobe and extensive cardiophrenic, mediastinal, and hilar lymphadenopathy as well as enlarged lymph nodes along the left arteria mammaria interna. An FDG PET/CT scan confirmed these findings, and the scan revealed a hypermetabolic activity in mesenteric lymph nodes and at the left pleura (**Figures 1A,B**). Thoracoscopy and biopsy of the parietal pleura were performed. Surprisingly, histopathological examination revealed a non-small cell carcinoma (**Figure 2A**) expressing CD5 (**Figure 2B**), CD117 (**Figure 2C**), and p63 all indicating a carcinoma of thymic origin (5). With no signs of a thymic pathology, the histopathological diagnosis of CASTLE was established, and as additional immunostainings for CD5 (**Figure 3B**) and CD117 (**Figure 3C**) in the specimen of the parotid cancer diagnosed 2008 were positive also, a rare case of a CASTLE tumor of the parotid healed at the primary and neck sites, but with late metastatic dissemination was diagnosed.

As CD117 was highly overexpressed in the tumor, exons 9, 11, 13, 14, and 17 of the C-KIT gene were analyzed after extraction of genomic DNA by PCR using specific primers, but no common mutation was found consistent with previous reports (11, 12). Anticancer immunity and potential response to immunotherapy were assessed by PD-L1 staining of the pleural tumor, which showed a high expression level of 60% (**Figure 2D**).

The patient underwent talc pleurodesis and left partial pleurectomy for recurrent pleural effusions. Systemically, disseminated metastatic disease was treated with the monoclonal PD-L1 inhibitor pembrolizumab at a dose 200 mg every 3 weeks. Four months after the start of immunotherapy a follow-up FDG PET/CT study showed a partial remission with a moderate morphologic reduction of the tumor load, but a markedly reduced metabolic activity at all tumor sites (**Figures 1C,D**). Pembrolizumab treatment continued at a dose of 200 mg IV every 3 weeks. The patient showed a mild skin rash treated with low dose prednisolone (20 mg with tapering) for 2 weeks. No other adverse events associated with pembrolizumab were observed, and the therapy was tolerated well. At the last follow-up, the patient was in good clinical condition and had gained 3 kg of weight. On March 28th, 2019, a second follow-up FDG PET/CT showed no residual pleural effusion (not shown) and a further regression of lesions in the right lung and lymph nodes. Residual focal FDG-Uptake was seen in the left pleura (**Figures 1E,F**).

DISCUSSION

CASTLE is a rare malignant tumor, and in the majority of cases, the tumor is localized in the thyroid gland (6). Histologically, CASTLE resembles thymic carcinoma, and the current postulation is that these tumors arise from remnants of the branchial pouches with thymic differentiation, or ectopic thymuses (3, 13). This hypothesis is further supported by the observation that these tumors show positive immunostaining for CD5, CD117, and p63 reminiscent of thymomas and thymic carcinomas (4, 5). As Gao et al. (6) suggested the low number of reported cases of this disease may be related to the variable, and non-specific clinical manifestation and a conclusive diagnosis can only be maid by postsurgical pathological examination including immunohistochemical studies. A few extrathyroidal cases of CASTLE have been reported, and one of them localized to the right parotid and was classified as WHO stage III, pT1pN1cM0, and expressed CD5, CD117, P40, and P63 (14). The patient was treated with right total parotidectomy and ipsilateral selective neck dissection followed by adjuvant radiotherapy and remained disease free for more than 1 year after completing treatment on follow-up with MRI scan (14). In the case reported here, the diagnosis of the primary tumor in the parotid was made in

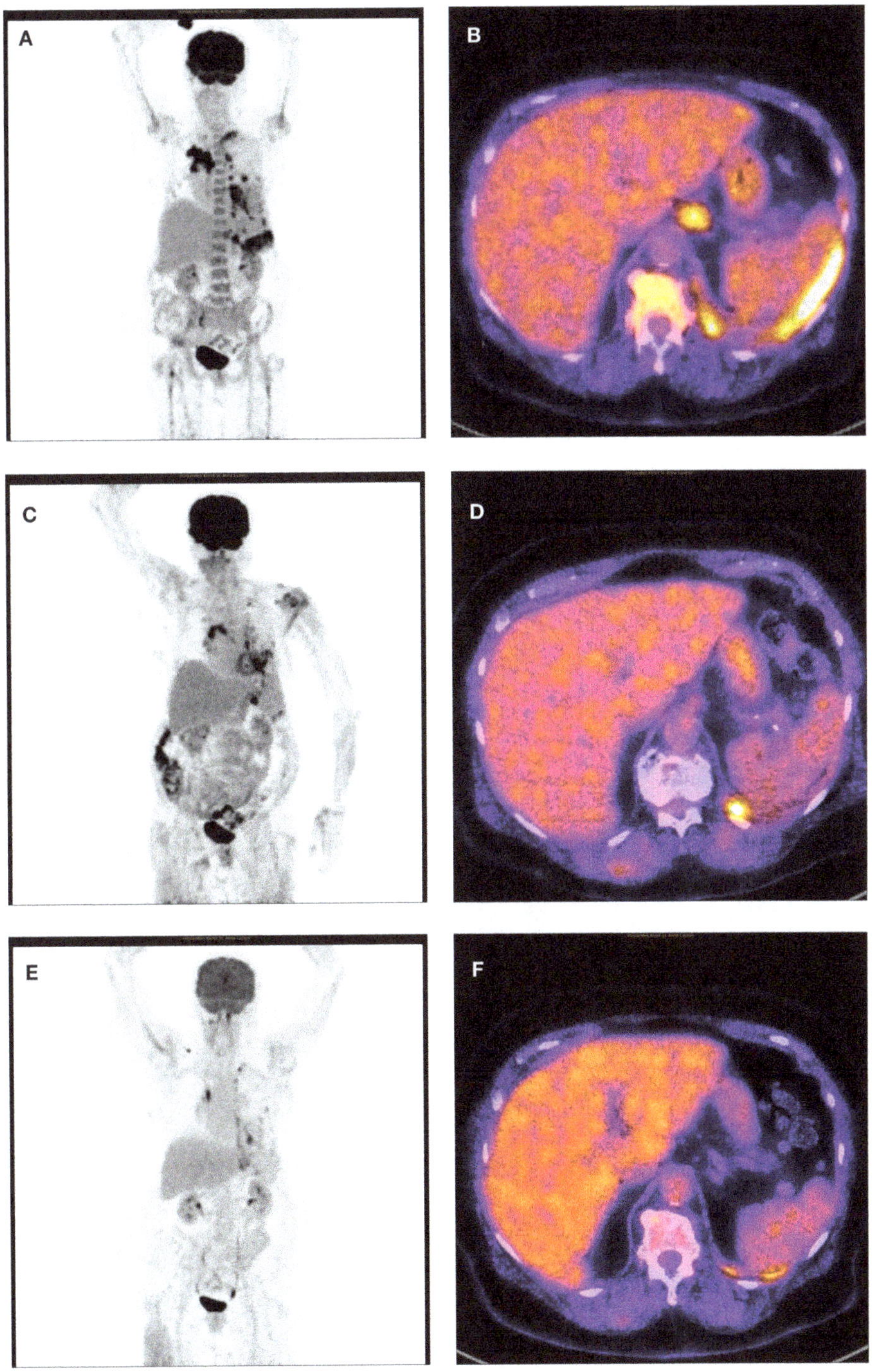

FIGURE 1 | Initial and follow-up FDG PET/CT: **(A)** Initial FDG-MIP with multiple hypermetabolic lesions in the upper lobe of the right lung, in mediastinal, hilar and upper mesenteric lymph nodes and at the left pleura. Increased turnover of the bone marrow. **(B)** Initial fusion FDG-PET/CT axial slice with pathologic high FDG-uptake in the left pleura, upper mesenteric lymph nodes, and bone marrow. Normal presentation of liver, spleen, and stomach. **(C)** Follow-up FDG-MIP after 4 months on pembrolizumab shows a generally reduced metabolism at all tumor locations. Normalization of the bone marrow turnover. Due to newly incipient traumatic injury at the left shoulder the patient could not lift up the left arm. **(D)** Fusion FDG-PET/CT axial slice after 4 months on pembrolizumab with residual FDG-uptake at the left pleura and in upper mesenteric lymph nodes. Normal presentation of the bone marrow. **(E)** Follow-up FDG-MIP after 11 months on pembrolizumab shows further regression of lesions in the upper lobe of the right lung as well as in mediastinal, hilar, and upper mesenteric lymph nodes (the focal lesions in the left mediastinum and supraclavicular right represent the central venous catheter). Residual focal FDG-Uptake in the left pleura. Normal turnover of the bone marrow. **(F)** Fusion FDG-PET/CT axial slice after 11 months on pembrolizumab with only little elevated FDG-uptake in the left pleura. The formerly upper mesenteric lymph node is healed up. Normal presentation of liver, spleen, stomach, and bone marrow.

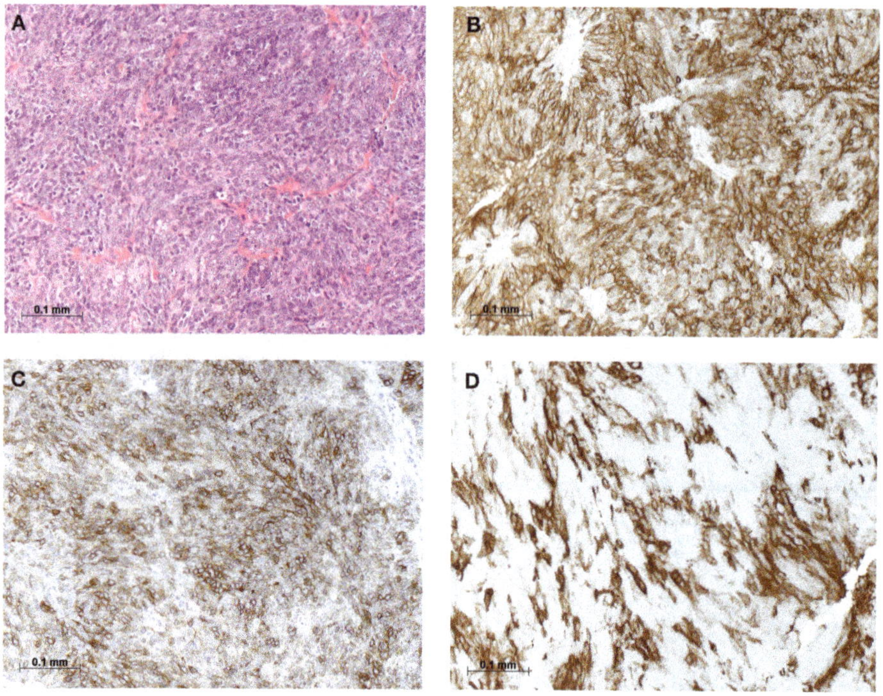

FIGURE 2 | Histomorphological and immunohistochemical analysis of parietal pleura, biopsy from 2018: **(A)** H & E staining, **(B)** Immunostaining for CD5, **(C)** Immunostaining for CD117, and **(D)** Immunostaining for PD-L1.

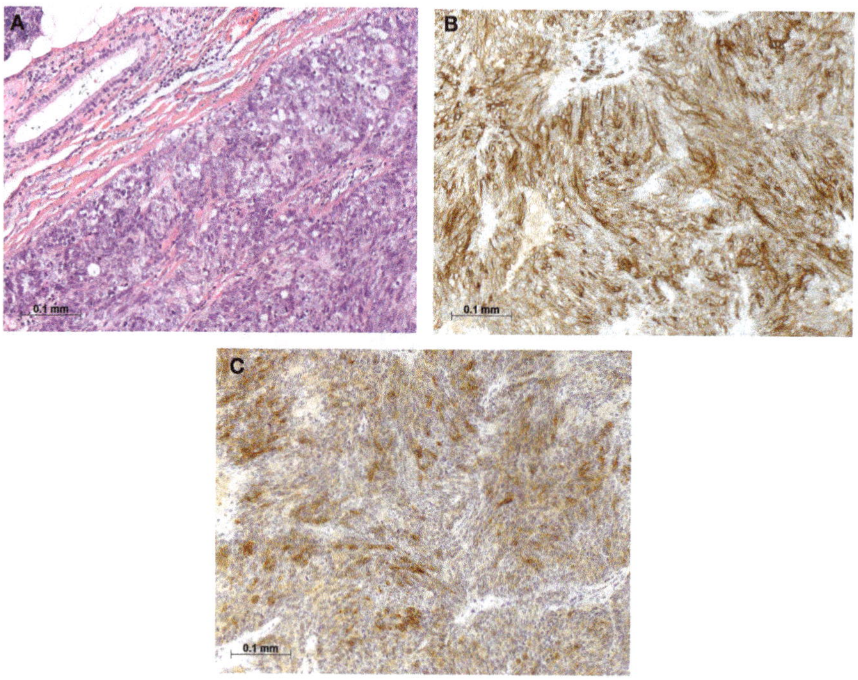

FIGURE 3 | Histomorphological and immunohistochemical analysis of parotid, tumor excisate from 2008: **(A)** H & E staining, **(B)** Immunostaining for CD5, and **(C)** Immunostaining for CD117.

retrospect after the disease was discovered in the pleural biopsy and after the parotid specimen was reanalyzed with additional staining for CD5 and CD117. We can not exclude the possibility of a metachronous CASTLE, but this seems unlikely due to the rarity of the disease. Also, we can not exclude with certainty that the lesion in the right upper lobe was a primary lung cancer with metastasis of the collateral, left-sided pleura. But, this alternative diagnosis seems less likely in this non-smoking patient presenting with weight loss over 6 months and dyspnea due to the process in the left pleura with large, left-sided pleural effusion. Expression of CD5 and CD117 strongly support CASTLE with metastatic dissemination, though a minority of NSCLC are known to express CD5 and CD117 (15).

The parotid tumor pT1pN2pM0 diagnosed 2008 was treated as undifferentiated cancer with a total parotidectomy and a selective neck dissection levels II-IV followed by radiotherapy, a therapeutic approach typically used for CASTLE as well.

Chemotherapeutic regimens for advanced, metastatic CASTLE have been used based on those designed for thymic carcinomas (16) with the assumption that the tumor biology of CASTLE is similar to thymic carcinomas, but available data is very limited, and the benefit for patient survival unknown (6). For metastatic thymic carcinomas, the response rate to chemotherapy is <50% (17), and new effective therapies are awaited. Importantly, thymic carcinomas express high levels of PD-L1 (18), and recently, a first prospective study with the anti-PD-L1 antibody pembrolizumab in patients with no response to chemotherapy or recurrent, progressive disease was encouraging showing a positive correlation between response, progression-free survival, overall survival, and PD-L1 expression (10). To the best of our knowledge, expression levels of PD-L1 in CASTLE has not been investigated. In our patient 60% of tumor cells expressed PD-L1, and after intensive discussion in our interdisciplinary tumor board, a first line systemic therapy with pembrolizumab was initiated, which resulted in a partial response documented in a follow-up FDG PET/CT at 4 months. Except a skin rash no other adverse event potentially related to pembrolizumab was observed. At the last follow-up in March 2019 the patient was in good condition and a second follow-up FDG-PET/CT showed a sustained partial response.

CASTLE tumors may be found also in the parotid, have a slow and indolent course in spite of their undifferentiated histopathology, express PD-L1 and are therefore good targets for complementary immunotherapy when needed for recurrent/metastatic disease.

ETHICS STATEMENT

We received a written informed consent of the patient for the publication of this case report.

AUTHOR CONTRIBUTIONS

LL collected all data. LL and JvR wrote the first draft of the manuscript. WA performed histological analyses, provided images, and reviewed the manuscript. NM treated the patient and reviewed the manuscript. US provided FDG PET/CT images and reviewed the manuscript. AS reviewed the manuscript. AJ wrote the manuscript. All authors read and approved the submitted version of the manuscript.

REFERENCES

1. Youens KE, Bean SM, Dodd LG, Jones CK. Thyroid carcinoma showing thymus-like differentiation (CASTLE): case report with cytomorphology and review of the literature. *Diagn Cytopathol.* (2011) 39:204–9. doi: 10.1002/dc.21399
2. Miyauchi A, Kuma K, Matsuzuka F, Matsubayashi S, Kobayashi A, Tamai H, et al. Intrathyroidal epithelial thymoma - an entity distinct from squamous-cell carcinoma of the thyroid. *World J Surg.* (1985) 9:128–34. doi: 10.1007/BF01656263
3. Chan JK, Rosai J. Tumors of the neck showing thymic or related branchial pouch differentiation: a unifying concept. *Hum Pathol.* (1991) 22:349–67. doi: 10.1016/0046-8177(91)90083-2
4. Marx A, Chan JK, Coindre JM, Detterbeck F, Girard N, Harris NL, et al. The 2015 world health organization classification of tumors of the thymus: continuity and changes. *J Thoracic Oncol.* (2015) 10:1383–95. doi: 10.1097/JTO.0000000000000654
5. Ge W, Yao YZ, Chen G, Ding YT. Clinical analysis of 82 cases of carcinoma showing thymus-like differentiation of the thyroid. *Oncol Lett.* (2016) 11:1321–6. doi: 10.3892/ol.2015.4055
6. Gao R, Jia X, Ji T, Feng J, Yang A, Zhang G. Management and prognostic factors for thyroid carcinoma showing thymus-like elements (CASTLE): a case series study. *Front Oncol.* (2018) 8:477. doi: 10.3389/fonc.2018.00477
7. Hargadon KM, Johnson CE, Williams CJ. Immune checkpoint blockade therapy for cancer: an overview of FDA-approved immune checkpoint inhibitors. *Int Immunopharmacol.* (2018) 62:29–39. doi: 10.1016/j.intimp.2018.06.001
8. Garon EB, Rizvi NA, Hui R, Leighl N, Balmanoukian AS, Eder JP, et al. Pembrolizumab for the treatment of non-small-cell lung cancer. *N Engl J Med.* (2015) 372:2018–28. doi: 10.1056/NEJMoa1501824
9. Fehrenbacher L, Spira A, Ballinger M, Kowanetz M, Vansteenkiste J, Mazieres J, et al. Atezolizumab versus docetaxel for patients with previously treated non-small-cell lung cancer (POPLAR): a multicentre, open-label, phase 2 randomised controlled trial. *Lancet.* (2016) 387:1837–46. doi: 10.1016/S0140-6736(16)00587-0
10. Giaccone G, Kim C, Thompson J, McGuire C, Kallakury B, Chahine JJ, et al. Pembrolizumab in patients with thymic carcinoma: a single-arm, single-centre, phase 2 study. *Lancet Oncol.* (2018) 19:347–55. doi: 10.1016/S1470-2045(18)30062-7
11. Pan Y, Zhao X, Yang J, Deng J, Zhan Z, Luo Y, et al. Absence of gene mutations in KIT-positive carcinoma showing thymus-like elements of the thyroid. *Hum Pathol.* (2012) 43:350–5. doi: 10.1016/j.humpath.2011.05.003
12. Wang YF, Liu B, Fan XS, Rao Q, Xu Y, Xia QY, et al. Thyroid carcinoma showing thymus-like elements: a clinicopathologic, immunohistochemical, ultrastructural, and molecular analysis. *Am J Clin Pathol.* (2015) 143:223–33. doi: 10.1309/AJCPB7PS6QHWEFRK
13. Reimann JD, Dorfman DM, Nose V. Carcinoma showing thymus-like differentiation of the thyroid (CASTLE): a comparative study: evidence of thymic differentiation and solid cell nest origin. *Am J Surg Pathol.* (2006) 30:994–1001. doi: 10.1097/00000478-200608000-00010
14. Wong EHC, Tetter N, Tzankov A, Muller L. CASTLE tumor of the parotid: First documented case, literature review, and genetic analysis of the cancer. *Head Neck.* (2018) 40:E1–4. doi: 10.1002/hed.24985
15. Nakagawa K, Matsuno Y, Kunitoh H, Maeshima A, Asamura H, Tsuchiya R. Immunohistochemical KIT (CD117) expression in thymic epithelial tumors. *Chest.* (2005) 128:140–4. doi: 10.1378/chest.128.1.140

16. Hanamura T, Ito K, Uehara T, Fukushima T, Sasaki S, Koizumi T. Chemosensitivity in carcinoma showing thymus-like differentiation: a case report and review of the literature. *Thyroid.* (2015) 25:969–72. doi: 10.1089/thy.2015.0155
17. Kelly RJ, Petrini I, Rajan A, Wang Y, Giaccone G. Thymic malignancies: from clinical management to targeted therapies. *J Clin Oncol.* (2011) 29:4820–7. doi: 10.1200/JCO.2011.36.0487
18. Weissferdt A, Fujimoto J, Kalhor N, Rodriguez J, Bassett R, Wistuba, II, et al. Expression of PD-1 and PD-L1 in thymic epithelial neoplasms. *Modern Pathol.* (2017) 30:826–33. doi: 10.1038/modpathol.2017.6

18

Weekly Paclitaxel, Carboplatin and Cetuximab as First-Line Treatment of Recurrent and/or Metastatic Head and Neck Squamous Cell Carcinoma for Patients Ineligible to Cisplatin-Based Chemotherapy: A Retrospective Monocentric Study in 60 Patients

Hélène Carinato[1], Mickaël Burgy[1], Régine Ferry[2†], Cathie Fischbach[1], Michal Kalish[1], Sébastien Guihard[3], Youssef Brahimi[3], Henri Flesch[4], Guy Bronner[4], Philippe Schultz[5], Véronique Frasie[6], Alicia Thiéry[7], Martin Demarchi[1], Thierry Petit[1], Alain C. Jung[8,9], Pierre Wagner[10], Pierre Coliat[11] and Christian Borel[1]*

[1] Institut de Cancérologie Strasbourg Europe, Department of Medical Oncology, Strasbourg, France, [2] Centre Paul Strauss, Department of Medical Oncology, Strasbourg, France, [3] Institut de Cancérologie Strasbourg Europe, Department of Radiation Oncology, Strasbourg, France, [4] Clinique Sainte Barbe, Head and Neck Surgery Unit, Strasbourg, France, [5] Hôpitaux Universitaires de Strasbourg, Department of Otorhinolaryngology and Head and Neck Surgery, Strasbourg, France, [6] Institut de Cancérologie Strasbourg Europe, Supportive Care Unit, Strasbourg, France, [7] Institut de Cancérologie Strasbourg Europe, Department of Biostatistics, Strasbourg, France, [8] Institut de Cancérologie Strasbourg Europe, Laboratoire de Biologie Tumorale, Strasbourg, France, [9] Université de Strasbourg, Inserm, UMR_S1113, Strasbourg, France, [10] Centre Paul Strauss, Department of Radiology, Strasbourg, France, [11] Institut de Cancérologie Strasbourg Europe, Pharmacy Department, Strasbourg, France

***Correspondence:**
Christian Borel
c.borel@icans.eu

†Present Address:
Régine Ferry, Hematology Department, CHRU de Nancy Hôpital Brabois, Vandoeuvre les Nancy, France

Objective: For most patients suffering from recurrent and/or metastatic head and neck squamous cell carcinoma (R/M HNSCC), chemotherapy is the main option after considering surgery and reirradiation. Cetuximab combined with a platinum-fluorouracil regimen (EXTREME) has been the standard of care for over a decade. Nevertheless, a significant number of patients remain unfit for this regimen because of age, severe comorbidities, or poor performance status. The aim of this study is to investigate an alternative regimen with sufficient efficacy and safety.

Methods: We reviewed retrospectively the medical charts of all patients treated with paclitaxel, carboplatin, and cetuximab (PCC) at our institution. Eligibility criteria were as follows: first-line R/M-HNSCC of the oral cavity, oropharynx, hypopharynx, or larynx not suitable for local therapy, cisplatin, and/or 5-FU ineligibility, ECOG-PS: 0–2. PCC consisted of paclitaxel 80 mg/m^2, carboplatin AUC 2, and cetuximab at an initial dose of 400 mg/m^2 then 250 mg/m^2, for 16 weekly administrations followed by cetuximab maintenance for patients for whom a disease control was obtained. The primary endpoint was overall survival (OS), and secondary endpoints were overall response rate (ORR), progression free survival (PFS), and safety.

Results: We identified 60 consecutive patients treated with PCC between 2010 and 2016 at our institution. Thirty-one patients (52%) were ECOG-PS 2. Fifty-five patients (92%) were cisplatin ineligible. ORR was 43.3% (95% CI, 30.8–55.8), and disease control rate was 65% (95% CI, 52.9–77.1). With a median follow-up of 35.7 months (IQR 28.6–48.8), median PFS was 5.8 months (95% CI, 4.5–7.2), and median OS was 11.7 months (95% CI, 7.5-14.8). For ECOG-PS 0–1 patients, median OS was 14.8 months (95% CI, 12.2–21.7) while it was only 7.5 months (95%CI: 5.5-12.7) for ECOG-PS 2 patients ($p < 0.04$). Grades III–IV toxicities occurred in 30 patients (50%). Most toxicities were hematologic. Six patients (10%) had febrile neutropenia. Nonhematologic toxicities were reported such as cutaneous toxicities, neuropathy, infusion-related reactions, or electrolyte disorders.

Conclusion: The weekly PCC regimen seems to be an interesting option in cisplatin-unfit patients. This study shows favorable PFS and OS when compared with what is achieved with the EXTREME regimen and a high controlled disease rate with predictable and manageable toxicities even in the more fragile population.

Keywords: head and neck squamous cell carcinoma, recurrent or metastatic, chemotherapy, cetuximab, paclitaxel, carboplatin, first-line

INTRODUCTION

Head and neck squamous cell carcinoma (HNSCC) represent more than 90% of the head and neck tumors. In Europe, approximately 140,000 new cases were diagnosed in 2014, corresponding to an annual incidence of 43/100,000. The main risk factors of HNSSC are tobacco with alcohol heavy/frequent consumption and HPV infection (1). In France, most patients are active or former smokers frequently in association with a high consumption of alcohol. Thus, they are likely to suffer from several active tobacco/alcohol-related comorbidities, undernourishment, and other active carcinomas. Considering significant concomitant nonmalignant diseases, age and general condition are crucial in oncological decision-making because a vast majority of patients turns out to be ineligible for clinical trial or standard of care (2).

Concerning recurrent and/or metastatic squamous cell carcinoma of head and neck (R/M HNSCC), palliative chemotherapy is the standard of care if local treatment (surgery or radiotherapy) cannot be curative. There is a need to find an optimal strategy to achieve the highest possible overall survival and patient's quality of life. In 2008, the EXTREME trial (3) showed the benefits of adding cetuximab to a platinum-5-FU chemotherapy in R/M HNSCC first-line treatment. An overall response rate (ORR) of 36% was achieved, median progression free survival (PFS) was 5.6 months, and median overall survival (OS) was 10.1 months. The EXTREME regimen has emerged as the standard of care for fit R/M HNSCC patients. Nevertheless, numerous patients remain unfit for this regimen because of frailties such as age, ECOG-PS >1, or heavy comorbidities, as evidenced by 82% of grades III–IV toxicities (3).

Other treatments consisting of a platinum-based chemotherapy associated with taxanes (docetaxel or paclitaxel) were investigated for HNSCC including R/M HNSCC (4). In a phase II trial (5), docetaxel combined with a cisplatin and cetuximab regimen (TPEx) achieved promising outcomes with a 44.4% ORR and a 79.6% disease control rate (DCR). Thus, the same authors carried out a phase II randomized trial (TPExtreme), comparing TPEx with EXTREME in terms of efficacy and safety (6). Results suggest that taxanes are an option in first-line treatment. However, this regimen should be used exclusively in cisplatin fit patients.

Therefore, some studies investigated alternative polychemotherapies in nonfit patients. Carboplatin with weekly paclitaxel is a safe and recommended option in the elderly population affected by advanced nonsmall cell lung cancer (7). In R/M HNSCC as well, some smaller nonrandomized studies demonstrated that first-line weekly carboplatin and paclitaxel could be safely used and improved efficacy when compared with monotherapy schedules in unfit patients (8). The paclitaxel, carboplatin, and cetuximab (PCE) regimen showed a 40% ORR, 5.2 months median PFS, and a 14.7-month median OS as first-line treatment in R/M HNSCC patients (9). The weekly paclitaxel, carboplatin, and cetuximab (PCC) regimen was first reported with promising results by Kies et al. in the locally advanced setting with a high dose of paclitaxel (10). The aim of this study is to provide a deeper insight into the weekly PCC efficacy and safety in the first-line R/M setting.

PATIENTS AND METHODS

Patient Selection

We retrospectively reviewed data from medical charts at our institution (Centre Paul Strauss, Strasbourg, France) between January 2010 and December 2016 to identify patients treated with paclitaxel, carboplatin, and cetuximab and suffering from histologically confirmed SCC of the oral cavity, oropharynx, larynx, hypopharynx, or cervical lymph node from assumed

HNSCC. Patients with skin SCC and sinus or nasopharynx carcinoma with poor differentiation were not selected.

Adult patients (aged 18 or older) in first-line treatment of a metastatic and/or recurrent HNSCC with no curative intent, ECOG-PS 0-2, and cisplatin and/or 5-FU ineligibility were included. Patients were considered cisplatin ineligible if at least one of the following criteria was met: age ≥70 or ECOG-PS 2 or creatinine clearance <60 ml/min or significant active comorbidities or cisplatin free interval <6 months. Patients were considered 5-FU ineligible in case of severe cardiovascular previous history including coronary insufficiency whether or not complicated by myocardial infarction, heart insufficiency, or lower limb arteriopathy of at least stage II. A treatment by radiotherapy or surgery for a previous locoregional relapse was permitted.

Induction regimen and palliative second-line or further treatment by PCC were excluded of the analysis.

The selection process is shown in **Figure 1**.

Treatment

From January 2010 to January 2012, we administered the PCC regimen as follows: carboplatin AUC 5 on day 1; paclitaxel 80 mg/m^2 on days 1, 8, and 15; and cetuximab 400 mg/m^2 loading dose then 250 mg/m^2 weekly. This pattern was repeated on day 22. A maximum of six cycles was administrated followed by a cetuximab maintenance given weekly or biweekly until progressive disease or unacceptable toxicities. However, administering carboplatin once every 3 weeks caused hematologic toxicity to such an extent that it became frequently impossible to administer paclitaxel on D15 and even sometime on D8.

Thus, from February 2012 to December 2016, the carboplatin infusion schedule was modified switching to a weekly administration: weekly carboplatin AUC 2 (maximum dose of 220 mg); paclitaxel 80 mg/m^2; and cetuximab 400 mg/m^2 loading dose then 250 mg/m^2. A maximum of 16 cycles was performed followed by a cetuximab maintenance given weekly (250 mg/m^2) or every 2 weeks (500 mg/m^2) until progressive disease or unacceptable toxicities.

Doses could be reduced initially or during treatment according to patient's comorbidities or toxicities.

Assessment

The efficacy of the protocol was assessed on the basis of response rate, progression-free survival and overall survival. A computed tomographic scan (or 18F-FDG PET/CT if needed) was performed at baseline, then every eight weeks. Measurements were compared between baseline and 8th-week CT scan (or 18F-FDG PET/CT) according to RECIST 1.1 criteria. The ORR is the complete response (CR) rate plus the partial response (PR) rate. The DCR is the ORR plus the stable disease (SD) rate. Radiologically, unevaluable patients were considered progressive if clinical reports mentioned it.

Toxicities were monitored weekly throughout the treatment and evaluated using the Common Terminology Criteria for Adverse Events version 4.0. Dose intensity data were calculated in order to assess regimen feasibility.

Statistical Analysis

PFS (time from first PCC infusion to progression or death) and OS (time from first PCC infusion to death) were estimated by the Kaplan-Meier method. If progression or death did not occur before the cutoff date, data were censored at the time of the last valid assessment.

The follow-up time is calculated from first PCC infusion to data cutoff (16 Jun 2018).

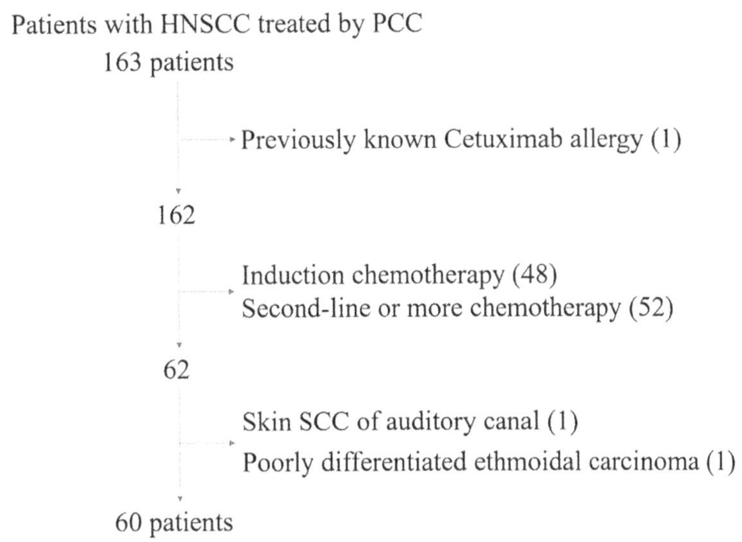

FIGURE 1 | Selection process.

RESULTS

Patient Characteristics

Sixty patients were treated with the first-line combination of paclitaxel and carboplatin plus cetuximab for a R/M HNSCC at our institution between January 2010 and December 2016. Median age was 61, with 10 patients (17%) aged 70 or more. Sex ratio was 5:1. In our study, the main risk factor was tobacco smoking as 80% of patients were former or current smokers. HPV infection was only assessed in two patients with oropharyngeal SCC by using p16 immunohistochemistry as a surrogate marker: one patient was p16 positive, the other one was not.

Five patients were diagnosed with distant metastases at the initial assessment and received PCC as a first treatment. Fifty-five patients had been pretreated with surgery and/or chemoradiotherapy. Fifteen patients in a recurrent setting had received locoregional treatments with a curative intent (such as surgery or reirradiation).

Forty-six patients (77%) were diagnosed with a locoregional relapse, among whom 38 patients in the field of an earlier irradiation. Twenty-nine patients (48%) had been already treated with platinum-based regimen in a neoadjuvant setting (18%) and/or with concurrent radiotherapy (32%) as a multimodality treatment of their initial tumor. Platinum-free interval was less than 3 months in 11 patients (18% of the whole patient population), between 3 and 6 months in three patients (5%) and longer than 6 months in 15 patients (25%). Because of a cisplatin-related kidney failure after a single course of TPEx, one patient received subsequently a PCC regimen. Patient characteristics are summarized in **Table 1**.

Twenty-nine patients (48%) were ECOG-PS 0–1 and 31 patients (52%) were ECOG-PS 2 at treatment onset. Frailty characteristics such as undernourishment and active comorbidities are reported in **Table 2**.

As defined in the inclusion criteria, 55 patients (92%) were ineligible to cisplatin. Thirty-four patients (57%) were ineligible to 5-FU because of severe cardiovascular comorbidities.

A second primary cancer arose in six patients during follow-up: two patients with a nonsmall cell lung cancer, one patient with a cutaneous melanoma and a nonsmall cell lung cancer, one patient with a hepatocellular carcinoma, one patient with a cutaneous squamous cell carcinoma, and one patient with a prostate adenocarcinoma.

PCC Delivery

Among the 60 patients included, six were treated with the first pattern to be used (carboplatin AUC 5 every 3 weeks, weekly paclitaxel 80 mg/m^2, and cetuximab 400 mg/m^2 initial dose, followed by weekly 250 mg/m^2). Starting in 2012, the 54 following patients were treated with weekly carboplatin AUC 2 (maximum dose of 220 mg: 49 patients were involved in dose limiting), paclitaxel 80 mg/m^2, and cetuximab 400 mg/m^2 loading dose then 250 mg/m^2. A maximum of 16 cycles was performed followed by a maintenance administration of cetuximab given weekly (250 mg/m^2) or biweekly (500 mg/m^2) until progressive disease or unacceptable toxicities.

A first clinical and radiological evaluation was done after eight cycles of PCC. As shown in **Table 3**, seven patients (12%) did not resume chemotherapy due to unacceptable toxicities and 16 patients (27%) because of progressive disease. A focal treatment (neck and/or metastasis) was carried out in seven patients (12%) because of a particularly good partial response. Cetuximab maintenance began after this assessment in eight patients (13%).

Median number of delivered cycles was 9.5 for chemotherapy and 10.5 for cetuximab. Twenty-four patients (40%) completed the 16 cycles of treatment, of whom 17 patients (28%) with the three drugs, while carboplatin or paclitaxel had to be stopped in seven patients.

Doses of paclitaxel and/or carboplatin and/or cetuximab had to be reduced in 19 patients, 37 patients, and three patients, respectively. Forty-five percent of patients experienced delayed chemotherapy due to side effects. PCC had to be stopped in 16 patients (27%) because of severe toxicities.

Toxicities are reported in **Table 4**. Thirty patients (50%) showed grades III–IV toxicities. Most toxicities were hematologic. Blood transfusions were required in 18 patients (30%). EPO and G-CSF were used as secondary prophylaxis in respectively nine (15%) and 30 patients (50%). Sixteen unexpected hospitalizations occurred due to infection, including six febrile neutropenia (10%). Four infections (6.6%), mostly pneumopathies, led to death which occurred only in ECOG-PS 2 patients. No other toxicity brought toxic death about. We observed 15 grades III–IV (25%) nonhematologic toxicities. Hypokalemia and hypomagnesemia are the most noticeable nonhematologic toxic effects in our study.

PCC Efficacy

PCC achieved a 43.3% (i.e., 26 responses) ORR (95% CI: 30.8–55.8) with three complete responses and 23 partial responses. Thirteen patients experienced stable disease. DCR came out at 65% (i.e., 39 controlled patients) (95% CI: 52.9–77.1). Progression occurred in 16 patients (26.7%): seven patients experienced clinical progression but could not be radiologically evaluated, six patients experienced CT-scan-proved disease progression, and three patients showed dissociated responses with appearance of new metastases despite partial responses on target lesions. Five patients were not evaluable because of nonmeasurable lesions (**Table 5**). The ORR is similar in the 38 patients with a locoregional relapse in a previously irradiated area; in this population, we observe 14 responses, i.e., a response rate of 36.8%. Among the 14 patients for whom the cisplatin free interval was less than 6 months, we observed three partial responses.

Change in target lesions was not evaluable in 12 patients: five patients died before evaluation (four due to progressive disease, one due to infection); one patient was not compliant; one patient could not be re-evaluated due to clinical deterioration; and five patients did not have any measurable lesion according to RECIST criteria. Change in target lesions is shown in **Figure 2**.

With a median follow-up of 35.7 months (IQR 28.6–48.8), we observed a median OS of 11.7 months (95% CI: 7.5–14.8) and a median PFS of 5.8 months (95% CI: 4.5–7.2). Kaplan-Meier curve-line estimate of PFS and OS are shown in **Figures 3, 4**.

TABLE 1 | Baseline characteristics of the patients.

Variable		N = 60
Gender [n (%)]	n	60
	Male	50 (83)
	Female	10 (17)
Age (years)	Median	61
	Range	23–79
Age [n (%)]	n	60
	<65 years	36 (60)
	65–69 years	14 (23)
	≥70 years	10 (17)
ECOG-PS [n (%)]	n	60
	0	9 (15)
	1	20 (33)
	2	31 (52)
Tobacco status [n (%)]	n	60
	Nonsmoker	12 (20)
	Current or former smoker	48 (80)
Primary tumor localization [n (%)]	n	60
	Oropharynx	23 (40)
	Oral cavity	17 (28)
	Hypopharynx	12 (20)
	Larynx	7 (12)
	Unknown	1 (2)
Histologic type [n (%)]	n (not specified or missing)	38 (22)
	Well differentiated	8 (21)
	Moderately differentiated	23 (60)
	Poorly differentiated	7 (18)
Initial treatment [n (%)]	n	60
	Neoadjuvant chemotherapy + Surgery	5 (8)
	Neoadjuvant chemotherapy + Surgery + CRT	1 (2)
	Neoadjuvant chemotherapy + CRT (cetuximab)	5 (8)
	Surgery	9 (15)
	Surgery + RT	6 (10)
	Surgery + CRT (platin-based)	15 (25)
	Surgery + CRT (other)	7 (12)
	RT alone	2 (3)
	CRT (cisplatin)	3 (5)
	CRT (cetuximab)	2 (3)
	No prior treatment	5 (8)
Local treatment for first relapse with a curative intent [n (%)]	Surgery	11 (18)
	Reirradiation	4 (7)
Tumor extension at baseline [n (%)]	n	60
	Loco regional only	33 (55)
	Loco regional and metastatic	13 (22)
	Metastatic only	14 (23)
Characteristics of relapse [n (%)]	n	60
	Relapse in RT field	38 (63)
	Relapse after platinum-based regimen (neoadjuvant, CRT)	29 (48)
Platinum free interval before baseline [n (%)]	n	29
	<3 months	11 (38)
	3–5.9 months	3 (10)
	≥6 months	15 (52)
Chemotherapy ineligibility [n (%)]	n	60
	Cisplatin	55 (92)
	5-FU	34 (57)

ECOG PS, Eastern Cooperative Oncology Group Performance Status; CRT, concurrent chemoradiotherapy; RT, radiotherapy.

In the ECOG-PS 0–1 population (i.e., 29 patients), median OS was 14.8 months (95% CI: 12.2–21.7) and median PFS was 7.1 months (95% CI: 6.3–9.0 months). In ECOG-PS 2 patients (i.e., 31 patients), median OS was 7.5 months (95% CI, 5.5–12.7; $p < 0.04$) and median PFS was 4.6 months (95% CI: 3.5–6.9; $p = 0.07$).

DISCUSSION

Our study shows that in first-line R/M HNSCC, a combination of paclitaxel, carboplatin, and cetuximab makes it possible to achieve results comparing favorably with what may be obtained through chemotherapies based on platinum-5-FU and

TABLE 2 | Frailty criteria of patients.

List of frailty criteria [*n* (%)]	*n*	60
	Age >70 years	10 (17)
	ECOG-PS = 2	31 (52)
	Undernourishment[a]	45 (75)
	Significant active associated comorbidities	
	Severe atheroma	32 (53)
	Heart insufficiency	10 (17)
	Chronic obstructive lung disease, ≥ stage 2	19 (32)
	Kidney insufficiency	2 (3)
	Pre-existing neuropathy	5 (8)
	Previously cured cancer	17 (28)
	Synchronous active cancer	6 (10)
	Others (psychiatric disorder, cirrhosis, organ transplant, etc.)	35 (58)
Number of criteria [*n* (%)]	*n*	60
	None	1 (2)
	1 criterion	10 (17)
	2 criteria	12 (20)
	3 or more criteria	37 (62)

[a]Undernourishment: albumin <30 g/L or weight loss over 5% in 6 months or weight loss over 2% if BMI >20 or BMI <18.5 or BMI <21 in 70 years and more aged patients.

TABLE 3 | PCC delivery before cetuximab maintenance.

Variable	*N* = 60	Paclitaxel 80 mg/m²/week	Carboplatin AUC2/week	Cetuximab 400 mg/m² then 250 mg/m²/week
Number of cycles	Median	9.5	9.5	10.5
	Range	1–19	1–21	1–21
Early discontinuation of treatment (≤8 cycles):			24 (40)	
- Due to unacceptable toxicities	*n* (%)		7 (12)	
- Due to progressive disease	*n* (%)		16 (27)	
- Change of treatment (local treatment, etc.)	*n* (%)		7 (12)	
Delivery completed (≥16 cycles)	*n* (%)		24 (40)	
Patients with dose reductions	*n* (%)	19 (32)	37 (62)	3 (5)
Patients with ≥1 dose held for ≥7 days	*n* (%)	27 (45)	27 (45)	23 (38)
Dose intensity[a]	Median	65	1.6	250
	Range	40–80	0.8–2	125–250

AUC, area under the curve. [a]Dose delivered per week, accounting for treatment delays and dose reductions. Units of measure are as follows: paclitaxel: mg/m²/week; carboplatin: AUC/week; cetuximab: mg/m²/week. The loading dose of cetuximab (i.e., 400[a]mg/m²) was not included in the calculation of dose density.

TABLE 4 | Maximal toxicity per patient.

	Grade I-II	Grade III		Grade IV
Overall toxicities [*n* (%)]	21 (35)		30 (50)	
Non hematologic toxicities [*n* (%)]	14 (23)		15 (25)	
Cutaneous	12 (20)	7 (12)		0
Neuropathy	3 (5)	2 (3)		0
Electrolytes disorders	3 (5)	5 (8)		2 (3)
Infusion reaction	3(5)	1 (2)		0
Nausea	5 (8)	0		0
Diarrhea	4 (7)	1 (2)		0
Hematologic toxicities [*n* (%)]	17 (28)		21 (35)	
Neutropenia	30 (50)	8 (13)		7 (12)
Anemia	26 (43)	7 (12)		0
Thrombopenia	7 (12)	1 (2)		0
Toxicity-related data [*n* (%)]				
Blood transfusion		18 (30)		
EPO (secondary prophylaxis)		9 (15)		
G-CSF (primary prophylaxis)		4 (7)		
G-CSF required (secondary prophylaxis)		30 (50)		
Febrile neutropenia		6 (10)		
Hospitalisation due to infection		16 (27)		
Hospitalisation		26 (43)		
Deaths in association with AEs		4 (6,6)		

TABLE 5 | Efficacy after 8 weeks of treatment.

	n = 60
Overall response rate (95% CI)	43.3% (30.8–55.8)
Complete response	3 (5%)
Partial response	23 (38.3%)
Disease control rate (95% CI)	65% (52.9–77.1)
Stable disease	13 (21.7%)
Progressive disease	16 (26.7%)
Non evaluable	5 (8.3%)

cetuximab (3) or cisplatin-docetaxel and cetuximab (5, 6), and this, with particularly frail patients.

Indeed, in our study, 55 patients (92%) are cisplatin ineligible: ECOG-PS 2: 52%, platinum free interval <6 months: 23%, at least three frailty criteria: 62%, age ≥70: 17%; however, a 43.3% ORR, a 5.8-month median PFS, and a 11.7-month median OS are achieved.

Although a 11.7-month median OS compares favorably with the 10.1 months obtained through the EXTREME regimen (3), it seems however shorter than the 14.5 months observed with the TPEx (6) and the 14.7 months with the PCE regimens (9). It should be noted however that these two latter studies concern a more favorable population of patients ECOG-PS 0 or 1 and that patients who were enrolled into the TPExtreme study were cisplatin fit and under age 70. In our study, when we consider the ECOG-PS 0–1 patients, the 14.8 months median OS is very similar to that reported with the TPEx or PCE regimens.

Pêtre et al. reported on a weekly paclitaxel and carboplatin combination in a particularly frail and heavily pretreated population that produced a 40% ORR, a median PFS of 4.7 months, and a median OS of 9.1 months (11). Interestingly, this study confirms the major impact of cisplatin eligibility and ECOG-PS on survival outcomes: median OS is 13.7 months for cisplatin-eligible patients whereas it is only 8 months for cisplatin-ineligible patients. For cisplatin-ineligible patients, median overall survival decreases from 11.5 to 3.6 months in patients ECOG-PS 0–1 and ECOG-PS 2–3, respectively (11).

The number of administered weekly PCC cycles, cetuximab maintenance, and subsequent treatments seem to be important factors of survival. Indeed, in the retrospective study reported by Narveson et al, where treatment is limited to six weekly cycles of PCC, although a similar ORR of 37% is reported, median PFS is 4.6 months and median OS is only 5.25 months (12).

Weekly paclitaxel is a well-established regimen which allows high dose intensity with low hematologic toxicity (13). Likewise, fractionated administration of carboplatin allows also to decrease the hematologic toxicity and thus to maintain continuous weekly administration of chemotherapy with as few toxicity-related interruptions as possible (9, 11). Nevertheless, in our study, although toxicity is noteworthy, it is however mostly hematologic and may be managed. It is caused to a large extent by the frailty of the treated population. We observed 10% of febrile neutropenia, 50% of secondary prophylaxis using G-CSF, and 27% of hospital readmission for sepsis which resulted in four deaths (6.6%). It should be noted however that deaths in association with adverse events are only observed in ECOG-PS 2 patients. Likewise, in the TPExtreme study, a 7.7% rate of deaths in association with adverse events is reported in the EXTREME arm and 5.9% in the TPEx arm (6). We are now proposing G-CSF as a primary prophylaxis which significantly reduces infectious toxicity. Indeed, weekly administration of G-CSF is safe and effective as reported by Kies et al. in the first publication of the weekly PCC (10).

Results of our study like these observed with the TPEx and the PCE regimens as well as in the CETMET trial show that it is possible to replace advantageously 5-FU by a taxane. The CETMET trial is a randomized phase II study which shows that the replacement of 5-FU by paclitaxel allows to decrease toxicity: 60% of the grades III–V reported toxicities being in the EXTREME arm (p = 0.034). Moreover, authors observed an increasing trend in the median PFS from 4.37 months in the EXTREME arm to 6.5 months in the paclitaxel, carboplatin, and cetuximab arm (p = 0.064) (14). The randomized phase II study TPExtreme did not show however any survival advantage when

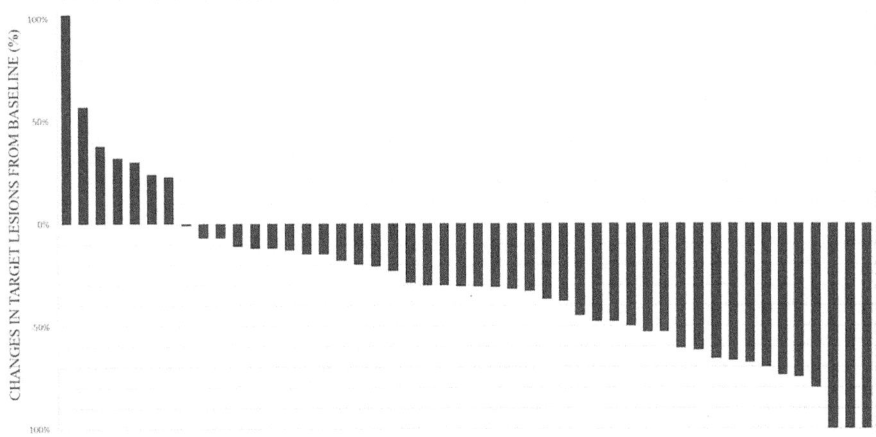

FIGURE 2 | Waterfall plot of 48 assessable patients for change in target lesions.

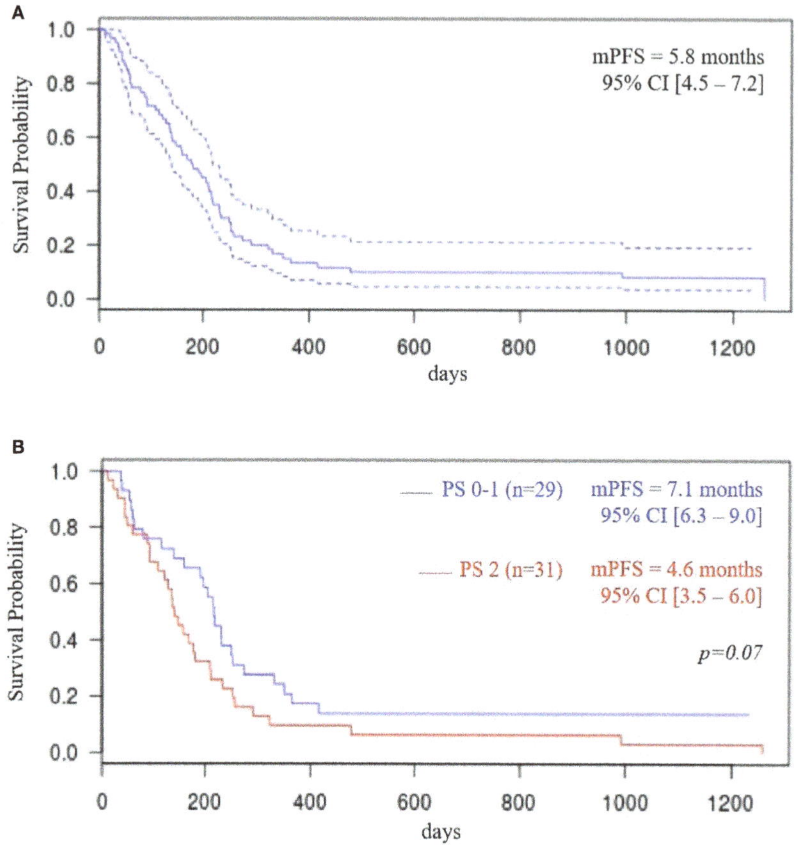

FIGURE 3 | Progression-free survival (PFS) total population **(A)**; PFS according to performance status (PS) **(B)**.

compared with the EXTREME protocol but confirms a high median survival of 14.5 months and a favorable safety profile in the TPEx arm (6).

The EXTREME protocol has remained the standard of care for first-line R/M until 2019 when the KEYNOTE-048 study has demonstrated, as far as survival is concerned, the superiority of immunotherapy by the anti-PD-1 pembrolizumab for the CPS ≥1 population and of the combination of pembrolizumab, platinum, and 5-FU in all patients (15). Nevertheless, platinum and cetuximab associations may remain relevant as first- or second-line R/M treatments in situations such as described hereunder. As first-line treatment, the association of platinum and cetuximab is appropriate when using an anti-PD-1 which is not suitable because of insufficient efficacy whenever the combined positive score (CPS) is inferior to 1 (which in Europe precludes its use in association with chemotherapy as well) or in case the patient is considered ineligible for immunotherapy particularly with an active autoimmune disease treated by immunosuppressive agents. In first-line treatment, there remains a need to address the problem of fragile patient, particularly cisplatin unfit or ECOG-PS 2 patients for whom the toxicity of the pembrolizumab combined to platinum/5-FU is too severe to be considered (85% of grades III–IV). Pembrolizumab alone may be proposed (55% of grades III–IV toxicity, 17% related to treatment), but the ORR is only 19% for the CPS ≥1 population (15) which appears inappropriate for severely symptomatic patients (16), whereas the response rate provided by the weekly PCC regimen is 43%. Moreover, the efficacy of pembrolizumab for ECOG-PS 2 patients has not been formally studied. As a second-line R/M treatment, following the administration of pembrolizumab alone, platinum and cetuximab combinations remain perfectly relevant and this especially since increased efficacy of chemotherapy following the use of anti-PD-1 agents has been reported (17). The weekly PCC may be then an interesting option for cisplatin-unfit patient, even for those who are ECOG-PS 2.

Despite its two main advantages (response duration and low toxicity), immunotherapy by pembrolizumab alone benefits only a minority of patients, and the determination of PD-L1 by combined positive score (CPS) remains an imperfect predictive factor (23% of response for CPS >20). Moreover, progression rate at first evaluation is high (around 40%) which makes it risky to propose immunotherapy alone to severely symptomatic patients. Combining pembrolizumab to chemotherapy makes it possible to improve results (ORR 36%, median OS of 13 months). There remain however two drawbacks: high toxicity (85% grades III–IV) and when compared with EXTREME, a survival benefit which is not clearly demonstrated for all subgroups (CPS <20) (18).

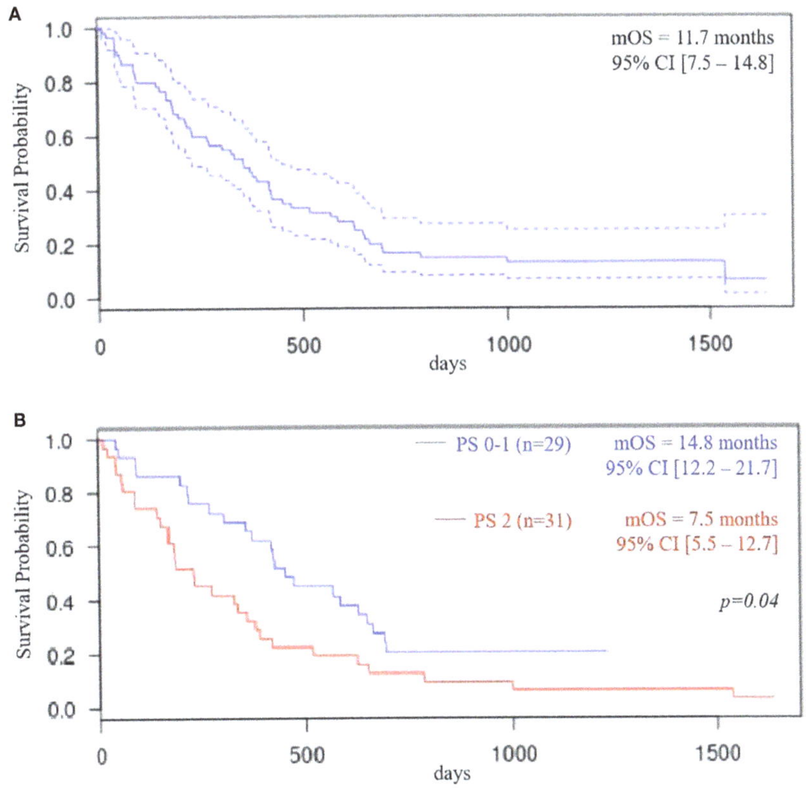

FIGURE 4 | Overall survival (OS) total population **(A)**; OS according to performance status (PS) **(B)**.

Considering the above, it remains clearly necessary to improve the immunotherapy combination or the associated chemotherapy. The combination of weekly paclitaxel, carboplatin, and durvalumab which is intended specifically for frail patients in first-line R/M is presently being studied in the frail-immune trial (19).

Combining monalizumab with cetuximab in at least second-line R/M patients pretreated with platinum, 45% of whom had also received an antiPD-1, has shown promising results which still remain to be confirmed in a randomized phase II study (20). A probable synergy of an anti-PD-1 with cetuximab (21) would justify the next step of studying a combination of PCC with an anti-PD-1 or also PCC with monalizumab.

In addition, the PCC regimen showed promising results in the neoadjuvant setting with an ORR ranging from 70% to 97% (10, 22, 23). Haddad et al. showed in a phase II randomized study, in the neoadjuvant setting, that weekly PCC is as effective and less toxic than cetuximab–Taxotere/platin/5-FU (C-TPF) making weekly PCC an option of choice for TPF-unfit patients (24).

ETHICS STATEMENT

Ethical review and approval was not required for the study on human participants in accordance with the local legislation and institutional requirements. Written informed consent for participation was not required for this study in accordance with the national legislation and the institutional requirements.

AUTHOR CONTRIBUTIONS

HC and CB conceptualized and drafted the study and the manuscript. MB and AJ critically reviewed the manuscript. HC, MB, RF, CF, and MK collected patients' data. CB and PW reviewed all CT scans. AT realized statistical analysis. All authors contributed to the article and approved the submitted version.

ACKNOWLEDGMENTS

Special thanks to Patrick Borel for his work of proofreading and correcting the text in English.

REFERENCES

1. Shaw R, Beasley N. Aetiology and Risk Factors for Head and Neck Cancer: United Kingdom National Multidisciplinary Guidelines. *J Laryngol Otol* (2016) 130(S2):S9–12. doi: 10.1017/S0022215116000360
2. Brom L, De Snoo-Trimp JC, Onwuteaka-Philipsen BD, Widdershoven GAM, Stiggelbout AM, Pasman HRW. Challenges in Shared Decision Making in Advanced Cancer Care: A Qualitative Longitudinal Observational and Interview Study. *Health Expect* (2017) 20(1):69–84. doi: 10.1111/hex.12434
3. Vermorken JB, Mesia R, Rivera F, Remenar E, Kawecki A, Rottey S, et al. Platinum-Based Chemotherapy Plus Cetuximab in Head and Neck Cancer. *N Engl J Med* (2008) 359(11):1116–27. doi: 10.1056/NEJMoa0802656
4. Gibson MK, Li Y, Murphy B, Hussain MHA, DeConti RC, Ensley J, et al. Randomized Phase III Evaluation of Cisplatin Plus Fluorouracil Versus Cisplatin Plus Paclitaxel in Advanced Head and Neck Cancer (E1395): An Intergroup Trial of the Eastern Cooperative Oncology Group. *J Clin Oncol* (2005) 23(15):3562–7. doi: 10.1200/JCO.2005.01.057
5. Guigay J, Fayette J, Dillies AF, Sire C, Kerger JN, Tennevet I, et al. Cetuximab, Docetaxel, and Cisplatin as First-Line Treatment in Patients With Recurrent or Metastatic Head and Neck Squamous Cell Carcinoma: A Multicenter, Phase II GORTEC Study. *Ann Oncol* (2015) 26(9):1941–7. doi: 10.1093/annonc/mdv268
6. Guigay J, Aupérin A, Fayette J, Saada-Bouzid E, Lafond C, Taberna M, et al. Cetuximab, Docetaxel, and Cisplatin Versus Platinum, Fluorouracil, and Cetuximab as First-Line Treatment in Patients With Recurrent or Metastatic Head and Neck Squamous-Cell Carcinoma (GORTEC 2014-01 TPExtreme): A Multicentre, Open-Label, Randomised, Phase 2 Trial. *Lancet Oncol* (2021) 22(4):463–75. doi: 10.1016/S1470-2045(20)30755-5
7. Quoix E, Zalcman G, Oster J-P, Westeel V, Pichon E, Lavolé A, et al. Carboplatin and Weekly Paclitaxel Doublet Chemotherapy Compared With Monotherapy in Elderly Patients With Advanced Non-Small-Cell Lung Cancer: IFCT-0501 Randomised, Phase 3 Trial. *Lancet Lond Engl* (2011) 378(9796):1079–88. doi: 10.1016/S0140-6736(11)60780-0
8. Moosmann P, Egli F, Stahel RA, Jost L. Weekly Paclitaxel and Carboplatin Combination Chemotherapy in Patients With Advanced Squamous Cell Carcinoma of the Head and Neck. *Onkologie* (2003) 26(6):568–72. doi: 10.1159/000074153
9. Tahara M, Kiyota N, Yokota T, Hasegawa Y, Muro K, Takahashi S, et al. Phase II Trial of Combination Treatment With Paclitaxel, Carboplatin and Cetuximab (PCE) as First-Line Treatment in Patients With Recurrent and/or Metastatic Squamous Cell Carcinoma of the Head and Neck (CSPOR-Hn02). *Ann Oncol* (2018) 29(4):1004–9. doi: 10.1093/annonc/mdy040
10. Kies MS, Jack Lee J, William WNJr., Glisson BS, Lin YH, Lewin JS, et al. Induction Chemotherapy and Cetuximab for Locally Advanced Squamous Cell Carcinoma of the Head and Neck: Results From a Phase II Prospective Trial. *J Clin Oncol* (2010) 28(1):8–14. doi: 10.1200/JCO.2009.23.0425
11. Pêtre A, Dalban C, Karabajakian A, Neidhardt E-M, Roux PE, Poupart M, et al. Carboplatin in Combination With Weekly Paclitaxel as First-Line Therapy in Patients With Recurrent/Metastatic Head and Neck Squamous Cell Carcinoma Unfit to EXTREME Schedule. *Oncotarget* (2018) 9(31):22038–46. doi: 10.18632/oncotarget.25157
12. Narveson L, Kathol E, Rockey M, Henry D, Grauer D, Neupane P. Evaluation of Weekly Paclitaxel, Carboplatin, and Cetuximab in Head and Neck Cancer Patients With Incurable Disease. *Med Oncol* (2016) 33(10):107. doi: 10.1007/s12032-016-0822-0
13. Tahara M, Minami H, Hasegawa Y, Tomita K, Watanabe A, Nibu K, et al. Weekly Paclitaxel in Patients With Recurrent or Metastatic Head and Neck Cancer. *Cancer Chemother Pharmacol* (2011) 68(3):769–76. doi: 10.1007/s00280-010-1550-3
14. Tsakonas G, Specht L, Kristensen CA, Herlestam Calero Moreno M, Haugen Cange H, Soderstrom K, et al. Randomized Phase II Study With Cetuximab in Combination With 5-FU and Cisplatin or Carboplatin Vs. Cetuximab in Combination With Paclitaxel and Carboplatin for Treatment of Patients With Relapsed or Metastatic Squamous Cell Carcinoma of the Head and Neck (CETMET Trial). *Cancers (Basel)* (2020) 12(11):3110. doi: 10.3390/cancers12113110
15. Burtness B, Harrington KJ, Greil R, Soulières D, Tahara M, de Castro G, et al. Pembrolizumab Alone or With Chemotherapy Versus Cetuximab With Chemotherapy for Recurrent or Metastatic Squamous Cell Carcinoma of the Head and Neck (KEYNOTE-048): A Randomised, Open-Label, Phase 3 Study. *Lancet* (2019) 394(10212):1915–28. doi: 10.1016/S0140-6736(19)32591-7
16. Peyrade F, Borel C, Daste A, Even C, Saada-Bouzid E, Guigay J. Systemic Treatment of Metastatic Squamous Cell Carcinoma of the Head and Neck: Proposal for Management Changes. *Curr Opin Oncol* (2021) 33(3):160–7. doi: 10.1097/CCO.0000000000000738
17. Saleh K, Daste A, Martin N, Pons-Tostivint E, Auperin A, Herrera-Gomez RG, et al. Response to Salvage Chemotherapy After Progression on Immune Checkpoint Inhibitors in Patients With Recurrent and/or Metastatic Squamous Cell Carcinoma of the Head and Neck. *Eur J Cancer* (2019) 121:123–9. doi: 10.1016/j.ejca.2019.08.026
18. Borel C, Jung AC, Burgy M. Immunotherapy Breakthroughs in the Treatment of Recurrent or Metastatic Head and Neck Squamous Cell Carcinoma. *Cancers (Basel)* (2020) 12(9):2691. doi: 10.3390/cancers12092691
19. *FRAIL-IMMUNE (GORTEC 2018-03) - Combination of Durvalumab With Carboplatin/Paclitaxel - Full Text View - ClinicalTrials.Gov*. Available at: https://clinicaltrials.gov/ct2/show/NCT03723967 (Accessed on 26 Apr 2020).
20. Cohen RB, Lefebvre G, Posner MR, Bauman JR, Salas S, Even C, et al. 1134p-Monalizumab in Combination With Cetuximab in Patients (Pts) With Recurrent or Metastatic (R/M) Head and Neck Cancer (SCCHN) Previously Treated or Not With PD-(L)1 Inhibitors (IO): 1-Year Survival Data. *Ann Oncol* (2019) 30(Suppl. 5):v460. doi: 10.1093/annonc/mdz252.026
21. Sacco AG, Chen R, Ghosh D, Wong DJL, Worden FP, Adkins D, et al. An Open Label, Nonrandomized, Multi-Arm, Phase II Trial Evaluating Pembrolizumab Combined With Cetuximab in Patients With Recurrent/Metastatic (R/M) Head and Neck Squamous Cell Carcinoma (HNSCC): Results of Cohort 1 Interim Analysis. *J Clin Oncol* (2019) 37 (Suppl.15):6033. doi: 10.1200/JCO.2019.37.15_suppl.6033
22. Bauman J, Langer C, Quon H, Algazy K, Lin A, Desai A, et al. Induction Chemotherapy With Cetuximab, Carboplatin and Paclitaxel for the Treatment of Locally Advanced Squamous Cell Carcinoma of the Head and Neck. *Exp Ther Med* (2013) 5(4):1247–53. doi: 10.3892/etm.2013.948
23. Wanebo HJ, Lee J, Burtness BA, Ridge JA, Ghebremichael M, Spencer SA, et al. Induction Cetuximab, Paclitaxel, and Carboplatin Followed by Chemoradiation With Cetuximab, Paclitaxel, and Carboplatin for Stage III/IV Head and Neck Squamous Cancer: A Phase II ECOG-ACRIN Trial (E2303). *Ann Oncol* (2014) 25(10):2035–41. doi: 10.1093/annonc/mdu248
24. Haddad RI, Massarelli E, Lee JJ, Lin HY, Hutcheson K, Lewis J, et al. Weekly Paclitaxel, Carboplatin, Cetuximab, and Cetuximab, Docetaxel, Cisplatin, and Fluorouracil, Followed by Local Therapy in Previously Untreated, Locally Advanced Head and Neck Squamous Cell Carcinoma. *Ann Oncol* (2019) 30 (3):471–7. doi: 10.1093/annonc/mdy549

19

Analysis of Genetic Alteration Signatures and Prognostic Values of m6A Regulatory Genes in Head and Neck Squamous Cell Carcinoma

Xuanchen Zhou[1], Jie Han[2]*, Xiaoyue Zhen[3], Yiqing Liu[1], Zhaoyang Cui[1], Zhiyong Yue[1], Ling Ding[1] and Shuai Xu[2]*

[1] Department of Otorhinolaryngology Head and Neck Surgery, Shandong Provincial Hospital Affiliated to Shandong First Medical University, Jinan, China, [2] Department of Otorhinolaryngology Head and Neck Surgery, Shandong Provincial Hospital Affiliated to Shandong University, Jinan, China, [3] Minimally Invasive Urology Center, Shandong Provincial Hospital Affiliated to Shandong First Medical University, Jinan, China

***Correspondence:**
Xuanchen Zhou
xuanchenzhou@163.com
Jie Han
hanjie64@sohu.com

Genetic alteration involving N6-methyladenosine (m6A) regulatory genes is a frequent characteristic of multiple tumors. Nevertheless, little is known regarding their genetic alteration signatures and prognostic values in head and neck squamous cell carcinoma (HNSCC). In this study, RNA sequence profiles and copy number variation (CNV) data of 506 HNSCC patients were downloaded from The Cancer Genome Atlas (TCGA) database. Correlation analysis involving alteration of m6A regulatory genes, clinicopathological characteristics, and patient survival was performed using R language. The results suggest that alteration of m6A regulatory genes was correlated with clinical staging. Patients with high expression of *ALKBH5*, *FTO*, *METTL14*, *WTAP*, *YTHDC1*, *YTHDF1*, and *YTHDF2* had poor overall survival (OS) than those with low expression. Univariate and multivariate Cox regression analyses showed that *ALKBH5* and *YTHDC2* were independent risk factors for OS. However, patients with high YTHDC2 expression had better OS. Moreover, according to machine learning results, *YTHDC2* was found to be the most important gene among the 10 m6A regulators. Additionally, high expression of *YTHDC2* was correlated with activation of apoptosis and ubiquitin-mediated proteolysis. Here, we identified alterations to m6A regulatory genes in HNSCC for the first time and found that seven m6A regulators were associated with poor prognosis, especially *ALKBH5*, whereas *YTHDC2* was associated with better prognosis. These m6A-related regulators could act as novel prognostic biomarkers for HNSCC. Our findings provide clues for understanding RNA epigenetic modifications in HNSCC.

Keywords: N6-Methyladenosine, head and neck squamous cell carcinoma, ALKBH5, YTHDC2, prognosis, biomarkers

INTRODUCTION

Head and neck squamous cell carcinoma (HNSCC) is a common clinically malignant tumor that mainly occurs on the mucous surface of the upper respiratory digestive tract, such as the nasal cavity, paranasal sinuses, nasopharynx, hypopharynx, larynx, trachea, oral cavity, and oropharynx. According to statistics, there are > 550,000 new cases of squamous cell carcinoma of the head and neck worldwide every year (1, 2). According to "Cancer statistics in China, 2015," the incidence of new lip, oral, and oropharyngeal cancer in 2015 was 48.1/100,000, and the mortality rate was 22.1/100,000. The incidence of new nasopharyngeal carcinoma (NPC) was 60.6/100,000, and the mortality rate was 34.1/100,000; the incidence of new laryngeal cancer was 26.4/100,000, and the mortality rate was 14.5/100,000 (3). The latest statistics show that, in the United States, HNSCC accounts for 3% of all cancer patients with 60,000 new cases per year and 12,000 deaths per year (4). The five-year survival rate of patients with HNSCC is approximately 40–50%.

At present, tobacco use and alcohol consumption are still the most important risk factors for development of HNSCC (5). There is relatively little information concerning the molecular mechanisms underlying HNSCC progression. However, in order to improve outcomes in HNSCC cases, identifying molecular genetic events during tumor progression is crucial to understanding mechanisms underlying malignancy.

The important role of RNA in biological systems is not only through the flow of genetic information from DNA to protein, but also through the regulation of various biological processes (6). The multiple functions of RNA are accompanied by more than 100 chemical modifications although the functions of most of these RNA modifications remain unclear (6). Among these modifications, adenosine N6 methylation (m6A) is considered to be the most common and conservative internal transcriptional modification in eukaryotic mRNAs (7). RNA m6A is thought to affect RNA transcription, processing, translation, and metabolism (7). The deposition of m6A is encoded by a methyltransferase complex, which involves three homologous factors, namely "writer," "eraser," and "reader" (7).

The "writers" (*METTL3*, *METTL14*, *WTAP*, and *RBM15/15B*) can catalyze the formation of m6A; "erasers" (*FTO* and *ALKBH5*) can selectively remove the methyl code from target mRNAs; "readers" (*YTHDF1*, *YTHDF2*, *YTHDF3*, *YTHDC1*, and *YTHDC2*) can decode methylation of m6A and produce a functional signal (7). m6A RNA modification is a dynamic and reversible process, which involves several biological functions in mammals, such as RNA transcription, processing events, splicing, RNA stability, and translation (8). To date, m6A has been reported to be associated with a variety of disorders, such as infectious diseases, nervous system development, obesity (9), infertility, inflammation, and cancer (10). Emerging evidence shows that m6A modification is related to tumor proliferation, differentiation, occurrence, invasion, and metastasis and plays the role of oncogene or antioncogenes in malignant tumors (7). In acute myeloid leukemia (AML), mimicking FTO depletion, an FTO inhibitor FB23-2 significantly inhibited the proliferation of human AML cell lines and primary cells *in vitro* and promoted cell differentiation/apoptosis (11). HNRNPC has been reported to control the invasiveness of glioblastoma (GBM) cells by regulating PDCD4 (12). In lung cancer, FTO enhances the expression of MZF1 by reducing the mA level and mRNA stability of MZF1 mRNA transcription, then leading to carcinogenic function (13). The deletion of m6A methyltransferase METTL3 leads to selective splicing and gene expression alteration of >20 genes involved in the TP53 signaling pathway in hepatocellular carcinoma (HCC) (14). In breast cancer (BRC), by inhibiting let-7g to upregulate METTL3, HBXIP forms a positive feedback loop of HBXIP/let-7g/METTL3/HBXIP, leading to accelerated proliferation of breast cancer cells (15). Although m6A has been found to be associated with tumorigenesis in various types of cancer, little is known regarding the relationship between m6A regulators and HNSCC. Therefore, we performed a retrospective analysis based on The Cancer Genome Atlas (TGCA) database to analyze genetic alterations involving m6A-related genes, their relationship with clinicopathological characteristics of HNSCC, and the prognostic value.

Abbreviations: m6A, N6-methyladenosine; HNSCC, head and neck squamous cell carcinoma; CNV, copy number variation; TCGA, The Cancer Genome Atlas; GEO, Gene Expression Omnibus; ccRCC, clear cell renal cell carcinoma; AML, acute myeloid leukemia; OS, overall survival; GSEA, gene set enrichment analysis; IHC, immunohistochemistry.

MATERIALS AND METHODS

All TCGA clinical data, copy number variations (CNVs), mutations, and mRNA expression data were retrieved using the UCSC Xena program, which is available to the public under certain guidelines. Therefore, written informed consent was obtained.

SNP and CNV Analysis of 506 HNSCC Samples

All of the TCGA RNA-sequencing data, single nucleotide polymorphisms (SNPs) and CNV data, clinical phenotypes, and survival data of 506 samples from patients with HNSCC were preliminarily integrated and standardized and could then be directly used for subsequent analysis. SNP analysis was based on VarScan2 variant aggregation and masking data in TCGA, in particular for mutation analysis of 10 m6A regulatory genes. These 10 m6A genes were *METTL3*, *METTL14*, *WTAP*, *FTO*, *ALKBH5*, *YTHDF1*, *YTHDF2*, *YTHDF3*, *YTHDC1*, and *YTHDC2*. SNP mutation analysis and results of visualization in this study were performed using the R maftools package (16).

CNV analysis of the 10 m6A regulatory genes was performed using GISTIC 2.0 (17) software with default parameters, and the results were visualized using the R programing language.

Relationship Involving CNVs, m6A Gene Expression, and Clinical Phenotypes

To investigate the relationship between CNVs and gene expression, we used the R package "ggpubr" to visualize the expression levels of the 10 m6A regulatory genes with or without CNVs and performed Kruskal–Wallis *H* tests between different CNV event groups. Here, expression results are represented as box plots.

To study relationships involving CNVs and clinical phenotypes, we performed analysis based on age, gender, clinical stage, tumor node metastasis (TNM) stage, and sample

CNV information. Chi-square testing was performed after grouping the clinical phenotype and CNV information.

Survival Analysis

We performed survival analysis based on regulatory gene expression levels of 10 m6A loci (log2 normalized) and overall survival time (OS) to determine the prognostic value of these 10 genes. Before survival analysis, we removed the gene expression level from the normal control sample from the original data. Samples with survival status of zero (survival) and survival time of <30 days were considered as follow-up failures in this study, and the remaining HNSCC samples were included in the subsequent survival analysis. The optimal cutoff point for gene expression was obtained based on the R package "survminer" (18). After high-low expression ranking of the samples using the optimal cutoff point, survival analysis was performed using the R package "survival" (19), and survival analysis results were visualized by the "ggsurvplot" method.

Construction of an m6A Regulatory Gene Network

We used the geneMANIA (20) database as the main analytical tool to explore the interaction between 10 m6A regulatory genes and other genes using default parameters. Ten m6A regulatory genes were used as analytical background genes, and the functions of the genes enriched in the visualization network results were further analyzed to study the potential main cellular roles of the 10 regulatory genes.

Machine Learning and Gene Set Enrichment Analysis (GSEA)

Based on the R package "caret," we constructed two different machine learning models to investigate features of importance involving 10 m6A regulatory genes. Random forest and neural network models were used to rank the 10 genes by their expression levels in two disease states (tumor and normal). Results were also visualized using R language, and the most important feature of the two models was selected as the key gene. We then used GSEA software (version 4.0.1) to perform GSEA analysis of key genes and other mRNAs. The Kyoto Encyclopedia of Genes and Genomes (KEGG).v7.0 was used as a gene sets database, and the Pearson method was selected as a metric for ranking genes while other parameters were used at default settings. Among the final enrichment results, $p < 0.05$ was used as the statistically significant cutoff to analyze optimal pathway enrichment results.

Immunohistochemistry (IHC)

According to the Abcam manufacturer's instructions, the *YTHDC2* and *ALKBH5* genes were analyzed by IHC using formalin-fixed, paraffin-embedded tissue blocks. Briefly, paraffin sections were dewaxed, and endogenous peroxidase activity was blocked with 0.3% hydrogen peroxide for 10 min at 37°C. Following antigen retrieval, the tissue sections were incubated with primary antibody *YTHDC2* (1:500; EPR21820-49, AB220160; Abcam, Inc., Cambridge, MA, USA) or *ALKBH5* (1:2000; EPR18958, ab195377, Abcam, Inc.) at 4°C overnight and then with a secondary antibody at room temperature (25°C) overnight. The sections were counterstained with hematoxylin.

RESULTS

SNP Mutation and CNV Results of m6A Regulatory Genes in HNSCC Samples

Of the 506 patients with sequencing data used for SNP mutation analysis, only 41 (8.1%) of the samples had mutation events in any of the 10 m6A regulatory genes as shown in **Figure 1**. For HNSCC samples, the mutation frequency involving the 10 m6A regulatory genes was not high, and each gene was mutated only in several samples (<8), where most of the mutation events were missense mutations. However, it was found that the 10 m6A regulatory genes had different levels of CNV events though analysis using GISTIC, ranging from 23.58 to 57.36%. "Reader" gene *YTHDF3* (57.36%) harbored the most CNV events among the 10 m6A genes (**Figure 2A**). CSMD1 (66.56%) and TP53 (31.61%) were non-m6A genes found to be mutated while

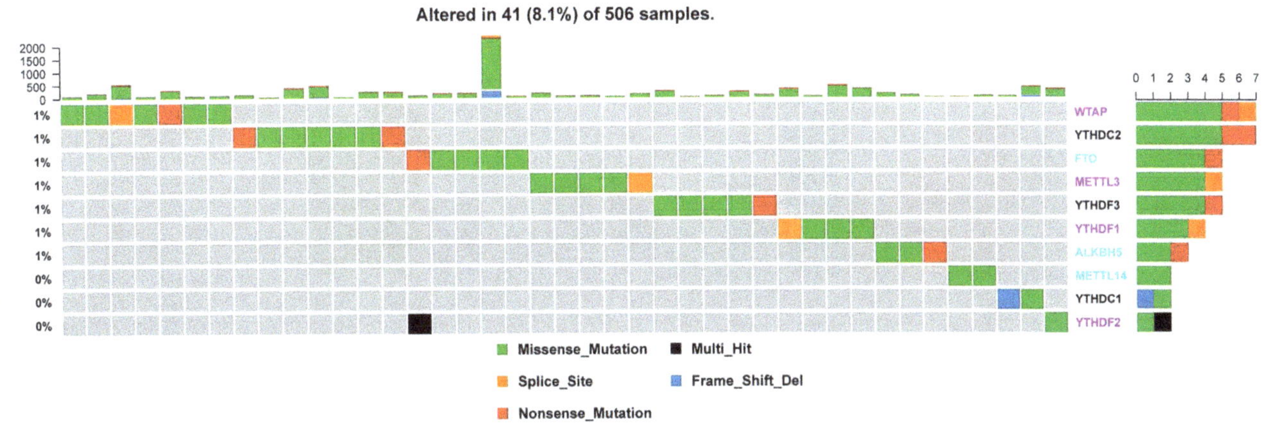

FIGURE 1 | Alteration frequency of m6A regulatory genes in the HNSCC sample based on the TCGA database.

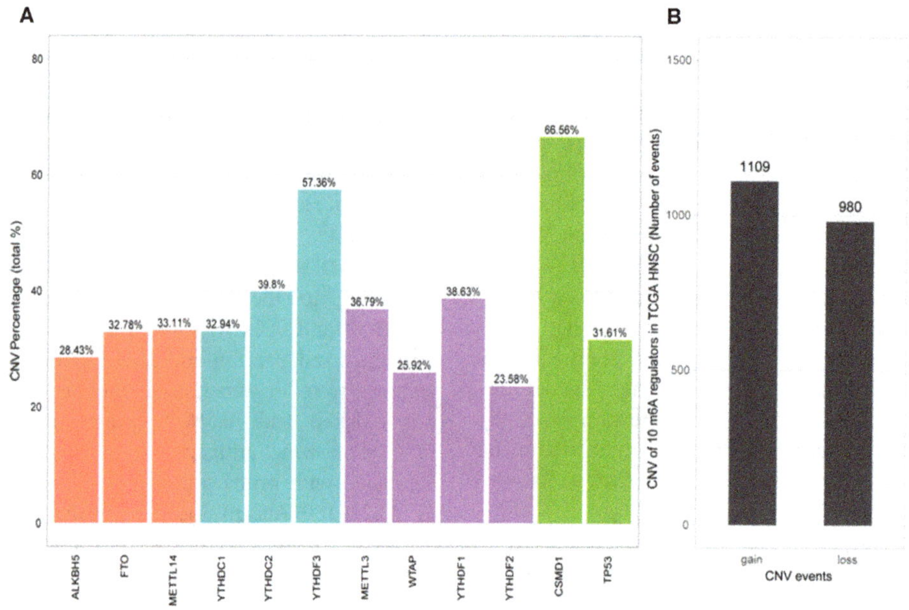

FIGURE 2 | Analysis of 10 m6A regulatory gene mutation data in the TCGA HNSCC sample. **(A)** Percentage of HNSCC samples with CNVs of the m6A regulatory genes from TCGA. **(B)** CNV events of gain or loss of m6A regulators in HNSCCC samples.

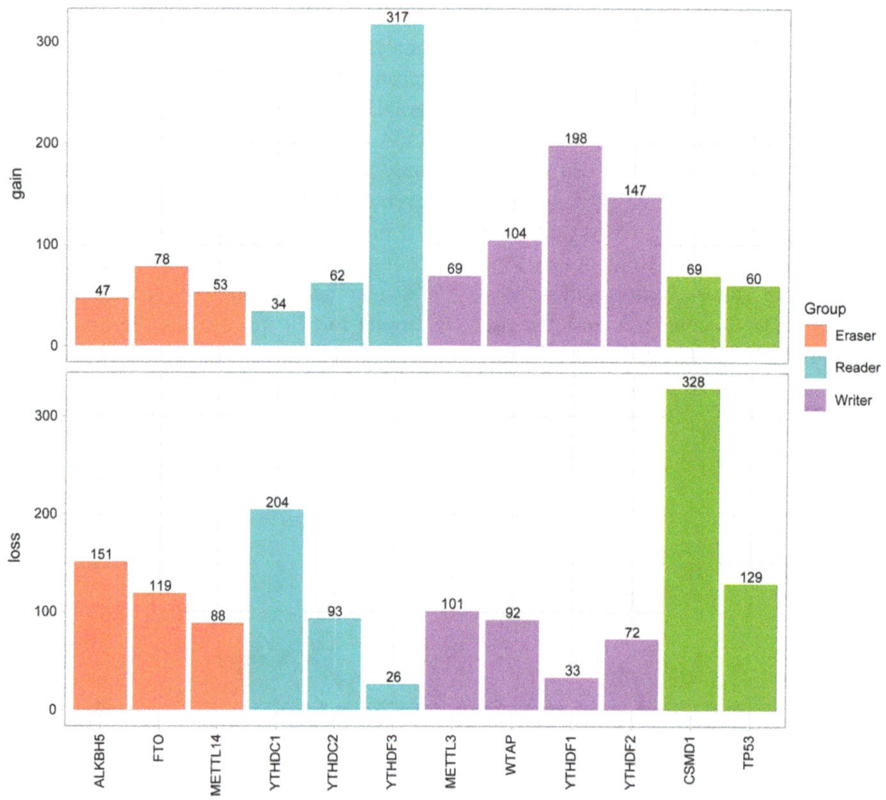

FIGURE 3 | Results of CNV analysis of 10 m6A regulatory genes in the HNSCC cohort.

CSMD1 was the most CNV events and TP53 was the most SNP events in all HNSCC samples. They were analyzed together with 10 m6A regulatory genes as references.

Next, the CNV patterns of the 10 m6A genes in the HNSCC samples were analyzed. It was found that the number of the CNV gain event was larger than that of loss events (1109 > 980) in the 10 m6A regulatory genes (**Figure 2B**). Unlike AML (21) and clear cell renal cell carcinoma (ccRCC) (22), among these 10 m6A regulatory genes, *YTHDF3* exhibited the highest number (317) of CNV gain events. *YTHDC1* had the most CNV loss events with 204 cases (**Figure 3**). Both *YTHDF3* and *YTHDC1* are m6A regulatory "reader" genes.

Additionally, SNP analysis revealed that the most frequent variant classification of m6A regulatory gene mutation was missense mutation, and the largest number of variant types was SNP (**Figure S1**). For SNPs, the most common SNV type was C > T, and the median number of variants per sample was 78. The most obvious mutations involved *TP53* as mentioned before (66%) and *TTN* (35%).

Association Involving CNV Alterations, Clinicopathological Characteristics, and Gene Expression

We then evaluated the relationship between CNV alterations in 10 m6A regulatory genes and clinicopathological features of HNSCC patients. Clinical staging was divided into I–IV according to the HNSCC guidelines of the American Joint Committee on Cancer (23). The results showed that alterations to m6A regulatory genes were significantly related to age, gender, and clinical stage ($P < 0.05$) (**Table 1**). In other words, being aged <60 years, male, with high-grade clinical staging were factors more related to CNV events involving 10 m6A regulatory genes.

Next, we analyzed relationships between CNV patterns and gene expression of the 10 m6A regulatory genes. As can be seen from **Figure 4**, there was a statistically significant relationship between CNV patterns and gene expression. With CNV events from deletion to amplification, gene expression of the 10 m6A regulatory genes also showed an upward trend; that is, gene expression increased with increased CNV amplification and decreased with CNV deletion.

TABLE 1 | Clinical pathological parameters of HNSCC patients with or without CNV of m6A regulatory genes.

Variable		With CNV events	Without CNV events	Total	chi-square value	*P*
Age	<=60	223	13	236	4.205	**0.0402**
	>60	216	27	243		
Gender	Male	329	22	351	6.462	**0.0110**
	Female	110	18	128		
Clinical Stage	Stage I	14	5	19	9.623	**0.0220**
	Stage II	83	9	92		
	Stage III	93	9	102		
	Stage IV	249	17	266		
Stage M	M0	424	39	463	1.63E-29	1
	M1	5	0	5		
	MX	10	1	11		
Stage N	N0	209	26	235	4.620	0.2018
	N1	74	6	80		
	N2	141	8	149		
	N3	7	0	7		
	NX	8	0	8		
Stage T	T1	28	5	33	4.369	0.2243
	T2	125	15	140		
	T3	118	9	127		
	T4	167	11	178		
	TX	1	0	1		

With or without CNV events: Cases have CNV or do not have CNV, confirmed by TCGA database. Ambiguous variables (Nx and Mx) were excluded from chi-square test. Bold values indicate P < 0.05 with significantly statistical difference.

Association Between m6A Regulatory Gene CNVs and HNSCC Patient Survival

We previously studied relationships between CNV patterns and m6A regulatory gene expression. The more extensive the CNV, the more the gene was expressed. We studied relationships between expression levels of m6A regulatory genes and the survival rate of HNSCC patients and explored the prognostic value of m6A regulatory genes. Our analysis revealed that expression of the 10 m6A regulatory genes was mostly related to the prognosis of HNSCC patients. Patients with high expression of *ALKBH5*, *FTO*, *METTL14*, *WTAP*, *YTHDC1*, *YTHDF1*, and *YTHDF2* had lower OS (**Figures 5A–H**), and patients with higher *YTHDC2* expression showed greater OS (**Figure 6A**). Furthermore, when HNSCC patients were grouped with or without CNV events for survival analysis, no statistically significant results were obtained (**Figure 6B**). It could be speculated that the occurrence of CNV events does not directly affect the prognosis of HNSCC patients, but rather that they affect the prognosis of HNSCC patients by influencing the expression of genes. Meanwhile, univariate and multivariate analyses demonstrated that increased expression of *ALKBH5* and *YTHDC2* were independent risk factors for OS in patients with HNSCC (**Table 2**).

Next, by further analysis, no significant differences were observed between different subgroups based on the CNVs of the 10 m6A regulatory genes (**Figure S2**).

Machine Learning and IHC Analysis

To study the important characteristics of the 10 genes, we used a neural network and random forest to build predictive models. As can be seen from **Figure 7**, in both models, the *YTHDC2* gene was consistently ranked the highest among the 10 genes. Combined with the results of the previous analysis (**Figure 2A**), among the 10 genes, the incidence of CNV events involving *YTHDC2* was second only to *YTHDF3*, and *YTHDC2* gene expression and survival prognosis results were also significant. However, association between the expression level of *YTHDF3* and survival prognosis was not statistically significant (**Figure 5I**). Therefore, *YTHDC2* was selected as the most prognostically important locus of the 10 m6A regulatory genes in HNSCC.

Furthermore, we performed IHC staining for *YTHDC2* and *ALKBH5* proteins in 20 pairs of normal and oral squamous cell carcinoma tissues to confirm such findings (**Figure 8**). These

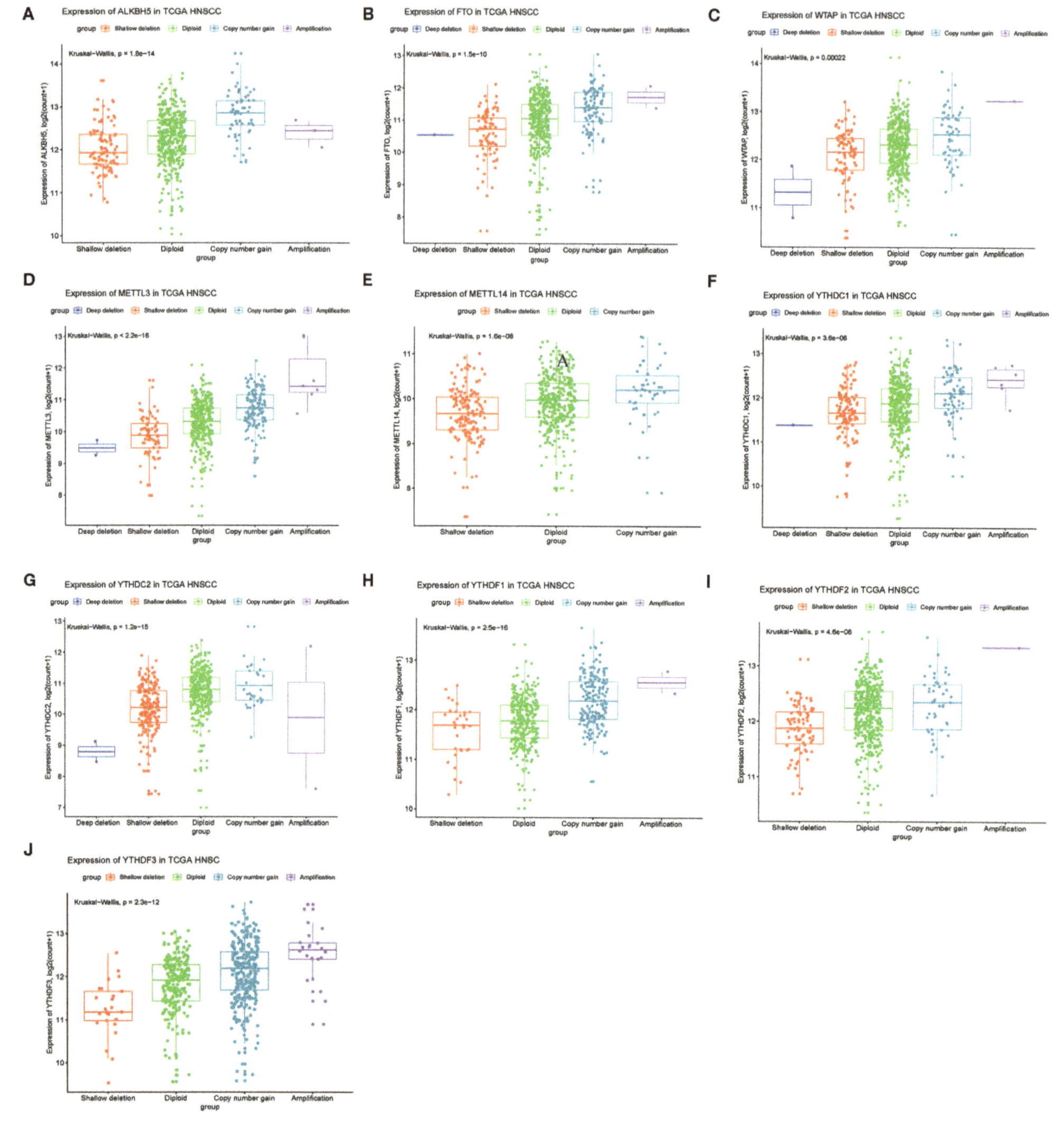

FIGURE 4 | Association between m6A regulatory gene CNV patterns and genetic expression. **(A)** ALKBH5, **(B)** FTO, **(C)** WTAP, **(D)** METTL3, **(E)** METTL14, **(F)** YTHDC1, **(G)** YTHDC2, **(H)** YTHDF1, **(I)** YTHDF2, **(J)** YTHDF3.

results were consistent with our predictions, indicating that *YTHDC2* and *ALKBH5* were expressed more highly in malignant HNSCC tissues than in normal oral tissues.

GSEA Analysis

Considering the importance of *YTHDC2* in the methylation process, we decided to explore the role of *YTHDC2* dysfunction in the pathogenesis of HNSCC. We examined enriched gene sets in samples with different *YTHDC2* mRNA expression levels. GSEA analysis implied that high expression of *YTHDC2* is associated with certain key pathways, such as apoptosis, ubiquitin-mediated proteolysis, long-term potentiation, and rig-i-like receptor signaling pathways, revealing the underlying mechanisms involved in HNSCC pathogenesis (**Figure 9**). To validate our findings, we examined the expression of several genes associated with these pathways. We found that apoptosis-related genes *caps3, 6, 8, 9, Bcl-2, Bid, UBE2S,* and *HERC3* associated with ubiquitin-mediated proteolysis were significantly

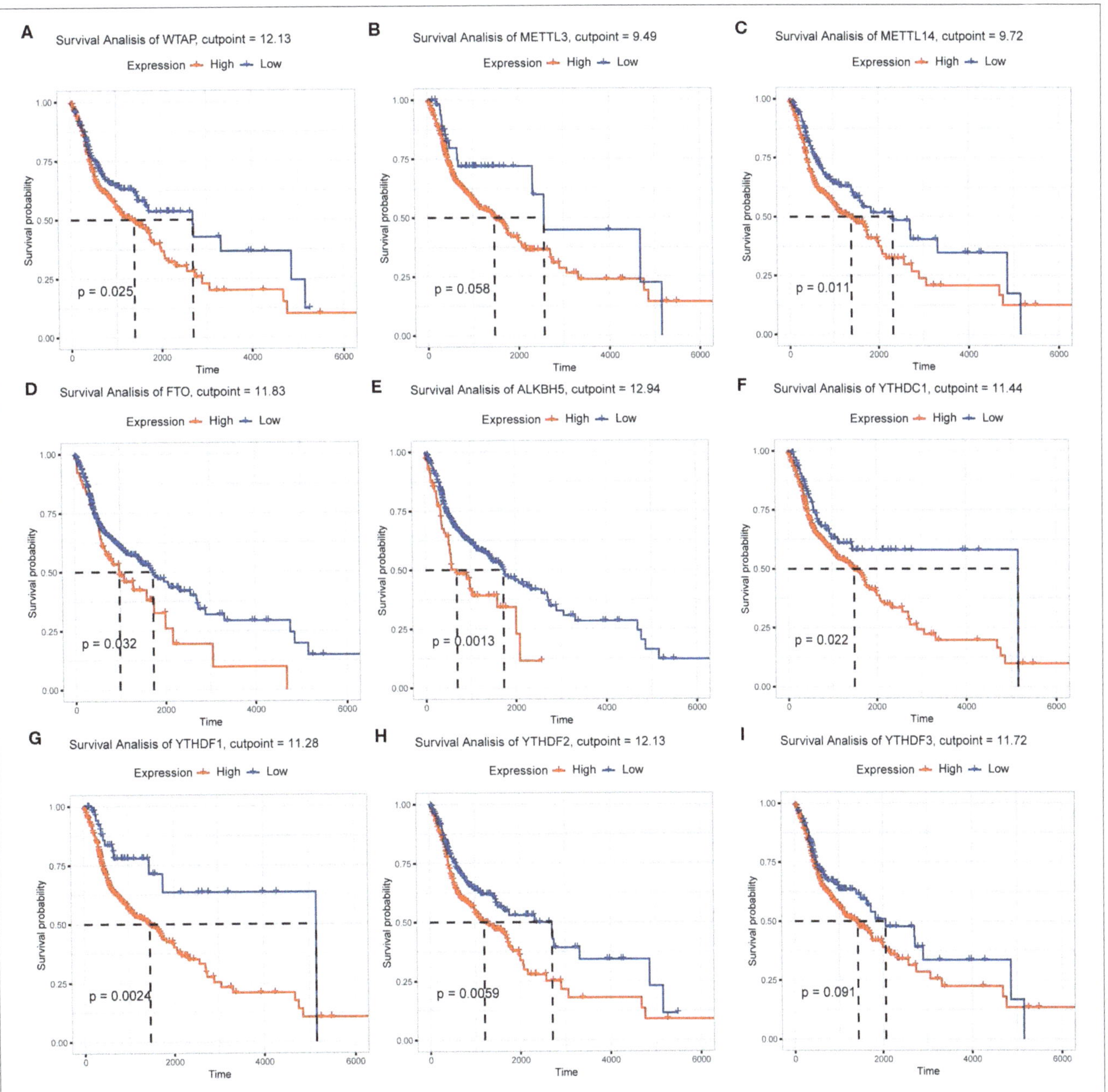

FIGURE 5 | Relationship between expression of nine m6A regulatory genes and overall survival. **(A)** WTAP, **(B)** METTL3, **(C)** METTL14, **(D)** FTO, **(E)** ALKBH5, **(F)** YTHDC1, **(G)** YTHDF1, **(H)** YTHDF2, **(I)** YTHDF3.

different in HNSCC tumor tissues compared to normal tissues (**Figure 10**). The GSEA results were partially validated.

DISCUSSION

m6A is the most abundant chemical modification of mRNA, which is regulated by m6A "writer," "eraser," and "reader" proteins (8, 24, 25). As an important complement to the central dogma, the study of m6A-mediated RNA methylation and its role in cancer has only just commenced. To date, little is known regarding the role of m6A in HNSCC. Only a single study has reported that m6A is associated with nasopharyngeal carcinoma in which m6A-mediated ZNF750 repression facilitates NPC progression (26). Due to the complexity of m6A-Seq and m6A-methylated RNA immunoprecipitation technologies, many studies have chosen alterative methods to assess genetic alterations to m6A regulatory genes, indirectly exploring relationships between m6A status and human disease. In this study, we applied bioinformatics methods to analyze genetic alteration in 10 m6A genes, their relationships with the clinical

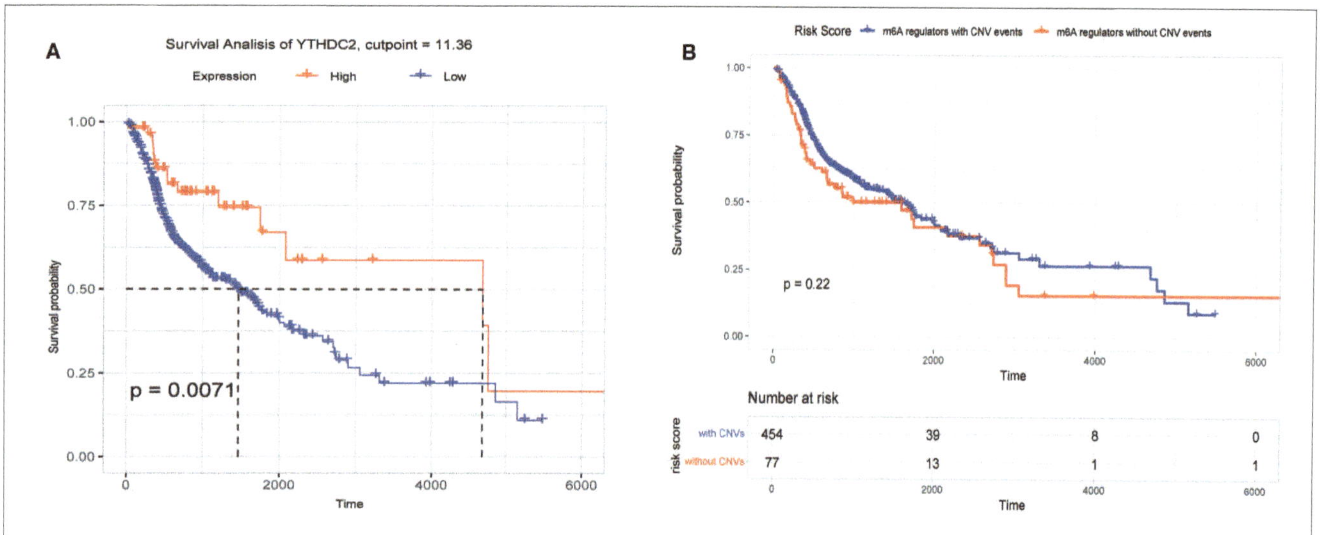

FIGURE 6 | Overall survival of HNSCC patients with or without CNV of m6A regulatory genes and YTHDC2 expression. **(A)** Relation between YTHDC2 expression and overall survival. **(B)** Relation between with or without CNVs and overall survival.

TABLE 2 | Univariate and multivariate COX regression analysis of various prognostic parameters for HNSCC cohort.

Risk factors	Univariate		Multivariate	
	HR(95% CI)	*P*	HR(95% CI)	*P*
Age	1.02(1.01-1.03)	**0.00123**	1.02(1.012-1.0404)	**0.000268**
Gender(male/female)	0.765(0.57-1.03)	0.0747	0.8668(0.6336-1.1858)	0.371157
Clinical M(M0/M1)	4.63(1.71-12.6)	**0.00263**	4.8295(1.744-13.3741)	**0.002444**
Clinical N(N0/N1-N3)	1.24(0.945-1.63)	0.12		
Clinical T(T1-T2/T3-T4)	1.31(0.97-1.76)	**0.0783**	0.7723(0.9535-1.7586)	0.097974
Clinical stage(stage i-ii/stage iii-iv)	1.24(0.889-1.74)	0.203		
METTL3(high/low)	1.617(0.371-1.031)	**0.0655**	1.1450(0.5020-1.5194)	0.631672
WTAP(high/low)	1.478(0.5028-0.9104)	**0.00987**	0.9995(0.6687-1.4971)	0.998031
METTL14(high/low)	1.552(0.4774-0.8693)	**0.00402**	1.3650(0.4864-1.1036)	0.136612
ALKBH5(high/low)	1.726(0.4062-0.8264)	**0.0026**	1.7626(0.3845-0.8371)	**0.004286**
FTO(high/low)	1.437(0.4907-0.9875)	**0.0423**	1.0381(0.6568-1.4128)	0.848160
YTHDF1(high/low)	2.554(0.2183-0.7019)	**0.00164**	1.7128(0.3056-1.1156)	0.103340
YTHDF2(high/low)	1.489(0.5073-0.8896)	**0.00549**	1.0431(0.6480-1.4183)	0.832774
YTHDF3(high/low)	1.251(0.5915-1.08)	0.144		
YTHDC1(high/low)	1.592(0.4346-0.9073)	**0.0132**	1.2575(0.4966-1.2734)	0.340161
YTHDC2(high/low)	0.4903(1.204-3.456)	**0.00806**	0.3896(1.4864-4.4323)	**0.000720**

Ambiguous variables (Nx, Mx, N/A and discrepancy) were deleted. Bold values indicate P < 0.05 with significantly statistical difference.

features of HNSCC, and their prognostic value based on a TCGA database.

In our cohort of 506 HNSCC cases, the CNV frequency involving the 10 m6A regulatory genes was similar to that reported in ccRCC (22), but much higher in AML (21), suggesting that m6A dysfunction may play a more important role in the carcinogenesis of HNSCC than that of AML. Furthermore, "reader" genes *YTHDC2* and *YTHDC3* exhibited higher incidences of CNVs than other genes in our HNSCC samples, which is different from that of ccRCC (22). This suggests that "readers" may be more important than "writers" and "erasers" in HNSCC. However, "erasers" *FTO* and *ALKBH5* have been shown to be more important in glioblastoma (27), AML (28), and BRC (29). This implies tissue specificity of the "writers," "erasers," and "readers" in different tumors. Unlike in AML (21) and ccRCC (22), the CNV events in the HNSCC samples here led to gains in copy number (1109/980). The most obvious gain and loss genes were "readers," which further demonstrated the importance of "reader" genes in m6A processing.

Mutations in CNV are usually associated with different clinicopathological features. In the ccRCC cohort, m6A regulatory gene alterations were significantly related to higher Fuhrman nuclear grading. In AML patients, bone marrow blast numbers, white blood cell count, and cytogenetic risk

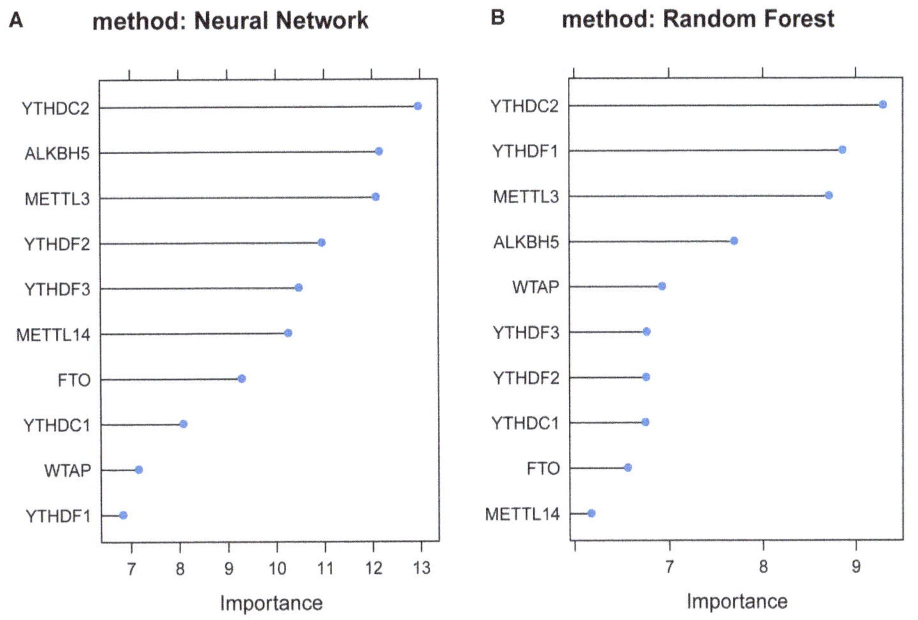

FIGURE 7 | Plots of neural network and random forest for 10 m6A regulatory genes. **(A)** Rank chart for the 10 m6A regulatory genes by Neural network. **(B)** Rank chart of the 10 m6A regulatory genes by Random Forest.

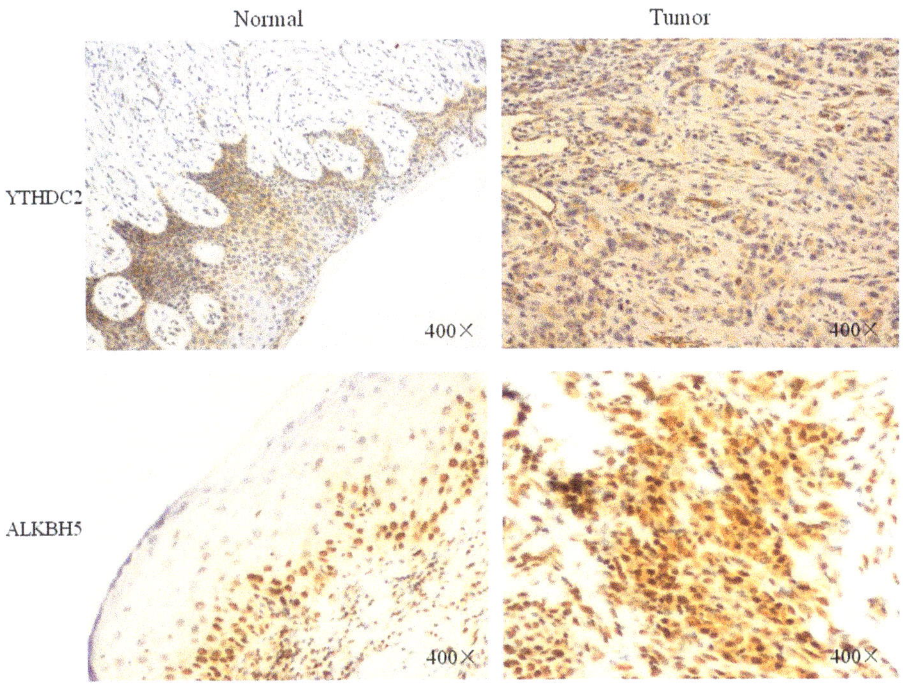

FIGURE 8 | The protein expression of YTHDC2 and ALKBH5 in oral squamous cell carcinoma and normal oral tissues.

are significantly associated with m6A gene alterations. In our HNSCC samples, the alterations to m6A regulatory genes were significantly correlated with age, sex, and clinical stage. This indicated that alterations in m6A CNV may show different clinical characteristics in different tumors. In the future, it will be necessary to study the characteristics of m6A mutations in different malignancies. Similar to ccRCC samples, in our study, copy number gains were correlated with higher mRNA expression and vice versa.

We evaluated the role of m6A regulatory genes in the survival of patients with HNSCC. In contrast toccRCC samples and BRC samples with only two and three m6A genes

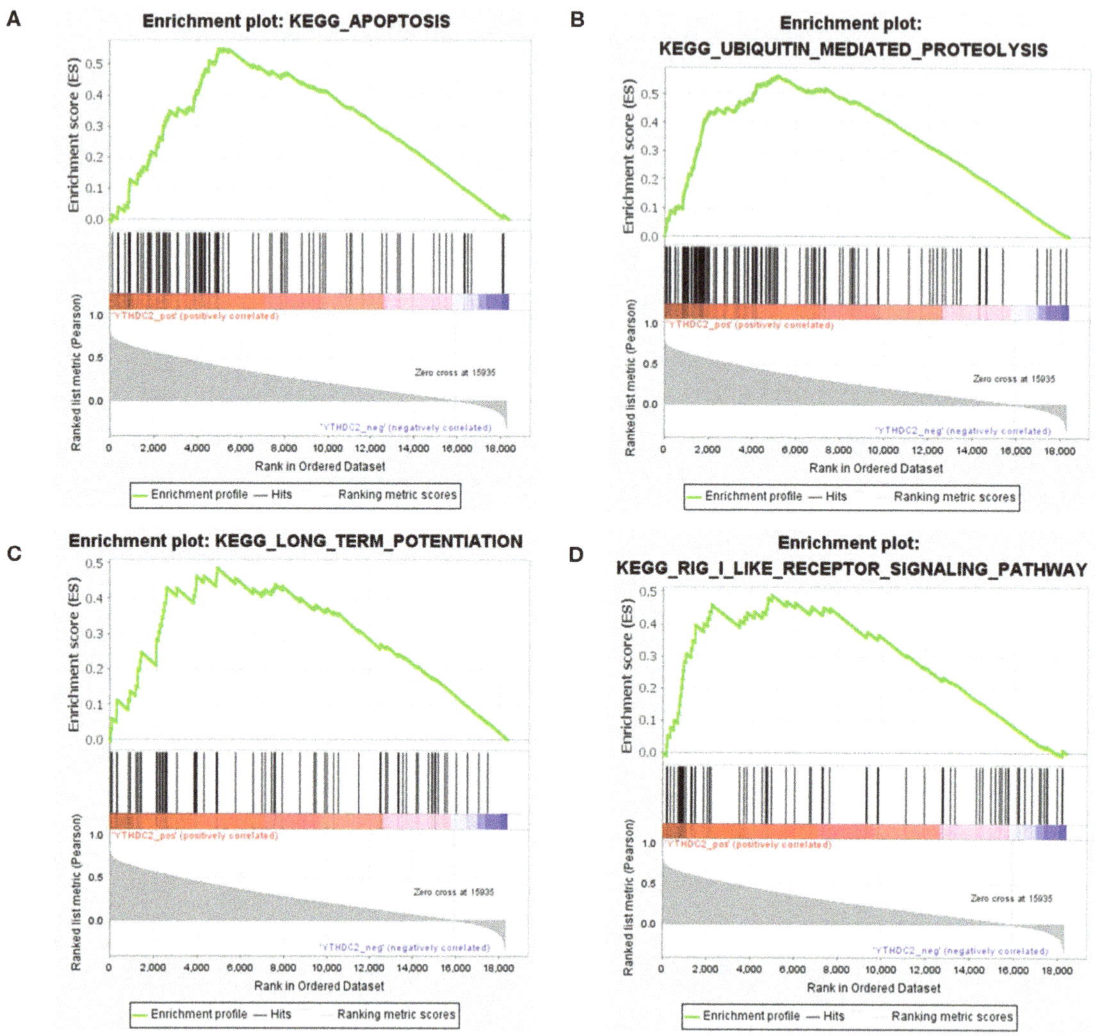

FIGURE 9 | GSEA results of different expression levels of YTHDC2. Gene set enrichment plots of **(A)** apoptosis, **(B)** ubiquitin-mediated proteolysis, **(C)** long-term potentiation, and **(D)** rig-i-like receptor signaling pathways related to low METTL3 mRNA level in the HNSCC samples.

associated with OS, here there were eight m6A regulatory genes that were significantly correlated with patient OS. In our study, patients with high expression of *ALKBH5*, *FTO*, *METTL14*, *WTAP*, *YTHDC1*, *YTHDF1*, and *YTHDF2* predicted poor patient prognosis. In BRC cohort, high expression levels of *YTHDF1*, *YTHDF3*, and *KIAA1429* predicted unfavorable patient prognosis. The two populations presented almost completely different prognostic genes. In the AML cohort, patients without m6A mutation had longer survival times. In HNSCC cases, we observed longer OS with diploid or copy number gain, which is different from the situation in AML but similar to that of ccRCC. These results showed that survival of patients with different types of tumors is related to different CNV patterns and different m6A regulatory gene abundance, which is a very attractive feature of m6A epigenetics.

In addition, the expression level of *ALKBH5* is a promising independent prognostic factor for HNSCC, suggesting that *ALKBH5* can be used as a new biomarker of HNSCC. In agreement with our study, some groups have reported that *ALKBH5* could serve as a novel prognostic biomarker that predicts a poor prognosis in colorectal (30) and pancreatic cancers (31).

Finally, we observed another interesting phenomenon. The HNSCC samples with higher *YTHDC2* expression were associated with longer-term survival, which is in contrast to the other m6A genes. *YTHDC2* has been identified as a frequently mutated gene in pancreatic cancer patients and plays a role in tumor metastasis by increasing the translational efficiency of HIF-1α (32, 33). Our IHC staining showed that the expression of *YTHDC2* in tumors was higher than that in normal tissues (**Figure 8**). Furthermore, by neural network and random forest methods, we found that *YTHDC2* was the most important gene among the 10 m6A regulatory genes. These results suggest that *YTHDC2* might play an

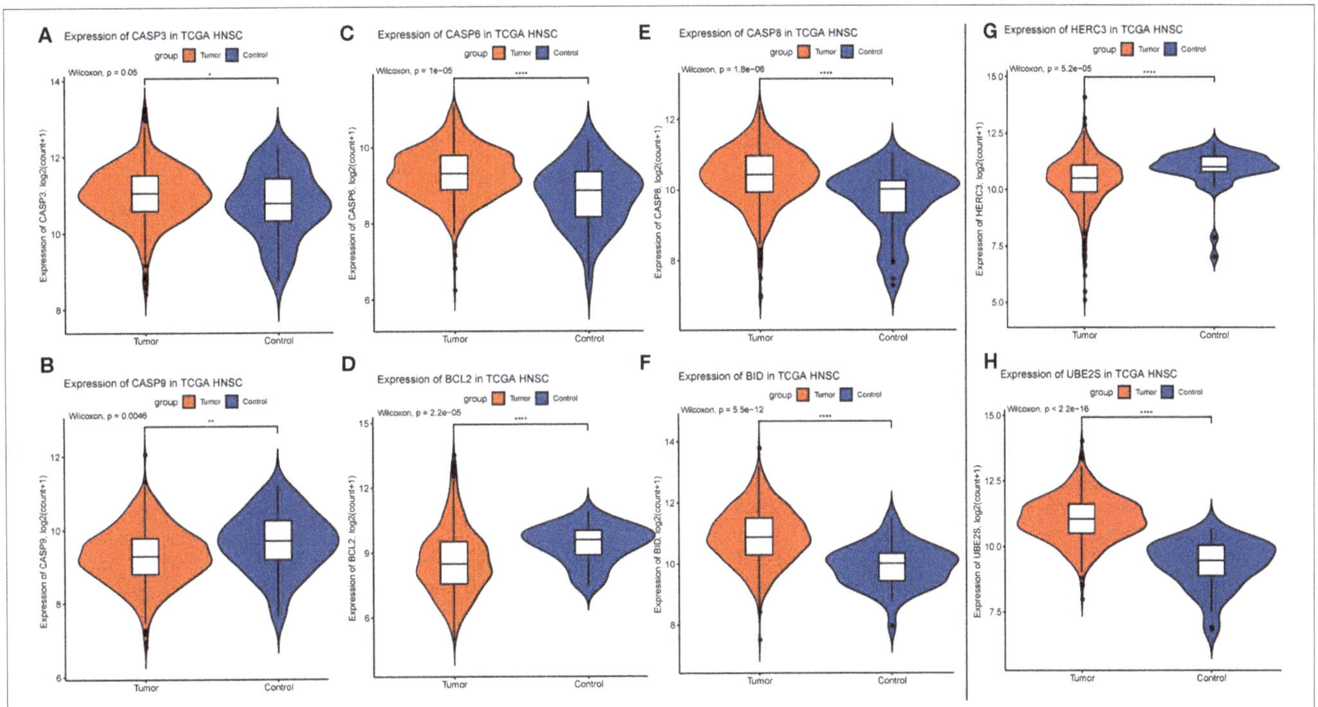

FIGURE 10 | Expression of genes related to apoptosis and ubiquitin-mediated proteolysis. **(A)** CASP3, **(B)** CASP9, **(C)** CASP6, **(D)** BCL2, **(E)** CASP8, **(F)** BID, **(G)** HERC3, **(H)** UBE2S.

important role in HNSCC. However, why did patients with higher *YTHDC2* expression have better prognoses? It has been found that *YTHDC2* is an m6A-binding protein that plays critical roles during spermatogenesis (34). The translation efficiency of *Smc3* (target *YTHDC2* in spermatogenesis) is significantly decreased in *YTHDC2-/-* mice compared to *YTHDC2 +/+* animals. In addition, the testes and epididymis from adult *YTHDC2-/-* mice are smaller in size than wild type (*YTHDC2 +/+*). These results show that high *YTHDC2* expression is beneficial for spermatogenesis, which might partly explain why high expression of *YTHDC2* was associated with prolonged OS. However, more work is needed to explore such a mechanism.

The development of HNSCC is related to a series of cancer-related pathways that become uncontrolled. In our HNSCC population, we found that high levels of *YTHDC2* mRNA expression are related to apoptotic activation and the ubiquitin-mediated proteolysis pathway, which are two very important cellular processes in the development of HNSCC. *METTL3* and *METTL14* are the most widely studied m6A regulatory genes in various cancers (24, 35). To date, only one study has reported that m6A is associated with HNSCC, in which *METTL3*-mediated *ZNF750* repression facilitates NPC progression. *METTL3* can promote apoptosis in gastric (36) and breast cancer cells (37) and is associated with ubiquitin-dependent process in pancreatic cancer cells (38). These pathways are similar to those involving *YTHDC2*. Due to the lack of research concerning *YTHDC2*, further studies are needed to verify our findings. However, there is no doubt that our results point out a new direction for the study of m6A in the pathogenesis and progression of HNSCC.

CONCLUSION

In HNSCC patients, a majority of highly expressed m6A regulatory genes is associated with poor OS, in particular *ALKBH5*, whereas *YTHDC2* was associated with better prognosis. We identified, for the first time, the expression characteristics and prognosis of m6A regulatory genes in patients with HNSCC. Our results will provide a direction for further exploration of the pathogenesis of HNSCC.

ETHICS STATEMENT

All clinical data, sequence profiles, and CNV data were extracted using UCSC-XENA and the TCGA database, which is open to the public under certain conditions. Therefore, it can be confirmed that all written informed consent forms are available. The study using human oral squamous cell carcinoma tissue and oral mucosa samples for IHC staining was approved by the Ethics Committee of Shandong Provincial Hospital affiliated to Shandong First Medical University. We obtained written informed consent from all participants.

AUTHOR CONTRIBUTIONS

XCZ and XYZ mainly performed experiments and data analysis. LD performed IHC of clinical specimens. JH and YL provided intellectual support and expertise in the field of cancer pathology. XCZ, ZC, and SX wrote the manuscript. JH and ZY designated all experiments in this study. All authors contributed to the critical review of the manuscript.

REFERENCES

1. Haddad RI, Shin DM. Recent advances in head and neck cancer. *The New England journal of medicine.* (2008) 359:1143–54. doi: 10.1056/NEJMra0707975
2. Bray F, Ferlay J, Soerjomataram I, Siegel RL, Torre LA, Jemal A. Global cancer statistics. *Cancer J Clin.* (2011) 61:69–90. doi: 10.3322/caac.20107
3. Chen W, Zheng R, Baade PD, Zhang S, Zeng H, Bray F, et al. Cancer statistics in China 2015. *Cancer J Clin.* (2016) 66:115–32. doi: 10.3322/caac.21338
4. Siegel RL, Miller KD, Jemal A. Cancer statistics, 2015. *CA Cancer J Clin.* (2015) 65:5–29. doi: 10.3322/caac.21254
5. Hashibe M, Brennan P, Chuang SC, Boccia S, Castellsague X, Chen C, et al. Interaction between tobacco and alcohol use and the risk of head and neck cancer. Pooled analysis in the International Head and Neck Cancer Epidemiology Consortium. *Cancer Epidemiol Biomarkers Prev.* (2009) 18:541–50. doi: 10.1158/1055-9965
6. Fu Y, Dominissini D, Rechavi G, He C. Gene expression regulation mediated through reversible m(6)A RNA methylation. *Nat Rev Genet.* (2014) 15:293–306. doi: 10.1038/nrg3724
7. Chen XY, Zhang J, Zhu JS. The role of m(6)A RNA methylation in human cancer. *Mol Cancer.* (2019) 18:103. doi: 10.1186/s12943-019-1033-z
8. Cao G, Li HB, Yin Z, Flavell RA. Recent advances in dynamic m6A RNA modification. *Open Biol.* (2016) 6:160003. doi: 10.1098/rsob.160003
9. Gallagher EJ, LeRoith D. Obesity and diabetes. The increased risk of cancer and cancer-related mortality. *Physiol Rev.* (2015) 95:727–48. doi: 10.1152/physrev.00030.2014
10. Wei W, Ji X, Guo X, Ji S. Regulatory role of N(6) -methyladenosine (m(6) A) methylation in RNA processing and human diseases. *J Cell Biochem.* (2017) 118:2534–43. doi: 10.1002/jcb.25967
11. Huang Y, Su R, Sheng Y, Dong L, Dong Z, Xu H, et al. Small-Molecule targeting of oncogenic FTO demethylase in acute myeloid leukemia. *Cancer Cell.* (2019) 35:677–91.e610. doi: 10.1016/j.ccell.2019.03.006
12. Cui Q, Shi H, Ye P, Li L, Qu Q, Sun G, et al. m(6)A RNA methylation regulates the self-renewal and tumorigenesis of glioblastoma stem cells. *Cell Rep.* (2017) 18:2622–34. doi: 10.1016/j.celrep.2017.02.059
13. Liu J, Ren D, Du Z, Wang H, Zhang H, Jin Y. m(6)A demethylase FTO facilitates tumor progression in lung squamous cell carcinoma by regulating MZF1 expression. *Biochem Biophys Res Commun.* (2018) 502:456–64. doi: 10.1016/j.bbrc.2018.05.175
14. Ma JZ, Yang F, Zhou CC, Liu F, Yuan JH, Wang F, et al. METTL14 suppresses the metastatic potential of hepatocellular carcinoma by modulating N(6) -methyladenosine-dependent primary MicroRNA processing. *Hepatology.* (2017) 65:529–43. doi: 10.1002/hep.28885
15. Cai X, Wang X, Cao C, Gao Y, Zhang S, Yang Z, et al. HBXIP-elevated methyltransferase METTL3 promotes the progression of breast cancer via inhibiting tumor suppressor let-7g. *Cancer Lett.* (2018) 415:11–19. doi: 10.1016/j.canlet.2017.11.018
16. Mayakonda A, Lin DC, Assenov Y, Plass C, Koeffler HP. Maftools: efficient and comprehensive analysis of somatic variants in cancer. *Genome Res.* (2018) 28:1747–56. doi: 10.1101/gr.239244.118
17. Mermel CH, Schumacher SE, Hill B, Meyerson ML, Beroukhim R, Getz G. GISTIC2.0 facilitates sensitive and confident localization of the targets of focal somatic copy-number alteration in human cancers. *Genome Biol.* (2011) 12:R41. doi: 10.1186/gb-2011-12-4-r41
18. Kassambara. A, Kosinski M. *survminer: Drawing Survival Curves using 'ggplot2'.* R package version 0.4.3. (2018). Available online at: https://CRAN.R-project.org/package=survminer.
19. *A Package for Survival Analysis in S_. version 2.38.* (2015). Available online at: https://CRAN.R-project.org/package=survival.
20. Warde-Farley D, Donaldson SL, Comes O, Zuberi K, Badrawi R, Chao P, et al. The GeneMANIA prediction server. biological network integration for gene prioritization and predicting gene function. *Nucleic acids Res.* (2010) 38(Web Server issue):W214–220. doi: 10.1093/nar/gkq537
21. Kwok CT, Marshall AD, Rasko JE, Wong JJ. Genetic alterations of m(6)A regulators predict poorer survival in acute myeloid leukemia. *J Hematol Oncol.* (2017) 10:39. doi: 10.1186/s13045-017-0410-6
22. Zhou J, Wang J, Hong B, Ma K, Xie H, Li L, et al. Gene signatures and prognostic values of m6A regulators in clear cell renal cell carcinoma - a retrospective study using TCGA database. *Aging.* (2019) 11:1633–47. doi: 10.18632/aging.101856
23. Sridharan S, Thompson LDR, Purgina B, Sturgis CD, Shah AA, Burkey B, et al. Early squamous cell carcinoma of the oral tongue with histologically benign lymph nodes. A model predicting local control and vetting of the eighth edition of the American Joint Committee on Cancer pathologic T stage. *Cancer.* (2019) 125:3198–207. doi: 10.1002/cncr.32199
24. Liu J, Yue Y, Han D, Wang X, Fu Y, Zhang L, et al. A METTL3-METTL14 complex mediates mammalian nuclear RNA N6-adenosine methylation. *Nat Chem Biol.* (2014) 10:93–5. doi: 10.1038/nchembio.1432
25. Ping XL, Sun BF, Wang L, Xiao W, Yang X, Wang WJ, et al. Mammalian WTAP is a regulatory subunit of the RNA N6-methyladenosine methyltransferase. *Cell Res.* (2014) 24:177–89. doi: 10.1038/cr.2014.3
26. Zhang P, He Q, Lei Y, Li Y, Wen X, Hong M, et al. m(6)A-mediated ZNF750 repression facilitates nasopharyngeal carcinoma progression. *Cell Death Dis.* (2018) 9:1169. doi: 10.1038/s41419-018-1224-3
27. Zhang S, Zhao BS, Zhou A, Lin K, Zheng S, Lu Z, et al. m(6)A demethylase ALKBH5 maintains tumorigenicity of glioblastoma stem-like cells by sustaining FOXM1 expression and cell proliferation program. *Cancer Cell.* (2017) 31:591–606 e596. doi: 10.1016/j.ccell.2017.02.013
28. Li Z, Weng H, Su R, Weng X, Zuo Z, Li C, et al. FTO plays an oncogenic role in acute myeloid leukemia as a N(6)-methyladenosine RNA demethylase. *Cancer Cell.* (2017) 31:127–41. doi: 10.1016/j.ccell.2016.11.017
29. Zhang C, Zhi WI, Lu H, Samanta D, Chen I, Gabrielson E, et al. Hypoxia-inducible factors regulate pluripotency factor expression by ZNF217- and ALKBH5-mediated modulation of RNA methylation in breast cancer cells. *Oncotarget.* (2016) 7:64527–42. doi: 10.18632/oncotarget.11743
30. Liu X, Liu L, Dong Z, Li J, Yu Y, Chen X, et al. Expression patterns and prognostic value of m(6)A-related genes in colorectal cancer. *Am J Trans Res.* (2019) 11:3972–91.
31. Cho SH, Ha M, Cho YH, Ryu JH, Yang K, Lee KH, et al. ALKBH5 gene is a novel biomarker that predicts the prognosis of pancreatic cancer: A retrospective multicohort study. *Ann Hepato—Pancr Surg.* (2018) 22:305–9. doi: 10.14701/ahbps.2018.22.4.305
32. Fanale D, Iovanna JL, Calvo EL, Berthezene P, Belleau P, Dagorn JC, et al. Germline copy number variation in the YTHDC2 gene: does it have a role in finding a novel potential molecular target involved in pancreatic adenocarcinoma susceptibility? *Exp Opin Thera Targ.* (2014) 18:841–50. doi: 10.1517/14728222.2014.920324
33. Tanabe A, Tanikawa K, Tsunetomi M, Takai K, Ikeda H, Konno J, et al. RNA helicase YTHDC2 promotes cancer metastasis via the enhancement of the efficiency by which HIF-1alpha mRNA is translated. *Cancer Lett.* (2016) 376:34–42. doi: 10.1016/j.canlet.2016.02.022
34. Hsu PJ, Zhu Y, Ma H, Guo Y, Shi X, Liu Y, et al. Ythdc2 is an N(6)-methyladenosine binding protein that regulates mammalian spermatogenesis. *Cell Res.* (2017) 27:1115–27. doi: 10.1038/cr.2017.99
35. Bokar JA, Shambaugh ME, Polayes D, Matera AG, Rottman FM. Purification and cDNA cloning of the AdoMet-binding subunit of the human mRNA (N6-adenosine)-methyltransferase. *RNA.* (1997) 3:1233–47.

36. He H, Wu W, Sun Z, Chai L. MiR-4429 prevented gastric cancer progression through targeting METTL3 to inhibit m(6)A-caused stabilization of SEC62. *Biochem Biophys Res Commun.* (2019) 517:581–7. doi: 10.1016/j.bbrc.2019.07.058
37. Wang H, Xu B, Shi J. N6-methyladenosine METTL3 promotes the breast cancer progression via targeting Bcl-2. *Gene.* (2020) 722:144076. doi: 10.1016/j.gene.2019.144076
38. Taketo K, Konno M, Asai A, Koseki J, Toratani M, Satoh T, et al. The epitranscriptome m6A writer METTL3 promotes chemo- and radioresistance in pancreatic cancer cells. *Int J Oncol.* (2018) 52:621–9. doi: 10.3892/ijo.2017.4219

20

Susceptibility of Multiple Primary Cancers in Patients with Head and Neck Cancer: Nature or Nurture?

Wei-long Zhang [1†], Zhuo-li Zhu [1†], Mei-chang Huang [1], Ya-Jie Tang [2], Ya-ling Tang [1] and Xin-hua Liang [1*]*

[1] State Key Laboratory of Oral Diseases, National Clinical Research Center for Oral Diseases, West China Hospital of Stomatology, Sichuan University, Chengdu, China, [2] State Key Laboratory of Microbial Technology, Shandong University, Qingdao, China

***Correspondence:**
Ya-ling Tang
tangyaling@scu.edu.cn
Xin-hua Liang
lxh88866@scu.edu.cn*

† These authors have contributed equally to this work

Multiple primary cancers (MPCs) are major obstacles to long-term survival in head and neck cancer (HNSCC), however, the molecular mechanism underlying multiple carcinogenesis remains unclear. "Field cancerization" is a classical theory to elaborate the malignant progression of MPCs. Apart from environmental and immune factors, genetic factors may have great potential as molecular markers for MPCs risk prediction. This review focuses on inherited and acquired gene mutations in MPCs, including germ-line mutation, single-nucleotide polymorphism, chromosomal instability, microsatellite instability and DNA methylation. And definition and prognosis of MPCs have also been discussed. These may pave the way for the early detection, prevention and effective treatment of MPCs in HNSCC.

Keywords: head and neck cancer, multiple primary cancer, field cancerization, cancer-associated fibroblasts, genetic factor, biomarker

INTRODUCTION

Head and neck squamous cancer (HNSCC) ranks sixth among the most prevalent malignancies in the world (1). It is estimated that HNSCC accounts for 64,690 new cases and 13,740 deaths in the United states in 2018 (2). Although significant improvements have been made in the therapeutic modalities, the prognosis of HNSCC remains stagnant in the past decades, with a 5-year survival of only 50% (3). The dismal prognosis has always been attributed to local recurrences, distant metastasis, and development of multiple primary cancers (MPCs).

MPCs are defined as two or more primary cancers occurring in an individual synchronously or metachronously, neither extensions, recurrences nor metastases of each other (International Agency for Research on Cancer), which accounts for approximately one-third of deaths in HNSCC (4, 5). MPCs are also named as second primary malignancies (SPMs), secondary primary tumors (SPTs), second primary cancers (SPCs), and multiple primary tumors (MPTs) (6). Several risk factors, including smoking exposure, alcohol consumption, human papilloma virus (HPV), and hepatitis C virus (HCV), have been suggested to be associated with the development of MPCs (7–10). However, researches revealed that a major proportion of MPCs could not be fully explained by these environmental factors, and genetic factors, such as single-nucleotide polymorphism (SNP), chromosomal instability (CIN), microsatellite instability (MSI), and epigenetic alterations, may contribute to the susceptibility of MPCs in HNSCC (11).

MPCs have been considered to be a clinical quandary both in diagnosis and treatment. It is challenging for the oncologists to distinguish MPCs from a metastasis or local recurrence merely on the basis of clinical and pathological information. Furthermore, this classification leaves a profound effect on the choice of treatment as well as patients' prognosis. Recently, there are a number of novel screening strategies for MPCs prediction, such as genetic markers, and the role of genetic alterations in the development of MPCs after index HNSCC were not fully elucidated (12). Here, we conducted this review to summarize the mechanisms and relevant genetic alterations of MPCs, which might provide benefit in the detection, prevention, and treatment of MPCs in HNSCC.

DEFINITION AND PROGNOSIS OF MPCs

In 1932, Warren and Gates published the classical clinical criteria of SPT, being (1) each of the malignancies must have been verified by histologic examination, (2) the malignancies must be anatomical separate by normal mucosa, and (3) exclude the possibility that the second malignancy represents a metastasis of the index tumor (13). However, this clinical definition carries the risk of misclassification and inability to differentiate between an SPT, a recurrence and a metastasis (14). For example, what distance should lie between the malignancies? How to define the normal mucosa, by naked eye or histologic examination? How to distinguish the SPT from a metastasis or a recurrence? To solve this dilemma, Braakhuis et al. proposed a new classification on the basis of molecular profiles of the tumors and the genetically altered mucosal field between the tumors (14). Tumors displaying distinct molecular profiles or sharing a common pattern attributed to chance are defined as SPTs, while those possessing similar molecular aberration are defined as local recurrences (14).

It is widely accepted that MPCs are the leading obstacle to long-term survival among HNSCC patients (15). According to a retrospective study conducted by Shiga et al., patients with synchronous SPMs displayed a poorer 5-year overall survival rate than those with metachromous SPMs in Japan (16). In line with this result, Bugter et al. claimed that the 5-yearsurvival rate for synchronous and metachronous primary cancer patients was 25 and 85%, respectively (17). The higher proportion of high-stage tumor in the synchronous primary cancer patients and unadjusted treatment protocol may account for this discrepancy.

However, accumulating evidence has demonstrated that HPV-positive HNSCC patients were accompanied by a decreased risk for SPT than HPV-negative HNSCC patients (18–20). HPV has been established as an emerging carcinogen in a subset of HNSCCs, particularly in the oropharynx (21). HPV-positive HNSCCs differ from HPV-negative HNSCCs induced by tobacco and alcohol epidemiologically, clinically, and biologically (22–24). The putative reasons for this phenomenon are as follows: (1) HPV-positive HNSCCs exhibited higher sensitivity to radiotherapy and chemotherapy (25); (2) HPV-positive HNSCCs often arise in an environment with lower exposure to tobacco and displayed fewer smoking-related genetic abnormalities, which is less associated with smoking-related SPTs (26–28); (3) Saito et al. suggested that field cancerization effect would not be observed in HPV-positive HNSCCs, since HPV viral DNA integration was limited to the cancerous tissue (29). However, the concrete mechanisms between HPV-positive HNSCCs and SPTs are remained to be elucidated in the future.

The dismal clinical outcome of MPCs in HNSCC emphasizes on the importance of early diagnosis and prevention. These genetic alterations could serve as molecular makers to guide the early diagnosis, prevention and treatment of HNSCC patients in several aspects. Firstly, these molecular markers could be readily obtained by the primary tumor samples without bringing additional invasion to patients (30). Secondly, genetic markers could select the high-risk individuals for MPCs, which should be under strict cancer surveillance and proper preventive procedures. Given the discrepancies between HPV-positive and HPV-negative HNSCC, Jain et al. proposed that future screening procedures for MPCs may be adjusted by HPV and smoking status (31). Thirdly, in-depth understanding of the role of these molecular markers in MPCs may pave the way for targeted gene therapies. In addition, genetic markers could be utilized to distinguish MPCs from a local recurrence or a metastasis. For example, Mercer et al. showed that microsatellite PCR facilitated the discrimination between second primary cancer and metastatic HNSCC (32). Daher et al. employed combined HPV typing and TP53 mutational profiling successfully identified the accurate origin of lung tumors in 32 HNSCC patients, in which only 13 cases were diagnosed correctly on the basis of clinical and morphological data alone (33). Apart from physical and pathological information, genetic profiles analysis could be an effective tool to distinguish MPCs from a recurrence. Gasparotto et al. suggested that 3 clinically diagnosed recurrences and 2 lung lesions were actually MPTs by comparing the p53 mutation status of primary tumors and corresponding recurrences/metastases in HNSCC patients (34). Microsatellite analysis indicated that 6 tumors showing clonally-related patterns with primary tumors were recurrences, while 17 tumors with clonally-unrelated patterns were SPTs in 23 HNSCC patients with genetic changes (35).

MECHANISM OF MPCs

The concrete molecular mechanism underlying multiple carcinogenesis remains unclear. "Field cancerization" theory has often been applied to explain the occurrence of MPCs (**Figure 1**). The stem cell receives one (or more) genetic hit (**Figure 1A**), probably a mutation of *p53* gene, and gives rise to a patch with genetically altered daughter cells [(36); **Figure 1B**]. Then a subsequent genetic alteration induces the patch to spread in a lateral direction and substitutes the normal epithelial cells to form a field [(36); **Figure 1C**]. As the field expands at the expense of normal epithelial cells, additional genetic alterations take place and promote the progression from field to an overt carcinoma (**Figure 1D**). The second tumor of monoclonal origin develops by implantation, intraepithelial migration or sub-mucosal spread of primary cancer cells (**Figure 1E**), while the polyclonal

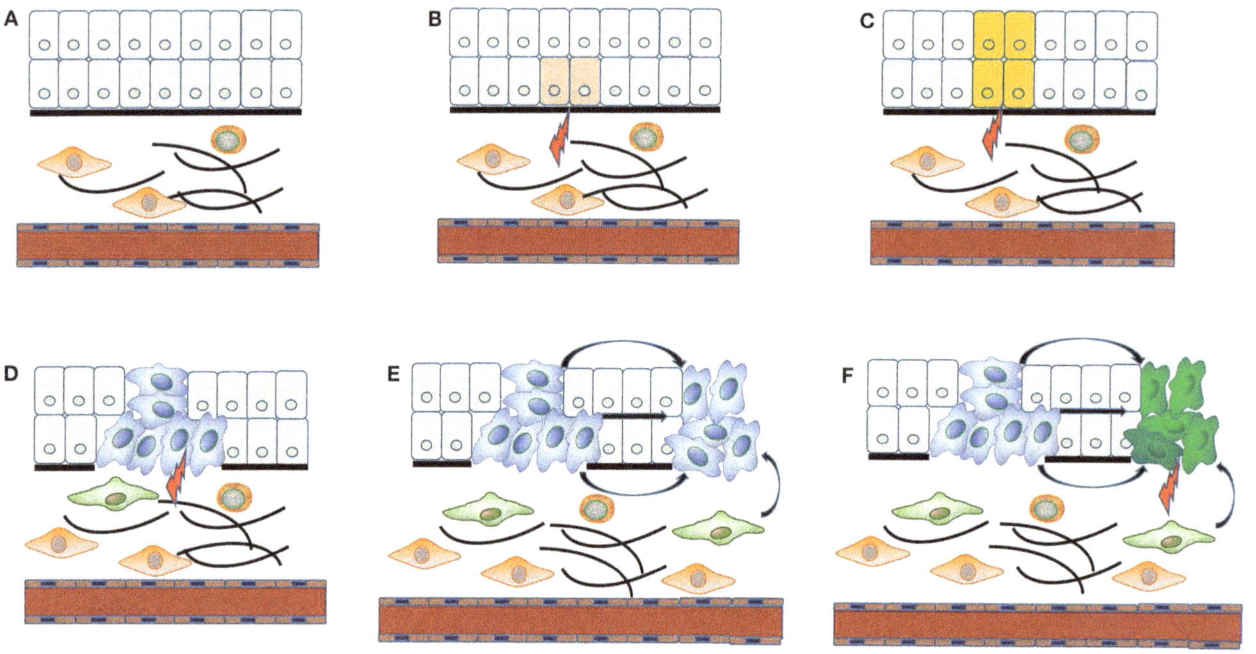

FIGURE 1 | "Field cancerization" theory in the MPCs of HNSCC. The stem cell receives first genetic hit **(A)**, and gives rise to a patch with genetically altered daughter cells **(B)**. Then a patch develops into a field by expanding in a lateral direction under the indduction of a second genetic hit **(C)**. Additional genetic alterations take place and convert the field to an overt carcinoma **(D)**. The implantation, intraepithelial migration or sub-mucosal spread of primary cancer cells lead to the development of a SPT with monoclonal origin **(E)**, while the final genetic hit induces the occurrence of a SPT with polyclonal origin **(F)**.

second tumor forms under the induction of final genetic hit [(14, 37); **Figure 1F**].

Failure of immune surveillance also contributed to the occurrence of SPTs in HNSCC (**Figure 2**). Patients with decreased T-cell numbers in the circulation were predisposed to infections, disease recurrence, or a second malignancy (38). Kuss et al. reported that CD4+ and CD8+ T cells were significantly reduced in the SPT group relative to normal control group in HNSCCs (38). And patients with recurrences or SPTs showed a 25% lower number of CD4+ T cells than those with primary disease (38). The TCR associated CD3 zeta chain plays a critical role in the signal transduction of T-cell activation, the absence of which impairs T-cell signaling and consequently leads to immune dysfunction (39). Kuss et al. concluded that individuals with SPTs or recurrences exhibited lowest zeta-chain expression, which might exert long-lasting negative effects on the anti-tumor immune response (40). Decreased expression of HLA class I molecules is considered to be an effective strategy for malignant cells to evade host immunosurveillance (41). Grandis et al. suggested that the number of HLA allelic loss increased the risk of developing a new primary tumor (41). Collectively, decreased T-cell numbers, CD3 zeta chain and HLA class I molecules may be associated with the development of SPT, which may provide new opportunities for cancer immunotherapy in HNSCC.

In addition, cancer-associated fibroblasts (CAFs) may play an unneglectable role in the development of field cancerization [(42); **Figure 2**]. Ge et al. proposed that migratory cancer-associated fibroblasts (CAFs), also named myofibroblast, may appear beneath the cluster of genetic altered epithelial cells, and ultimately lead to the malignant transformation of these cells (42). Angadi et al. demonstrated that myofibroblasts were present in the stroma around the oral squamous cell carcinoma (OSCC) cell as well as the connective tissue below the histologically normal mucosa adjacent to OSCC by immunochemistry, which validates Ge's hypothesis further (43). Chan et al. indicated that cancer-associated fibroblasts promoted field cancerization by elevating the expression of reactive oxygen species (ROS) in the microenvironment (44). CAFs from squamous cell carcinoma reduced the expression of Smad3 and cJUN to suppress the activity of glutathione peroxidase 1 (GPX1), one key enzyme affecting hydrogen peroxide detoxification. Suppression of GPX1 leads to elevation of extracellular hydrogen peroxide, which facilitates the conversion of normal fibroblast to CAF phenotype, and promotes the tumor-forming capacity and invasiveness. Till now, there is no more available evidences on the role of tumor microenvironment in MPCs, including macrophages, myeloid-derived suppressor cells (MDSCs) and etc., which warrants further investigation in the future.

MPCs AND INHERITED MUTATIONS

MPCs and Germ-Line Mutations

Germ-line mutation of tumor suppressor genes has been considered to be a potential driver of MPCs. *p53* gene, known as the "the guardian of the genome," is an well-known tumor

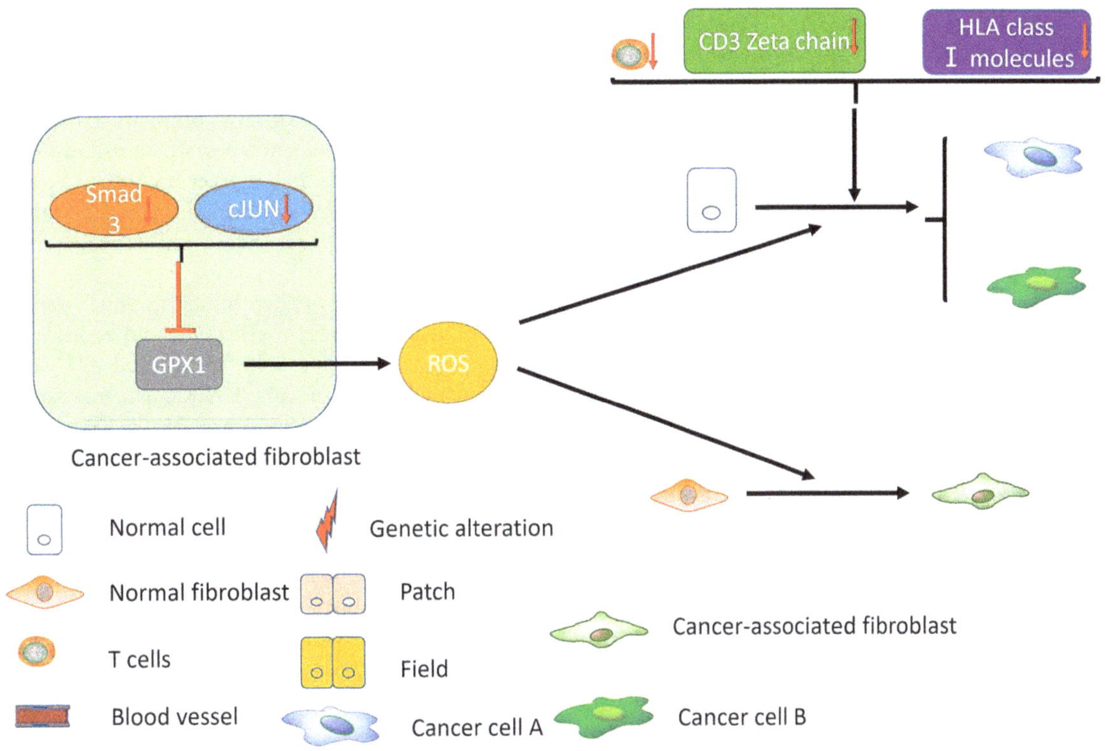

FIGURE 2 | Immune factors and CAFs contribute to the development of MPCs. Decreased T-cell numbers, CD3 zeta chain and HLA class I molecules may promote the development of MPCs by inducing immunosuppression. In the CAFs, reduced expression of Smad3 and cJUN suppress the activity of GPX1, leading to the elevation of extracellular hydrogen peroxide. High hydrogen peroxide level in the microenvironment induces the conversion of normal fibroblast to CAF phenotype, and promotes the occurrence of MPCs.

suppressor gene which has been involved in the cell cycle control and DNA repair (45). It is estimated that *p53* gene was mutated in approximately 50% of HNSCC patients (46). In 1999, Gallo and his colleagues employed polymerase chain reaction single-strand conformation polymorphism (PCR-SSCP) analysis and DNA sequencing to examine the *p53* germ-line mutations in 24 HNSCC patients who developed MPCs and their first-degree relatives. As a consequence, only one missense mutation in exon 6 as well as two same-sense mutations in exon 6 and 8 have been detected (47). So the authors proposed that *p53* gene might not be the only target responsible for the multiple genetic alterations of field cancerization (47).

CDKN2A, a tumor suppressor gene exerting an important role in the regulation of cell cycle, is associated with the occurrence of HNSCC. Cabanillas et al. proposed that germ-line mutations of *CDKN2A* gene may serve as a common feature of HNSCC (30). However, Jefferies et al. screened full coding sequence of *CDKN2A* gene and failed to detect any germ-line mutations in 40 HNSCC patients with a SPC, which suggested that germ-line mutations of *CDKN2A* contributed less to the susceptibility of MPCs (48).

Mismatch genes, such as *hMLHI*, contribute greatly to the MPCs of gastrointestinal cancers. Nevertheless, its germ-lime mutations don't seem to be an major event in the carcinogenesis of HNSCC or MPTs (49). Piccinin et al. analyzed the mutations of *hMLHI* gene by PCR-SSCP and sequencing in 67 HNSCC patients, 22 MPTs and 45 controls, and no somatic or germ-lime mutations of hMLHI have been identified (49).

Based on the above, it seems that germ-line mutations of certain tumor suppressor genes and DNA repair genes, including *p53*, *CDKN2A*, and *hMLHI*, exert a minor influence on the genetic predisposition of MPCs after index HNSCC.

MPCs and SNPs

It is estimated that SNP accounts for up to 90% of genetic variability (50). Researchers have demonstrated that genetic polymorphisms of various genes were correlated with the risk of MPCs in HNSCC. Based on their functions, these genes could be classified into four categories: tumor suppressor genes, oncogenes, DNA repair genes and carcinogen metabolism-related genes, which were listed in detail as follows.

SNPs of Tumor Suppressor Genes

p53 makes a substantial contribution to the regulation of cell cycle, cellular apoptosis and anti-cancer properties (45). *p53* mutations have been shown to be correlated with the occurrence of primary HNSCC as well as SPMs (51). The polymorphism of *p53* commonly occurred at the codon 72, with a substitution of proline for arginine, which might promote the carcinogenesis by disturbing the apoptosis process and cell cycle (52). Several studies indicated that *p53* codon 72 polymorphism may play a minor role in the development of HNSCC (53, 54). However, Li et al. showed that patients with *p53* 72Arg/Pro and the combined *p53* 72Arg/Pro + Pro/Pro genotypes exhibited a significantly greater risk of SPMs in a cohort of 1271 HNSCC patients, compared with *p53* 72Arg/Arg genotype (51). The authors speculated that *p53* codon 72 polymorphism may influence the SPM risk by modifying the response to DNA-damaging treatments (51). Despite the inherited limitations of patient selection and clinical outcome collection, these results indicated that *p53* codon 72 polymorphism could serve as a genetic marker to evaluate the risk of SPMs in HNSCC.

Functionally, tumor suppressor gene *p14* and *p73* belong to the *p53*-related gene family. $p14^{ARF}$ gene maps to 9p21 and encodes proteins of $p16^{INK4a}$ and $p14^{ARF}$, thus playing an important role in maintaining genomic stability via *p53* and *Rb* pathways (6). Direct interaction between $p14^{ARF}$ and *MDM2* impedes the protesomal degradation of p53, resulting in an abnormal cell cycle regulation and cellular apoptosis (55). Genetic Alterations of $p14^{ARF}$ have been considered to be rare in the development of HNSCC. Gruttgen et al. evaluated the p14 expression with immunochemistry, and concluded that loss of $p14^{ARF}$ merely occurred in 15 of 100 HNSCC patients (56). Zhang et al. stated that $p14^{\mathrm{ARF}}$-rs3088440 and rs3731217 polymorphisms were correlated with a moderately increased risk of SPMs in HNSCC (6). Compared with those without $p14^{ARF}$ variant genotypes, HNSCC patients with both variant genotypes had a 3-fold increased risk for developing SPMs (6). Therefore, $p14^{ARF}$ polymorphisms could serve as a risk marker for SPMs in HNSCC patients (6).

p73 displays a similar function as *p53* in the regulation of cell cycle, apoptosis and DNA repair by inducing apoptosis or G1 cell cycle arrest (57). It has been assumed that *p73* compensated for the absence of *p53* induced by mutations (58). Previous studies have revealed that genetic abnormalities of *p73*, such as its G4C14-to-A4T14 polymorphism, were associated the risk of HNSCC (59, 60). Li et al. investigated the role of *p73* G4C14-to-A4T14 polymorphism in SPMs in a cohort of 1384 HNSCC patients, and advocated that patients carrying *p73* GC/AT heterozygotes or the combined *p73* GC/AT+AT/AT genotypes had a significantly lower SPM susceptibility, compared to those with *p73* GC/GC genotype. The *p73* GC/AT+AT/AT genotypes conferred a pronounced protection over SPMs in several subgroups, for example, older patients, men, minorities, ever smoker, and ever drinkers, further supporting the role of *p73* polymorphism as a genetic marker of MPCs in HNSCC patients (61).

FAS belongs to the death receptor family and interacts with its ligand, *FASLG*, to modulate the extrinsic apoptosis pathway, cellular homeostasis and immune escape of tumor cells (62, 63). Genetic alterations of the *FAS/FASLG* signaling pathway may lead to immune evasion, thus facilitating tumorigenesis including SPM (64). *FAS*-1377G>A, *FAS*−670A>G, *FASLG*-844C>T, and *FASLG*-124 A>G are four well-known SNPs in the FAS/FASLG signaling pathway. Zhang et al. reported that subjects with both the *FAS*-1377 AA and *FAS*-670 (GG + AG) genotypes were associated with an increased risk of HNSCC, but not for those with *FASLG* variant genotypes (65). But things are really different when it comes to the incidence of MPCs. It has been demonstrated that patients carrying *FAS*-670 AG+GG genotypes or *FASLG*-844 CT+TT genotypes were significantly associated with mounting risk of SPMs compared with the wild-type homozygous genotypes, which makes *FAS* and *FASLG* polymorphisms a potential marker for HNSCC patients at high SPM risk (64). Additionally, the risk of SPM was augmented in a dose-response manner for those with increasing number of risk genotypes (64).

p21 and p27 are two CDK inhibitors which participate in the regulation of DNA repair, cell cycle, and apoptosis (66). It has been demonstrated that SNPs in *p21* and *p27* were associated with risk of HNSCC (67, 68). HNSCC patients carrying *p27* 109 TG/GG, *p21* 98 CA/AA, and *p21* 70 CT/TT variant genotypes had a worse survival and an increased SPM risk than those with *p27*109 TT, *p21* 98 CC, and *p21* 70 CC genotypes, respectively (69). Moreover, patients with *p27* (T109G) and *p21* (C98A and C70T) polymorphisms were 2.4 times more susceptible to develop MPCs than those without variant genotypes (69). These results indicated that *p27* T109G and *p21* (C98A and C70T) polymorphisms seem to modulate the susceptibility of SPMs in HNSCC.

Accumulating evidences have established that SNPs of tumor suppressor genes made a considerable contribution to the formation of MPCs in HNSCC, which makes SNPs of tumor suppressor genes a potential molecular marker to predict the risk of MPCs in HNSCC.

SNPs of Oncogenes

Murine double minute 2 (*MDM2*), also known as an E3 ubiquitin ligase, is the central antagonist of the tumor suppressor *p53* (70). MDM2 negatively regulates the activity of *p53* by suppressing its transcriptional activity and promoting its degradation, thus contributing to the carcinogenic process (71). The overexpression and genetic alterations of *MDM2* have been commonly reported in HNSCC (72). Two SNPs in its promoter region, *MDM2*-rs2279744 and *MDM2*-rs937283, may alter MDM2 expression at transcriptional level and subsequently modulate the risk of HNSCC (71). With respect to SPM, Jin et al. reported that *MDM2*-rs2279744 and *MDM2*-rs937283 increased the susceptibility of SPM in HNSCC by 90 and 20%, respectively (73).

Analogous to *MDM2* in structure, murine double minute 4 (*MDM4*) is also a negative regulator of *p53*. Several studies suggested that high *MDM4* expression may substitute for *p53* mutations, and *MDM4* overexpression was a common event in the HNSCC patients (74). Three *MDM4* SNPs, rs11801299G>A, rs1380576C>G, and rs10900598G>T, have been identified in HNSCC patients. Yu et al. proposed that individuals with combined 1-3 risk genotypes of *MDM4* SNPs exhibited significantly increased risk of oropharyngeal cancer (75). In a cohort of 1283 HNSCC patients, Jin et al. concluded that *MDM4*-rs11801299, *MDM4*-rs1380576, and *MDM4*-rs10900598 enhanced the incidence of SPMs in index HNSCC cases by 10, 10, and 40%, respectively (73). Collectively, *MDM2* and *MDM4* polymorphisms may increase the susceptibility of SPMs in HNSCC to some extent, which may improve the precision of risk estimates of SPMs.

SNPs of DNA Repair Genes

The MRN complex, composed of *MRE11*, *RAD50*, and *Nbs1*, plays a critical role in the double-strand break repair and telomere maintenance (76). To evaluate the role of *MRE11* and *RAD50* genes in HNSCC, Ziółkowska-Suchanek et al. conducted a case and control study of 358 HNSCC patients. Their results suggested that common variants of *MRE11* and *RAD50* genes contributed little to the occurrence of HNSCC and SPTs located in the head and neck region (77). *XRCC3*, short for X-ray repair cross-complementing group 3, is another important gene which participates in the double-strand break repair (78). Several studies revealed that *XRCC3* C18067T polymorphism may play a minor role in the etiology of primary HNSCC as well as MPTs. (78, 79).

The X-ray repair cross-complementing group 1 (*XRCC1*) exerts on a vital role in the DNA single-strand break repair pathway (80). *XRCC1* Arg194Trp, *XRCC1* Arg280His, and *XRCC1* Arg399Gln are the three most common examined SNPs in the *XRCC1* gene (81, 82). Lou et al. suggested that *XRCC1* Arg194Trp, *XRCC1* Arg280His, and *XRCC1* Arg399Gln posed limited effect on the HNSCC risk in a meta-analysis with 29 studies (83). Similarly, no significant associations have been presented between *XRCC1* gene SNPs and the incidence of MPT in the HNSCC patients (79).

Apart from double-strand and single-strand repair pathway, the host can protect the genome from damage induced by various environmental carcinogens by means of nucleotide excision repair (NER) pathway (84). Seven SNPs of the *NER* genes involved in the HNSCC are listed as follows: *XPC* Ala499Val, *XPC* Lys939Gln, *XPD* Asp312Asn, *XPD* Lys751Gln, *XPG* His1104Asp, *ERCC1* C8092A, and *XPA* G23A. Zafereo et al. declared that no significant association between aforementioned seven SNPs and the SPM susceptibility, independently or collectively, has been found in a recessive model (84).

All in all, no significant associations between SNPs of DNA repair genes and MPC risk have been found so far. On the basis of above evidences, it is plausible that SNPs of DNA repair genes might not play a major role in the development of MPCs in the HNSCC subjects.

SNPs of Carcinogen Metabolism-Related Genes

Glutathione peroxidase I (GPX1), a selenium-dependent enzyme, participates in the detoxification of activated oxygen species (85). Genetic alterations or polymorphism in the coding region of *GPX1* gene might be involved in the development of cancer. A significant correlation has been observed between *GPX1* expression and T-stage as well as index tumor sites in HNSCC patients (86). The *GPX1* polymorphism represents three possible alleles, namely ALA5, ALA6, and ALA7. Jefferies et al. evaluated the association between *GPX1* genetic polymorphisms and HNSCC patients who developed SPTs in a case-control study. A significant difference in allele frequencies of *GPX1* ALA*6 and ALA*7 was observed between the SPT cases and controls, which indicated that polymorphisms of *GPX1* gene may be a molecular marker for the development of SPTs in HNSCC (85).

CYP1A1 and *CYP2E1* are two main genes associated with the carcinogen metabolic activation. Rydzanicz et al. reported that HNSCC patients with *CYP1A1* genotype *1/*4 and allele *4 represented a 4.1- and 2.6-fold risk of developing MPT, respectively (79). However, no significant correlations has been established between SNPs of *CYP2E1* gene and the incidence of MPT, which suggested a limited role of *CYP2E1* in the susceptibility of MPTs in HNSCC (79).

Glutathione S transferase (GST) plays a critical role in the detoxication and elimination of various carcinogens (87). *GSTM1*, *GSTT1*, and *GSTM3* gene are three members of the GST family in human (87). Studies reported that the *GSTT1* null genotype and polymorphism in *GSTM3* gene were not correlated with a statistically significant increased risk for SPTs or tobacco-related SPTs (79, 88). Inversely, a significant association was observed between the polymorphism in *GSTM1* gene and development of SPTs or tobacco-related SPTs (88).

N-acetyltransferase 2 (*NAT2*) gene participates in the metabolism of aromatic, heterocyclic amines and hydrazines (89). Evidence from 23 case and control studies indicated that *NAT2* polymorphisms could increase the incidence of HNSCC by 23% and serve as a risk factor of HNSCC in Asians (90). With respect to MPCs, *NAT2**7B was significantly correlated with an increased risk for SPTs in patients after index HNSCC (79).

According to the available evidences, a significant association has been observed between MPCs and SNPs of carcinogen metabolism-related genes, such as *CYP1A1*, *GSTM1*, and *NAT2*. However, well-designed, large-scale, multi-center studies are still warranted to verify these conclusions in the future.

MPCs AND ACQUIRED MUTATIONS

MPCs and CIN

CIN comprises altered DNA copy number and loss or rearrangement of the chromosomes, resulting in the loss or gain of function of certain genes (91). Piccinin et al. evaluated the LOH status at 1p, 3p, 9p, 13q, and 19p. However, no significant differences have been observed between the MPCs group and single cancer group, which suggested that chromosomal instability may not account for the propensity to develop SPMs in the upper aerodigestive tract (49).

MPCs and MSI

MSI, a major hallmark of genetic instability, originates from deficient DNA mismatch repair (92). It is mostly observed and studied in the hereditary non-polyposis colorectal cancer, which is characterized by MPCs of different organs, such as gastrointestinal, endometrial and urinary tract (93). So, MSI is considered to be a major determinant in the development of MPCs. Piccinin et al. analyzed the MSI on five chromosomes in 67 HNSCC patients, 22 MPCs and 45 controls, and revealed that no significant differences existed between MSI and MPCs cases (49). This implied that except for MSI, other systems concerning the genome integrity might be responsible for the

TABLE 1 | Genetic factors, genes, and potential biomarkers of multiple primary cancer of HNSCC.

Factors	Genes	Potential biomarkers
Germline mutation	*p53, CDKN2A, hMLHI*	Unidentified
SNP	Tumor suppressor genes: *p53, p1p14, p73, FAS/FASLG, p21, p27*	*p53, p1p14, p73, FAS/FASLG, p21, p27*
	Oncogenes: *MDM2, MDM4*	*MDM2, MDM4*
	DNA repair genes: *MRE11, RAD50, NBN, XRCC3, XRCC1, XPC, XPD, XPG, ERCC1, XPA*	Unidentified
	Carcinogen Metabolism-related genes: *GPX1, CYP1A1, CYP2E1, GSTT1*, GSTM1, *GSTM3, NAT2*	*GPX1, CYP1A1, GSTM1, NAT2*
CIN	Unidentified	Unidentified
MSI	Unidentified	Unidentified
Epigenetic alterations	*CCNA1, DCC, TIMP3*	*CCNA1, TIMP3*

carcinogenesis of HNSCC and tumor multiplicity of the head and neck region (49).

MPCs and DNA Methylation

DNA methylation is a well-categorized change of epigenetic alterations in tumors, which is capable of silencing the classic tumor suppressor genes (94). DNA methylation could disrupt the tumor suppressor gene function by obstructing its promoter region and impeding the transcriptional process (95). Longo et al. have detected *CCNA1*, *DCC*, and *TIMP3* hypermethylation in the exfoliated cell samples of HNSCC patients (96). To investigate the relationship between hypermethylation and MPCs in HNSCC, Rettori et al. examined the methylation patterns of 19 genes in 70 HNSCC cases (97), revealing that *CCNA1* and *TIMP3* hypermethylation were significantly connected with formation of SPT in HNSCC. Hypermethylation of *CCNA1* and *TIMP3* might be a promising genetic marker to predict the incidence of SPT in HNSCC subjects, providing the basis for the use of preventive measures and adjuvant treatment.

CONCLUSIONS

The dismal prognosis of HNSCC has always been attributed to the occurrence of MPCs. "Field cancerization," induced by carcinogens and CAFs, is proposed to elaborate the development of MPCs. Apart from environmental and immune factors, genetic factors may play a major role in the risk of MPCs. In summary, SNPs of tumor suppressor genes, oncogenes and carcinogen metabolism-related genes, together with DNA methylation, may serve as potential molecular markers of MPCs risk (**Table 1**). SNP chips and next-generation sequencing technology will enables us to access the strength of these "nature" components of MPCs, resulting in early diagnosis and better survival in HNSCC patients. However, there is still a long way to go before the clinical application of these genetic markers. HNSCC is a genetically heterogeneous disease with a wide range of genetic alterations (98), so a panel of genetic markers with the most accuracy and specificity need to be selected. On the other hand, large-scale, well-designed, and multi-center studies are warranted to examine their clinical relevance.

AUTHOR CONTRIBUTIONS

All authors listed have made a substantial, direct and intellectual contribution to the work, and approved it for publication.

REFERENCES

1. Whaley JT, Indelicato DJ, Morris CG, Hinerman RW, Amdur RJ, Mendenhall WM, et al. Ewing tumors of the head and neck. *Am J Clin Oncol.* (2010) 33:321–6. doi: 10.1097/COC.0b013e3181aaca71
2. Siegel RL, Miller KD, Jemal A. Cancer statistics, 2018. *CA Cancer J Clin.* (2018) 68:7–30. doi: 10.3322/caac.21442
3. Leemans CR, Braakhuis BJ, Brakenhoff RH. The molecular biology of head and neck cancer. *Nat Rev Cancer.* (2011) 11:9–22. doi: 10.1038/nrc2982
4. Simpson MC, Massa ST, Boakye EA, Antisdel JL, Stamatakis KA, Varvares MA, et al. Primary cancer vs competing causes of death in survivors of head and neck cancer. *JAMA Oncol.* (2018) 4:257–9. doi: 10.1001/jamaoncol.2017.4478
5. van der Schroeff MP, van de Schans SA, Piccirillo JF, Langeveld TP, Baatenburg de Jong RJ, Janssen-Heijnen ML. Conditional relative survival in head and neck squamous cell carcinoma: permanent excess mortality risk for long-term survivors. *Head Neck.* (2010) 32:1613–8. doi: 10.1002/hed.21369
6. Zhang Y, Sturgis EM, Zafereo ME, Wei Q, Li G. p14ARF genetic polymorphisms and susceptibility to second primary malignancy in patients with index squamous cell carcinoma of the head and neck. *Cancer.* (2011) 117:1227–35. doi: 10.1002/cncr.25605
7. Do KA, Johnson MM, Lee JJ, Wu XF, Dong Q, Hong WK, et al. Longitudinal study of smoking patterns in relation to the development of smoking-related secondary primary tumors in patients with upper aerodigestive tract malignancies. *Cancer.* (2004) 101:2837–42. doi: 10.1002/cncr.20714
8. Leon X, Del Prado Venegas M, Orus C, Kolanczak K, Garcia J, Quer M. Metachronous second primary tumours in the aerodigestive tract in patients with early stage head and neck squamous cell carcinomas. *Eur Arch Otorhinolaryngol.* (2005) 262:905–9. doi: 10.1007/s00405-005-0922-5
9. Nagao Y, Sata M. High incidence of multiple primary carcinomas in HCV-infected patients with oral squamous cell carcinoma. *Med Sci Monit.* (2009) 15:CR453–9.
10. Xu CC, Biron VL, Puttagunta L, Seikaly H. HPV status and second primary tumours in oropharyngeal squamous cell carcinoma. *J Otolaryngol Head Neck Surg.* (2013) 42:36. doi: 10.1186/1916-0216-42-36
11. Foulkes WD, Brunet JS, Sieh W, Black MJ, Shenouda G, Narod SA. Familial risks of squamous cell carcinoma of the head and neck: retrospective case-control study. *BMJ.* (1996) 313:716–21. doi: 10.1136/bmj.313.7059.716

12. Bunbanjerdsuk S, Vorasan N, Saethang T, Pongrujikorn T, Pangpunyakulchai D, Mongkonsiri N, et al. Oncoproteomic and gene expression analyses identify prognostic biomarkers for second primary malignancy in patients with head and neck squamous cell carcinoma. *Mod Pathol.* (2019) 32:943–56. doi: 10.1038/s41379-019-0211-2
13. Warren S, Gates O. Multiple primary malignant tumors: a survey of the literature and statistical study. *Am J Cancer.* (1932) 16:1358–414.
14. Braakhuis BJ, Tabor MP, Leemans CR, van der Waal I, Snow GB, Brakenhoff RH. Second primary tumors and field cancerization in oral and oropharyngeal cancer: molecular techniques provide new insights and definitions. *Head Neck.* (2002) 24:198–206. doi: 10.1002/hed.10042
15. León X, Quer M, Orús C, Venegas MdP. Can cure be achieved in patients with head and neck carcinomas? The problem of second neoplasm. *Expert Rev Anticancer Ther.* (2001) 1:125–33. doi: 10.1586/14737140.1.1.125
16. Shiga K, Tateda M, Katagiri K, Nakanome A, Ogawa T, Asada Y, et al. Distinct features of second primary malignancies in head and neck cancer patients in Japan. *Tohoku J Exp Med.* (2011) 225:5–12. doi: 10.1620/tjem.225.5
17. Bugter O, van Iwaarden DLP, Dronkers EAC, de Herdt MJ, Wieringa MH, Verduijn GM, et al. Survival of patients with head and neck cancer with metachronous multiple primary tumors is surprisingly favorable. *Head Neck.* (2019) 41:1648–55. doi: 10.1002/hed.25595
18. Ang KK, Harris J, Wheeler R, Weber R, Rosenthal DI, Nguyen-Tan PF, et al. Human papillomavirus and survival of patients with oropharyngeal cancer. *N Engl J Med.* (2010) 363:24–35. doi: 10.1056/NEJMoa0912217
19. Huang SF, Li HF, Liao CT, Wang HM, Chen IH, Chang JT, et al. Association of HPV infections with second primary tumors in early-staged oral cavity cancer. *Oral Dis.* (2012) 18:809–15. doi: 10.1111/j.1601-0825.2012.01950.x
20. Martel M, Alemany L, Taberna M, Mena M, Tous S, Bague S, et al. The role of HPV on the risk of second primary neoplasia in patients with oropharyngeal carcinoma. *Oral Oncol.* (2017) 64:37–43. doi: 10.1016/j.oraloncology.2016.11.011
21. Weinberger PM, Yu Z, Haffty BG, Kowalski D, Harigopal M, Brandsma J, et al. Molecular classification identifies a subset of human papillomavirus–associated oropharyngeal cancers with favorable prognosis. *J Clin Oncol.* (2006) 24:736–47. doi: 10.1200/JCO.2004.00.3335
22. D'Souza G, Kreimer AR, Viscidi R, Pawlita M, Fakhry C, Koch WM, et al. Case-control study of human papillomavirus and oropharyngeal cancer. *N Engl J Med.* (2007) 356:1944–56. doi: 10.1056/NEJMoa065497
23. Benson E, Li R, Eisele D, Fakhry C. The clinical impact of HPV tumor status upon head and neck squamous cell carcinomas. *Oral Oncol.* (2014) 50:565–74. doi: 10.1016/j.oraloncology.2013.09.008
24. Rampias T, Sasaki C, Psyrri A. Molecular mechanisms of HPV induced carcinogenesis in head and neck. *Oral Oncol.* (2014) 50:356–63. doi: 10.1016/j.oraloncology.2013.07.011
25. Fakhry C, Westra WH, Li S, Cmelak A, Ridge JA, Pinto H, et al. Improved survival of patients with human papillomavirus-positive head and neck squamous cell carcinoma in a prospective clinical trial. *J Natl Cancer Inst.* (2008) 100:261–9. doi: 10.1093/jnci/djn011
26. Licitra L, Perrone F, Bossi P, Suardi S, Mariani L, Artusi R, et al. High-risk human papillomavirus affects prognosis in patients with surgically treated oropharyngeal squamous cell carcinoma. *J Clin Oncol.* (2006) 24:5630–6. doi: 10.1200/JCO.2005.04.6136
27. Klussmann JP, Mooren JJ, Lehnen M, Claessen SM, Stenner M, Huebbers CU, et al. Genetic signatures of HPV-related and unrelated oropharyngeal carcinoma and their prognostic implications. *Clin Cancer Res.* (2009) 15:1779–86. doi: 10.1158/1078-0432.CCR-08-1463
28. Martinez I, Wang J, Hobson KF, Ferris RL, Khan SA. Identification of differentially expressed genes in HPV-positive and HPV-negative oropharyngeal squamous cell carcinomas. *Eur J Cancer.* (2007) 43:415–32. doi: 10.1016/j.ejca.2006.09.001
29. Saito Y, Ebihara Y, Ushiku T, Omura G, Kobayashi K, Ando M, et al. Negative human papillomavirus status and excessive alcohol consumption are significant risk factors for second primary malignancies in Japanese patients with oropharyngeal carcinoma. *Jpn J Clin Oncol.* (2014) 44:564–9. doi: 10.1093/jjco/hyu042
30. Cabanillas R, Astudillo A, Valle M, de la Rosa J, Álvarez R, Durán NS, et al. Novel germline CDKN2A mutation associated with head and neck squamous cell carcinomas and melanomas. *Head Neck.* (2013) 35:E80–4. doi: 10.1002/hed.21911
31. Jain KS, Sikora AG, Baxi SS, Morris LG. Synchronous cancers in patients with head and neck cancer: risks in the era of human papillomavirus-associated oropharyngeal cancer. *Cancer.* (2013) 119:1832–7. doi: 10.1002/cncr.27988
32. Mercer RR, Lucas NC, Simmons AN, Zander DS, Tsongalis GJ, Funkhouser WK, et al. Molecular discrimination of multiple primary versus metastatic squamous cell cancers of the head/neck and lung. *Exp Mol Pathol.* (2009) 86:1–9. doi: 10.1016/j.yexmp.2008.11.003
33. Daher T, Tur MK, Brobeil A, Etschmann B, Witte B, Engenhart-Cabillic R, et al. Combined human papillomavirus typing and TP53 mutation analysis in distinguishing second primary tumors from lung metastases in patients with head and neck squamous cell carcinoma. *Head Neck.* (2018) 40:1109–19. doi: 10.1002/hed.25041
34. Gasparotto D, Maestro R, Barzan L, Vukosavljevic T, Doglioni C, Sulfaro S, et al. Recurrences and second primary tumours in the head and neck region: differentiation by p53 mutation analysis. *Ann Oncol.* (1995) 6:933–9. doi: 10.1093/oxfordjournals.annonc.a059362
35. Ronchetti D, Arisi E, Neri A, Pruneri G, Digiuni B, Sambataro G, et al. Microsatellite analyses of recurrence or second primary tumor in head and neck cancer. *Anticancer Res.* (2005) 25:2771–5.
36. Braakhuis BJ, Tabor MP, Kummer JA, Leemans CR, Brakenhoff RH. A genetic explanation of Slaughter's concept of field cancerization: evidence and clinical implications. *Cancer Res.* (2003) 63:1727–30.
37. Simple M, Suresh A, Das D, Kuriakose MA. Cancer stem cells and field cancerization of oral squamous cell carcinoma. *Oral Oncol.* (2015) 51:643–51. doi: 10.1016/j.oraloncology.2015.04.006
38. Kuss I, Hathaway B, Ferris RL, Gooding W, Whiteside TL. Decreased absolute counts of T lymphocyte subsets and their relation to disease in squamous cell carcinoma of the head and neck. *Clin Cancer Res.* (2004) 10:3755–62. doi: 10.1158/1078-0432.CCR-04-0054
39. Atienza JA, Dasanu CA. Incidence of second primary malignancies in patients with treated head and neck cancer: a comprehensive review of literature. *Curr Med Res Opin.* (2012) 28:1899–909. doi: 10.1185/03007995.2012.746218
40. Kuss I, Saito T, Johnson JT, Whiteside TL. Clinical significance of decreased zeta chain expression in peripheral blood lymphocytes of patients with head and neck cancer. *Clin Cancer Res.* (1999) 5:329–34.
41. Grandis JR, Falkner DM, Melhem MF, Gooding WE, Drenning SD, Morel PA. Human leukocyte antigen class I allelic and haplotype loss in squamous cell carcinoma of the head and neck: clinical and immunogenetic consequences. *Clin Cancer Res.* (2000) 6:2794–802.
42. Ge L, Meng W, Zhou H, Bhowmick N. Could stroma contribute to field cancerization? *Med Hypotheses.* (2010) 75:26–31. doi: 10.1016/j.mehy.2010.01.019
43. Angadi PV, Patil PV, Kale AD, Hallikerimath S, Babji D. Myofibroblast presence in apparently normal mucosa adjacent to oral squamous cell carcinoma associated with chronic tobacco/areca nut use: evidence for field cancerization. *Acta Odontol Scand.* (2014) 72:502–8. doi: 10.3109/00016357.2013.871648
44. Chan JS, Tan MJ, Sng MK, Teo Z, Phua T, Choo CC, et al. Cancer-associated fibroblasts enact field cancerization by promoting extratumoral oxidative stress. *Cell Death Dis.* (2017) 8:e2562. doi: 10.1038/cddis.2016.492
45. Lane DP. Cancer. p53, guardian of the genome. *Nature.* (1992) 358:15–6. doi: 10.1038/358015a0
46. Brachman DG, Graves D, Vokes E, Beckett M, Haraf D, Montag A, et al. Occurrence of p53 gene deletions and human papilloma virus infection in human head and neck cancer. *Cancer Res.* (1992) 52:4832–6.
47. Gallo O, Sardi I, Pepe G, Franchi A, Attanasio M, Giusti B, et al. Multiple primary tumors of the upper aerodigestive tract: is there a role for constitutional mutations in the p53 gene? *Int J Cancer.* (1999) 82:180–6. doi: 10.1002/(SICI)1097-0215(19990719)82:2<180::AID-IJC5>3.0.CO;2-P
48. Jefferies S, Edwards S, Hamoudi R, A'Hern R, Foulkes W, Goldgar D, et al. No germline mutations in CDKN2A (p16) in patients with squamous cell cancer of the head and neck and second primary tumours. *Br J Cancer.* (2001) 85:1383. doi: 10.1054/bjoc.2001.2068
49. Piccinin S, Gasparotto D, Vukosavljevic T, Barzan L, Sulfaro S, Maestro R, et al. Microsatellite instability in squamous cell carcinomas of the head and neck

related to field cancerization phenomena. *Br J Cancer.* (1998) 78:1147–51. doi: 10.1038/bjc.1998.644
50. Skierucha M, Milne AN, Offerhaus GJ, Polkowski WP, Maciejewski R, Sitarz R. Molecular alterations in gastric cancer with special reference to the early-onset subtype. *World J Gastroenterol.* (2016) 22:2460–74. doi: 10.3748/wjg.v22.i8.2460
51. Li F, Sturgis EM, Chen X, Zafereo ME, Wei Q, Li G. Association of p53 codon 72 polymorphism with risk of second primary malignancy in patients with squamous cell carcinoma of the head and neck. *Cancer.* (2010) 116:2350–9. doi: 10.1002/cncr.25072
52. Bergamaschi D, Samuels Y, Sullivan A, Zvelebil M, Breyssens H, Bisso A, et al. iASPP preferentially binds p53 proline-rich region and modulates apoptotic function of codon 72-polymorphic p53. *Nat Genet.* (2006) 38:1133–41. doi: 10.1038/ng1879
53. Mojtahedi Z, Hashemi SB, Khademi B, Karimi M, Haghshenas MR, Fattahi MJ, et al. p53 codon 72 polymorphism association with head and neck squamous cell carcinoma. *Braz J Otorhinolaryngol.* (2010) 76:316–20. doi: 10.1590/S1808-86942010000300008
54. Hamel N, Black MJ, Ghadirian P, Foulkes WD. No association between P53 codon 72 polymorphism and risk of squamous cell carcinoma of the head and neck. *Br J Cancer.* (2000) 82:757–9. doi: 10.1054/bjoc.1999.0993
55. Lowe SW, Sherr CJ. Tumor suppression by Ink4a-Arf: progress and puzzles. *Curr Opin Genet Develop.* (2003) 13:77–83. doi: 10.1016/S0959-437X(02)00013-8
56. Gruttgen A, Reichenzeller M, Junger M, Schlien S, Affolter A, Bosch FX. Detailed gene expression analysis but not microsatellite marker analysis of 9p21 reveals differential defects in the INK4a gene locus in the majority of head and neck cancers. *J Pathol.* (2001) 194:311–7. doi: 10.1002/path.906
57. Flores ER, Tsai KY, Crowley D, Sengupta S, Yang A, McKeon F, et al. p63 and p73 are required for p53-dependent apoptosis in response to DNA damage. *Nature.* (2002) 416:560–4. doi: 10.1038/416560a
58. Zheng T, Wang J, Chen X, Meng X, Song X, Lu Z, et al. Disruption of p73-MDM2 binding synergizes with gemcitabine to induce apoptosis in HuCCT1 cholangiocarcinoma cell line with p53 mutation. *Tumour Biol.* (2010) 31:287–95. doi: 10.1007/s13277-010-0035-7
59. Li G, Sturgis EM, Wang LE, Chamberlain RM, Amos CI, Spitz MR, et al. Association of a p73 exon 2 G4C14-to-A4T14 polymorphism with risk of squamous cell carcinoma of the head and neck. *Carcinogenesis.* (2004) 25:1911–6. doi: 10.1093/carcin/bgh197
60. Galli P, Cadoni G, Volante M, De Feo E, Amore R, Giorgio A, et al. A case-control study on the combined effects of p53 and p73 polymorphisms on head and neck cancer risk in an Italian population. *BMC Cancer.* (2009) 9:137. doi: 10.1186/1471-2407-9-137
61. Li F, Sturgis EM, Zafereo ME, Liu Z, Wang LE, Wei Q, et al. p73 G4C14-to-A4T14 polymorphism and risk of second primary malignancy after index squamous cell carcinoma of head and neck. *Int J Cancer.* (2009) 125:2660–5. doi: 10.1002/ijc.24570
62. Blaes J, Thome CM, Pfenning PN, Rubmann P, Sahm F, Wick A, et al. Inhibition of CD95/CD95L (FAS/FASLG) signaling with APG101 prevents invasion and enhances radiation therapy for glioblastoma. *Mol Cancer Res.* (2018) 16:767–76. doi: 10.1158/1541-7786.MCR-17-0563
63. Reichmann E. The biological role of the Fas/FasL system during tumor formation and progression. *Semin Cancer Biol.* (2002) 12:309–15. doi: 10.1016/S1044-579X(02)00017-2
64. Lei D, Sturgis EM, Wang LE, Liu Z, Zafereo ME, Wei Q, et al. FAS and FASLG genetic variants and risk for second primary malignancy in patients with squamous cell carcinoma of the head and neck. *Cancer Epidemiol Biomarkers Prev.* (2010) 19:1484–91. doi: 10.1158/1055-9965.EPI-10-0030
65. Zhang Z, Wang LE, Sturgis EM, El-Naggar AK, Hong WK, Amos CI, et al. Polymorphisms of FAS and FAS ligand genes involved in the death pathway and risk and progression of squamous cell carcinoma of the head and neck. *Clin Cancer Res.* (2006) 12:5596–602. doi: 10.1158/1078-0432.CCR-05-1739
66. Llanos S, Garcia-Pedrero JM, Morgado-Palacin L, Rodrigo JP, Serrano M. Stabilization of p21 by mTORC1/4E-BP1 predicts clinical outcome of head and neck cancers. *Nat Commun.* (2016) 7:10438. doi: 10.1038/ncomms10438
67. Li G, Liu Z, Sturgis EM, Shi Q, Chamberlain RM, Spitz MR, et al. Genetic polymorphisms of p21 are associated with risk of squamous cell carcinoma of the head and neck. *Carcinogenesis.* (2005) 26:1596–602. doi: 10.1093/carcin/bgi105
68. Li G, Sturgis EM, Wang LE, Chamberlain RM, Spitz MR, El-Naggar AK, et al. Association between the V109G polymorphism of the p27 gene and the risk and progression of oral squamous cell carcinoma. *Clin Cancer Res.* (2004) 10:3996–4002. doi: 10.1158/1078-0432.CCR-04-0089
69. Wang Z, Sturgis EM, Zhang F, Lei D, Liu Z, Xu L, et al. Genetic variants of p27 and p21 as predictors for risk of second primary malignancy in patients with index squamous cell carcinoma of head and neck. *Mol Cancer.* (2012) 11:17. doi: 10.1186/1476-4598-11-17
70. Li Q, Lozano G. Molecular pathways: targeting Mdm2 and Mdm4 in cancer therapy. *Clin Cancer Res.* (2013) 19:34–41. doi: 10.1158/1078-0432.CCR-12-0053
71. Yu H, Huang YJ, Liu Z, Wang LE, Li G, Sturgis EM, et al. Effects of MDM2 promoter polymorphisms and p53 codon 72 polymorphism on risk and age at onset of squamous cell carcinoma of the head and neck. *Mol Carcinog.* (2011) 50:697–706. doi: 10.1002/mc.20806
72. Whibley C, Pharoah PD, Hollstein M. p53 polymorphisms: cancer implications. *Nat Rev Cancer.* (2009) 9:95–107. doi: 10.1038/nrc2584
73. Jin L, Sturgis EM, Zhang Y, Huang Z, Wei P, Guo W, et al. Genetic variants in p53-related genes confer susceptibility to second primary malignancy in patients with index squamous cell carcinoma of head and neck. *Carcinogenesis.* (2013) 34:1551–7. doi: 10.1093/carcin/bgt096
74. Valentin-Vega YA, Barboza JA, Chau GP, El-Naggar AK, Lozano G. High levels of the p53 inhibitor MDM4 in head and neck squamous carcinomas. *Hum. Pathol.* (2007) 38:1553–62. doi: 10.1016/j.humpath.2007.03.005
75. Yu H, Wang LE, Liu Z, Wei S, Li G, Sturgis EM, et al. Polymorphisms of MDM4 and risk of squamous cell carcinoma of the head and neck. *Pharmacogenet Genomics.* (2011) 21:388–96. doi: 10.1097/FPC.0b013e32834632e4
76. Lamarche BJ, Orazio NI, Weitzman MD. The MRN complex in double-strand break repair and telomere maintenance. *FEBS Lett.* (2010) 584:3682–95. doi: 10.1016/j.febslet.2010.07.029
77. Ziolkowska-Suchanek I, Mosor M, Wierzbicka M, Rydzanicz M, Baranowska M, Nowak J. The MRN protein complex genes: MRE11 and RAD50 and susceptibility to head and neck cancers. *Mol Cancer.* (2013) 12:113. doi: 10.1186/1476-4598-12-113
78. Shen H, Sturgis EM, Dahlstrom KR, Zheng Y, Spitz MR, Wei Q. A variant of the DNA repair gene XRCC3 and risk of squamous cell carcinoma of the head and neck: a case-control analysis. *Int J Cancer.* (2002) 99:869–72. doi: 10.1002/ijc.10413
79. Rydzanicz M, Wierzbicka M, Gajecka M, Szyfter W, Szyfter K. The impact of genetic factors on the incidence of multiple primary tumors (MPT) of the head and neck. *Cancer Lett.* (2005) 224:263–78. doi: 10.1016/j.canlet.2005.01.015
80. Whitehouse CJ, Taylor RM, Thistlethwaite A, Zhang H, Karimi-Busheri F, Lasko DD, et al. XRCC1 stimulates human polynucleotide kinase activity at damaged DNA termini and accelerates DNA single-strand break repair. *Cell.* (2001) 104:107–17. doi: 10.1016/S0092-8674(01)00195-7
81. Laantri N, Jalbout M, Khyatti M, Ayoub WB, Dahmoul S, Ayad M, et al. XRCC1 and hOGG1 genes and risk of nasopharyngeal carcinoma in North African countries. *Mol Carcinog.* (2011) 50:732–7. doi: 10.1002/mc.20754
82. Csejtei A, Tibold A, Koltai K, Varga Z, Szanyi I, Gobel G, et al. Association between XRCC1 polymorphisms and head and neck cancer in a Hungarian population. *Anticancer Res.* (2009) 29:4169–73.
83. Lou Y, Peng WJ, Cao DS, Xie J, Li HH, Jiang ZX. DNA repair gene XRCC1 polymorphisms and head and neck cancer risk: an updated meta-analysis including 16344 subjects. *PLoS ONE.* (2013) 8:e74059. doi: 10.1371/journal.pone.0074059
84. Zafereo ME, Sturgis EM, Liu Z, Wang LE, Wei Q, Li G. Nucleotide excision repair core gene polymorphisms and risk of second primary malignancy in patients with index squamous cell carcinoma of the head and neck. *Carcinogenesis.* (2009) 30:997–1002. doi: 10.1093/carcin/bgp096
85. Jefferies S, Kote-Jarai Z, Goldgar D, Houlston R, Frazer-Williams M-J, A'Hern R, et al. Association between polymorphisms of the GPX1 gene and second primary tumours after index squamous cell cancer of the head and neck. *Oral Oncol.* (2005) 41:455–61. doi: 10.1016/j.oraloncology.2004.09.012

86. Dequanter D, Dok R, Koolen L, Vander Poorten V, Nuyts S. Prognostic significance of glutathione peroxidase levels (GPx1) in head and neck cancers. *Front Oncol.* (2017) 7:84. doi: 10.3389/fonc.2017.00084
87. Singh H, Sachan R, Devi S, Pandey SN, Mittal B. Association of GSTM1, GSTT1, and GSTM3 gene polymorphisms and susceptibility to cervical cancer in a North Indian population. *Am J Obstet Gynecol.* (2008) 198:303 e1–6. doi: 10.1016/j.ajog.2007.09.046
88. Minard CG, Spitz MR, Wu X, Hong WK, Etzel CJ. Evaluation of glutathione S-transferase polymorphisms and mutagen sensitivity as risk factors for the development of second primary tumors in patients previously diagnosed with early-stage head and neck cancer. *Cancer.* (2006) 106:2636–44. doi: 10.1002/cncr.21928
89. Walker K, Ginsberg G, Hattis D, Johns DO, Guyton KZ, Sonawane B. Genetic polymorphism in N-Acetyltransferase (NAT): population distribution of NAT1 and NAT2 activity. *J Toxicol Environ Health B Crit Rev.* (2009) 12:440–72. doi: 10.1080/10937400903158383
90. Zhang L, Xiang Z, Hao R, Li R, Zhu Y. N-acetyltransferase 2 genetic variants confer the susceptibility to head and neck carcinoma: evidence from 23 case-control studies. *Tumour Biol.* (2014) 35:3585–95. doi: 10.1007/s13277-013-1473-9
91. McClelland SE. Role of chromosomal instability in cancer progression. *Endocr Relat Cancer.* (2017) 24:T23–31. doi: 10.1530/ERC-17-0187
92. Yamamoto H, Imai K. Microsatellite instability: an update. *Arch Toxicol.* (2015) 89:899–921. doi: 10.1007/s00204-015-1474-0
93. Yamashita K, Arimura Y, Kurokawa S, Itoh F, Endo T, Hirata K, et al. Microsatellite instability in patients with multiple primary cancers of the gastrointestinal tract. *Gut.* (2000) 46:790–4. doi: 10.1136/gut.46.6.790
94. Jones PA, Baylin SB. The fundamental role of epigenetic events in cancer. *Nat Rev Genet.* (2002) 3:415–28. doi: 10.1038/nrg816
95. Garinis GA, Patrinos GP, Spanakis NE, Menounos PG. DNA hypermethylation: when tumour suppressor genes go silent. *Hum Genet.* (2002) 111:115–27. doi: 10.1007/s00439-002-0783-6
96. Longo AL, Rettori MM, de Carvalho AC, Kowalski LP, Carvalho AL, Vettore AL. Evaluation of the methylation profile of exfoliated cell samples from patients with head and neck squamous cell carcinoma. *Head Neck.* (2014) 36:631–7. doi: 10.1002/hed.23345
97. Rettori MM, de Carvalho AC, Longo AL, de Oliveira CZ, Kowalski LP, Carvalho AL, et al. TIMP3 and CCNA1 hypermethylation in HNSCC is associated with an increased incidence of second primary tumors. *J Transl Med.* (2013) 11:316. doi: 10.1186/1479-5876-11-316
98. Wiseman SM, Stoler DL, Anderson GR. The role of genomic instability in the pathogenesis of squamous cell carcinoma of the head and neck. *Surg Oncol Clin N Am.* (2004) 13:1–11. doi: 10.1016/S1055-3207(03)00118-2

Comparison Between PET-CT–Guided Neck Dissection and Elective Neck Dissection in cT1-2N0 Tongue Squamous Cell Carcinoma

Fengjie Zhu [1]*, *Shuhan Sun* [2] *and Kai Ba* [1]*

[1] Department of Oral Medicine, The First Affiliated Hospital of Zhengzhou University, Zhengzhou, China, [2] Department of Oral Medicine, The Third Affiliated Hospital of Zhengzhou University, Zhengzhou, China

***Correspondence:**
Fengjie Zhu
zhfjhappy@163.com
Kai Ba
k.ba@msn.com

Objective: Neck management in cT1-2N0 tongue squamous cell carcinoma (SCC) remains controversial. Our goal was to compare the survival difference between PET-CT–guided neck dissection and elective neck dissection (END) for the treatment of cT1-2 tongue SCC.

Methods: Patients with surgically treated cT1-2N0 tongue SCC were retrospectively enrolled. These patients were divided into two groups. Group A: The decision of whether to perform neck dissection was mainly based on the results of preoperative PET-CT examinations. Group B: Patients received END treatment without preoperative PET-CT examinations. The study endpoints were regional control (RC) and disease-specific survival (DSS). The Kaplan–Meier method was used to calculate the survival rates.

Results: Group A consisted of 66 patients, and 16 patients underwent neck dissection owing to positive PET-CT results. Group B consisted of 169 patients. The 5-year RC rates in group A and group B were 86 and 87%, respectively, and the difference was not significant ($p = 0.731$). The 5-year DSS rates in group A and group B were 93 and 90%, respectively, and the difference was not significant ($p = 0.583$).

Conclusions: Neck dissection can be safely avoided when the PET-CT scan reveals no neck lymph node involvement.

Keywords: PET-CT, elective neck dissection, survival analysis, early stage tongue cancer, tongue squamous cell carcinoma

INTRODUCTION

Tongue squamous cell carcinoma (SCC) is the most common malignancy in the oral cavity, and surgery is usually the first choice of treatment. For cT1-2N0 tongue SCC, its occult metastasis rate varies with different countries and races (1–3). Usually, neck dissection is required if the metastasis rate is greater than 20%. Although current high-quality research has described that routine neck dissection improves the prognosis by distinguishing patients who need adjuvant radiotherapy (1, 4, 5), researchers argue that most patients with cT1-2N0 disease do not have pathologic lymph node metastasis, and they are over-treated and exposed to possible neck dissection–related complications (2, 3); more importantly, the survival benefit associated with routine neck dissection could be contributed to by the late treatment of the metastatic necks at initial treatment. Owing to the development of individualized treatment concepts, it is very important for us to identify patients with pathologic lymph node metastasis preoperatively to achieve both oncologic and functional outcomes. A number of scholars support the predictive value of the depth of invasion (DOI), perineural invasion (PNI), and lymphovascular invasion (LVI) (6–8). However, these data are not always able to be obtained preoperatively.

PET-CT has been widely used for detecting primary cancer disease and possible metastasis sites. Zhang et al. (9) describe that the overall sensitivity and specificity of PET-CT for predicting lymph node metastasis in cT1-2 oral SCC was 21.4% and 98.4%, respectively, with a negative predictive value of 99.1%. Myers et al. (10) presented an estimated overall sensitivity of PET-CT for the N0 neck of 78% with a specificity of 100%. Similar results were also reported by Zheng et al. (11), Lee et al. (12), and Wong et al. (13). All these findings suggest that there might be high reliability for PET-CT in assessing neck status in cT1-2 tongue SCC. Therefore, our goal was to compare the survival difference between PET-CT–guided neck dissection and elective neck dissection (END) for the treatment of cT1-2 tongue SCC.

PATIENTS AND METHODS

Ethnic Consideration

The Zhengzhou University Institutional Research Committee approved our study, and all patients signed informed consent agreements for medical research before the initial treatment. All methods were performed in accordance with the relevant guidelines and regulations.

Patient Selection

From January 2010 to December 2016, patients with surgically treated primary cT1-2N0 tongue SCC were retrospectively enrolled. Patients without follow-up information were excluded from the analysis. Data regarding demographic and pathologic information as well as follow-up data were extracted. There was no consensus on the standard treatment of a cN0 neck in cT1-2 tongue SCC in China; therefore, in our cancer center, PET-CT was selectively suggested for patients with early stage oral SCC considering the patient's demand and the surgeon's preference from 2008, and our medical team had verified the feasibility of PET-CT in treating early stage tongue SCC (14). Therefore, enrolled patients were divided into two groups. Group A: The decision of whether to perform neck dissection was mainly based on the results of preoperative PET-CT examinations; if a positive result was reported by PET-CT, a neck dissection was performed, and if not, a wait-and-see policy was conducted. Group B: Patients received END treatment without preoperative PET-CT examinations.

Important Variable Definition

Smokers/drinkers were defined as patients who smoked/drank at diagnosis or who had stopped for <1 year prior to diagnosis (15, 16). All pathological sections were re-reviewed by at least two pathologists. PNI was considered to be present if tumor cells were identified within the perineural space and/or nerve bundle; LVI was positive if tumor cells were noted within the lymphovascular channels (17). The pathologic DOI was measured from the level of the adjacent normal mucosa to the deepest point of tumor infiltration regardless of the presence or absence of ulceration (18). The cT1-2 status was defined according to the AJCC 2018 classification, and the cN0 status was defined as no doubt of metastatic lymph nodes after palpation and ultrasound, CT, and MRI examinations.

Treatment Proposal

All patients underwent complete tumor resection with a margin of at least 1 cm, and the sublingual gland as well as the adipose tissue in the floor of the mouth was simultaneously resected. The neck dissection field included levels 1–3. Patients were followed every 3 months within 2 years after the operation and every 6 months for 2 years after the operation until the fifth year after the operation. Immediate interference was performed if disease recurrence was suspected. Adjuvant radiotherapy was suggested if there was pathologic lymph node metastasis, positive margins, PNI, or LVI.

Pathologic Analysis

Surgical specimens were immediately fixed in 10% formalin and then cut into pieces with a thickness of 5 mm and a side length of 1 cm by embedding in paraffin. Sections of a thickness of 5 um were obtained at 0.5-mm intervals and stained with haematoxylin and eosin. All pathologic sections had been reviewed by at least two pathologists. Immunohistochemistry was performed if there was difficulty in identifying malignant disease.

PET-CT Examination

The PET-CT scans (GE Healthcare, Milwaukee, WI) were performed by several technicians. Patients had an empty stomach for at least 6 hours before examination with glucose levels <200 mg/dL, and 10–20 mCi of [^{18}F] FDG dosed according to the weight was given to each patient. Diagnostic CT images and axial PET were obtained from the calvarial vertex through the upper thighs. Emission images were obtained after radiopharmaceutical injection 60 min later. During the CT scan, no contrast medium was used. The images were reconstructed with a 2.5-mm thickness slice. For every suspicious lesion, the isocontour region of interest centered on the maximum value pixel was drawn automatically with workstation tools generating the SUV max of the region. An SUV max cutoff of 2.5 MBq/g was used for FDG-avid primary tumors and lymph nodes on PET-CT.

Statistic Analysis

Student's t-tests and chi-square tests were used to compare the clinical and pathologic variables between the two groups, and the Kaplan–Meier method was used to calculate the regional control (RC) rate and disease-specific survival (DSS) rate. The survival time was calculated from the date of surgery to the last follow-up, the date of the first regional recurrence, or the date of cancer-caused death. All statistical analyses were performed using SPSS 20.0, and $p < 0.05$ was considered to be significant.

RESULTS

Demography and Pathologic Data

A total of 235 patients (172 males and 63 females) were included in the analysis, and the mean age was 54.8 (range: 31–79) years. There were 66 patients in group A and 169 patients in group B.

In group A, there were 52 (78.8%) males and 14 (21.2%) females, and the mean age was 55.7 years. A total of 42 (63.6%) and 29 (43.9%) patients were smokers and drinkers, respectively. cT1 and cT2 tumors were present in 25 (37.9%) and 41 (62.1%) patients, respectively. PNI and LVI were reported in eight (12.1%) and seven (10.6%) patients, respectively. The mean pathologic DOI was 4.8 mm. pT1 and pT2 tumors were present in 20 (30.3%) and 46 (69.7%) patients, respectively. Tumor differentiation was well distributed in 22 (33.3%) patients, moderately distributed in 35 (53.0%) patients, and poorly distributed in nine (13.6%) patients. Negative margins were achieved in all patients. Fourteen (21.2%) patients received postoperative radiotherapy (**Table 1**).

In group B, there were 120 (71.0%) males and 49 (29.0%) females, and the mean age was 54.4 years. A total of 111 (65.6%) and 58 (34.3%) patients were smokers and drinkers, respectively. cT1 and cT2 tumors were present in 45 (26.6%) and 124 (73.4%) patients, respectively. PNI and LVI were reported in 22 (13.0%) and 17 (10.1%) patients, respectively. The mean pathologic DOI was 4.7 mm. pT1 and pT2 tumors were present in 40 (23.7%) and 129 (76.3%) patients, respectively. Pathologic lymph node metastasis occurred in 30 (17.8%) patients, and in these patients, N1 was present in 25 cases, and N2a was present in five cases. Tumor differentiation was well distributed in 53 (31.4%) patients, moderately distributed in 99 (58.6%) patients, and poorly distributed in 17 (10.1%) patients. Negative margins were achieved in all patients. Thirty (17.8%) patients received postoperative radiotherapy (**Table 1**).

The two groups had similar distributions regarding age, sex, smoking status, drinking status, clinical, and pathologic tumor stage, PNI, LVI, tumor differentiation, and postoperative radiotherapy (**Table 1**, all $p > 0.05$).

TABLE 1 | Demographic and pathologic information in the two groups.

Variables	Group A ($n = 66$)	Group B ($n = 169$)	p
Age	55.7	54.4	0.884
Sex			
Male	52 (78.8%)	120 (71.0%)	
Female	14 (21.2%)	49 (29.0%)	0.170
Smoker	42 (63.6%)	111 (65.7%)	0.768
Drinker	29 (43.9%)	58 (34.3%)	0.170
Clinical tumor stage			
cT1	25 (37.9%)	45 (26.6%)	
cT2	41 (62.1%)	124 (73.4%)	0.090
Perineural invasion	8 (12.1%)	22 (13.0%)	0.853
Lymphovascular invasion	7 (10.6%)	17 (10.1%)	0.901
Pathologic tumor stage			
pT1	20 (30.3%)	40 (23.7%)	
pT2	46 (69.7%)	129 (76.3%)	0.295
Tumor differentiation			
Well	22 (33.3%)	53 (31.4%)	
Moderate	35 (53.0%)	99 (58.6%)	
Poor	9 (13.6%)	17 (10.1%)	0.649
Postoperative radiotherapy	14 (21.2%)	30 (17.8%)	0.541

PET-CT–Guided Neck Dissection

In group A, 16 (9.5%) patients underwent neck dissection owing to positive PET-CT results, and postoperative pathology confirmed occult metastasis in 14 patients. Of the 14 patients, N1 was present in 12 patients, and N2a was present in two patients.

Survival Analysis

During our follow-up with a mean time of 48.5 months, in group A of the 66 patients, regional recurrence occurred in nine patients: level I occurrence in four patients, level II in three patients, and level III in two patients (**Table 2**). Among these nine patients, seven had a pathologic N+ neck at the initial treatment, two patients had not previously received neck dissection owing to previous negative PET-CT results, there was no local recurrence or distant metastasis, the 5-year RC rate was 86%, recurrent disease was successfully salvaged in six patients with radical operations, four patients died of the disease, and the 5-year DSS rate was 93%. In group B, local recurrence occurred in five patients, and regional recurrence occurred in 20 patients: level I recurrence in nine patients, level II in six patients, level IV in three patients, and level V in two patients (**Table 2**). Among these 20 patients, 14 had a pathologic N+ neck at the initial treatment, there was no distant metastasis, the 5-year RC rate was 87%, patients with local recurrence were all successfully salvaged with radial operations, regional recurrent disease was successfully salvaged in eight patients with radial operations, 14 patients died of the disease, and the 5-year DSS rate was 90%. The two groups had similar RC ($p = 0.731$) and DSS ($p = 0.583$) rates (**Figures 1, 2**, both $p > 0.05$).

TABLE 2 | Neck recurrence pattern in the two groups.

Metastatic level	Group A ($n = 9$)	Group B ($n = 20$)
Ipsilateral		
I	4 (44.4%)	8 (40.0%)
II	2 (22.2%)	6 (20.0%)
III	2 (22.2%)	0
IV	0	3 (15.0%)
V	0	1 (5.0%)
Contralateral		
I	1 (11.1%)	1 (5.0%)
II	2 (22.2%)	2 (10.0%)
III	0	0
IV	0	1 (5.0%)
V	0	1 (5.0%)

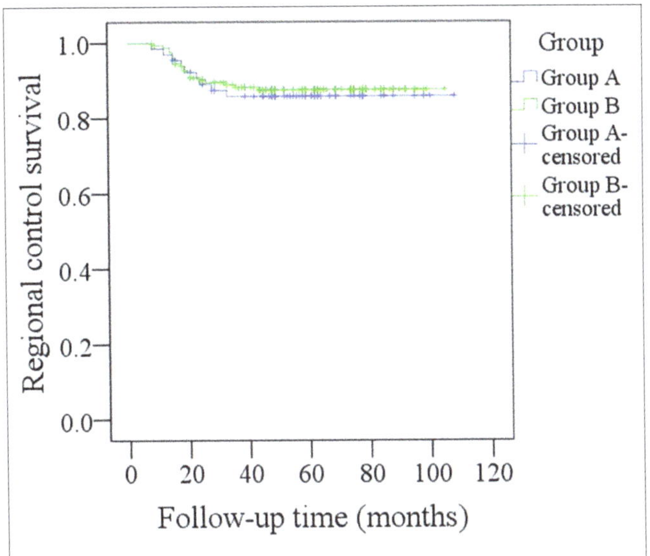

FIGURE 1 | Comparison of regional control between the two groups (p = 0.731).

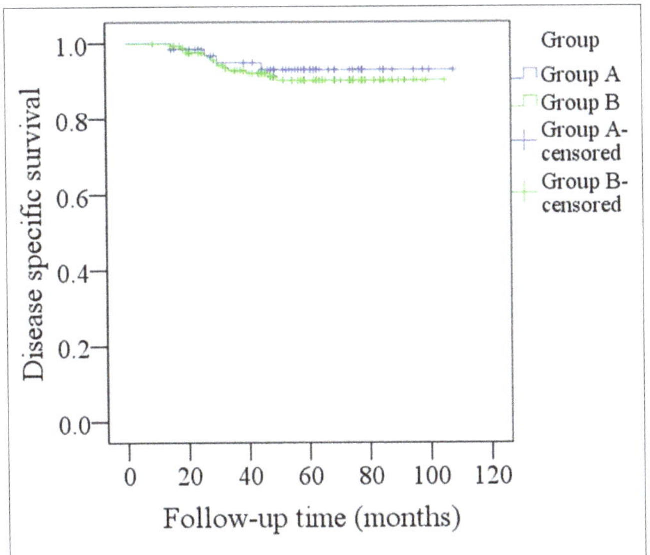

FIGURE 2 | Comparison of disease-specific survival between the two groups (p = 0.583).

DISCUSSION

The most significant finding in the current study was that, compared to elective neck dissection, PET-CT–guided neck dissection obtained similar disease control of cT1-2N0 tongue SCC; moreover, there was a higher possibility of successful salvage with PET-CT–guided neck dissection than with elective neck dissection. Our study may provide more suggestions for neck management during early stage tongue SCC treatment, and it provides the first evidence for the high reliability of PET-CT–guided neck dissection.

Neck lymph node status is the most important prognostic factor; usually, the survival rate decreases by half if lymph node metastasis is present (19–21). It is important that surgeons correctly address the neck. However, owing to the varying occult metastasis rates, there is still substantial controversy regarding the best neck management. Canis et al. (4) studied early stage SCC of the upper aerodigestive tract, and the 5-year recurrence-free survival rate was 95% in the neck dissection group and 96% in the wait-and-see group; the authors concluded that a wait-and-see approach was justified in patients with early stage disease. Deganello et al. (22) described that the occult neck disease rate was only 12.5% for laryngeal SCC, and the findings indicated the need to refine the treatment strategy, restricting elective neck dissection only to advanced stage disease. However, tongue SCC was significantly different from SCC in other sites, and the conclusions based on the overall sample of head and neck SCC or laryngeal SCC might not be suitable for tongue SCC. Moratin et al. (23) depicted that regional metastases occurred in 29 of the 97 patients with early stage tongue SCC, and although rare, bilateral cervical metastases could be detected in 2.1% of T1 and 11.8% of T2 disease; therefore, the authors suggested that neck dissection was required in all tongue SCC patients irrespective of tumor stage. Recent evidence showed that, after matched analysis in 1,234 patients, the 5-year overall survival rates were 87.1% in the neck dissection group and 76.2% in the wait-and-see group ($p = 0.0051$), and the DSS rates were 89.2% and 82.2% ($p = 0.0335$), respectively. This finding suggests that routine neck dissection was beneficial for cT1-2N0 tongue SCC (24). A similar viewpoint was also demonstrated by Gad et al. (25), Orabona et al. (26), and D'Cruz et al. (1). However, at least two aspects must be considered seriously when comprehending the conclusions: First, the occult metastasis rate was variable in early stage tongue SCC, and most of the patients would have been over-treated if routine neck dissection was performed; second, the so-called survival difference between elective neck dissection and the wait-and-see policy would have been mainly explained by the undetected real metastatic lymph nodes at the first visit in the wait-and-see group. This raised the point that, if we could identify patients who had real metastatic lymph nodes preoperatively, we might avoid unnecessary neck dissection and achieve similar survival compared to routine neck dissection.

A number of authors have aimed to assess the predictors of occult lymph node metastasis in cT1-2N0 tongue SCC. Jiang et al. (6) introduced a nomogram including the site of the primary lesion, depth of invasion, size of the tumor, and histopathological grade with high consistency for predicting the probability of occult cervical metastasis before surgery. Tam et al. (7) demonstrated that a DOI of 7.25 mm was most predictive for occult nodal disease. Other predictors included PNI and LVI (1). However, the data were always unavailable preoperatively, which greatly limited the clinical application.

PET-CT has been widely used to detect occult lymph node disease in the clinic. Slightly conflicting results have been reported by previous researchers. Stoeckli et al. (27) assessed the value of PET-CT for the staging of cN0 necks in oral and oropharyngeal SCC using sentinel lymph node biopsy and elective neck dissection as the "gold standard" for comparison, and sentinel lymph node biopsy was accurately feasible in all 12 patients and correctly diagnosed five cases of occult metastasis; however, PET-CT only suggested that two patients had occult metastasis, of whom one turned out to be a false positive case. A similar finding was also reported by Krabbe et al. (28), but both studies did not specifically focus on tongue SCC, which is significantly different from SCC in other sites, and HPV infection might also affect the accuracy of PET-CT. Increasing evidence supports the high reliability of PET-CT for identifying cervical nodal disease. Zhang et al. (9) described that the overall sensitivity and specificity of PET-CT for predicting lymph node metastasis in cT1-2 oral SCC was 21.4 and 98.4%, respectively, with a negative predictive value of 99.1%. Myers et al. (10) presented an estimated overall sensitivity of PET-CT for the N0 neck of 78% with a specificity of 100%. Similar results were also reported by Zheng et al. (11), Lee et al. (12), and Wong et al. (13). A recent important study by Lowe et al. (29) described that PET-CT had a highly negative predictive value for the N0 neck in T2 to T4 SCC of the head and neck and that PET/CT might assist clinicians with the decision of the best therapy for the clinically N0 neck in SCC of the head and neck. Our results supported most of those of other researchers and verified the high reliability of PET-CT for predicting occult metastasis in cT1-2 disease, which could result in similar oncologic outcomes as routine neck dissection. The two groups had comparable important variables except the clinical tumor stage; patients undergoing a PET-CT–guided neck dissection tended to have a smaller tumor, it indicated that we selectively suggested a PET-CT for a small tumor to avoid unnecessary neck dissection and obtain a better functional result previously. Additionally, the tending difference of clinical tumor stage might have led to survival difference between the two groups, but in fact, it was not. It brought some puzzle in comprehending our finding; more high quality research is needed to clarify these questions.

Another heated debated tool of detecting occult metastasis was sentinel lymph node biopsy (SLNB). Moya-Plana et al. (30) compared the reliability between SLNB and END in 229 cT1-2N0 oral SCC patients; the authors reported negative predictive value of SLNB was as high as 92.7%, and the two groups had similar recurrence-free survival and overall survival. Riese et al. (31) described in 36 patients with early oral and oropharynx SCC, all the 12 patients with pathologic metastasis were detected in SLNB, and it showed a sensitivity of 94.4% and a specificity of 100%. All these findings as well as recent research (32–34) confirmed SLNB was a precise diagnostic procedure in oral SCC and superior to PET-CT in melanoma and anal cancer for assessing nodal status. However, comparison between SLNB and PET-CT in oral SCC was never reported, and also application of SLNB in oral cancer was not widely accepted in China. More high-quality studies are needed to clarify these questions.

Salvage operations are important for improving survival, but the rate of successful salvage operations is usually <50% in tongue SCC patients (1–3). A similar finding was also noted in our END group. However, in group A, our salvage operation rate was as high as 66.7%, and it tended to be higher than that in group B. This finding was interesting: The high salvage operation rate might have resulted in improved DSS, but owing to our limited sample size, we could not draw any persuasive conclusions.

It was interesting to note the occult metastasis rate of Group B was just 17.8%; it was a little lower than those of similar studies (35, 36). The difference might be partially explained by different pathologic DOI and races. On the other hand, micrometastasis disease was also partially responsible during standard haematoxylin and eosin; van den Brekel et al. (37) previously presented that 25% of patients with positive lymph nodes had micrometastasis and were at high risk for undetected disease. Similar findings were also reported by Barrera et al. (38) and Rhee et al. (39).

There are some limitations that must be acknowledged. First, this was a retrospective study, it lacked of randomization, and the inherent bias could decrease the statistical power. In our future work, we will perform a prospective study with additional data regarding patient characteristics, especially other preoperative investigations, which could increase the predictive value of negative or positive PET-CT results. Second, our sample size was small, and a study with a larger sample size is needed. Third, some confounding factors might not have been taken into consideration, such as oral hygiene.

In summary, neck dissection could be safely avoided when the PET-CT scan reveals no neck lymph node involvement.

ETHICS STATEMENT

The Zhengzhou University Institutional Research Committee approved our study, and all patients signed informed consent agreements for medical research before initial treatment.

AUTHOR CONTRIBUTIONS

All the authors make the contribution in data collection, data analysis, and manuscript writing.

ACKNOWLEDGMENTS

This study was supported by National Natural Science Foundation of China (Grant No. 81500826).

REFERENCES

1. D'Cruz AK, Vaish R, Kapre N, Dandekar M, Gupta S, Hawaldar R, Agarwal JP, et al. Elective versus therapeutic neck dissection in node-negative oral cancer. *N Engl J Med.* (2015) 373:521–9. doi: 10.1056/NEJMoa1506007
2. Abu-Ghanem S, Yehuda M, Carmel NN, Leshno M, Abergel A, Gutfeld O, et al. Elective neck dissection vs observation in early-stage squamous cell carcinoma of the oral tongue with no clinically apparent lymph node metastasis in the neck: a systematic review and meta-analysis. *JAMA Otolaryngol Head Neck Surg.* (2016) 142:857–65. doi: 10.1001/jamaoto.2016.1281
3. Liu JY, Chen CF, Bai CH. Elective neck dissection versus observation in early-stage (cT1/T2N0) Oral squamous cell carcinoma. *Laryngoscope Investig Otolaryngol.* (2019) 4:554–61. doi: 10.1002/lio2.301
4. Canis M, Plüquett S, Ihler F, Matthias C, Kron M, Steiner W. Impact of elective neck dissection vs observation on regional recurrence and survival in cN0-staged patients with squamous cell carcinomas of the upper aerodigestive tract. *Arch Otolaryngol Head Neck Surg.* (2012) 138:650–5. doi: 10.1001/archoto.2012.1026
5. Borgemeester MC, van den Brekel MW, van Tinteren H, Smeele LE, Pameijer FA, van Velthuysen ML, et al. Ultrasound-guided aspiration cytology for the assessment of the clinically N0 neck: factors influencing its accuracy. *Head Neck.* (2008) 30:1505–13. doi: 10.1002/hed.20903
6. Jiang Q, Tang A, Long S, Qi Q, Song C, Xin Y, et al. Development and validation of a nomogram to predict the risk of occult cervical lymph node metastases in cN0 squamous cell carcinoma of the tongue. *Br J Oral Maxillofac Surg.* (2019) 57:1092–7. doi: 10.1016/j.bjoms.2019.09.024
7. Tam S, Amit M, Zafereo M, Bell D, Weber RS. Depth of invasion as a predictor of nodal disease and survival in patients with oral tongue squamous cell carcinoma. *Head Neck.* (2019) 41:177–84. doi: 10.1002/hed.25506
8. Faisal M, Abu Bakar M, Sarwar A, Adeel M, Batool F, Malik KI, et al. Depth of invasion (DOI) as a predictor of cervical nodal metastasis and local recurrence in early stage squamous cell carcinoma of oral tongue (ESSCOT). *PLoS ONE.* (2018) 13:e0202632. doi: 10.1371/journal.pone.0202632
9. Zhang H, Seikaly H, Biron VL, Jeffery CC. Utility of PET-CT in detecting nodal metastasis in cN0 early stage oral cavity squamous cell carcinoma. *Oral Oncol.* (2018) 80:89–92. doi: 10.1016/j.oraloncology.2018.04.003
10. Myers LL, Wax MK, Nabi H, Simpson GT, Lamonica D. Positron emission tomography in the evaluation of the N0 neck. *Laryngoscope.* (1998) 108:232–6. doi: 10.1097/00005537-199802000-00014
11. Zheng D, Niu L, Liu W, Zheng C, Yan R, Gong L, et al. Relationship between the maximum standardized uptake value of fluoro-2-deoxyglucose-positron emission tomography/computed tomography and clinicopathological characteristics in tongue squamous cell carcinoma. *J Cancer Res Ther.* (2019) 15:842–8. doi: 10.4103/jcrt.JCRT_855_18
12. Lee SJ, Choi JY, Lee HJ, Baek CH, Son YI, Hyun SH, et al. Prognostic value of volume-based (18)F-fluorodeoxyglucose PET/CT parameters in patients with clinically node-negative oral tongue squamous cell carcinoma. *Korean J Radiol.* (2012) 13:752–9. doi: 10.3348/kjr.2012.13.6.752
13. Wong WL, Sonoda LI, Gharpurhy A, Gollub F, Wellsted D, Goodchild K, et al. 18F-fluorodeoxyglucose positron emission tomography/computed tomography in the assessment of occult primary head and neck cancers–an audit and review of published studies. *Clin Oncol.* (2012) 24:190–5. doi: 10.1016/j.clon.2011.11.001
14. Zhao G, Sun J, Zhang Y, Ba K. Significance of PET-CT for detecting occult lymph node metastasis and affecting prognosis in early-stage tongue squamous cell carcinoma. *Front Oncol.* (2020) 10:368. doi: 10.3389/fonc.2020.00386
15. Ouyang PY, Su Z, Mao YP, Liang XX, Liu Q, Xie FY. Prognostic impact of family history in southern Chinese patients with undifferentiated nasopharyngeal carcinoma. *Br J Cancer.* (2013) 109:788–94. doi: 10.1038/bjc.2013.343
16. Fang QG, Shi S, Liu FY, Sun CF. Squamous cell carcinoma of the oral cavity in ever smokers: a matched-pair analysis of survival. *J Craniofac Surg.* (2014) 25:934–7. doi: 10.1097/SCS.0000000000000710
17. Skulsky SL, O'Sullivan B, McArdle O, Leader M, Roche M, Conlon PJ, et al. Review of high-risk features of cutaneous squamous cell carcinoma and discrepancies between the American Joint Committee on cancer and NCCN clinical practice guidelines in oncology. *Head Neck.* (2017) 39:578–94. doi: 10.1002/hed.24580
18. Lydiatt WM, Patel SG, O'Sullivan B, Brandwein MS, Ridge JA, Migliacci JC, et al. Head and Neck cancers-major changes in the American Joint Committee on cancer eighth edition cancer staging manual. *Cancer J Clin.* (2017) 67:122–37. doi: 10.3322/caac.21389
19. Fang Q, Li P, Qi J, Luo R, Chen D, Zhang X. Value of lingual lymph node metastasis in patients with squamous cell carcinoma of the tongue. *Laryngoscope.* (2019) 129:2527–30. doi: 10.1002/lary.27927
20. Dai L, Fang Q, Li P, Liu F, Zhang X. Oncologic outcomes of patients with sarcomatoid carcinoma of the hypopharynx. *Front Oncol.* (2019) 9:950. doi: 10.3389/fonc.2019.00950
21. Du W, Fang Q, Wu Y, Wu J, Zhang X. Oncologic outcome of marginal mandibulectomy in squamous cell carcinoma of the lower gingiva. *BMC Cancer.* (2019) 19:775. doi: 10.1186/s12885-019-5999-0
22. Deganello A, Gitti G, Meccariello G, Parrinello G, Mannelli G, Gallo O. Effectiveness and pitfalls of elective neck dissection in N0 laryngeal cancer. *Acta Otorhinolaryngol Ital.* (2011) 31:216–221.
23. Moratin J, Metzger K, Engel M, Hoffmann J, Freudlsperger C, Freier K, et al. The occurrence of cervical metastases in squamous cell carcinoma of the tongue: Is there a rationale for bilateral neck dissection in early-stage tumors? *J Craniomaxillofac Surg.* (2019) 47:1134–8. doi: 10.1016/j.jcms.2019.03.003
24. Otsuru M, Ota Y, Yanamoto S, Okura M, Umeda M, Kirita T, et al. A multicenter retrospective study of elective neck dissection for T1-2N0M0 tongue squamous cell carcinoma: analysis using propensity score-matching. *Ann Surg Oncol.* (2019) 26:555–63. doi: 10.1245/s10434-018-07089-7
25. Gad ZS, El-Malt OA, El-Sakkary MAT, Abdal Aziz MM. Elective neck dissection for management of early- stage oral tongue cancer. *Asian Pac J Cancer Prev.* (2018) 19:1797–803. doi: 10.22034/APJCP.2018.19.7.1797
26. Orabona GD, Bonavolontà P, Maglitto F, Friscia M, Iaconetta G, Califano L. Neck dissection versus "watchful-waiting" in early squamous cell carcinoma of the tongue our experience on 127 cases. *Surg Oncol.* (2016) 25:401–4. doi: 10.1016/j.suronc.2016.09.005
27. Stoeckli SJ, Steinert H, Pfaltz M, Schmid S. Is there a role for positron emission tomography with 18F-fluorodeoxyglucose in the initial staging of nodal negative oral and oropharyngeal squamous cell carcinoma. *Head Neck.* (2002) 24:345–9. doi: 10.1002/hed.10057
28. Krabbe CA, Balink H, Roodenburg JL, Dol J, de Visscher JG. Performance of 18F-FDG PET/contrast-enhanced CT in the staging of squamous cell carcinoma of the oral cavity and oropharynx. *Int J Oral Maxillofac Surg.* (2011) 40:1263–70. doi: 10.1016/j.ijom.2011.06.023
29. Lowe VJ, Duan F, Subramaniam RM, Sicks JD, Romanoff J, Bartel T, et al. Multicenter trial of [18F]fluorodeoxyglucose positron emission tomography/computed tomography staging of head and neck cancer and negative predictive value and surgical impact in the N0 Neck: results from ACRIN 6685. *J Clin Oncol.* (2019) 37:1704–12. doi: 10.1200/JCO.18.01182
30. Moya-Plana A, Aupérin A, Guerlain J, Gorphe P, Casiraghi O, Mamelle G, et al. Sentinel node biopsy in early oral squamous cell carcinomas: Long-term follow-up and nodal failure analysis. *Oral Oncol.* (2018) 82:187–94. doi: 10.1016/j.oraloncology.2018.05.021
31. Riese CGU, Karstadt JA, Schramm A, Güleryüz S, Dressel G, Lorenz KJ, et al. Validity of sentinel node biopsy in early oral and oropharyngeal carcinoma. *J Craniomaxillofac Surg.* (2018) 46:1748–52. doi: 10.1016/j.jcms.2018.07.021
32. Schilling C, Shaw R, Schache A, McMahon J, Chegini S, Kerawala C, et al. Sentinel lymph node biopsy for oral squamous cell carcinoma. Where are we now? *Br J Oral Maxillofac Surg.* (2017) 55:757–62. doi: 10.1016/j.bjoms.2017.07.007
33. El-Maraghi RH, Kielar AZ. PET vs sentinel lymph node biopsy for staging melanoma: a patient intervention, comparison, outcome analysis. *J Am Coll Radiol.* (2008) 5:924–31. doi: 10.1016/j.jacr.2008.02.022
34. De Nardi P, Guarneri G, Canevari C, Tamburini A, Slim N, Passoni P, et al. Prognostic value of fluorodeoxyglucose positron emission tomography/computed tomography and inguinal sentinel lymph node biopsy in patients with anal cancer. *Colorectal Dis.* (2019) 21:1017–24. doi: 10.1111/codi.14691
35. Ahmed SQ, Junaid M, Awan S, Kazi M, Khan HU, Halim S. Frequency of cervical nodal metastasis in early-stage squamous

cell carcinoma of the tongue. *Int Arch Otorhinolaryngol.* (2018) 22:136–40. doi: 10.1055/s-0037-1603626

36. Abbate V, Dell'Aversana Orabona G, Salzano G, Bonavolontà P, Maglitto F, Romano A, et al. Pre-treatment neutrophil-to-lymphocyte ratio as a predictor for occult cervical metastasis in early stage (T1-T2 cN0) squamous cell carcinoma of the oral tongue. *Surg Oncol.* (2018) 27:503–7. doi: 10.1016/j.suronc.2018.06.002
37. van den Brekel MW, van der Waal I, Meijer CJ, Freeman JL, Castelijns JA, Snow GB. The incidence of micrometastases in neck dissection specimens obtained from elective neck dissections. *Laryngoscope.* (1996) 106:987–91. doi: 10.1097/00005537-199608000-00014
38. Barrera JE, Miller ME, Said S, Jafek BW, Campana JP, Shroyer KR. Detection of occult cervical micrometastases in patients with head and neck squamous cell cancer. *Laryngoscope.* (2003) 113:892–6. doi: 10.1097/00005537-200305000-00022
39. Rhee D, Wenig BM, Smith RV. The significance of immunohistochemically demonstrated nodal micrometastases in patients with squamous cell carcinoma of the head and neck. *Laryngoscope.* (2002) 112:1970–4. doi: 10.1097/00005537-200211000-00011

22

Defining a Standard Set of Health Outcomes for Patients with Squamous Cell Carcinoma of the Head and Neck in Spain

Virginia Arrazubi[1†], *Gerardo Cajaraville*[2†], *David Cantero*[3†], *Jordi Giralt*[4†], *Ricard Mesia*[5†], *Florencio Monje*[6†], *Antonio Rueda*[7†], *Alexander Sistiaga*[8†], *Jorge Suarez*[9], *Alejandro Mut*[9], *Marta Comellas*[10] and *Luis Lizán*[10,11*]

[1] *Oncology, Complejo Hospitalario de Navarra, Pamplona, Spain,* [2] *Hospital Pharmacy, Fundación Onkologikoa, San Sebastián, Spain,* [3] *Quality and Innovation, Organización Sanitaria Integrada (Integrated Health Organisation) (OSI) Barrualde Galdakao, Galdakao, Spain,* [4] *Radiation Oncology, Hospital Universitari Vall d'Hebrón, Barcelona, Spain,* [5] *Medical Oncology, Institut Català d'Oncología, Group Badalona Applied Research Group in Oncology (B-ARGO) Group, Institut d'Investigació Germans Trias i Pujol (IGTP), Badalona, Spain,* [6] *Oral and Maxillofacial Surgery, Hospital Universitario de Badajoz, Badajoz, Spain,* [7] *Oncology, Hospital Regional Universitario de Málaga, Málaga, Spain,* [8] *Otolaryngology, Hospital Universitario Donostia, San Sebastián, Spain,* [9] *Bristol Myers Squibb, Madrid, Spain,* [10] *Outcomes'10, Castellón de la Plana, Spain,* [11] *Medicine Department, Jaume I University, Castellón de la Plana, Spain*

Correspondence:
Luis Lizán
lizan@outcomes10.com

†These authors have contributed equally to this work and share first authorship

Purpose: A systematic, standardized collection of health outcomes during patient treatment and follow-up, relevant from the perspective of all stakeholders, is a crucial step toward effective and efficient disease management. This project aimed to define a standard set of health outcomes for patients with squamous cell carcinoma of the head and neck (SCCHN).

Methods: The project was led and coordinated by a scientific committee (SC). It comprised: (1) a literature review (to identify variables used during SCCHN management); (2) 1st-SC meeting (to select the variables for presentation during nominal groups-NG); (3) five NG (n=42 experts) and four interviews with patients (to reach consensus on the variables for inclusion); and (4) final-SC meeting (to review the results of NG ensuring consensus on the variables where consensus was not reached).

Results: Experts agreed to include the following variables in the standard set: treatment-related (treatment intent and type, response to treatment, treatment toxicity/complication, treatment completion), degree of health (performance status, patient-reported health status, pain, dysphonia, feeding and speech limitations, body image alteration, tracheotomy), survival (overall and progression-free survival, cause of death), nutritional (weight, nutritional intervention), other variables (smoking status, alcohol consumption, patient satisfaction with aftermath care, employment status), and case-mix variables (demographic, tumor-related, clinical and nutritional factors).

Conclusions: This project may pave the way to standardizing the collection of health outcomes in SCCHN and promote the incorporation of patients' perspective in its management. The information provided through the systematic compilation of this standard set may define strategies to achieve high-quality, patient-centered care.

Keywords: head and neck cancer, patient-centered care, outcome measurement, patient-reported outcomes, patient centricity, quality of life

1 INTRODUCTION

Head and neck cancer includes a group of neoplasms of various anatomical sites that differ in terms of etiology, diagnostic and treatment approaches (1). It was the seventh most common cancer worldwide in 2020 accounting for 932,000 new cases and 466,500 deaths (2). In Spain, it was estimated that 14,200 new cases of head and neck cancer would be diagnosed in 2020 (3). More than 90% of cases are squamous cell carcinomas of the head and neck (SCCHN) (4) and more than 60% of patients with SCCHN present with stage III or IV disease (5). SCCHN is typically diagnosed in older patients, with smoking and alcohol consumption being two of the main risk factors for its development (1). Moreover, human papilloma virus (HPV) infection has emerged as a new risk factor, especially in oropharyngeal cancer (6).

Treatment for SCCHN is complex and requires a multidisciplinary approach since it differs according to the stage of the disease, anatomical site, and surgical accessibility. It may require intricate surgery, radiation, chemotherapy, and/or targeted therapy, and/or immunotherapy (7, 8). Some of these treatment options involve changes to critical structures for speaking, eating and breathing, which can lead to functionality problems. Therefore, as a result of treatment, patients with SCCHN face long-term challenges beyond surveillance for recurrent or secondary cancer, including adapting to disfigurement, managing dysphagia and developing alternative speech (9, 10).

In addition to curative intention, structural and functional preservation, amelioration of morbidities when feasible, and long-term maintenance of health-related quality of life (HRQoL) are the principal treatment objectives. Therefore, treatment selection based on a multidisciplinary tumor board decision is essential (11, 12). There is growing evidence supporting the routine collection of patient-reported outcomes (PROs) to enable improved, patient-centered care. The systematic collection of PROs in oncology has a positive effect on patient-physician communication, improves the monitoring of disease progression and response to therapy, helps identify unrecognized problems (physical, emotional and/or social problems), contributes to detecting adverse effects of treatment, and enhances patients' experience and satisfaction (13). Despite the collection of PROs being considered the cornerstone for achieving the best results and preserving patients' HRQoL, their systematic collection using standardized and validated instruments is mostly limited to clinical research environment, with scarce use in clinical practice.

To move toward an effective and efficient patient-centered system, a holistic approach is required, integrating evidence from clinical outcomes and PROs. Experience gained from other fields shows that the systematic and standardized collection of outcomes is the *sine qua non* to improve the quality of any process (14). During the last few years, pioneer initiatives such as the one performed by the International Consortium for Health Outcomes Measurements (ICHOM) (15) have focused on the development of standard sets of health outcomes for various diseases, among which SCCHN is not included. The long-term goal of these initiatives is to promote consistency in data collection between different institutions within the same country or among different countries. A systematic, standardized compilation of health outcomes, relevant from the perspective of all stakeholders, during patient treatment and follow-up, is a key step toward effective and efficient disease management. This project aimed to define a standard set of health outcomes and the most appropriate instruments to measure them for managing patients diagnosed with SCCHN. This is the first step to ensure to standardize the collection of health outcomes in SCCHN.

2 MATERIALS AND METHODS

The project comprised four phases: (1) a literature review; (2) first scientific committee meeting; (3) five nominal groups (described in greater detail below) and four semi-structured interviews with patients, and; (4) final scientific committee meeting (**Figure 1**). The scientific committee and nominal group meetings were conducted between June 2019 and December 2020. The project was led and coordinated by a scientific committee consisting of healthcare professionals who are experts in the management of SCCHN, and/or have experience in implementing strategies to standardize health outcomes (three specialists in medical oncology [VA, RM, AR], one specialist in radiation oncology [JG], one specialist in otolaryngology [AS], one specialist in oral and maxillofacial surgery [FM], one specialist in quality and innovation [DC], one hospital pharmacist [GC]) and one representative of a

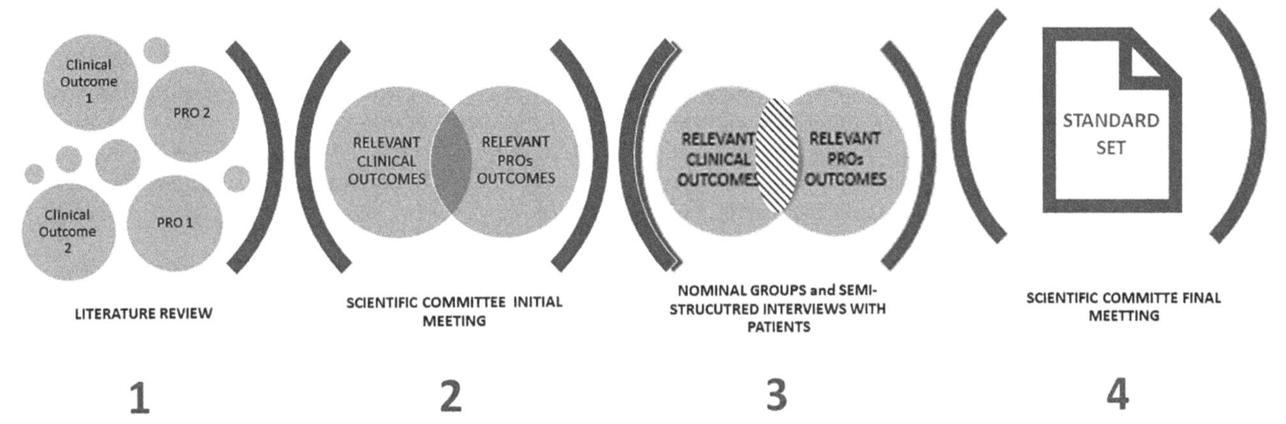

FIGURE 1 | Project phases.

Spanish patient advocacy group (*Grupo Español de Pacientes con Cancer*, GEPAC).

2.1 Literature Review

To identify health outcomes [clinical and patient-reported outcomes (PROs)], instruments, and frequency of measurement to be used during SCCHN patient follow-up, a systematic literature review according to the Cochrane Handbook for Systematic Reviews of Interventions (16) (**Supplementary Table S1**), was carried out in Medline/PubMed. Clinical trials or systematic reviews that include clinical trials in SCCHN, published in English and/or Spanish between 01/01/2016 and 03/31/2019 were reviewed.

2.2 First Scientific Committee Meeting

The first meeting with the members of the scientific committee aimed to present the project, define the target population and, based on the results of the literature review, select the health outcomes for presenting during the nominal groups.

During the discussion group, the scientific committee screened health outcomes (variable/instrument/frequency of measurement) identified in the literature review and selected them according to their relevance for patient follow-up and availability in the Spanish setting. Moreover, the scientific committee proposed new health outcomes not previously identified in the literature review, but relevant from their perspective.

2.3 Nominal Group Meetings and Semi-Structured Interviews With Patient Representatives

Five nominal multidisciplinary groups were conducted to reach a consensus on the health outcomes for inclusion in the standard set. Nominal group meetings took place either face-to-face (n=4 meetings) or online (n=1 meeting), depending on participants' availability to meet.

A nominal group is a qualitative methodology that allows reaching a consensus and ensuring balanced participation among group members, giving them equal opportunities to share their opinions (17). Following the methodological recommendation (18), nominal groups involved five main steps: 1) Introduction and explanation: welcome and description of the purpose and procedure of the meeting; 2) Silent generation of ideas: each participant individually (without consulting or discussing with others) evaluated the health outcomes proposed; 3) Sharing ideas: separately, participants shared the health outcomes they had selected; 4) Group discussion: participants could seek a verbal explanation or further details about any of the health outcomes that other participants had proposed; 5) Voting and ranking: during this phase, participants were asked to prioritize the health outcomes proposed. Health outcomes were included if $\geq$ 75% of participants agreed on their inclusion. The five nominal groups worked on the same standard set (based on scientific committee proposal). An individual consensus on specific standard set was reached in each of the nominal group.

The participation in each nominal group was limited to a maximum of 12 experts. Nominal groups consisted of experts from different geographic areas of Spain, including medical oncologists, radiation oncologists, otolaryngologists, oral and maxillofacial surgeons, a phoniatrician, primary care specialists, hospital pharmacists, hospital managers, psycho-oncologists, nutritionists, speech therapists, and dentists. Members of the nominal groups were identified by the scientific committee, in collaboration with the study coordinator. They were selected based on their experience in SCCHN management, PRO measurement, implementing strategies to standardize health outcomes, as well as their availability and interest in the project.

To gain patients' perspectives on the impact of the disease and its treatment on their day-to-day lives, semi-structured telephone interviews (**Supplementary Table S2**) were conducted with four patient representatives.

2.4 Second Scientific Committee Meeting

The main objective of the last meeting of the scientific committee was to define the final standard set for SCCHN. For this purpose, the agreed health outcomes (clinical and PROs) in each nominal group were presented to the scientific committee. The scientific committee reviewed the individual results of the five nominal groups, ensuring consensus on the health outcomes for which no agreement was reached among the nominal groups. Therefore, if a health outcome did not reach the consensus of inclusion in the five nominal groups, the scientific committee members assessed its inclusion or exclusion from the final standard set. The consensus was reached if ≥ 75% of the members of the scientific committee agreed on the inclusion/exclusion of the health outcome.

Additionally, results from semi-structured interviews with patients were also presented to confirm that the most relevant health outcomes from the patients' perspective were included in the standard set.

Based on the meeting results, the health outcomes for inclusion in the standard set for SCCHN were defined.

3 RESULTS

3.1 Literature Review

The database search yielded 66 references of which 30 were excluded as their title and abstract contained detailed reviews that did not report health outcomes for patient follow-up. The remaining 36 publications were assessed for eligibility. All of them were selected to be reviewed for qualitative synthesis and identification of health outcomes, measuring instrument, and frequency (**Figure 2**).

A total of 47 health outcomes were identified in the literature review. They were categorized into case-mix variables (baseline factors that may affect the health outcomes but cannot be controlled as part of the management of the condition and enable patient characterization) (n=27) and 20 outcomes variables (variables for patient follow-up) (n=20) (**Supplementary Table S3**).

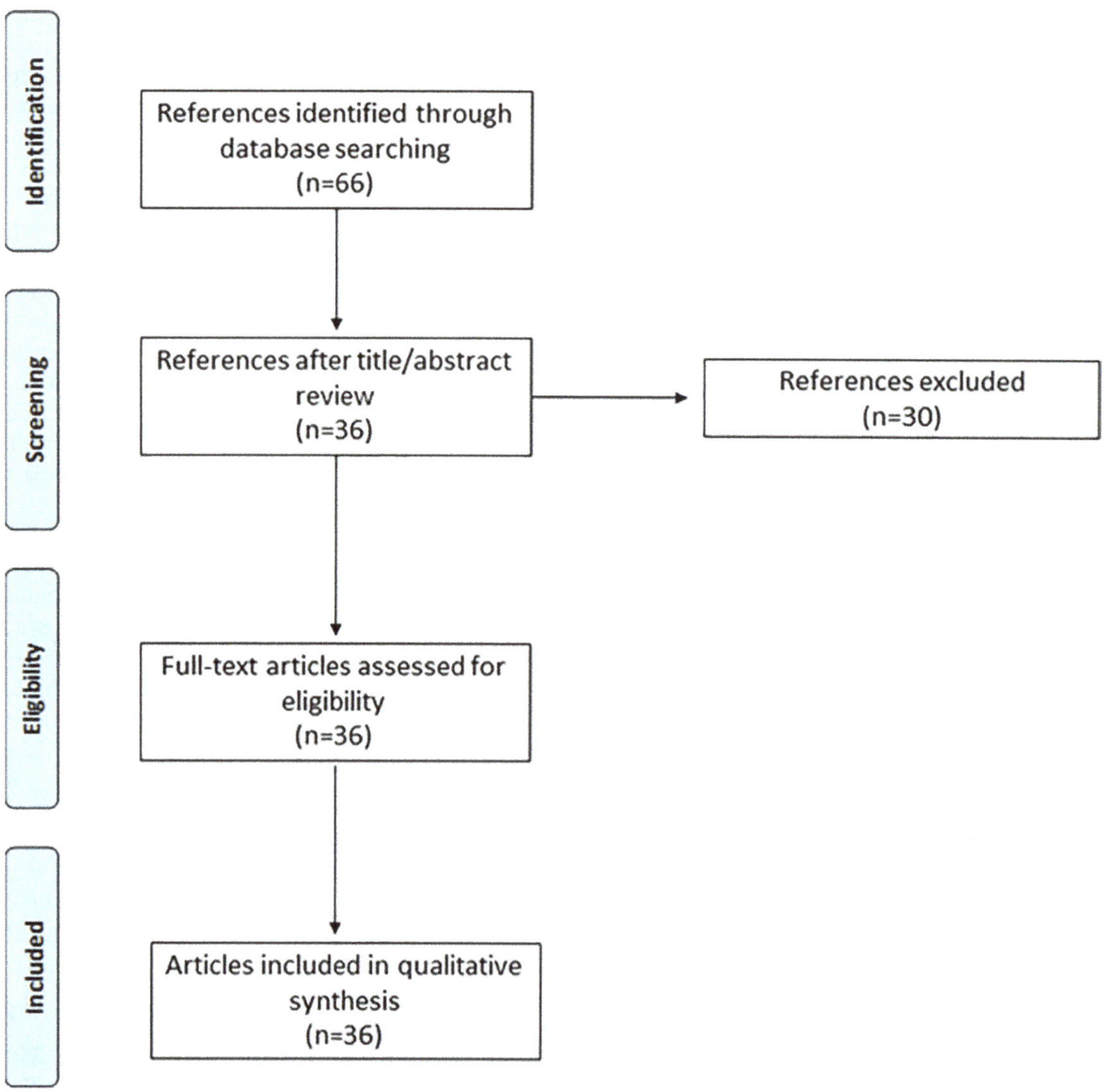

FIGURE 2 | PRISMA flow diagram.

3.2 First Scientific Committee Meeting

The scientific committee considered 18 out of 27 case-mix and 11 out of 20 outcomes variables previously identified in the literature as being relevant. Moreover, two additional case-mix and nine outcomes variables were proposed. Thus, 20 case-mix and 20 outcomes variables were selected by the scientific committee for presentation and evaluation during the nominal groups (**Supplementary Table S4**).

The target population of the standard set was also defined. The scientific committee agreed to include all patients with newly-diagnosed SCCHN originating from the oral cavity, oropharynx, hypopharynx and larynx. Head and neck cancers originating from salivary glands, nasopharynx, paranasal sinuses and nasal cavity, and those with a histological type other than squamous, have special characteristics and are subject to specific recommendations and were therefore not included in the target population of this standard set.

3.3 Nominal Group Meetings

A total of 42 experts on SCCHN from different specialties (n=12 medical oncologists, n=4 radiation oncologists, n=6 otolaryngologists, n=2 oral and maxillofacial surgeons, n=1 phoniatrician, n=1 primary care specialist, n=10 hospital pharmacists, n=1 hospital manager, n=2 psycho-oncologists, n=1 nutritionist, n=1 speech therapist, and n=1 dentist) and geographical areas of Spain participated in four nominal group meetings.

The experts agreed to include twelve case-mix and thirteen outcomes variables proposed by the scientific committee in the standard set. Additionally, thirteen new case-mix and thirteen outcomes variables were proposed during the nominal groups (**Supplementary Table S5**).

3.4 Semi-Structured Interviews With Patients

Four patient representatives participated in the semi-structured interviews (100% men, age range: 54-82 years).

Patients described the impact of the disease and its treatment on HRQoL, mainly due to disease aftermath. The most common symptoms and side effects reported by patients included dry mouth, oral pain, fatigue and loss of taste and smell. Moreover, several dysfunctions such as speech or voice and swallowing problems were also pointed out.

The disease also harmed patients' working lives, as most of the patients who were active at the time of diagnosis were unable to return to work.

3.5 Second Scientific Committee Meeting

Based on the consensus reached among nominal groups, the scientific committee assessed the inclusion or exclusion of the new health outcomes proposed and those for which the nominal groups did not reach a consensus.

3.5.1 Case-Mix Variables

Case-mix variables are defined as factors that may affect the health outcomes but cannot be controlled as part of the management of the condition. The experts agree to collect at baseline the main sociodemographic factors (age, gender, and social/familiar support), tumor-related factors (tumor localization and sublocalization, cancer staging based on TNM status, and date of diagnosis), clinical factors (alcohol consumption; smoking status, performance status, comorbidities, global patient health status, pain, dysphagia, dysphonia, p16 expression, PD-L1 expression, fragility, and referral to dentistry), and nutritional factors (unintentional weight loss, and dental problem) at the time of diagnosis, before initiating treatment (baseline visits) (**Table 1**).

Social/familial support was defined as a proxy for predicting whether the patient would be able to cope with the disease and complete treatment from the physician's perspective (yes/no).

To standardize the assessment of alcohol consumption, a consensus was reached to classify patients as consumers (regular or occasional) or non-consumers from the patient's perspective. Similarly, to collect smoking status at diagnosis in a standardized way, the experts agreed to report if the patient was a never-smoker, an ex-smoker (defined as a patient who has stopped at least one year before diagnosis), or a current smoker. For ex-smoker and current smoker patients, it was agreed to record whether the patient's pack-year index (calculated by multiplying the number of packs of cigarettes smoked per day by the number of years the person has smoked) was < or ≥10.

To systematically report patients' comorbidities, a list of diseases that can influence treatment and/or clinical practice was developed to select patient comorbidities. The list includes: vasculopathy, renal failure, liver failure, anemia, neuropathy, deafness, diagnosed mental illness, other primary cancer, diabetes, COPD, heart disease, and autoimmune disease.

The experts agreed to use validated questionnaires to assess and collect some of these case-mix variables. To describe patients' performance status, experts agreed on the use of the Eastern Cooperative Oncology Group (ECOG) scale, which assesses patients' level of functioning in terms of self-care, carrying out daily activities, and physical ability (19). A generic HRQoL questionnaire (EQ-5D) (20, 21) and head and neck cancer-specific HRQoL questionnaire [EORTC QL-Q H&N43 (22)] were proposed to assess patients' global health status and the impact of the disease on their social, working and personal function. The use of EORTC QL-Q H&N43 also allows gathering information about patients' perspective of pain, dysphagia, and dysphonia. And finally, to evaluate patients' fragility, the experts agreed to complete the G8 questionnaire (23) in patients over 70 years of age.

3.5.2 Outcomes Variables

Outcomes variables establish the evolution of patients' health status and determine the response (success) in managing the medical condition (**Table 2**). They are collected during patient follow-up.

3.5.2.1 Treatment-Related Variables

It was agreed to collect, prior to initiating treatment, data on treatment intention and type. For patients that receive curative treatment, the experts reached a consensus on the inclusion of

TABLE 1 | Spanish standard set of patient-centered outcomes in SCCHN.

Patient profile	Variable	Supporting information	Measurement instrument	Timing	Data sources
Sociodemographic factors					
All patients	Age		Date of birth	Baseline (before treatment begins)	Clinical report
	Gender		F: female; M: male		Clinical report
	Family support	Assessment of patient's environment/support as a proxy for predicting whether he/she will be able to cope with the disease and complete treatment	(1) Yes; (2) No		Physician-reported
Baseline tumor factors					
All patients	TNM status		TNM scale	Baseline (before treatment begins)/ after pathological anatomy results (if available)	Clinical report
	Tumor localization and sub localization		NA		Clinical report
	Date of diagnosis		NA		Clinical report
Baseline clinical factors					
Patients with oropharyngeal cancer	p16 expression		(1) positive; (2) negative		Clinical report
Recurrent metastatic cancer	PD-L1 expression		(1) positive; (2) negative		Clinical report
Patients >70 years	Fragility		G8 questionnaire		Physician-reported
All patients	Alcohol consumption	Alcohol consumption at diagnosis	(1) Consumer (regular or occasional consumer); (2) Non-consumer	Baseline (before treatment begins)	Physician-reported according to patient-notification
	Smoking status	Smoking status at diagnosis	1) Never-smoker; (2) Ex-smoker (stopped >1 year before diagnosis): years + PYI <10 or PYI ≥10; (3) Current smoker: PYI <10 or PYI ≥10		Physician-reported according to patient-notification
	Performance status		ECOG scale		Physician-reported
	Comorbidities		Comorbidities list*		Clinical report
	Patient-reported health status	Global health and impact of the disease on physical, social and emotional function	Tracked *via* generic questionnaire EQ5D and H&N specific questionnaire EORTC QL-Q H&N43		Patient-reported
	Pain		Tracked *via* items 31,32, 34, 63 of EORTC QL-Q H&N43		Patient-reported
	Referral to dentistry		(1) Yes; (2) No		Physician-reported
	Dysphagia	Swallowing problems	Tracked *via* items 35-38 of EORTC QL-Q H&N43		Patient-reported
	Dysphonia		Tracked *via* items 47, of 55-58 EORTC QL-Q H&N43		Patient-reported
Baseline nutritional factors					
All patients	Unintentional weight loss	Unintentional weight loss during the previous 3 months	Yes/No/I don't know	Baseline (before treatment begins)	Patient-reported
	Dental problems	Loss of teeth or dental problems	Tracked *via* items 39, 40 and 73 of EORTC QL-Q H&N43		Clinical report

*PYI, Pack-year index; NA, not applicable; ECOG, Eastern Cooperative Oncology Group; PD-L1, Programmed death-ligand; EQ-5D, EuroQol; EORTC, quality of life core questionnaire; H&N, head and neck cancer; *includes: vasculopathy, renal failure, liver failure, anemia, neuropathy, deafness, diagnosed mental illness, other primary cancer, diabetes, COPD, heart disease, and autoimmune disease.*
Case-mix variables.

treatment response at three months after end of treatment. For patients receiving palliative treatment, it was agreed to assess response to treatment using RECIST criteria every three cycles of treatment.

The experts agreed to report if the patient had developed treatment toxicity or any surgical complication interfering with or modifying the treatment plan. Finally, the experts considered it relevant to indicate if the patient had completed

TABLE 2 | Spanish standard set of patient-centered outcomes in SCCHN.

Patient profile	Measure	Supporting information	Measurement instrument	Timing	Data sources
Treatment variables					
All patients	Treatment intent		(1) curative; (2) palliative	Baseline (before treatment begins)	Physician-reported
	Type of treatment		(1) Surgery; (2) Radiotherapy; (3) Chemotherapy: (4) Immunotherapy; (5) Targeted therapy; (6) Supportive therapy	Baseline (before treatment begins)	Physician-reported
	Response to curative treatment		(1) Disease-free; (2) Persists; (3) Progress	At 3 months after treatment ends	Clinical report
	Response to palliative treatment	Using RECIST criteria	(1) Complete response; (2) Partial response; (3) Progressive disease; (4) Stable disease	Every 3 cycles of treatment	Clinical report
	Treatment toxicity or surgical complication	Development of treatment toxicity or surgical complications that have interfered with or modified treatment plan	(1) Yes; (2) No	During treatment or surgery	Physician-reported (according to clinical report or patient's perspective)
	Treatment plan completed		(1) Yes; (2) No; due to lack of efficiency; (3) No, due to toxicity; (4) No, due to patient's death; (5) No, due to intermittent cause	At treatment end	Physician-reported
Degree of health					
All patients	Performance status		ECOG scale	1st year: every 3 m/2nd-3rd years: every 6 m/later: every year	Clinical report
	Patient-reported health status	Global health status, physical and emotional function	Tracked *via* generic questionnaire EQ5D and SCCHN specific questionnaire EORTC QL-Q H&N43	1st year: every 6 m/later: every year	Patient-reported
	Pain		Tracked *via* items 31-34, 63 of EORTC QL-Q H&N43		Patient-reported
	Dysphonia		Tracked *via* items 47, of 55-58 of EORTC QL-Q H&N43		Patient-reported
	Feeding limitations	Includes: dysphagia, dental problems, xerostomia, taste/smell alteration, chewing/eating problems	Tracked *via* items 35-45, 51-54, 73 of EORTC QL-Q H&N43		Patient-reported
	Oral communication limitations	Includes hoarseness and problems talking	Tracked *via* items 47, 55-58 EORTC QL-Q H&N43		Patient-reported
	Body image alteration	Include body image and sexual limitation	Tracked *via* items 48-50, 59-61 of EORTC QL-Q H&N43		Patient-reported
	A requirement for permanent tracheotomy		(1) Yes; (2) No	When tracheotomy is required	Clinical report
Survival					
All patients	Overall survival		Date of death	NA	Administrative data (death registry)
	Progression-free survival		NA	1st year: every 3 m/2nd-3rd years: every 6 m/later: every year	
	Cause of death	Tumor/treatment-related or not	NA	NA	Administrative data (death registry)
Nutritional variables					
All patients	Weight		NA	1st year: every 3 m/2nd-3rd years: every 6 m/later: every year	Clinical report
	Nutritional intervention	Nutritional intervention required during treatment or follow-up	(1) Yes, oral supplementation; (2) Yes, tube enteral nutrition tube; (3) yes, enteral nutrition by ostomy; (4) Not required	When nutritional intervention is required	Clinical report
Others					
All patients	Smoking status	Reported if patient still smokes:	(1) Yes; (2) No; (3) Patient did not smoke prior to diagnosis	1st year: every 3 m/2nd-3rd years: every 6 m/later: every year	Physician-reported according to patient-notification
	Alcohol consumption	Reported if patient still consumes alcohol	(1) Yes; (2) No; 3) Patient did not drink alcohol prior to diagnosis		

(Continued)

TABLE 2 | Continued

Patient profile	Measure	Supporting information	Measurement instrument	Timing	Data sources
				1st year: every 3 m/2nd-3rd years: every 6 m/later: every year	Physician-reported according to patient notification
	Patient satisfaction with aftermath care		(1) Satisfied;(2) Not satisfied; (3) Patient does not have an aftermath	After hospital discharge or 5 years after treatment ends	Patient-reported
	Employment status	Record whether the patient has been able to return to their previous job in the same conditions	(1) Yes;(2) No; (3) Patient did not work prior to diagnosis	After oncology department discharge or 5 years after treatment ends	Patient-reported

NA, not applicable; ECOG, Eastern Cooperative Oncology Group; EQ-5D: EuroQol; EORTC, quality of life core questionnaire; H&N: head and neck cancer. Outcomes variables.

the treatment plan and, when applicable, record the reason for not doing so.

3.5.2.2 Degree of Health

SCCHN has a negative impact on patients' performance and health status. Therefore, it was agreed to collect both sets of variables during patient follow-up. As previously indicated, the ECOG scale (19) was selected to assess patients' performance status, while the EQ-5D (20, 21) and EORTC QL-Q H&N43 (22) were chosen for the assessment of patients' HRQoL. The use of EORTC QL-Q H&N43 annually during patient follow-up allows the evaluation of the impact of the disease on patients' lives, including pain, dysphonia, feeding limitations, oral communication limitations, and body image alterations.

Given the significant impact that it can have on patients, it was also agreed to collect information on whether or not the patient requires a permanent tracheotomy.

3.5.2.3 Survival

Overall survival and progression-free survival were considered key variables for inclusion in the standard set for patient follow-up. Moreover, participants agreed on gathering information regarding cause of death, indicating whether it was tumor- or treatment-related.

3.5.2.4 Nutritional Variables

The disease and its treatment have a negative impact on patients' nutritional status. For this reason, it was agreed to collect patients' weight at each visit, and record whether the patient had required nutritional intervention during treatment or follow-up.

It is important to note that the use of EORTC QL-Q H&N43 allows the physician to assess dysphagia, dental problems, xerostomia, taste/smell alterations, and chewing/eating problems that may impact patients' nutritional status.

3.5.2.5 Others

Alcohol and tobacco consumption are the main risk factors for SCCHN development, and their maintenance during and/or after treatment is related with recurrence, second neoplasms and tobacco/alcohol-related death. Consequently, it was agreed to record whether the patient continued smoking or consuming alcohol after diagnosis.

SCCHN may also affect patients' employment status; therefore, the experts agreed to report whether patients can return to their previous job under similar conditions after discharge from the oncology department or five years after end of treatment.

Most patients with SCCHN reported difficulty in access to aftermath care. Therefore, it was agreed to record whether patients were satisfied with the aftermath care received after being discharged from the oncology department and five years after treatment end.

4 DISCUSSION

A systematic and standardized collection of health outcomes during follow-up of patients with SCCHN is a crucial step toward a more effective and efficient healthcare system. A holistic approach, integrating all stakeholders' perspectives, is necessary to ensure the best quality care. To this end, a standard set that includes relevant health outcomes from the perspective of both patients and healthcare professionals is required. The SCCHN standard set defined herein is an excellent opportunity to promote patient-centered care and optimize SCCHN management.

The SCCHN standard set includes 21 outcomes variables. In addition to traditional variables regarding survival or treatment, eight are included related to patients' degree of health (performance status, patient-reported health status, pain, dysphonia, feeding limitations, oral communication limitations, body image alteration, and need for permanent tracheostomy). Six of them are proposed for tracking *via* HRQoL questionnaires, EQ-5D-3L and EORTC QL-Q H&N43. SCCHN and its treatment can compromise vital functions, such as breathing, swallowing, and speech. Therefore, the disease can lead to significant physical, emotional, and social problems, reducing patients' HRQL. Although the collection of HRQoL and other PROs is scarce in clinical practice, the inclusion of these variables in the standard set was considered key to establishing the impact of the disease from the patients' perspective (24, 25). Due to the lack of resources and the limited knowledge of these questionnaires in clinical practice (26), it was proposed to complete these questionnaires every six months during the first year and then annually. Moreover, by using the EORTC QL-Q H&N43 questionnaire, information about the impact of the disease and its treatment on nutritional status, such as dysphagia, dental problems, dry mouth, sensory problems, taste/smell alterations, problems with chewing, and weight loss, can also be gathered.

Although some healthcare professionals perceive the use of PROs in clinical practice as time-consuming, a one-year pilot study conducted in the Netherlands demonstrated that the ICHOM standard set could be implemented during routine SCCHN treatment without significantly disturbing the everyday workflow (27, 28). The authors concluded that the collection of PROs is not overly time-consuming; however, it requires *ad hoc* tools and dedicated staff (27, 28).

Providing patient-centered care is essential to move toward high-quality integrated care. Therefore, the inclusion of PROs in the standard set is crucial. Other initiatives have been conducted to promote the use of PROs and patient-reported experiences (PREs) to measure the quality of care, showing that PROs and PREs are promising for measuring and improving the quality and personalization of healthcare in patients with SCCHN (29, 30).

In addition to defining the essential variables for patient follow-up, the experts agreed on those necessary to characterize the patient, the case-mix. The inclusion of these variables is beneficial for benchmarking purposes and for comparing results based on patient profiles.

Data from the implementation of other standard sets in clinical practice has shown benefits from patients' and clinicians' perspectives. On the one hand, the inclusion of PROs in the standard set will allow clinicians to focus on the aspects of the disease that most matter to the patient, and therefore encourage better patient engagement in disease management. Moreover, clinicians can learn from the outcomes data they gather, and from the experience of other healthcare professionals in different settings, the standard set thus becoming a valuable tool for benchmarking (31–34).

This project presents several limitations. This standard set reflects the opinion of a group of 50 experts on the management of SCCHN, four patient representatives (all men) and one patient advocacy group representative. Although no significant differences are expected, different groups of experts and patients, including women, could have agreed on various other recommendations. To minimize this potential bias and ensure national representativeness, participants from four broad geographic areas were involved in the project. Secondly, some health outcomes, for instead data regarding surgical details are finally excluded from the standard set. In this regard, it is important to bear in mind that we aim to achieve a minimum, standard set to ensure that at a minimum these health outcomes are collected. In third place, some relevant variables, such as biomarkers may not have been considered when elaborating on the standard set. To minimize this limitation, and due to the continuing advances in both the knowledge and treatment of this disease, we recommend periodically updating the list of biomarkers for evaluation during patient follow-up. We also suggest that the present standard set be regularly updated.

Although this standard set for SCCHN marks a starting point, several barriers need to be overcome on the road to its successful implementation in the Spanish setting. Namely, the time required for the collection of the health outcomes proposed, the lack of digital tools allowing systematic and automatic PRO measurements (PROMs) compilation, together with limited education and information of patients and clinicians about PROs, have been identified as the main barriers to the implementation of the present standard set (35). Newer platforms for data collection, based on information and communication technologies, may reduce the burden on both patient and clinician, as well as data processing time, thus facilitating the use of PROs in clinical practice (36). It is important to notice that, regardless of the platform used to collect the health outcomes of the standard set, they will be included in the patient's medical record; therefore, the protection of personal data will be guaranteed and will follow the same procedure as the rest of the data in the medical record. Other barriers that must be overcome to ensure the widespread use of this standard set are inherent to the structure of the Spanish national healthcare system (SNHS). Indeed, one of the main characteristics of the SNHS is its heterogeneity: healthcare processes, organizational models as well as information systems differ widely both among and within regions.

Besides addressing these barriers, a further step to promote the integration of the defined standard set into the Spanish healthcare model may involve conducting a pilot implementation study. A pilot study may help establish the feasibility of introducing the standard set in the routine clinical practice, providing insights into the leading resource requirements and organizational challenges to be tackled during implementation.

5 CONCLUSION

The standard set defined may pave the way to standardizing the collection of variables in SCCHN and contribute to promoting the incorporation of patient perspective in SCCHN management. In turn, the information provided through the systematic compilation of this set of health outcomes may allow both clinicians and health policymakers to define strategies aimed at achieving high-quality, patient-centered care.

AUTHOR CONTRIBUTIONS

VA, GC, DC, JG, RM, FM, AR, and AS: contributed equally to this work with data acquisition and data interpretation. JS, AM, and LL contributed to the conceptualization and design of the study. JS and AM did not participate either as members of Scientific Committee or on the selection of members of the Scientific Committee. MC contributed to the conceptualization and design of the study, data acquisition, data analysis, data interpretation and wrote the first draft of the manuscript. All authors contributed to manuscript revision, read and approved the submitted version.

ACKNOWLEDGMENTS

The authors would like to thank to all participants in the nominal groups and to the following Spanish Scientific Societies for endorsing the Project: Sociedad Española de Oncología Médica (SEOM), Sociedad Española de Oncología Radioterápica (SEOR), Grupo Español de oncología Radioterápica de Cabeza y Cuello (GEORCC), Sociedad Española de Cabeza y Cuello (SECyC), Sociedad Española de Cirugía Oral y Maxilofacial de Cabeza y Cuello (SECOM-CyC), Sociedad Española de Otorrinolaringología y Cirugía de Cabeza y Cuello (SEORL-CCC), Grupo Español de Tratamiento de Tumores de Cabeza y cuello (TTCC), Fundación para la Excelencia y la Calidad de la Oncología (ECO), Sociedad Española de Medicina Oral (SEMO), Sociedad Española de Farmacia Hospitalaria (SEFH)] and to Spanish patient advocacy group Grupo Español de Pacientes con Cáncer (GEPAC)].

REFERENCES

1. Orlandi E, Alfieri S, Simon C, Trama A, Licitra L, Group RW. Treatment Challenges in and Outside a Network Setting: Head and Neck Cancers. *Eur J Surg Oncol* (2019) 45:40–5. doi: 10.1016/j.ejso.2018.02.007
2. Sung H, Ferlay J, Siegel RL, Laversanne M, Soerjomataram I, Jemal A, et al. Global Cancer Statistics 2020: GLOBOCAN Estimates of Incidence and Mortality Worldwide for 36 Cancers in 185 Countries. *CA Cancer J Clin* (2021) 71:209–49. doi: 10.3322/caac.21660
3. Sociedad Española de Oncología Médica. Las Cifras del Cáncer en España 2020. *Soc Española Oncol Médica* (2020) 36.
4. Vigneswaran N MDW. Epidemiological Trends in Head and Neck Cancer and Aids in Diagnosis. *Oral Maxillofac Surg Clin North Am* (2014) 26:123–41. doi: 10.1016/j.coms.2014.01.001
5. Chow LQM. Head and Neck Cancer. *N Engl J Med* (2020) 382:60–72. doi: 10.1056/NEJMra1715715
6. Hayes DN, Van Waes C, Seiwert TY. Genetic Landscape of Human Papillomavirus-Associated Head and Neck Cancer and Comparison to Tobacco-Related Tumors. *J Clin Oncol* (2015) 33:3227–34. doi: 10.1200/JCO.2015.62.1086
7. Iglesias Docampo L, Arrazubi Arrula V, Baste Rotllan N, Carral Maseda A, Cirauqui Cirauqui B, Escobar Y, et al. SEOM Clinical Guidelines for the Treatment of Head and Neck Cancer (2017). *Clin Transl Oncol* (2017) 20:75–83. doi: 10.1007/s12094-017-1776-1
8. Bonner JA, Harari PM, Giralt J, Azarnia N, Shin DM, Cohen RB, et al. Radiotherapy Plus Cetuximab for Squamous-Cell Carcinoma of the Head and Neck. *N Engl J Med* (2006) 354:567–78. doi: 10.1056/NEJMoa053422
9. Roman B, Goldenberg D, Givi B. AHNS. Adult Height and Head and Neck Cancer: A Pooled Analysis Within the INHANCE Consortium. *Head Neck* (2016) 38:168–74. doi: 10.1002/hed.24100
10. Nelke KH, Pawlak W, Gerber H, Leszczyszyn J. Head and Neck Cancer Patients' Quality of Life. *Adv Clin Exp Med* (2014) 23:1019–27. doi: 10.17219/acem/37361
11. Mañós M, Giralt J, Rueda A, Cabrera J, Martinez-Trufero J, Marruecos J, et al. Multidisciplinary Management of Head and Neck Cancer: First Expert Consensus Using Delphi Methodology From the Spanish Society for Head and Neck Cancer (Part 1). *Oral Oncol* (2017) 70:58–64. doi: 10.1016/j.oraloncology.2017.04.004
12. Rueda A, Giralt J, Mañós M, Lozano A, Sistiaga A, García-Miragall E, et al. Multidisciplinary Management of Head and Neck Cancer: First Expert Consensus Using Delphi Methodology From the Spanish Society for Head and Neck Cancer (Part 2). *Oral Oncol* (2017) 70:65–72. doi: 10.1016/j.oraloncology.2017.04.005
13. Chen J, Ou L, Hollis SJ. A Systematic Review of the Impact of Routine Collection of Patient Reported Outcome Measures on Patients, Providers and Health Organisations in an Oncologic Setting. *BMC Health Serv Res* (2013) 13:211. doi: 10.1186/1472-6963-13-211
14. Porter M, Larsson S, Lee T. Standardizing Patient Outcomes Measurement Michael. *N Engl Med* (2016) 374:504–6. doi: 10.1056/NEJMp1511701
15. *International Consortium for Health Outcomes Measurement (ICHOM)* (2019).
16. Higgins J, Green S, editors. *Cochrane Handbook for Systematic Reviews of Interventions Version 5.1.0 [updated March 2011]*. The Cochrane Collaboration (2011). Available from handbook.cochrane.org.
17. Gallagher M, Hares T, Spencer J, Bradshaw C, Webb I. The Nominal Group Technique: A Research Tool for General Practice? *Fam Pract* (1993) 10:76–81. doi: 10.1093/fampra/10.1.76
18. Potter M, Gordon S, Hamer P. The Nominal Group Technique: A Useful Consensus Methodology in Physiotherapy Research. *New Zeal J Physiother* (2004) 32:126–30.
19. Oken MM, Creech R, Tormey DC, Horton J, Davis TE, McFadden ET, et al. Toxicity and Response Criteria of the Eastern Cooperative Oncology Group. *Am J Clin Oncol* (1982) 5:649–55. doi: 10.1097/00000421-198212000-00014
20. Tsang HHL, Cheung JPY, Wong CKH, Cheung PWH, Lau CS, Chung HY. Psychometric Validation of the EuroQoL 5-Dimension (EQ-5D) Questionnaire in Patients With Spondyloarthritis. *Arthritis Res Ther* (2019) 21:41. doi: 10.1186/s13075-019-1826-x
21. Badia X, Roset M, Montserrat S, Herdman M, Segura A. The Spanish Version of EuroQol: A Description and Its Applications. European Quality of Life Scale. *Med Clin (Barc)* (1999) 112 Suppl:79–85.
22. Singer S, Amdal CD, Hammerlid E, Tomaszewska IM, Castro Silva J, Mehanna H, et al. International Validation of the Revised European Organisation for Research and Treatment of Cancer Head and Neck Cancer Module, the EORTC QLQ-HN43: Phase Iv. *Head Neck* (2019) 41:1725–37. doi: 10.1002/hed.25609
23. Bellera CA, Rainfray M, Mathoulin-Pélissier S, Mertens C, Delva F, Fonck M, et al. Screening Older Cancer Patients: First Evaluation of the G-8 Geriatric Screening Tool. *Ann Oncol* (2012) 23:2166–72. doi: 10.1093/annonc/mdr587
24. Silveira A, Monteiro E, Sequeira T. Head and Neck Cancer: Improving Patient-Reported Outcome Measures for Clinical Practice. *Curr Treat Options Oncol* (2018) 19(11):59. doi: 10.1007/s11864-018-0578-1
25. Porter I, Gonçalves-Bradley D, Ricci-Cabello I, Gibbons C, Gangannagaripalli J, Fitzpatrick R, et al. Framework and Guidance for Implementing Patient-Reported Outcomes in Clinical Practice: Evidence, Challenges and Opportunities. *J Comp Eff Res* (2016) 5:507–19. doi: 10.2217/cer-2015-0014
26. McHorney CA, Earl Bricker D. A Qualitative Study of Patients' and Physicians' Views About Practice-Based Functional Health Assessment. *Med Care* (2002) 40:1113–25. doi: 10.1097/00005650-200211000-00012
27. van Meerbeeck J, De Backer L, Hiddinga B, Janssens A. Pilot Trial of the ICHOM Lung Cancer Standard Set, European Respiratory Society (ERS). (2017) 50:PA4234. doi: 10.1183/1393003.congress-2017.PA4234
28. Van Meerbeeck J, De Backer L, Janssens A, Hiddinga B, Vanhoutte G. P1.04-028 Collection of ICHOM-Defined Patient-Reported Outcome Measures (PROMs) During Routine Lung Cancer Treatment: A Pilot Study. *J Thorac Oncol* (2017) 12:S612. doi: 10.1016/j.jtho.2016.11.784
29. Van Overveld LFJ, Takes RP, Braspenning JCC, Smeele LE, Merkx MAW, Hermens RPM. Quality of Dutch Integrated Head and Neck Cancer Care: Measurements and Evaluation. *J Clin Oncol* (2017) 35:209–9. doi: 10.1200/JCO.2017.35.8_suppl.209
30. *Head and Neck Audit (HANA Project)*. Available at: https://HanaKillermultimediaCom/n.d.
31. Arora J, Haj M. *Implementing Ichom'S Standard Sets of Outcomes: Cleft Lip and Palate at Erasmus University Medical Centre in the Netherlands*. London, UK: International Consortium for Health Outcomes Measurement (ICHOM) (2016). Available at: www.ichom.org.
32. Arora J, Tavella R. *Implementing Ichom's Standard Sets of Outcomes: Coronary Artery Disease in the Coronary Angiogram Database of South Australia (CADOSA)*. London, UK: International Consortium for Health Outcomes Measurement (ICHOM) (2017). Available at: www.ichom.org.

33. Arora J, Lewis S, Cahill MA, Arora J. *Implementing Ichom's Standard Set of Outcomes: Parkinson's Disease at Aneurin Bevan University Health Board in South Walles, Uk.* London, UK: International Consortium for Health Outcomes Measurement (ICHOM) (2017). Available at: www.ichom.org.
34. Ackerman IN, Cavka B, Lippa J, Bucknill A. The Feasibility of Implementing the ICHOM Standard Set for Hip and Knee Osteoarthritis: A Mixed-Methods Evaluation in Public and Private Hospital Settings. *J Patient Rep Outcomes* (2018) 2:32. doi: 10.1186/s41687-018-0062-5
35. Alonso-Caballero J, Ferrer-Fores M. *Monografías de Política Y Gestión. Resultados Reportados Por Los Pacientes (PROs). 1a ed.* Madrid: Ergon (2017).
36. Wildevuur SE, Wl Simonse L. Information and Communication Technology–Enabled Person-Centered Care for the &Quot; Big Five &Quot; Chronic Conditions: Scoping Review. *J Med Internet Res J Med Internet Res* (2015) 17 (3):e77. doi: 10.2196/jmir.3687.

23

Targeting the Immune Microenvironment in the Treatment of Head and Neck Squamous Cell Carcinoma

Hui-Ching Wang[1,2], *Leong-Perng Chan*[1,3] *and Shih-Feng Cho*[2,4*]

[1] *Graduate Institute of Clinical Medicine, College of Medicine, Kaohsiung Medical University, Kaohsiung, Taiwan,* [2] *Division of Hematology and Oncology, Department of Internal Medicine, Kaohsiung Medical University Hospital, Kaohsiung Medical University, Kaohsiung, Taiwan,* [3] *Department of Otolaryngology-Head and Neck Surgery, Kaohsiung Medical University Hospital, Kaohsiung Medical University, Kaohsiung, Taiwan,* [4] *Faculty of Medicine, College of Medicine, Kaohsiung Medical University, Kaohsiung, Taiwan*

***Correspondence:**
Shih-Feng Cho
sifong96@gmail.com

Head and neck squamous cell carcinoma (HNSCC) is a highly aggressive solid tumor, with a 5-year mortality rate of ~50%. The development of immunotherapies has improved the survival of patients with HNSCC, but, the long-term prognosis of patients with recurrent or metastatic HNSCC remains poor. HNSCC is characterized by intratumoral infiltration of regulatory T cells, dysfunctional natural killer cells, an elevated Treg/CD8$^+$ T cell ratio, and increased programmed cell death ligand 1 protein on tumor cells. This leads to an immunocompromised niche in favor of the proliferation and treatment resistance of cancer cells. To achieve an improved treatment response, several potential combination strategies, such as increasing the neoantigens for antigen presentation and therapeutic agents targeting components of the tumor microenvironment, have been explored and have shown promising results in preclinical studies. In addition, large-scale bioinformatic studies have also identified possible predictive biomarkers of HNSCC. As immunotherapy has shown survival benefits in recent HNSCC clinical trials, a comprehensive investigation of immune cells and immune-related factors/cytokines and the immune profiling of tumor cells during the development of HNSCC may provide more insights into the complex immune microenvironment and thus, facilitate the development of novel immunotherapeutic agents.

Keywords: head and neck cancer, microenvironment, biomarkers, immunotherapy, immunoresistance

INTRODUCTION

Head and neck cancer, 90% of which is squamous cell carcinoma (HNSCC), is the sixth most common cancer globally (1). HNSCC is composed of a heterogeneous group of tumors developing from the mucosa of the nasal and oral cavity, oropharynx, hypopharynx, or larynx (2). The major risk factors for HNSCC are smoking and alcohol consumption. Other risk factors include high risk human papillomavirus (HPV) infection, which is associated with oropharyngeal cancer increasingly worldwide (3). The areca nut chewing is linked to development of oral cancer in south Asia, Taiwan, and Pacific islanders. Treatment of HNSCC involves a multidisciplinary approach composed of surgery, radiotherapy, chemotherapy, and targeted therapy. However, the prognosis of metastatic HNSCC remains extremely poor. A combination of cetuximab and chemotherapy (cisplatin and 5-fluorouracil) shows better clinical efficacy than conventional chemotherapy; however, the median overall survival time is ~10 months (4). In recent years, the introduction of immune checkpoint inhibitors (ICIs) targeting the programmed death 1-programmed death ligand 1 (PD1-PDL1) pathway has resulted in further improvements in the outcome of patients with metastatic HNSCC, but the results remain unsatisfactory when compared with other malignancies, like melanoma and lung cancer (5, 6).

Accumulating data suggest that the tumor microenvironment (TME) plays an important role in the pathogenesis and development of treatment resistance in a variety of malignancies, including HNSCC. Several cell subtypes, including regulatory T cells (Tregs), cancer-associated fibroblasts, and macrophages, together with non-cellular components, like extracellular matrix (ECM), have been shown to be associated with immunocompromised status and the dysfunction of normal immune cells, like cytotoxic T cells or dendritic cells in the TME of HNSCC (7). HPV infection status and smoking are also related with distinct immune TMEs (8, 9).

To achieve improved treatment responses and clinical outcomes in the immunotherapy era, it is important to understand the complex immune TME of HNSCC. In this review, we describe major cell subtypes and cellular components and discuss their function. In addition, we summarize potential strategies to overcome TME-mediated treatment resistance.

TUMOR MICROENVIRONMENT OF HNSCC

The heterogeneity of molecular and cellular components has been reported in the TME of HNSCC (10, 11). However, the HNSCC TME is still characterized by some unique features, leading to immunosuppression and diminished anticancer immunity (**Table 1**). The TME is composed of stromal cells, immune cells, tumor cells, and cytokines, which mediate the interactions between these cells. HNSCC patients have decreased absolute T cell counts in the tumor and the circulation and the T cells have apoptotic features via the Fas/FasL signaling pathway and defective function (12, 16). The functional defects of tumor-infiltrating lymphocytes (TIL) include decreased expression of the CD3 zeta chain, decreased cytokine secretion, and loss of the ability to kill cancer cells (13–15). Tregs account for the major proportion of T cell components, which construct an immunosuppressive barrier, thus hindering the activity of effector T cells (Teffs) in the TME and interfering with the antitumor response to immunotherapy (26). A decrease in the number of immune cells with antigen-presenting machinery (such as dendritic cells) and in cytotoxic ability (such as natural killer cells) results in a profoundly immunodeficient tumor, which is common in HNSCC (16, 19, 27). Moreover, HNSCC tumors are characterized by desmoplastic stromal fibroblasts, which promote tumor invasion and progression via autocrine and paracrine factors (28, 29).

Communication within cancer cells, immune cells, and stromal cells via extracellular vesicles (EVs) is increasingly thought to be important (30). EVs not only deliver oncogenic proteins and non-coding RNA molecules to modulate tumor progression, but also modulate immune responses by inhibiting T cell proliferation and Th1 and Th17 differentiation (31). EVs promote suppressive immunity by activating Fas ligand (FasL), to induce $CD8^+$ T cell apoptosis and the polarization of THP-1 to tumor-associated macrophages (TAMs) of the M2 phenotype (32, 33). Although several studies have analyzed the TME, it remains difficult to define HNSCC as an immune-inflamed, immune-excluded, or immune-desert tumor, due to diverse intratumor/peritumor expression patterns and the distribution of immune cells and cytokines (34, 35). The antitumor immune response to immunotherapy in the TME depends on the balance of stromal components, intratumoral Teffs, and immune-suppressive cell populations.

Cellular Component of the HNSCC TME

Regulatory T Cells

Tregs are a subset of T cells that contribute to the immunosuppressive TME in HNSCC (21). Treg recruitment is mediated by chemokines and associated receptors, such as CCL28-CCR10 and CXCL12-CXCR4 (36, 37). Tregs are characterized by specific markers, such as of CD4; CD25; and the transcription factor, forkhead box P3 (FOXP3) (22). Tregs express high levels of cytotoxic T-lymphocyte-associated protein 4 (CTLA-4), which binds to CD80 and CD86 on antigen-presenting cells (APCs), leading to a reduced capacity to activate Teffs. Tregs exhibit their suppressor function by the consumption of interleukin-2 (IL-2), the secretion of granzyme and/or perforin to damage effector cells, and the production of immune-inhibitory cytokines and molecules, such as IL-10, IL-35, and transforming growth factor-β (38, 39). Tregs release large amounts of ATP and provide inhibitory signals to Teffs and APCs via the engagement of adenosine A_{2A} receptor ($A_{2A}R$) (40). In HNSCC, as in other malignancies, large numbers of Tregs infiltrate the TME. Intratumoral Tregs are more immunosuppressive than circulating Tregs, as evidenced by an increased expression of immune checkpoint molecules (23). A recent study identified a subset of Tregs with high levels of T-cell immunoglobulin and mucin domain-3 (TIM-3) expression from a population of $CD4^+CTLA\text{-}4^+CD25^{high}$ Treg cells. These high TIM-3-expressing Tregs are more immunosuppressive than Tregs with low levels of TIM-3 expression. After the administration of an anti-PD-1 monoclonal antibody, the expression of TIM-3 on this subgroup of T cells decreased (41). Another recent study demonstrated that Tregs are related to resistance to radiotherapy. The incorporation of an anti-CD25 antibody can overcome Treg-related treatment resistance (42). Several studies have demonstrated a negative prognostic impact of large numbers of Tregs in HNSCC (43, 44).

Myeloid-Derived Suppressor Cells

Myeloid-derived suppressor cells (MDSCs) can be divided into three major subtypes, $Ly6C^+$ monocytic MDSCs (M-MDSCs); $Ly6G^+$ granulocytic polymorphonuclear myeloid-derived suppressor cells (PMN-MDSCs); and early stage e-MDSCs, which consist of the former two subsets deficient in

TABLE 1 | Immune profilings of tumor microenvironment in HNSCC.

Characteristics	Functions and mechanisms	References
Decrease absolute T cell counts in tumor and circulation	Activation of Fas/FasL signaling pathway, leading to apoptosis of T cells	(12)
Dysregulation of T cell functions	1. Decreased HLA-DR expression on DCs and defective functions to stimulate allogeneic T cells 2. Decreased expression of the CD3 zeta chain (CD3ζ) 3. Decreased response to mitogens or IL-2 4. Absence of IL-2 and/or IFN-γ production	(13–15)
Downregulation of antigen processing machinery	Myeloid DCs is lower than lymphoid DCs	(16)
Increased Treg cell	1. Induce apoptosis of $CD8^+$ T cells 2. Inhibition of the proliferation of $CD4^+$ T cells	(12)
Increased MDSCs	Increased arginase-1 and iNOS driving immunosuppression partially by inactivating effector T cells	(17, 18)
Decreased NK cells	Impaired NK cell activity	(19)
Increased Activated, antigen-presenting and memory B cells		(20)
Increased expression of immune checkpoint ligand and receptors	A series of inhibitory immune checkpoints including PD-1, CTLA-4, TIM3, IDO, KIR, and TIGIT	(21–23)
Deficiencies or alterations of tumor HLA class I expression	Causing T-cell tolerance	(21)
Increased TGF-β, IL-6, and IL-10	Secreted by Tregs and MDSCs	(24, 25)
Aberrant activation of the transcription factors STAT3 and NF-kB	Related to IL-6 and TGF-β signaling, respectively	(24, 25)
Increase enzymes IDO-mediated degradation of the amino acid tryptophan	1. Deprivation of the tumor microenvironment of essential nutrients for T cell function 2. Activate Tregs to overcome immunogenic responses and promote tumorigenesis	(17, 18)

HLA, human leukocyte antigen; DC, dendritic cells; IL, interleukin; IFN, Interferon; DC, dendritic cells; MDSC, myeloid-derived suppressor cells; iNOS, inducible nitric oxide synthase; PD-1, Programmed death-1; CTLA-4, cytotoxic T-lymphocyte–associated antigen 4; TIM3, T-cell immunoglobulin and mucin domain-3; IDO, indoleamine 23-dioxygenase; KIR, killer cell immunoglobulin-like receptors; TIGIT, T cell immunoreceptor with Ig and ITIM domains; TGF, transforming growth factor; STAT3, Signal transducer and activator of transcription 3; NF-kB, nuclear factor kappa light chain enhancer of activated B cells.

myeloid lineage markers (45). The accumulation of MDSCs in the TME is associated with cancer progression and the inhibition of T cell activity and function (46). Various factors in the TME can induce the accumulation of MDSCs, including vascular endothelial growth factor (VEGF), IL-6, and granulocyte-macrophage colony-stimulating factor (GM-CSF) (20). In addition, MDSCs regulate the TME by increasing the production of nitric oxide, reactive oxygen species, inducible NO synthase, and arginase-1; depleting various amino acids, such as L-arginine, L-tryptophan, and L-cystein; inducing pro-angiogenic factors; and elevating the expression of PD-L1 (17, 18). In HNSCC, a recent study demonstrated that a higher frequency of PMN-MDSCs is associated with poorer survival. Specifically, a subset of $CD66b^+/CD11b^+/CD16^+$ mature PMN-MDSCs showed higher expression and activity of arginase I and demonstrated a greater suppressing effect on T cell proliferation and cytokine production than other MDSC subtypes. Moreover, high levels of $CD11b^+/CD16^+$ PMN-MDSCs, but not other PMN-MDSC subsets, are strongly correlated with adverse outcomes in HNSCC patients (47).

Cancer-Associated Fibroblasts

Cancer-associated fibroblasts (CAFs) construct the stroma of the TME to promote the growth of cancer cells. CAFs possess different characteristics dependent on their status. For example, the active form of CAFs displays typical markers, such as α-smooth muscle actin and fibroblast activation protein and promotes tumor proliferation, invasion, and metastasis (48–50). CAFs regulate the TME via secretion of various cytokines and growth factors, such as VEGF, epidermal growth factor, C-X-C motif chemokine ligands, and C-C motif chemokine ligands (CCLs) (51, 52). Most importantly, CAFs secrete matrix-metalloproteinases (MMPs), which are crucial regulators of the TME and are responsible for degradation of the ECM (53). CAFs can be transformed from diverse progenitor cells, including endothelial cells, resting fibroblasts, and epithelial cells, via mesothelial-mesenchymal transition or epithelial-mesenchymal transition (EMT) (54, 55). In the TME of HNSCC, CAFs can promote the proliferation, migration, and invasion of tumor cells (29). CAFs also have a metabolic relationship with tumor cells. CAFs secrete hepatocyte growth factor (HGF), which then activates c-met to promote the progression of HNSCC (56). Additionally, HNSCCs secrete basic fibroblast growth factor (bFGF) which increases the phosphorylation of p44/42 mitogen-activated protein kinase, leading to the secretion of HGF from CAFs. Notably, the secretion of bFGF is also mediated by CAF-secreted HGF. Inhibition of c-met and the FGF receptor can reduce tumor volume. CAFs are also associated with the development of cancer stem cells, which is associated with treatment resistance (57). CAF secretes periostin, which promotes a cancer stem cell-like phenotype via interaction with protein tyrosine kinase 7 (58). Another study also showed that CAFs secrete several proteins that promote the expression of stemness-associated genes in HNSCC cells.

Inhibition of these protein-associated pathways can suppress tumor growth (59).

Tumor-Associated Macrophages

TAMs have two distinct phenotypes, M1 and M2, with different morphological and biological characteristics (60, 61). The activated M1 phenotype promotes Th1 response and displays pro-inflammatory behaviors, whereas the activated M2 phenotype enhances Th2 response and mediates anti-inflammatory functions, which are more associated with tumor progression, invasion, metastasis, and the suppression of T cell immunity (61–63). Activated M2 macrophages demonstrate upregulated levels of IL-10, arginase-1, and peroxisome proliferator-activated receptor γ, which are known as markers of M2 TAMs (64–66). The M2 phenotype is induced by several cytokines, such as IL-4, IL-10, and IL-13. Activated M2 macrophages inhibit M1 TAMs and promote tissue remodeling through the production and secretion of anti-inflammatory cytokines, including IL-1 receptor antagonist, IL-10, transforming growth factor-β (TGF-β), VEGF, and tumor necrosis factor-α (TNF-α) (24, 25). In HNSCC, TAMs are recruited to the TME and directly contact SCC cells. A recent study showed that CCL18 derived from M2 macrophages is able to promote tumor metastasis by inducing EMT and stemness (67). Regarding clinical significance, a meta-analysis showed that high $CD68^+$ and $CD163^+$ TAM density is associated with poor cell differentiation and advanced disease status (68). Another meta-analysis showed that high stromal levels of $CD163^+$ TAMs are associated with poorer overall and progression-free survival (69).

Other Cellular Subtypes

Human natural killer (NK) cells are important in the innate immune system and can be classified into two subgroups according to the surface expression of CD56 and CD16. $CD56^{dim}/CD16^{bright}$ NK cells are predominantly responsible for natural cytotoxicity, whereas $CD56^{bright}/CD16^{dim}$ NK cells regulate immune reactions through the secretion of cytokines, such as interferon-γ and TNF-α (70, 71). The activation of NK cells induces the apoptosis of target cancer cell, through the exocytosis of perforin and granzymes, FasL and TNF-related apoptosis-inducing ligand (TRAIL) activation, or antibody-dependent cellular cytotoxicity (ADCC) (72, 73). The natural killer group 2D (NKG2D) receptors on immune cells, including NK and several T cell subsets, play an important role in immunosurveillance. By identifying and engaging the NKG2D ligand (NKG2DL) on tumor cells, NK and T cells can exert anti-tumor effects. In HNSCC, high plasma levels of shed NKG2DLs correlate with NK cell inhibition and disease progression (74).

Neutrophils are involved in the adaptive immunity response. Tumor-associated neutrophils (TANs) exhibit both pro- and anti-tumor characteristics. Similar to TAMs, TANs are also divided into two subgroups, N1 and N2 (75). Neutrophils eradicate cancer cells by releasing the antimicrobial and cytotoxic contents of their granules or by secreting immune mediators to recruit other antitumor effector cells. However, other factors from the tumor can shift neutrophils into a pro-tumor phenotype (76). Neutrophils with the pro-tumor N2 phenotype possess CXCR4, VEGF, and MMP-9 markers, which facilitate tumorigenesis, promote tumor growth, stimulate angiogenesis, and mediate immunosuppression (75).

Non-cellular Components in the TME

The ECM contains large composites of non-cellular factors, including structural proteins, growth factors, proteoglycans, and glycoproteins, which form the main structure of the TME (77). MMPs, which are mainly produced by the ECM, are a large family of proteins and peptide hydrolases that mediate the degradation of the ECM and facilitate the migration of cancer cells (78). MMPs also activate bFGF, VEGF, and TGF-β and promote angiogenesis (79, 80). Fibronectin is the major glycoprotein in the ECM and it plays a crucial role in interactions between other molecules, such as integrins, collagens, and fibrin (81, 82). Increased levels of fibronectin are associated with tumor invasion, progression, and resistance to treatment (83, 84). Other molecules are also involved in cell adhesion and proliferation and assist in supporting the surrounding TME.

HPV Infection and Smoking Are Associated With a Distinct Immune TME

HPV Infection

HPV infection plays a pivotal role in the immune modulation of HNSCC. In general, HPV-positive HNSCCs demonstrate relatively inflamed immunity compared with HPV-negative HNSCCs (**Table 2**). A TME with a prolonged viral infection induces anti-tumor immunity via the expression of tumor-associated antigens (TAAs) and tumor-specific antigens in immune cells and tumor cells (8). After cytotoxic therapies (radiotherapy or chemotherapy), the antigen-processing machinery (APM) promotes the expression of major histocompatibility complex (MHC) class I molecules to present the antigen peptide from dying tumor cells to T cells (89). In addition, an increase in the infiltration of NK cells and T cells, including $CD3^+$, $CD4^+$, and $CD8^+$ TILs, creates a vigorous TME that stimulates cellular immunity in HPV-positive HNSCCs (85, 86). Interestingly, HPV-positive oropharyngeal cancer demonstrates higher $CD4^+$, higher $CD8^+$, and lower $CD4^+/CD8^+$ ratio compared with HPV-negative HNSCC (85). Humoral immunity is also induced by the recruitment of $CD19^+/CD20^+$ B cells (87). Antigen presentation and cytotoxicity are promoted by gathering dendritic cells (DCs) and APCs (86). An increase in the number of intratumor and peritumor infiltrating immune cells results in a favorable prognosis and enhances the response to radiotherapy and immunotherapy (34). The interaction between HPV-negative oropharyngeal cancer cells and CAFs results in the secretion of chemokines via an IL-1/IL-1R-mediated mechanism, which is less prominent within the HPV-positive TME (88). Thus, the metabolic profiles are quite different between HPV-positive and HPV-negative HNSCCs.

The communication vesicles, EVs, also display different features depending on viral status. In HPV-positive cancers, exosomes carry viral proteins, genes, and TAAs (90, 91).

TABLE 2 | Different immune modulations between HPV-negative and HPV-positive HNSCC.

HPV negative HNSCC	HPV positive HNSCC	References
Lower CD3+ T cells	Higher CD3+ T cells	(85, 86)
Lower CD4+ T cells	Higher CD4+ T cells	(85, 86)
Lower CD8+ T cells	Higher CD8+ T cells	(85, 86)
Increased CD4+/ CD8+ ratio	Decreased CD4+/ CD8+ ratio	(85, 86)
Lower CD45+ cells, CD8+ cells, CD8+ IFNγ+ cells, and CD8+IL-17+ cells	Higher CD45+ cells, CD8+ cells, CD8+ IFNγ+ cells, and CD8+IL-17+ cells	(85, 86)
Lower CD45+ lymphocytes and CD19+/CD20+ B cells	Higher CD45+ lymphocytes and CD19+/CD20+ B cells	(87)
Higher Treg cells	Lower Treg cells	(85, 86)
Low CD56dim NK cells	High CD56dim NK cells	(85, 86)
Lower tumor-infiltrating APCs	higher tumor-infiltrating APCs	(86)
Lower myeloid and plasmacytoid DCs	Higher myeloid and plasmacytoid DCs	(86)
Lower DC signatures, including CD103, and CD11C	Higher DC signatures	(86)
Lower levels of chemokines	Higher levels of chemokines	(88)
Higher levels of Cox-2 and Tim-3 mRNA	Lower levels of Cox-2 and Tim-3 mRNA	(86)
Lower levels of PD-1 mRNA	Higher levels of PD-1 mRNA	(86)
Lower "T-cell exhaustion markers," including LAG3, PD-1, TIGIT, TIM3, and CD39	Higher "T-cell exhaustion markers"	(87)
Lower levels of cytotoxic mediators, including granzyme A, granzyme B, and perforin	Higher levels of cytotoxic mediators	(87)
Exosomes suppressed DC maturation and expression of APM components	Exosomes promoted DC maturation and did not suppress expression of APM components in mature DCs	(89)
Increased MAGEA1 and MAGEA3 gene expression	Increased CDKN2A gene expression	(87)

IFN, interferon; IL, interleukin; NK cells, natural killer cells; APC, antigen-presenting cell; DC, dendritic cells; Cox-2, cyclooxygenase-2; Tim-3, T-cell immunoglobulin and mucin domain-3; LAG-3, lymphocyte-activation gene 3; PD-1, Programmed death-1; TIGIT, T cell immunoreceptor with Ig and ITIM domains; APM, antigen processing machinery; MAGEA, melanoma-associated antigen; CDKN2A, cyclin-dependent kinase Inhibitor 2A.

However, these differences in EVs do not occur by influencing the T cell response. The functions of both CD4+ and CD8+ T cells are suppressed by these exosomes. The expression of co-stimulatory CD80 and CD83 molecules on immature DCs is up-regulated, but the expression of APM components is not suppressed in HPV-positive exosomes. In contrast, HPV(−) exosomes inhibit DC maturation and APM component expression (8). Moreover, HPV-negative tumors have a more active metabolic signature, with elevated expression of genes associated with glycolysis and oxidative phosphorylation (92). HPV-negative tumors are also characterized by increased MCT1 expression, which indicates that the regulation of lactate homoeostasis is more significant in promoting the invasion of HPV-negative HNSCCs (93).

Smoking

Smoking is a risk factor for the development of HNSCC and it promotes pro-inflammatory and immunosuppressive effects, which impact the TME of HNSCCs, to facilitate tumor development (94, 95). Smoking results in enrichment of immunogenic neoantigens which cause both pro- and anti-immunity effects in smoking-associated cancers, including lung cancer and HNSCC. In lung cancer, smoking leads to increased neoantigens and constructs an inflamed TME, which suggests higher response rates to ICIs in smokers. In contrast, the enhancement of immunogenic neoantigens by smoking forms a more immunosuppressive in TME in HNSCC by increased T cell apoptosis which is mediated through reactive oxygen and nitrogen species (94). In the TCGA database, enrichment scores from two Gene Expression Omnibus cohorts were higher in never-smoker and never-drinker (NSND) patients compared with smoker and drinker (SD) patients. To identify biological differences, gene set enrichment analysis of the TCGA dataset was performed and immunity-associated pathways were found to predominantly involve T-cell activation and differentiation in NSND patients. The TME in NSND patients is more immunoactive than the TME of SD patients, including an increased number of CD8+ TIL cells; increased INF-γactivation; overexpression of immune checkpoint ligands and receptors, such as indoleamine 23-dioxygenase 1 (IDO1) and PD-L1; and higher scores in the pembrolizumab-response signature (96). Tobacco smoking attenuates the cytotoxicity of the TME by repressing CD8+ T cells, NK cells, and DCs (9). Overall, smoking has a negative impact on immune responses, regardless of alcohol consumption.

MECHANISMS OF TME-MEDIATED DRUG RESISTANCE IN HNSCC

The mechanisms of resistance to epidermal growth factor receptor (EGFR) inhibitors have been known for decades and they include nuclear localization of EGFR, activation of other ErbB family receptors, mutant forms of the receptor (EGFRvIII), or cross-talk with other signaling pathways (97, 98). However, issues of resistant mechanisms to immunotherapy have been gradually emphasized recently. These include a lack of production, editing, and presentation of neo-antigens;

impaired intratumoral immune infiltration; impaired IFNγ signaling; immune factors within the TME; upregulation of alternative immune checkpoints; severe T-cell exhaustion; and T-cell epigenetic changes (99–102).

The downregulation of human leukocyte antigen (HLA) class I molecules and loss of β2-microglobulin expression interferes with antigen presentation to cytotoxic T cells (103). Specific oncogenic signaling pathways change the TME. Loss of the PTEN induces the expression of CCL2 and VEGF and blocks T-cell infiltration, leading to resistance to ICIs (104). Alterations in β-catenin/WNT signaling decrease CCL4 production and hinder the infiltration of DCs (105). During the development of ICI resistance, the TME shows an increase in the number of effector memory CD8 T cells ($CCR7^-CD45RA^-$), a lower CD4/CD8 ratio, and upregulation of TIM-3 on CD4 and CD8 T cells (100). Moreover, the major regulators of therapeutic response and resistance are Tregs and TAMs. In preclinical HNSCC mouse models, the Treg population is elevated during tumor rebound after combined treatment with ICI and radiation (26). Depletion of major histocompatibility complex class II-low TAMs increases chemotherapy-related DNA damage and apoptosis (106). Depletion of tumor-infiltrating Tregs using an anti-CD25 antibody, enhances the binding ability of activating Fc gamma receptors, increases Teff:Treg ratios, and improves the response to ICIs (107). High levels of alternative co-inhibitory receptors on T cells (e.g., CTLA-4, TIM-3, lymphocyte-activation gene 3, and V-domain Ig suppressor of T cell activation) and high levels of immune-suppressive cytokines or metabolites, causes T cell exhaustion, which also induces ICI resistance (108).

POTENTIAL STRATEGIES TO OVERCOME TME-MEDIATED DRUG RESISTANCE

Novel Therapeutic Agents or Combination Therapies

Due to the insufficient response elicited by immunotherapy alone, several mechanisms for the regulation of immunoresistant niches have been proposed, including defective immunorecognition, tumor insensitivity to T cell effector molecules, an immunosuppressive TME, and the compensatory regulation of multiple inhibitory and costimulatory immune checkpoints (**Figure 1**) (109). Combinations of diverse agents targeting distinct mechanisms have been investigated in recent years (**Table 3**).

Defective immunorecognition involves dysfunction of antigen presentation in tumor cells, anergy of tumor-specific cytotoxic T lymphocyte, and immunoediting. Radiotherapy and cytotoxic therapy (NCT02318771, NCT03040999, NCT03894891, NCT03162731, NCT02764593, NCT02938273) induce cell death to promote antigen presentation and trigger activation of the cGAS-STING pathway to enhance the T-cell response. Moreover, radiation adjusts the stromal TME (110). Cetuximab (NCT02764593, NCT03082534, NCT02938273) binds to EGFR

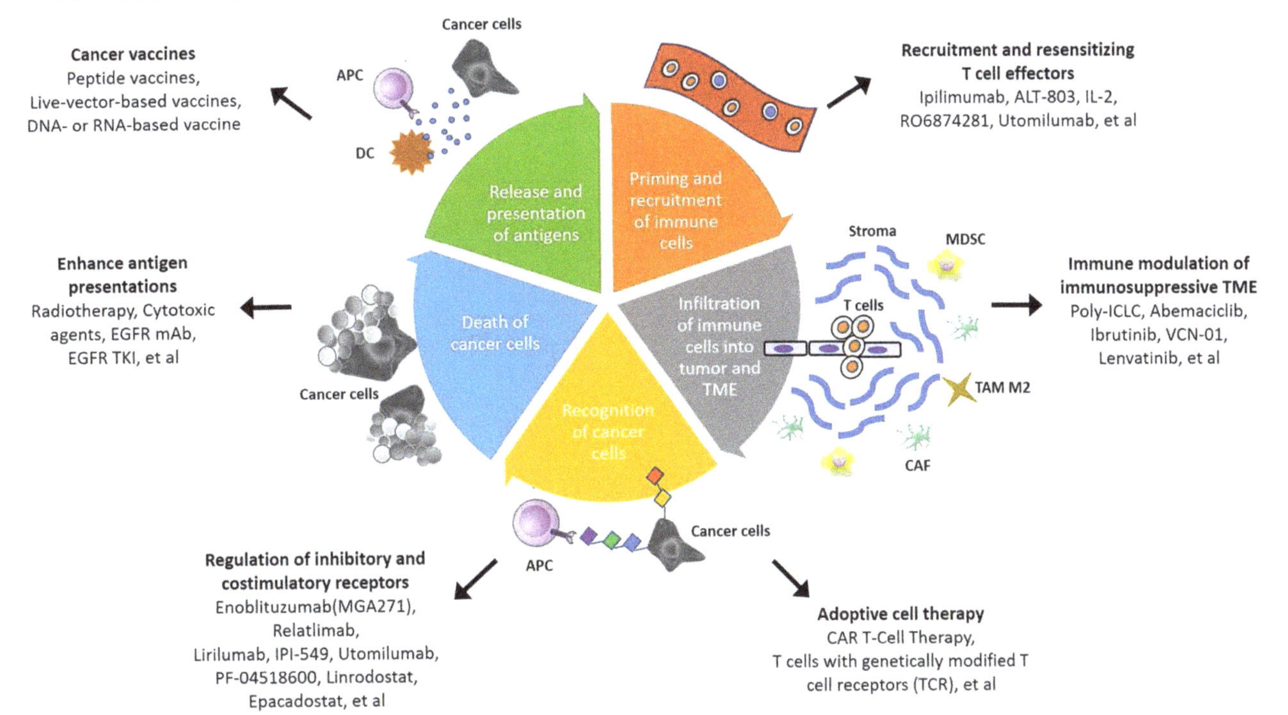

FIGURE 1 | Schematic summary of potential strategies to overcome immunosuppressive TME in head and neck squamous cell carcinoma (HNSCC). In cancer-immunity cycle, there are several therapeutic strategies that can be applied to overcome TME-mediated treatment resistance. The steps of immune responses involve priming and recruitment of immune cells, infiltration of immune cells into tumor, and TME, recognition and death of cancer cells, then release and presentation of antigen from cancer cells. Targeting different mechanism of immune response become more potential therapeutic approach in the future.

TABLE 3 | Combination therapy to enhance PD-1/PD-L1-based treatment efficacy.

Strategy	Treatments	Therapeutic modalities	Potential mechanisms	Phase	NCT ID status
Immunorecognition					
Enhance antigen presentations	Radiotherapy	• RT (1 fraction, 8 Gy) + Pembrolizumab • RT (5 fractions, 4 Gy) + Pembrolizumab • Pembrolizumab + RT (1 fraction, 8 Gy) + Pembrolizumab • Pembrolizumab + RT (5 fractions, 4 Gy) + Pembrolizumab	1. Induce cell death to promote antigen presentation 2. Trigger activation of cGAS-STING pathway to enhance T-cell response 3. Adjust stromal TME	1	NCT02318771 Active, not recruiting
	Radiotherapy Cytotoxic agents	• Pembrolizumab + Cisplatin + RT • Placebo + Cisplatin + RT		3	NCT03040999 Active, not recruiting
	Radiotherapy Cytotoxic agents	• Docetaxel + Cisplatin + Nivolumab + Radioimmunotherapy		2	NCT03894891 Recruiting
	Radiotherapy CTLA-4 inhibitor	• Nivolumab + Ipilimumab + RT		1	NCT03162731 Recruiting
	Radiotherapy Cytotoxic agents EGFR mAb	• Nivolumab + Cisplatin • Nivolumab + High-dose Cisplatin • Nivolumab + Cetuximab • Nivolumab + IMRT		1	NCT02764593 Active, not recruiting
	EGFR mAb	• Pembrolizumab + Cetuximab	1. Stimulate antibody-dependent cell-mediated cytotoxicity 2. Prime adaptive and innate cellular immunity 3. Competitively inhibit the binding of EGF and other ligands (TGF-α)	2	NCT03082534 Recruiting
		• Avelumab + Cetuximab + RT		1	NCT02938273 Active, not recruiting
	EGFR TKI	• Nivolumab + Afatinib	1. Downregulate PD-L1 expression 2. Reduce PD-L1 expression via inhibiting NF-κB 3. Block the immune escape by upregulating the expression of NKG2D ligands on tumor cells and NKG2D on NK cells 4. Enhance the susceptibility to NK cell-mediated lysis by induction of ULBP1 by inhibition of PKC pathwy	1	NCT03652233 Withdrawn
		• Pembrolizumab + Afatinib		2	NCT03695510 Not yet recruiting
Resensitizing T cell effectors	Interleukin	• ALT-803 + Pembrolizumab • ALT-803 + Nivolumab • ALT-803 + Atezolizumab • ALT-803 + Avelumab	1. IL-15 superagonist 2. promote $CD8^+$ T and NK cell expansion and function	2	NCT03228667 Recruiting
		• IL-2 + Pembrolizumab + Hypofractionated RT	1. Intralesional IL-2 2. increase PD-L1 expression and $CD8^+$ T cell infiltration	1/2	NCT03474497 Recruiting
		• RO6874281+ Atezolizumab	1. IL-2 Variant (IL-2v), engineered IL2v moiety with abolished binding to IL-2Ra 2. targeting Fibroblast Activation Protein-A 3. Activation of immune effector CD8 T and NK cells, reduce activity on Tregs	2	NCT03386721 Recruiting
Immune modulation of immunosuppressive TME					
DC/NK cells	Carboxymethylcellulose, polyinosinic-polycytidylic acid, and poly-L-lysine dsRNA	• IV Durvalumab + IV Tremelimumab + IT/IM Poly-ICLC	1. Synthetic dsRNA complex which directly activate DCs and trigger NK cells to kill tumor cells 2. Induce interferon-γ production	1/2	NCT02643303 Recruiting

(Continued)

TABLE 3 | Continued

Strategy	Treatments	Therapeutic modalities	Potential mechanisms	Phase	NCT ID status
Cell cycles	CDK4/6 inhibitor	• Abemaciclib + Nivolumab	Create an immune inflamed TMEs through T cell activation and tumor cell intrinsic effects	1/2	NCT03655444 Recruiting
Cytokines	BTK inhibitor	• Ibrutinib + Nivolumab • Ibrutinib + Cetuximab	1. Inhibit IL-2 inducible T-cell kinase (ITK) 2. Maintain balance between Th1/Th2 T cells	2	NCT03646461 Recruiting
HU	Stroma	• VCN-01 and Durvalumab	Tumor-selective replication-competent adenovirus expressing PH20 hyaluronidase	1	NCT03799744 Recruiting
VEGF	VEGF	• Lenvatinib + Pembrolizumab	1. Reduce tumor associated macrophages 2. Enhance the ratio of memory T cells	1b/2	NCT02501096 Recruiting
Regulation of inhibitory and costimulatory receptors					
Inhibitory receptor	B7-H3 (CD276)	• Enoblituzumab (MGA271) + Pembrolizumab	1. Synergistic antitumor activity 2. Engagement of both innate and adaptive immunity 3. Modulation of T-cell immunosuppression 4. Decrease the risk of auto-immune related AE	1	NCT02475213 Active, not recruiting
	LAG-3	• Relatlimab • Relatlimab + Nivolumab	1. Synergistic antitumor activity 2. Positively regulate effector T cell function	1/2	NCT01968109 Recruiting
	KIR	• Nivolumab • Nivolumab + Lirilumab • Nivolumab + Ipilimumab + Lirilumab	1. Block interaction between KIR2DL-1,-2,-3 inhibitory receptors and ligands 2. Promote effector T cell function 3. Reverse T cell exhaustion	1/2	NCT01714739 Active, not recruiting
	PI3K	• IPI-549 and Nivolumab	Transform macrophages from an immune-suppressive to an immune-activating phenotype	1	NCT02637531 Recruiting
	CTLA-4	• Nivolumab with Ipilimumab • Nivolumab	1. CTLA-4 inhibitor: induce a proliferative signature in a subset of memory T-cells 2. PD-1 inhibitor: modulate genes that are involved in T-cell or NK-cell effector functions 3. Increase in plasma cytokine or chemokine levels	2	NCT02919683 Recruiting
		• Nivolumab and Ipilimumab • Nivolumab and placebo		2	NCT02823574 Active, not recruiting
Stimulatory receptor	4-1BB (CD137) OX40 TLR9 agonist	• Cohort A5: Avelumab + Utomilumab (Human IgG2 4-1BB mAb) • Cohort F1: CMP-001(VLP-encapsulated TLR9 agonist) +Avelumab • Cohort F2: CMP-001 + Avelumab + Utomilumab • Cohort F3: CMP-001 + Avelumab+PF-04518600 (OX40 agonist)	1. Utomilumab: production of IFN-γ and IL-2; stimulate and increase NK cells and T cells 2. PF-04518600: co-stimulate effector T cells and deplete regulatory T cells, resulting in enhanced tumor immunity 3. CMP-001: release the oligonucleotide into APCs	1	NCT02554812 Recruiting
	4-1BB (CD137)	• PF-04518600 • PF-04518600 + Utomilumab (PF-05082566)		1	NCT02315066 Active, not recruiting
Other pathway	IDO1	• Nivolumab and Linrodostat (BMS986205) • Nivolumab	1. Inhibitor of indoleamine 2,3-dioxygenase 1, a cytosolic enzyme for oxidation of tryptophan into kynurenine. 2. Inhibition of IDO1–kynurenine–AhR signaling	2	NCT03854032 Recruiting

(Continued)

TABLE 3 | Continued

Strategy	Treatments	Therapeutic modalities	Potential mechanisms	Phase	NCT ID status
		• Nivolumab + Linrodostat • Cetuximab + Cisplatin/Carboplatin + Fluorouracil		3	NCT03386838 Withdrawn
		• Nivolumab + Epacadostat • Nivolumab + Epacadostat + Chemotherapy		1/2	NCT02327078 Active, not recruiting
		• Pembrolizumab + Epacadostat • Pembrolizumab • EXTREME regimen		3	NCT03358472 Active, not recruiting

RT, radiotherapy; Gy, gray; TME, tumor microenvironment; CTLA-4, cytotoxic T-lymphocyte–associated antigen 4; EGFR, epidermal growth factor receptor; mAb, monoclonal antibody; IMRT, intensity-modulated radiotherapy; EGF, epidermal growth factor; TGF, transforming growth factor; TKI, tyrosine kinase inhibitor; PD-L1, Programmed death-ligand 1; NK cells, Natural killer cells; IL, interleukin; DC, dendritic cells; IV, intravenous; IT, intratumoral; IM, intramuscular; dsRNA, double-stranded RNA; BTK, Bruton's tyrosine kinase; Th cells, T helper cells; HU, hyaluronidase; VEGF, vascular endothelial growth factor; AE, adverse event; LAG-3, lymphocyte-activation gene 3; KIR, killer cell immunoglobulin-like receptors; PI3K, phosphoinositide 3-kinases; IFN, Interferon; TLR9, Toll-like receptor 9; VLP, virus-like particle; APC, antigen-presenting cell; IDO1, indoleamine 23-dioxygenase 1; AhR, aryl hydrocarbon receptor.

and to the CD16 receptor on NK cells and DCs, resulting in innate and adaptive immune responses, including ADCC and T cell priming (111). Afatinib (NCT03652233, NCT03695510), an EGFR tyrosine kinase inhibitor, downregulates PD-L1 expression via the inhibition of NF-κB. However, afatinib hinders immune escape by increasing the expression of NKG2D ligands on tumor cells and NKG2D on NK cells (112). ALT-803 (NCT03228667), an IL-15 superagonist, promotes CD8^{+} T cell and NK cell expansion and function and has demonstrated anti-tumor efficacy in preclinical models (113). Intralesional IL-2 (NCT03474497) increases PD-L1 expression and promotes CD8^{+} T cell infiltration (114). RO6874281 (NCT03386721), an engineered IL2v moiety, maintains its affinity for IL-2Rβγ, thus activating effector CD8 T cells and NK cells and reducing Treg activity (115).

The immunosuppressive TME also contributes to the low sensitivity of HNSCC to ICIs. Modulating different components of the TME improves the efficacy of ICIs and enhances self-immunity. Poly-ICLC (NCT02643303), a carboxymethylcellulose, polyinosinic-polycytidylic acid, and poly-L-lysine dsRNA, is a synthetic dsRNA complex that directly activates DCs, triggers NK cells, and induces interferon-γ production (116). Abemaciclib (NCT03655444), a CDK4/6 inhibitor, creates an immune inflamed TME through T cell activation and intrinsic tumor cell effects (117). Ibrutinib (NCT03646461), a Bruton's tyrosine kinase inhibitor, inhibits IL-2 inducible T-cell kinase (ITK), to strengthen specific anti-tumor responses (118). ITK plays a crucial role in maintaining the balance between Th1 and Th2 T cells. VCN-01 (NCT03799744), a selective oncolytic adenovirus encoding the human glycosylphosphatidylinositol-anchored enzyme, PH20 hyaluronidase, shows potential anti-tumor effects. Replication of the injected adenovirus in tumor cells results in cell death and the infection of adjacent tumor cells. Hyaluronidase also degrades hyaluronic acid (HA), which is abundant in the ECM and inhibits tumor cell growth and metastasis (119). Lenvatinib (NCT02501096), a multikinase inhibitor of VEGFR 1–3, fibroblast growth factor receptors (FGFR) 1–4, platelet-derived growth factor α receptors, RET, and KIT, reduces the number of TAMs and increases the ratio of memory T cells (120).

The regulation of inhibitory and costimulatory receptors synergically enhances the immunological anti-tumor effect. Inhibitory receptors, including B7-H3, LAG-3, killer cell immunoglobulin-like receptors (KIRs), phosphoinositide 3-kinases (PI3Ks), and CTLA-4, are applied in combination therapies. Enoblituzumab (NCT02475213), an Fc optimized, humanized IgG1 monoclonal antibody, promotes binding to activating FcγR and recognizes B7-H3, which is highly expressed in HNSCC. Combination therapy may contribute to synergistic antitumor activity (121). Relatlimab (NCT01968109), an anti-LAG-3 monoclonal antibody, shows an additive antitumor effect when administered with ICIs. LAG3 negatively regulates Teff function and is a marker of T cell exhaustion (122). IPI-549 (NCT02637531), a selective PI3K-γ inhibitor, transforms macrophages from an immune-suppressive to an immune-activating phenotype, which may help overcome resistance to ICIs (123). The well-known dual blockade therapy consisting of anti-CTLA-4 and anti-PD-1 antibodies (NCT02919683, NCT02823574), stimulates distinct immune cells and results in an inflammatory TME to overcome cancer cells (124). Similarly, cooperation with stimulatory receptors increases clinical benefits and treatment efficacy. Utomilumab (NCT01307267, NCT02315066), a 4-1BB/CD137 agonist, stimulates the activity and number of NK cells and T cells (125). PF-04518600 (NCT01307267, NCT02315066), a selective anti-OX40 antibody, activates OX40 and increases the proliferation of memory and effector T-lymphocytes (126). CMP-001 (NCT01307267), a Toll-like receptor 9 (TLR9) agonist, comprises a CpG-A oligodeoxynucleotide packaged in particles. It activates tumor-associated plasmacytoid DCs, which construct an interferon-rich TME and results in anti-tumor CD8^{+} T cell responses (127). IDO1, a major enzyme in tryptophan catabolism, is a target in clinical development, in combination with PD-1 ICIs (NCT03854032, NCT03386838,

NCT02327078, NCT03358472). IDO1 converts tryptophan to kynurenine, which then activates aryl hydrocarbon receptor (AhR), a ligand-activated transcription factor, in Tregs, DCs, and NK cells. Activation of AhR induces subsequent cascades in three different cell types. In Tregs, AhR results in the nuclear translocation and enhancement of FoxP3 transcripts and IL10, eventually increasing Treg populations. In DCs, AhR promotes the production of IL-10 and inhibits IFNβ signaling. In NK cells, AhR induces the production of both IL-10 and IFNγ. The IDO1-kynurenine-AhR axis demonstrates a positive feedback loop. These effects on immune cells help establish an immunosuppressive TME. The inhibition of IDO reverses immunosuppression and enhances the response to ICIs (128).

Cancer Vaccines

Cancer vaccines targeting HPV antigens and tumor-associated antigens enhance the immune response in HNSCC. Therapeutic vaccines include peptide vaccines, live-vector-based vaccines, and DNA- or RNA-based vaccines. Peptide vaccines derived from HPV antigens are taken up by DCs and displayed by either MHC class I, class II, or both molecules, after which they induce a T-cell mediated immune response. Several trials have investigated such drugs, including DPX-E7 (NCT02865135), GL-0817/GL-0810 (NCT00257738), P16_37-63 peptide (NCT01462838, NCT02526316), and ISA 101(NCT02426892). However, the response rates have been variable in relatively small populations of patients (129, 130). Live-vector-based vaccines are more immunogenic and induce strong pathogen-derived CD8 epitopes (131). Recent cancer vaccine modalities include DNA and RNA vaccines encoding selected tumor antigens or synthetic long peptide (SLP) vaccines co-delivering CD4 and CD8 epitopes (132). DNA or peptide vaccines targeting HPV E6 and E7 oncoproteins have demonstrated specific clinical efficacy in precancerous lesions and have shown promise in the treatment of HPV-related HNSCC. However, the development of vaccines against HPV-independent HNSCC has been less successful due to the difficulty in identifying available targets (133). Additional vaccine modalities are required to overcome the immunosuppressive TME in HNSCC.

Cell-Based Therapy

T cells, including TILs, T cells with genetically modified T cell receptors (TCRs), and T cells transfected with chimeric antigen receptors (CAR), are the main types of cell-based therapy (134). Sufficient numbers of TILs overcome the immunosuppressive TME by removing other exhausted immune cells and inhibitory factors, such as cytokines. Adoptive immunotherapy using CAR T cells has displayed promising outcomes in hematological malignancies, such as leukemia and multiple myeloma. The process of CAR T cell therapy includes retrieving T cells from the patient's blood or tumor, training and stimulating their expansion in an *in vitro* system, and injecting the expanded cells back into the patient to promote cancer elimination. The development of tumor antigen-specific TCRs, for example HPV-targeted TCRs in genetically modify T cells, is another approach for adoptive immunotherapy. These modified T cells possess high levels of immune-signaling initiators and show rapid recognition of intracellular antigens, which can initiate an immune response against cancer cells. A phase I/II trial targeting the HLA-A*02:01-restricted epitope of E6 (E6 TCR T cells) enrolled patients with HPV-positive and HLA-A*02:01-positive metastatic epithelial cancers and showed that a dose up to 2×10^{11} cells was safe for patients. Partial responses in 2 of 12 patients (both with anal cancer) were reported (135). A phase I trial of T4 CAR T cell immunotherapy in HNSCC demonstrated safe intratumoral administration of T4 T-cells that co-express: (i) T1E28ζ, a CAR containing an ErbB ligand coupled to a $CD28^{+}CD3\zeta$ endodomain and (ii) 4αβ, an IL-4-responsive chimeric cytokine receptor. Although a lymphopenia rate of 62% was observed, T4 manufacture was successful in 13/13 cases, yielding 2.5–7.5 Bn T cells (69 ± 13% transduced) (136). However, the development of adoptive cell therapy for HNSCC is still immature. There are still numerous difficulties and challenges including the identification of more specific peptide and genetic profiles of HNSCC cells. More precise knowledge of intracellular and extracellular neoantigens would help to identify potentially novel targets for cell therapy in HNSCC.

POTENTIAL BIOMARKERS IN HNSCC IMMUNOTHERAPY

Potential biomarkers in HNSCC have been discussed for many years, but there is still no consensus. Recent studies have tended to focus on specific biomarkers, including PD-L1 expression, HPV status, tumor immune infiltration, immune-associated signatures, gene expression profiles (GEPs), tumor mutational burden (TMB), the status of DNA mismatch repair, and smoking-related signatures. PD-L1 immunohistochemistry is the most frequently used marker in clinical practice. However, there are several challenges in the clinical application of these biomarkers. For example, PD-L1 is a heterogeneous marker with different intratumoral/temporal and primary/metastatic variations in expression (137). Different immunohistochemistry assays have been used, with different thresholds for positivity and different scoring criteria, including a tumor proportional score (TPS) and a combined proportional score (CPS) (138). HPV status also influences immunity within the TME and affects responses to immunotherapy (6). TILs, defined as $CD8^{+}$ T cells and Tregs, have demonstrated a possible role in distinguishing ICI responders from ICI non-responders (139). GEP and TMB, analyzed by microarray or next-generation sequencing platforms, have been investigated as predictive biomarkers for biological phenotypes and clinical outcomes in HNSCC. Some analyses have shown that TMB, CPS, and GEP can serve as independent predictive biomarkers for responsiveness to anti-PD-1/PD-L1 antibodies (140). Tumors with more mutations influencing the DNA damage response, for example those with mismatch repair deficiency (dMMR), have a higher TMB and are more sensitive to ICIs. This contributed to the FDA approval of pembrolizumab for patients with dMMR or MSI-H tumors, regardless of histology (141–143). Overall, while the interactions between the tumor, the immune system, and the microenvironment are complex, more reliable predictive biomarkers are required to assess tumor responsiveness to immunotherapy.

PERSPECTIVES AND CONCLUSIONS

As ICI monotherapy shows a durable response in only a small subset of patients, combination therapy with anti-PD-1/PD-L1 antibodies has emerged as an alternative and has shown encouraging results in the treatment of HNSCC. In addition, the anti-tumor effects of ICIs can be reinforced by increasing antigen presentation via radiation or chemotherapy/target therapy, modulating TME, or collaborating with costimulatory and inhibitory receptors on tumor cells or immune cells. The niches around cancer cells are crucial for interference with the efficacy of checkpoint inhibitors and they determine whether a tumor is "immunoactive" or "immunosuppressive." Methods to overcome the immunotherapy resistance of the TME will become more crucial in the future. Multimodalities of treatment strategies aid in strengthening immunosurveillance and immunoediting. Studies to identify more specific targets for adoptive T cell therapies are ongoing. In addition, further studies designed to identify ideal biomarkers of individual tumors and to elucidate the mechanisms of immune escape are warranted.

AUTHOR CONTRIBUTIONS

H-CW, L-PC, and S-FC substantially contributed to the conception, drafting, editing, and final approval of this manuscript.

REFERENCES

1. Parkin DM, Bray F, Ferlay J, Pisani P. Global cancer statistics, 2002. *CA Cancer J Clin.* (2005) 55:74–108. doi: 10.3322/canjclin.55.2.74
2. Haddad RI, Shin DM. Recent advances in head and neck cancer. *N Engl J Med.* (2008) 359:1143–54. doi: 10.1056/NEJMra0707975
3. Hsu WL, Yu KJ, Chiang CJ, Chen TC, Wang CP. Head and neck cancer incidence trends in Taiwan, 1980 ~ 2014. *Int J Head Neck Sci.* (2017) 1:180–9. doi: 10.6696/IJHNS.2017.0103.05
4. Vermorken JB, Mesia R, Rivera F, Remenar E, Kawecki A, Rottey S, et al. Platinum-based chemotherapy plus cetuximab in head and neck cancer. *N Engl J Med.* (2008) 359:1116–27. doi: 10.1056/NEJMoa0802656
5. Ferris RL, Blumenschein GR, Fayette J, Guigay J, Colevas AD, Licitra LF, et al. Further evaluations of nivolumab (nivo) versus investigator's choice (IC) chemotherapy for recurrent or metastatic (R/M) squamous cell carcinoma of the head and neck (SCCHN): CheckMate 141. *Am Soc Clin Oncol.* (2016) doi: 10.1200/JCO.2016.34.15_suppl.6009
6. Chow LQ, Haddad R, Gupta S, Mahipal A, Mehra R, Tahara M, et al. Antitumor activity of pembrolizumab in biomarker-unselected patients with recurrent and/or metastatic head and neck squamous cell carcinoma: results from the phase Ib KEYNOTE-012 expansion cohort. *J Clin Oncol.* (2016) 34:3838–45. doi: 10.1200/JCO.2016.68.1478
7. Peltanova B, Raudenska M, Masarik M. Effect of tumor microenvironment on pathogenesis of the head and neck squamous cell carcinoma: a systematic review. *Mol Cancer.* (2019) 18:63. doi: 10.1186/s12943-019-0983-5
8. Ludwig S, Sharma P, Theodoraki MN, Pietrowska M, Yerneni SS, Lang S, et al. Molecular and functional profiles of exosomes from HPV (+) and HPV (-) head and neck cancer cell lines. *Front Oncol.* (2018) 8:445. doi: 10.3389/fonc.2018.00445
9. Stämpfli MR, Anderson GP. How cigarette smoke skews immune responses to promote infection, lung disease and cancer. *Nat Rev Immunol.* (2009) 9:377–84. doi: 10.1038/nri2530
10. Keck MK, Zuo Z, Khattri A, Stricker TP, Brown CD, Imanguli M, et al. Integrative analysis of head and neck cancer identifies two biologically distinct HPV and three non-HPV subtypes. *Clin Cancer Res.* (2015) 21:870–81. doi: 10.1158/1078-0432.CCR-14-2481
11. Hanna GJ, Liu H, Jones RE, Bacay AF, Lizotte PH, Ivanova EV, et al. Defining an inflamed tumor immunophenotype in recurrent, metastatic squamous cell carcinoma of the head and neck. *Oral Oncol.* (2017) 67:61–9. doi: 10.1016/j.oraloncology.2017.02.005
12. Duray A, Demoulin S, Hubert P, Delvenne P, Saussez S. Immune suppression in head and neck cancers: a review. *Clin Dev Immunol.* (2010) 2010:701657. doi: 10.1155/2010/701657
13. Reichert TE, Rabinowich H, Johnson JT, Whiteside TL. Mechanisms responsible for signaling and functional defects. *J Immunother.* (1998) 21:295–306. doi: 10.1097/00002371-199807000-00007
14. Whiteside TL. Immunobiology of head and neck cancer. *Cancer Metastasis Rev.* (2005) 24:95–105. doi: 10.1007/s10555-005-5050-6
15. Sakakura K, Chikamatsu K, Takahashi K, Whiteside TL, Furuya N. Maturation of circulating dendritic cells and imbalance of T-cell subsets in patients with squamous cell carcinoma of the head and neck. *Cancer Immunol Immunother.* (2006) 55:151–9. doi: 10.1007/s00262-005-0697-y
16. Pitt JM, Vétizou M, Daillère R, Roberti MP, Yamazaki T, Routy B, et al. Resistance mechanisms to immune-checkpoint blockade in cancer: tumor-intrinsic and-extrinsic factors. *Immunity.* (2016) 44:1255–69. doi: 10.1016/j.immuni.2016.06.001
17. Corzo CA, Cotter MJ, Cheng P, Cheng F, Kusmartsev S, Sotomayor E, et al. Mechanism regulating reactive oxygen species in tumor-induced myeloid-derived suppressor cells. *J Immunol.* (2009) 182:5693–701. doi: 10.4049/jimmunol.0900092
18. Noman MZ, Desantis G, Janji B, Hasmim M, Karray S, Dessen P, et al. PD-L1 is a novel direct target of HIF-1α, and its blockade under hypoxia enhanced MDSC-mediated T cell activation. *J Exp Med.* (2014) 211:781–90. doi: 10.1084/jem.20131916
19. Echarri M, Lopez-Martin A, Hitt R. Targeted therapy in locally advanced and recurrent/metastatic head and neck squamous cell carcinoma (LA-R/M HNSCC). *Cancers.* (2016) 8:27. doi: 10.3390/cancers8030027
20. Lechner MG, Liebertz DJ, Epstein AL. Characterization of cytokine-induced myeloid-derived suppressor cells from normal human peripheral blood mononuclear cells. *J Immunol.* (2010) 185:2273–84. doi: 10.4049/jimmunol.1000901
21. Lahl K, Loddenkemper C, Drouin C, Freyer J, Arnason J, Eberl G, et al. Selective depletion of Foxp3+ regulatory T cells induces a scurfy-like disease. *J Exp Med.* (2007) 204:57–63. doi: 10.1084/jem.20061852
22. Sakaguchi S, Miyara M, Costantino CM, Hafler DA. FOXP3+ regulatory T cells in the human immune system. *Nat Rev Immunol.* (2010) 10:490–500. doi: 10.1038/nri2785
23. Jie H, Gildener-Leapman N, Li J, Srivastava R, Gibson S, Whiteside T, et al. Intratumoral regulatory T cells upregulate immunosuppressive molecules in head and neck cancer patients. *Br J Cancer.* (2013) 109:2629–35. doi: 10.1038/bjc.2013.645
24. Sica A, Mantovani A. Macrophage plasticity and polarization: *in vivo* veritas. *J Clin Invest.* (2012) 122:787–95. doi: 10.1172/JCI59643
25. El-Rouby DH. Association of macrophages with angiogenesis in oral verrucous and squamous cell carcinomas. *J Oral Pathol Med.* (2010) 39:559–64. doi: 10.1111/j.1600-0714.2010.00879.x

26. Oweida A, Hararah MK, Phan A, Binder D, Bhatia S, Lennon S, et al. Resistance to radiotherapy and PD-L1 blockade is mediated by TIM-3 upregulation and regulatory T-cell infiltration. *Clin Cancer Res.* (2018) 24:5368–80. doi: 10.1158/1078-0432.CCR-18-1038
27. Kather JN, Suarez-Carmona M, Charoentong P, Weis CA, Hirsch D, Bankhead P, et al. Topography of cancer-associated immune cells in human solid tumors. *Elife.* (2018) 7:e36967. doi: 10.7554/eLife.36967
28. Kunz-Schughart LA, Knuechel R. Tumor-associated fibroblasts (part I): active stromal participants in tumor development and progression? *Histol Histopathol.* (2002) 17:599–621. doi: 10.14670/HH-17.599
29. Wheeler SE, Shi H, Lin F, Dasari S, Bednash J, Thorne S, et al. Tumor associated fibroblasts enhance head and neck squamous cell carcinoma proliferation, invasion, and metastasis in preclinical models. *Head Neck.* (2014) 36:385–92. doi: 10.1002/hed.23312
30. Xie C, Ji N, Tang Z, Li J, Chen Q. The role of extracellular vesicles from different origin in the microenvironment of head and neck cancers. *Mol Cancer.* (2019) 18:83. doi: 10.1186/s12943-019-0985-3
31. Whiteside TL. Immune modulation of T-cell and NK (natural killer) cell activities by TEXs (tumour-derived exosomes). *Biochem Soc Trans.* (2013) 41:245–51. doi: 10.1042/BST20120265
32. Kim JW, Wieckowski E, Taylor DD, Reichert TE, Watkins S, Whiteside TL. Fas ligand–positive membranous vesicles isolated from sera of patients with oral cancer induce apoptosis of activated T lymphocytes. *Clin Cancer Res.* (2005) 11:1010–20.
33. Al-Samadi A, Awad SA, Tuomainen K, Zhao Y, Salem A, Parikka M, et al. Crosstalk between tongue carcinoma cells, extracellular vesicles, and immune cells in *in vitro* and *in vivo* models. *Oncotarget.* (2017) 8:60123–34. doi: 10.18632/oncotarget.17768
34. Hegde PS, Karanikas V, Evers S. The where, the when, and the how of immune monitoring for cancer immunotherapies in the era of checkpoint inhibition. *Clin Cancer Res.* (2016) 22:1865–74. doi: 10.1158/1078-0432.CCR-15-1507
35. Canning M, Guo G, Yu M, Myint C, Groves M, Byrd K, et al. Heterogeneity of the head and neck squamous cell carcinoma immune landscape and its impact on immunotherapy. *Front Cell Dev Biol.* (2019) 7:52. doi: 10.3389/fcell.2019.00052
36. Facciabene A, Peng X, Hagemann IS, Balint K, Barchetti A, Wang LP, et al. Tumour hypoxia promotes tolerance and angiogenesis via CCL28 and T reg cells. *Nature.* (2011) 475:226–30. doi: 10.1038/nature10169
37. Zou L, Barnett B, Safah H, LaRussa VF, Evdemon-Hogan M, Mottram P, et al. Bone marrow is a reservoir for CD4+ CD25+ regulatory T cells that traffic through CXCL12/CXCR4 signals. *Cancer Res.* (2004) 64:8451–5. doi: 10.1158/0008-5472.CAN-04-1987
38. Togashi Y, Shitara K, Nishikawa H. Regulatory T cells in cancer immunosuppression—implications for anticancer therapy. *Nat Rev Clin Oncol.* (2019) 16:356–71. doi: 10.1038/s41571-019-0175-7
39. Jarnicki AG, Lysaght J, Todryk S, Mills KH. Suppression of antitumor immunity by IL-10 and TGF-beta-producing T cells infiltrating the growing tumor: influence of tumor environment on the induction of CD4+ and CD8+ regulatory T cells. *J Immunol.* (2006) 177:896–904. doi: 10.4049/jimmunol.177.2.896
40. Maj T, Wang W, Crespo J, Zhang H, Wang W, Wei S, et al. Oxidative stress controls regulatory T cell apoptosis and suppressor activity and PD-L1-blockade resistance in tumor. *Nat Immunol.* (2017) 18:1332–41. doi: 10.1038/ni.3868
41. Liu Z, McMichael EL, Shayan G, Li J, Chen K, Srivastava R, et al. Novel effector phenotype of Tim-3+ regulatory T cells leads to enhanced suppressive function in head and neck cancer patients. *Clin Cancer Res.* (2018) 24:4529–38. doi: 10.1158/1078-0432.CCR-17-1350
42. Oweida AJ, Darragh L, Phan A, Binder D, Bhatia S, Mueller A, et al. STAT3 Modulation of regulatory T cells in response to radiation therapy in head and neck cancer. *J Natl Cancer Inst.* (2019). doi: 10.1093/jnci/djz036. [Epub ahead of print].
43. Strauss L, Bergmann C, Gooding W, Johnson JT, Whiteside TL. The frequency and suppressor function of CD4+ CD25highFoxp3+ T cells in the circulation of patients with squamous cell carcinoma of the head and neck. *Clin Cancer Res.* (2007) 13:6301–11. doi: 10.1158/1078-0432.CCR-07-1403
44. Al-Qahtani D, Anil S, Rajendran R. Tumour infiltrating CD25+ FoxP3+ regulatory T cells (Tregs) relate to tumour grade and stromal inflammation in oral squamous cell carcinoma. *J Oral Pathol Med.* (2011) 40:636–42. doi: 10.1111/j.1600-0714.2011.01020.x
45. Ribechini E, Greifenberg V, Sandwick S, Lutz MB. Subsets, expansion and activation of myeloid-derived suppressor cells. *Med Microbiol Immunol.* (2010) 199:273–81. doi: 10.1007/s00430-010-0151-4
46. Gabrilovich DI. Myeloid-derived suppressor cells. *Cancer Immunol Res.* (2017) 5:3–8. doi: 10.1158/2326-6066.CIR-16-0297
47. Lang S, Bruderek K, Kaspar C, Höing B, Kanaan O, Dominas N, et al. Clinical relevance and suppressive capacity of human myeloid-derived suppressor cell subsets. *Clin Cancer Res.* (2018) 24:4834–44. doi: 10.1158/1078-0432.CCR-17-3726
48. Lim KP, Cirillo N, Hassona Y, Wei W, Thurlow JK, Cheong SC, et al. Fibroblast gene expression profile reflects the stage of tumour progression in oral squamous cell carcinoma. *J Pathol.* (2011) 223:459–69. doi: 10.1002/path.2841
49. Park JE, Lenter MC, Zimmermann RN, Garin-Chesa P, Old LJ, Rettig WJ. Fibroblast activation protein, a dual specificity serine protease expressed in reactive human tumor stromal fibroblasts. *J Biol Chem.* (1999) 274:36505–12. doi: 10.1074/jbc.274.51.36505
50. Wonganu B, Berger BW. A specific, transmembrane interface regulates fibroblast activation protein (FAP) homodimerization, trafficking and exopeptidase activity. *Biochim Biophys Acta.* (2016) 1858:1876–82. doi: 10.1016/j.bbamem.2016.05.001
51. Bello IO, Vered M, Dayan D, Dobriyan A, Yahalom R, Alanen K, et al. Cancer-associated fibroblasts, a parameter of the tumor microenvironment, overcomes carcinoma-associated parameters in the prognosis of patients with mobile tongue cancer. *Oral Oncol.* (2011) 47:33–8. doi: 10.1016/j.oraloncology.2010.10.013
52. Lotti F, Jarrar AM, Pai RK, Hitomi M, Lathia J, Mace A, et al. Chemotherapy activates cancer-associated fibroblasts to maintain colorectal cancer-initiating cells by IL-17A. *J Exp Med.* (2013) 210:2851–72. doi: 10.1084/jem.20131195
53. Glentis A, Oertle P, Mariani P, Chikina A, El Marjou F, Attieh Y, et al. Cancer-associated fibroblasts induce metalloprotease-independent cancer cell invasion of the basement membrane. *Nat Commun.* (2017) 8:924. doi: 10.1038/s41467-017-00985-8
54. Sandoval P, Jiménez-Heffernan JA, Rynne-Vidal Á, Pérez-Lozano ML, Gilsanz Á, Ruiz-Carpio V, et al. Carcinoma-associated fibroblasts derive from mesothelial cells via mesothelial-to-mesenchymal transition in peritoneal metastasis. *J Pathol.* (2013) 231:517–31. doi: 10.1002/path.4281
55. Iwano M, Plieth D, Danoff TM, Xue C, Okada H, Neilson EG. Evidence that fibroblasts derive from epithelium during tissue fibrosis. *J Clin Invest.* (2002) 110:341–50. doi: 10.1172/JCI0215518
56. Knowles LM, Stabile LP, Egloff AM, Rothstein ME, Thomas SM, Gubish CT, et al. HGF and c-Met participate in paracrine tumorigenic pathways in head and neck squamous cell cancer. *Clin Cancer Res.* (2009) 15:3740–50. doi: 10.1158/1078-0432.CCR-08-3252
57. Fiori ME, Di Franco S, Villanova L, Bianca P, Stassi G, De Maria R. Cancer-associated fibroblasts as abettors of tumor progression at the crossroads of EMT and therapy resistance. *Mol Cancer.* (2019) 18:70. doi: 10.1186/s12943-019-0994-2
58. Yu B, Wu K, Wang X, Zhang J, Wang L, Jiang Y, et al. Periostin secreted by cancer-associated fibroblasts promotes cancer stemness in head and neck cancer by activating protein tyrosine kinase 7. *Cell Death Dis.* (2018) 9:1082. doi: 10.1038/s41419-018-1116-6
59. Álvarez-Teijeiro S, García-Inclán C, Villaronga M, Casado P, Hermida-Prado F, Granda-Díaz R, et al. Factors secreted by cancer-associated fibroblasts that sustain cancer stem properties in head and neck squamous carcinoma cells as potential therapeutic targets. *Cancers.* (2018) 10:334. doi: 10.3390/cancers10090334
60. Murray PJ, Allen JE, Biswas SK, Fisher EA, Gilroy DW, Goerdt S, et al. Macrophage activation and polarization: nomenclature and experimental guidelines. *Immunity.* (2014) 41:14–20. doi: 10.1016/j.immuni.2014.06.008

61. Lin CN, Chien CY, Chuang HC. Are friends or foes? New strategy for head and neck squamous cell carcinoma treatment via immune regulation. *Int J Head Neck Sci.* (2017) 1:105–13. doi: 10.6696/IJHNS.2017.0102.03
62. Weber M, Büttner-Herold M, Hyckel P, Moebius P, Distel L, Ries J, et al. Small oral squamous cell carcinomas with nodal lymphogenic metastasis show increased infiltration of M2 polarized macrophages–an immunohistochemical analysis. *J Craniomaxillofac Surg.* (2014) 42:1087–94. doi: 10.1016/j.jcms.2014.01.035
63. Mantovani A, Biswas SK, Galdiero MR, Sica A, Locati M. Macrophage plasticity and polarization in tissue repair and remodelling. *J Pathol.* (2013) 229:176–85. doi: 10.1002/path.4133
64. Liu CY, Xu JY, Shi XY, Huang W, Ruan TY, Xie P, et al. M2-polarized tumor-associated macrophages promoted epithelial–mesenchymal transition in pancreatic cancer cells, partially through TLR4/IL-10 signaling pathway. *Lab Invest.* (2013) 93:844–54. doi: 10.1038/labinvest.2013.69
65. Rodriguez PC, Hernandez CP, Quiceno D, Dubinett SM, Zabaleta J, Ochoa JB, et al. Arginase I in myeloid suppressor cells is induced by COX-2 in lung carcinoma. *J Exp Med.* (2005) 202:931–9. doi: 10.1084/jem.20050715
66. Van Ginderachter JA, Meerschaut S, Liu Y, Brys L, De Groeve K, Ghassabeh GH, et al. Peroxisome proliferator-activated receptor gamma (PPARgamma) ligands reverse CTL suppression by alternatively activated (M2) macrophages in cancer. *Blood.* (2006) 108:525–35. doi: 10.1182/blood-2005-09-3777
67. She L, Qin Y, Wang J, Liu C, Zhu G, Li G, et al. Tumor-associated macrophages derived CCL18 promotes metastasis in squamous cell carcinoma of the head and neck. *Cancer Cell Int.* (2018) 18:120. doi: 10.1186/s12935-018-0620-1
68. Kumar AT, Knops A, Swendseid B, Martinez-Outschoorn UE, Harshyne L, Philp NJ, et al. Prognostic significance of tumor-associated macrophage content in head and neck squamous cell carcinoma: a meta-analysis. *Front Oncol.* (2019) 9:656. doi: 10.3389/fonc.2019.00656
69. Troiano G, Caponio VCA, Adipietro I, Tepedino M, Santoro R, Laino L, et al. Prognostic significance of CD68+ and CD163+ tumor associated macrophages in head and neck squamous cell carcinoma: a systematic review and meta-analysis. *Oral Oncol.* (2019) 93:66–75. doi: 10.1016/j.oraloncology.2019.04.019
70. Cooper MA, Fehniger TA, Caligiuri MA. The biology of human natural killer-cell subsets. *Trends Immunol.* (2001) 22:633–40. doi: 10.1016/S1471-4906(01)02060-9
71. Konjevic G, Jurisic V, Jovic V, Vuletic A, Martinovic KM, Radenkovic S, et al. Investigation of NK cell function and their modulation in different malignancies. *Immunol Res.* (2012) 52:139–56. doi: 10.1007/s12026-012-8285-7
72. Topham NJ, Hewitt EW. Natural killer cell cytotoxicity: how do they pull the trigger? *Immunology.* (2009) 128:7–15. doi: 10.1111/j.1365-2567.2009.03123.x
73. Wang W, Erbe AK, Hank JA, Morris ZS, Sondel PM. NK cell-mediated antibody-dependent cellular cytotoxicity in cancer immunotherapy. *Front Immunol.* (2015) 6:368. doi: 10.3389/fimmu.2015.00368
74. Weil S, Memmer S, Lechner A, Huppert V, Giannattasio A, Becker T, et al. Natural killer group 2D ligand depletion reconstitutes natural killer cell immunosurveillance of head and neck squamous cell carcinoma. *Front Immunol.* (2017) 8:387. doi: 10.3389/fimmu.2017.00387
75. Fridlender ZG, Sun J, Kim S, Kapoor V, Cheng G, Ling L, et al. Polarization of tumor-associated neutrophil phenotype by TGF-beta:"N1" versus "N2" TAN. *Cancer cell.* (2009) 16:183–94. doi: 10.1016/j.ccr.2009.06.017
76. Zhang X, Zhang W, Yuan X, Fu M, Qian H, Xu W. Neutrophils in cancer development and progression: roles, mechanisms, and implications. *Int J Oncol.* (2016) 49:857–67. doi: 10.3892/ijo.2016.3616
77. Levental KR, Yu H, Kass L, Lakins JN, Egeblad M, Erler JT, et al. Matrix crosslinking forces tumor progression by enhancing integrin signaling. *Cell.* (2009) 139:891–906. doi: 10.1016/j.cell.2009.10.027
78. Egeblad M, Werb Z. New functions for the matrix metalloproteinases in cancer progression. *Nat Rev Cancer.* (2002) 2:161–74. doi: 10.1038/nrc745
79. Bergers G, Brekken R, McMahon G, Vu TH, Itoh T, Tamaki K, et al. Matrix metalloproteinase-9 triggers the angiogenic switch during carcinogenesis. *Nat Cell Biol.* (2000) 2:737–44. doi: 10.1038/35036374
80. Tatti O, Vehviläinen P, Lehti K, Keski-Oja J. MT1-MMP releases latent TGF-beta1 from endothelial cell extracellular matrix via proteolytic processing of LTBP-1. *Exp Cell Res.* (2008) 314:2501–14. doi: 10.1016/j.yexcr.2008.05.018
81. Garcia AJ, Boettiger D. Integrin–fibronectin interactions at the cell-material interface: initial integrin binding and signaling. *Biomaterials.* (1999) 20:2427–33. doi: 10.1016/S0142-9612(99)00170-2
82. Brown AC, Dysart MM, Clarke KC, Stabenfeldt SE, Barker TH. Integrin $\alpha3\beta1$ binding to fibronectin is dependent on the ninth type III repeat. *J Biol Chem.* (2015) 290:25534–47. doi: 10.1074/jbc.M115.656702
83. Lou X, Han X, Jin C, Tian W, Yu W, Ding D, et al. SOX2 targets fibronectin 1 to promote cell migration and invasion in ovarian cancer: new molecular leads for therapeutic intervention. *OMICS.* (2013) 17:510–8. doi: 10.1089/omi.2013.0058
84. Knowles LM, Gurski LA, Engel C, Gnarra JR, Maranchie JK, Pilch J. Integrin $\alpha v\beta3$ and fibronectin upregulate Slug in cancer cells to promote clot invasion and metastasis. *Cancer Res.* (2013) 73:6175–84. doi: 10.1158/0008-5472.CAN-13-0602
85. Matlung SE, Wilhelmina van Kempen PM, Bovenschen N, Baarle DV, Willems SM. Differences in T-cell infiltrates and survival between HPV+ and HPV-oropharyngeal squamous cell carcinoma. *Future Sci OA.* (2016) 2:FSO88. doi: 10.4155/fso.15.88
86. Partlová S, Bouček J, Kloudová K, Lukešová E, Zábrodský M, Grega M, et al. Distinct patterns of intratumoral immune cell infiltrates in patients with HPV-associated compared to non-virally induced head and neck squamous cell carcinoma. *Oncoimmunology.* (2015) 4:e965570. doi: 10.4161/21624011.2014.965570
87. Lechner A, Schlößer HA, Thelen M, Wennhold K, Rothschild SI, Gilles R, et al. Tumor-associated B cells and humoral immune response in head and neck squamous cell carcinoma. *Oncoimmunology.* (2019) 8:1535293. doi: 10.1080/2162402X.2018.1535293
88. Al-Sahaf S, Hunter KD, Bolt R, Ottewell PD, Murdoch C. The IL-1/IL-1R axis induces greater fibroblast-derived chemokine release in human papillomavirus-negative compared to positive oropharyngeal cancer. *Int J Cancer.* (2019) 144:334–44. doi: 10.1002/ijc.31852
89. Bloy N, Garcia P, Laumont CM, Pitt JM, Sistigu A, Stoll G, et al. Immunogenic stress and death of cancer cells: contribution of antigenicity vs adjuvanticity to immunosurveillance. *Immunol Rev.* (2017) 280:165–74. doi: 10.1111/imr.12582
90. Honegger A, Leitz J, Bulkescher J, Hoppe-Seyler K, Hoppe-Seyler F. Silencing of human papillomavirus (HPV) E6/E7 oncogene expression affects both the contents and the amounts of extracellular microvesicles released from HPV-positive cancer cells. *Int J Cancer.* (2013) 133:1631–42. doi: 10.1002/ijc.28164
91. Harden ME, Munger K. Human papillomavirus 16 E6 and E7 oncoprotein expression alters microRNA expression in extracellular vesicles. *Virology.* (2017) 508:63–9. doi: 10.1016/j.virol.2017.05.005
92. Fleming JC, Woo J, Moutasim K, Mellone M, Frampton SJ, Mead A, et al. HPV, tumour metabolism and novel target identification in head and neck squamous cell carcinoma. *Br J Cancer.* (2019) 120:356–67. doi: 10.1038/s41416-018-0364-7
93. Halestrap AP, Wilson MC. The monocarboxylate transporter family—role and regulation. *IUBMB Life.* (2012) 64:109–19. doi: 10.1002/iub.572
94. Desrichard A, Kuo F, Chowell D, Lee KW, Riaz N, Wong RJ, et al. Tobacco smoking-associated alterations in the immune microenvironment of squamous cell carcinomas. *J Natl Cancer Inst.* (2018) 110:1386–92. doi: 10.1093/jnci/djy060
95. Hernandez CP, Morrow K, Velasco C, Wyczechowska DD, Naura AS, Rodriguez PC. Effects of cigarette smoke extract on primary activated T cells. *Cell Immunol.* (2013) 282:38–43. doi: 10.1016/j.cellimm.2013.04.005
96. Foy JP, Bertolus C, Michallet MC, Deneuve S, Incitti R, Bendriss-Vermare N, et al. The immune microenvironment of HPV-negative oral squamous cell carcinoma from never-smokers and never-drinkers patients suggests higher clinical benefit of IDO1 and PD1/PD-L1 blockade. *Ann Oncol.* (2017) 28:1934–41. doi: 10.1093/annonc/mdx210
97. Sok JC, Coppelli FM, Thomas SM, Lango MN, Xi S, Hunt JL, et al. Mutant epidermal growth factor receptor (EGFRvIII) contributes to head and neck cancer growth and resistance to EGFR targeting. *Clin Cancer Res.* (2006) 12:5064–73. doi: 10.1158/1078-0432.CCR-06-0913

98. Hama T, Yuza Y, Suda T, Saito Y, Norizoe C, Kato T, et al. Functional mutation analysis of EGFR family genes and corresponding lymph node metastases in head and neck squamous cell carcinoma. *Clin Exp Metastasis.* (2012) 29:19–25. doi: 10.1007/s10585-011-9425-5
99. Bhatia S, Oweida A, Lennon S, Darragh LB, Milner D, Phan AV, et al. Inhibition of EphB4–Ephrin-B2 signaling reprograms the tumor immune microenvironment in head and neck cancers. *Cancer Res.* (2019) 79:2722–35. doi: 10.1158/0008-5472.CAN-18-3257
100. Koyama S, Akbay EA, Li YY, Herter-Sprie GS, Buczkowski KA, Richards WG, et al. Adaptive resistance to therapeutic PD-1 blockade is associated with upregulation of alternative immune checkpoints. *Nat Commun.* (2016) 7:10501. doi: 10.1038/ncomms10501
101. Gubin MM, Zhang X, Schuster H, Caron E, Ward JP, Noguchi T, et al. Checkpoint blockade cancer immunotherapy targets tumour-specific mutant antigens. *Nature.* (2014) 515:577–81. doi: 10.1038/nature13988
102. Jenkins RW, Barbie DA, Flaherty KT. Mechanisms of resistance to immune checkpoint inhibitors. *Br J Cancer.* (2018) 118:9–16. doi: 10.1038/bjc.2017.434
103. Zaretsky JM, Garcia-Diaz A, Shin DS, Escuin-Ordinas H, Hugo W, Hu-Lieskovan S, et al. Mutations associated with acquired resistance to PD-1 blockade in melanoma. *N Engl J Med.* (2016) 375:819–29. doi: 10.1056/NEJMoa1604958
104. Peng W, Chen JQ, Liu C, Malu S, Creasy C, Tetzlaff MT, et al. Loss of PTEN promotes resistance to T cell–mediated immunotherapy. *Cancer Discov.* (2016) 6:202–16. doi: 10.1158/2159-8290.CD-15-0283
105. Spranger S, Bao R, Gajewski TF. Melanoma-intrinsic β-catenin signalling prevents anti-tumour immunity. *Nature.* (2015) 523:231–5. doi: 10.1038/nature14404
106. Olson OC, Kim H, Quail DF, Foley EA, Joyce JA. Tumor-associated macrophages suppress the cytotoxic activity of antimitotic agents. *Cell Rep.* (2017) 19:101–13. doi: 10.1016/j.celrep.2017.03.038
107. Vargas FA, Furness AJ, Solomon I, Joshi K, Mekkaoui L, Lesko MH, et al. Fc-optimized anti-CD25 depletes tumor-infiltrating regulatory T cells and synergizes with PD-1 blockade to eradicate established tumors. *Immunity.* (2017) 46:577–86. doi: 10.1016/j.immuni.2017.03.013
108. O'Donnell JS, Long GV, Scolyer RA, Teng MW, Smyth MJ. Resistance to PD1/PDL1 checkpoint inhibition. *Cancer Treat Rev.* (2017) 52:71–81. doi: 10.1016/j.ctrv.2016.11.007
109. Syn NL, Teng MW, Mok TS, Soo RA. De-novo and acquired resistance to immune checkpoint targeting. *Lancet Oncol.* (2017) 18:e731–41. doi: 10.1016/S1470-2045(17)30607-1
110. Wang Y, Deng W, Li N, Neri S, Sharma A, Jiang W, et al. Combining immunotherapy and radiotherapy for cancer treatment: current challenges and future directions. *Front Pharmacol.* (2018) 9:185. doi: 10.3389/fphar.2018.00185
111. Ferris RL, Lenz HJ, Trotta AM, García-Foncillas J, Schulten J, Audhuy F, et al. Rationale for combination of therapeutic antibodies targeting tumor cells and immune checkpoint receptors: Harnessing innate and adaptive immunity through IgG1 isotype immune effector stimulation. *Cancer Treat Rev.* (2018) 63:48–60. doi: 10.1016/j.ctrv.2017.11.008
112. Liang H, Liu X, Wang M. Immunotherapy combined with epidermal growth factor receptor-tyrosine kinase inhibitors in non-small-cell lung cancer treatment. *Onco Targets Ther.* (2018) 11:6189–96. doi: 10.2147/OTT.S178497
113. Knudson KM, Hicks KC, Alter S, Schlom J, Gameiro SR. Mechanisms involved in IL-15 superagonist enhancement of anti-PD-L1 therapy. *J Immunother Cancer.* (2019) 7:82. doi: 10.1186/s40425-019-0551-y
114. Langan EA, Kümpers C, Graetz V, Perner S, Zillikens D, Terheyden P. Intralesional interleukin-2: a novel option to maximize response to systemic immune checkpoint therapy in loco-regional metastatic melanoma. *Dermatol Ther.* (2019) 32:e12901. doi: 10.1111/dth.12901
115. Soerensen MM, Ros W, Rodriguez-Ruiz ME, Robbrecht D, Rohrberg KS, Martin-Liberal J, et al. Safety, PK/PD, and anti-tumor activity of RO6874281, an engineered variant of interleukin-2 (IL-2v) targeted to tumor-associated fibroblasts via binding to fibroblast activation protein (FAP). *Am Soc Clin Oncol.* (2018) 36(Suppl. 15):e15155. doi: 10.1200/JCO.2018.36.15_suppl.e15155
116. Rady P, Cadet P, Bui T, Tyring S, Baron S, Stanton G, et al. Production of interferon gamma messenger RNA by cells of non-immune origin. *Cytokine.* (1995) 7:793–8. doi: 10.1006/cyto.1995.0095
117. Schaer D, Beckmann R, Dempsey J, Huber L, Forest A, Amaladas N, et al. The CDK4/6 inhibitor abemaciclib induces a T cell inflamed tumor microenvironment and enhances the efficacy of PD-L1 checkpoint blockade. *Cell Rep.* (2018) 22:2978–94. doi: 10.1016/j.celrep.2018.02.053
118. Sagiv-Barfi I, Kohrt HE, Czerwinski DK, Ng PP, Chang BY, Levy R. Therapeutic antitumor immunity by checkpoint blockade is enhanced by ibrutinib, an inhibitor of both BTK and ITK. *Proc Natl Acad Sci USA.* (2015) 112:E966–72. doi: 10.1073/pnas.1500712112
119. Hidalgo M, Gil M, Garcia-Carbonero R, Alvarez R, Laquente B, Moreno R, et al. First-in-human dose-escalation study of VCN-01, a selective oncolytic adenovirus with hyaluronidase activity in patients with advanced or metastatic cancer. *Eur J Cancer.* (2016) 69:S99–100. doi: 10.1016/S0959-8049(16)32895-7
120. Taylor MH, Rasco DW, Brose MS, Vogelzang NJ, Richey SL, Cohn AL, et al. A phase 1b/2 trial of lenvatinib plus pembrolizumab in patients with squamous cell carcinoma of the head and neck. *Am Soc Clin Oncol.* (2018) 36(Suppl. 15):6016. doi: 10.1200/JCO.2018.36.15_suppl.6016
121. Rizvi NA, Loo D, Baughman JE, Yun S, Chen F, Moore PA, et al. A phase 1 study of enoblituzumab in combination with pembrolizumab in patients with advanced B7-H3-expressing cancers. *Am Soc Clin Oncol.* (2016) 34(Suppl. 15):TPS3104. doi: 10.1200/JCO.2016.34.15_suppl.TPS3104
122. Lipson E, Long G, Tawbi H, Schadendorf D, Atkinson V, Maurer M, et al. 1302TiP CA224–047: a randomized, double-blind, phase II/III study of relatlimab (anti–LAG-3) in combination with nivolumab (anti–PD-1) versus nivolumab alone in previously untreated metastatic or unresectable melanoma. *Ann Oncol.* (2018) 29:mdy289.058. doi: 10.1093/annonc/mdy289.058
123. Sullivan RJ, Hong DS, Tolcher AW, Patnaik A, Shapiro G, Chmielowski B, et al. Initial results from first-in-human study of IPI-549, a tumor macrophage-targeting agent, combined with nivolumab in advanced solid tumors. *Am Soc Clin Oncol.* (2018) 36(Suppl. 15):3013. doi: 10.1200/JCO.2018.36.15_suppl.3013
124. Das R, Verma R, Sznol M, Boddupalli CS, Gettinger SN, Kluger H, et al. Combination therapy with anti–CTLA-4 and anti–PD-1 leads to distinct immunologic changes *in vivo*. *J Immunol.* (2015) 194:950–9. doi: 10.4049/jimmunol.1401686
125. Chin SM, Kimberlin CR, Roe-Zurz Z, Zhang P, Xu A, Liao-Chan S, et al. Structure of the 4–1BB/4–1BBL complex and distinct binding and functional properties of utomilumab and urelumab. *Nat Commun.* (2018) 9:4679. doi: 10.2210/pdb6mgp/pdb
126. Diab A, El-Khoueiry A, Eskens F, Ros W, Thompson J, Konto C, et al. A first-in-human (FIH) study of PF-04518600 (PF-8600) OX40 agonist in adult patients (pts) with select advanced malignancies. *Ann Oncol.* (2016) 27:359–78. doi: 10.1093/annonc/mdw378.08
127. Milhem M, Gonzales R, Medina T, Kirkwood JM, Buchbinder E, Mehmi I, et al. Abstract CT144: intratumoral toll-like receptor 9 (TLR9) agonist, CMP-001, in combination with pembrolizumab can reverse resistance to PD-1 inhibition in a phase Ib trial in subjects with advanced melanoma. *Cancer Res.* (2018) 78(Suppl. 13):CT144. doi: 10.1158/1538-7445.AM2018-CT144
128. Labadie BW, Bao R, Luke JJ. Reimagining IDO pathway inhibition in cancer immunotherapy via downstream focus on the tryptophan–kynurenine–aryl hydrocarbon axis. *Clin Cancer Res.* (2019) 25:1462–71. doi: 10.1158/1078-0432.CCR-18-2882
129. Massarelli E, William W, Johnson F, Kies M, Ferrarotto R, Guo M, et al. Combining immune checkpoint blockade and tumor-specific vaccine for patients with incurable human papillomavirus 16-related cancer: a phase 2 clinical trial. *JAMA Oncol.* (2019) 5:67–73. doi: 10.1001/jamaoncol.2018.4051
130. Schneider K, Grønhøj C, Hahn CH, von Buchwald C. Therapeutic human papillomavirus vaccines in head and neck cancer: a systematic review of current clinical trials. *Vaccine.* (2018) 36:6594–605. doi: 10.1016/j.vaccine.2018.09.027
131. Rice J, Ottensmeier CH, Stevenson FK. DNA vaccines: precision tools for activating effective immunity against cancer. *Nat Rev Cancer.* (2008) 8:108–20. doi: 10.1038/nrc2326

132. Krieg AM. CpG motifs in bacterial DNA and their immune effects. *Annu Rev Immunol.* (2002) 20:709–60. doi: 10.1146/annurev.immunol.20.100301.064842
133. Wang C, Dickie J, Sutavani RV, Pointer C, Thomas GJ, Savelyeva N. Targeting head and neck cancer by vaccination. *Front Immunol.* (2018) 9:830. doi: 10.3389/fimmu.2018.00830
134. Qureshi HA, Lee SM. Immunotherapy approaches beyond PD-1 inhibition: the future of cellular therapy for head and neck squamous cell carcinoma. *Curr Treat Options Oncol.* (2019) 20:31. doi: 10.1007/s11864-019-0630-9
135. Hinrichs CS, Doran SL, Stevanovic S, Adhikary S, Mojadidi M, Kwong ML, et al. A phase I/II clinical trial of E6 T-cell receptor gene therapy for human papillomavirus (HPV)-associated epithelial cancers. *Am Soc Clin Oncol.* (2017) 35(Suppl. 15):3009. doi: 10.1200/JCO.2017.35.15_suppl.3009
136. Papa S, Adami A, Metoudi M, Achkova D, van Schalkwyk M, Parente Pereira A, et al. A phase I trial of T4 CAR T-cell immunotherapy in head and neck squamous cancer (HNSCC). *Am Soc Clin Oncol.* (2018) 36(Suppl. 15):3046. doi: 10.1200/JCO.2018.36.15_suppl.3046
137. Okada S, Itoh K, Ishihara S, Shimada J, Kato D, Tsunezuka H, et al. Significance of PD-L1 expression in pulmonary metastases from head and neck squamous cell carcinoma. *Surg Oncol.* (2018) 27:259–65. doi: 10.1016/j.suronc.2018.04.007
138. Hirsch FR, McElhinny A, Stanforth D, Ranger-Moore J, Jansson M, Kulangara K, et al. PD-L1 immunohistochemistry assays for lung cancer: results from phase 1 of the blueprint PD-L1 IHC assay comparison project. *J Thorac Oncol.* (2017) 12:208–22. doi: 10.1016/j.jtho.2016.11.2228
139. Hanna GJ, Lizotte P, Cavanaugh M, Kuo FC, Shivdasani P, Frieden A, et al. Frameshift events predict anti–PD-1/L1 response in head and neck cancer. *JCI Insight.* (2018) 3:98811. doi: 10.1172/jci.insight.98811
140. Cristescu R, Mogg R, Ayers M, Albright A, Murphy E, Yearley J, et al. Pan-tumor genomic biomarkers for PD-1 checkpoint blockade–based immunotherapy. *Science.* (2018) 362:eaar3593. doi: 10.1126/science.aar3593
141. Chalmers ZR, Connelly CF, Fabrizio D, Gay L, Ali SM, Ennis R, et al. Analysis of 100,000 human cancer genomes reveals the landscape of tumor mutational burden. *Genome Med.* (2017) 9:34. doi: 10.1186/s13073-017-0424-2
142. Le DT, Durham JN, Smith KN, Wang H, Bartlett BR, Aulakh LK, et al. Mismatch repair deficiency predicts response of solid tumors to PD-1 blockade. *Science.* (2017) 357:409–13. doi: 10.1126/science.aan6733
143. Yarchoan M, Hopkins A, Jaffee EM. Tumor mutational burden and response rate to PD-1 inhibition. *N Engl J Med.* (2017) 377:2500–1. doi: 10.1056/NEJMc1713444

Permissions

All chapters in this book were first published by Frontiers; hereby published with permission under the Creative Commons Attribution License or equivalent. Every chapter published in this book has been scrutinized by our experts. Their significance has been extensively debated. The topics covered herein carry significant findings which will fuel the growth of the discipline. They may even be implemented as practical applications or may be referred to as a beginning point for another development.

The contributors of this book come from diverse backgrounds, making this book a truly international effort. This book will bring forth new frontiers with its revolutionizing research information and detailed analysis of the nascent developments around the world.

We would like to thank all the contributing authors for lending their expertise to make the book truly unique. They have played a crucial role in the development of this book. Without their invaluable contributions this book wouldn't have been possible. They have made vital efforts to compile up to date information on the varied aspects of this subject to make this book a valuable addition to the collection of many professionals and students.

This book was conceptualized with the vision of imparting up-to-date information and advanced data in this field. To ensure the same, a matchless editorial board was set up. Every individual on the board went through rigorous rounds of assessment to prove their worth. After which they invested a large part of their time researching and compiling the most relevant data for our readers.

The editorial board has been involved in producing this book since its inception. They have spent rigorous hours researching and exploring the diverse topics which have resulted in the successful publishing of this book. They have passed on their knowledge of decades through this book. To expedite this challenging task, the publisher supported the team at every step. A small team of assistant editors was also appointed to further simplify the editing procedure and attain best results for the readers.

Apart from the editorial board, the designing team has also invested a significant amount of their time in understanding the subject and creating the most relevant covers. They scrutinized every image to scout for the most suitable representation of the subject and create an appropriate cover for the book.

The publishing team has been an ardent support to the editorial, designing and production team. Their endless efforts to recruit the best for this project, has resulted in the accomplishment of this book. They are a veteran in the field of academics and their pool of knowledge is as vast as their experience in printing. Their expertise and guidance has proved useful at every step. Their uncompromising quality standards have made this book an exceptional effort. Their encouragement from time to time has been an inspiration for everyone.

The publisher and the editorial board hope that this book will prove to be a valuable piece of knowledge for researchers, students, practitioners and scholars across the globe.

List of Contributors

Chia Ying Li
Department of Surgery, Show Chwan Memorial Hospital, Changhua, Taiwan
Ph.D. Program in Tissue Engineering and Regenerative Medicine, National Chung Hsing University, Taichung, Taiwan

Jia-Hua Cai, Jeffrey J. P. Tsai and Charles C. N. Wang
Department of Bioinformatics and Medical Engineering, Asia University, Taichung, Taiwan

Pao-Yu Tseng and Mu-Kuan Chen
Department of Otorhinolaryngology, Head and Neck Surgery, Changhua Christian Hospital, Changhua, Taiwan

Yen-Tze Liu
Department of Family Medicine, Changhua Christian Hospital, Changhua, Taiwan
Institute of Medicine, Chung Shan Medical University, Taichung, Taiwan
Department of Holistic Wellness, Mingdao University, Changhua, Taiwan
Oral Cancer Research Center, Changhua Christian Hospital, Changhua, Taiwan

Chia-Chieh Lin, Yi-Ching Chuang, Yu-Sheng Lo and Yi-Ting Hsi
Oral Cancer Research Center, Changhua Christian Hospital, Changhua, Taiwan

Ming-Ju Hsieh
Institute of Medicine, Chung Shan Medical University, Taichung, Taiwan
Department of Holistic Wellness, Mingdao University, Changhua, Taiwan
Oral Cancer Research Center, Changhua Christian Hospital, Changhua, Taiwan
Graduate Institute of Biomedical Sciences, China Medical University, Taichung, Taiwan

Lorena Arribas
Clinical Nutrition Unit, Catalan Institute of Oncology (ICO), L'Hospitalet de Llobregat, Barcelona, Spain
Bellvitge Biomedical Research Institute (IDIBELL), L'Hospitalet de Llobregat, Barcelona, Spain
Head and Neck Cancer Unit, Bellvitge University Hospital, Catalan Institute of Oncology (ICO), L'Hospitalet de Llobregat, Barcelona, Spain
University of Barcelona, Barcelona, Spain

Noelia Vilariño
Medical Oncology Department, Catalan Institute of Oncology (ICO), ONCOBELL, L'Hospitalet de Llobregat, Barcelona, Spain

Maria Plana
Head and Neck Cancer Unit, Bellvitge University Hospital, Catalan Institute of Oncology (ICO), L'Hospitalet de Llobregat, Barcelona, Spain
Medical Oncology Department, Catalan Institute of Oncology (ICO), ONCOBELL, L'Hospitalet de Llobregat, Barcelona, Spain

Miren Taberna and Marc Oliva
Bellvitge Biomedical Research Institute (IDIBELL), L'Hospitalet de Llobregat, Barcelona, Spain
Head and Neck Cancer Unit, Bellvitge University Hospital, Catalan Institute of Oncology (ICO), L'Hospitalet de Llobregat, Barcelona, Spain
Medical Oncology Department, Catalan Institute of Oncology (ICO), ONCOBELL, L'Hospitalet de Llobregat, Barcelona, Spain

Maria Sospedra
Unitat de Nutrició Clínica i Dietètica, Hospital Universitari Germans Trias i Pujol (HUGTiP), Barcelona, Spain

Natalia Pallarés
Unitat de Bioestadística (UBiDi), Bellvitge University Hospital, L'Hospitalet de Llobregat, Barcelona, Spain

Luis Miguel Del Rio
Grupo Ascires, CETIR Grupo Médico, Barcelona, Spain

Ricard Mesia
Bellvitge Biomedical Research Institute (IDIBELL), L'Hospitalet de Llobregat, Barcelona, Spain
Head and Neck Cancer Unit, Bellvitge University Hospital, Catalan Institute of Oncology (ICO), L'Hospitalet de Llobregat, Barcelona, Spain
Medical Oncology, Institut Català d'Oncología, Group Badalona Applied Research Group in Oncology (B-ARGO) Group, Institut d'Investigació Germans Trias i Pujol (IGTP), Badalona, Spain

Vickie Baracos
Division of Palliative Care Medicine, Department of Oncology, University of Alberta, Cross Cancer Institute, Edmonton, AB, Canada

Ana Regina González Tampán
Clinical Nutrition Unit, Catalan Institute of Oncology (ICO), L'Hospitalet de Llobregat, Barcelona, Spain
Head and Neck Cancer Unit, Bellvitge University Hospital, Catalan Institute of Oncology (ICO), L'Hospitalet de Llobregat, Barcelona, Spain

Silvia Giunco and Anita De Rossi
Department of Surgery, Oncology and Gastroenterology, Section of Oncology and Immunology, University of Padova, Padova, Italy
Immunology and Diagnostic Molecular Oncology Unit, Veneto Institute of Oncology (IOV), Istituto di Ricovero e Cura a Carattere Scientifico (IRCCS), Padova, Italy

Marzia Morello and Giovanni Esposito
Immunology and Diagnostic Molecular Oncology Unit, Veneto Institute of Oncology (IOV), Istituto di Ricovero e Cura a Carattere Scientifico (IRCCS), Padova, Italy

Giacomo Spinato
Department of Surgery, Oncology and Gastroenterology, Section of Oncology and Immunology, University of Padova, Padova, Italy
Department of Neurosciences, Section of Otolaryngology, University of Padova, Treviso, Italy

Anna Menegaldo, Enzo Emanuelli, Monica Mantovani and Marco Stellin
Department of Neurosciences, Section of Otolaryngology, University of Padova, Treviso, Italy

Giancarlo Tirelli and Margherita Tofanelli
Department of Medical, Surgical and Health Sciences, Section of Otolaryngology, University of Trieste, Trieste, Italy

Paolo Boscolo-Rizzo
Department of Neurosciences, Section of Otolaryngology, University of Padova, Treviso, Italy
Department of Medical, Surgical and Health Sciences, Section of Otolaryngology, University of Trieste, Trieste, Italy

Lara Alessandrini, Valentina Carraro and Angelo Paolo Dei Tos
Department of Medicine (DIMED), Section of Pathology, University of Padova, Padova, Italy

Roberto Di Carlo, Piero Nicolai and Luigia Bandolin
Department of Neurosciences, Section of Otolaryngology, University of Padova, Padova, Italy

Marco Rossi
Unit of Oral and Maxillofacial Surgery, Treviso Regional Hospital, Treviso, Italy

Rossana Bussani
Department of Medical, Surgical and Health Sciences, Section of Pathology, University of Trieste, Trieste, Italy

Maria Guido
Department of Medicine (DIMED), Section of Pathology, University of Padova, Treviso, Italy

Jonathan Fussey
Department of ENT/Head and Neck Surgery, Queen Elizabeth University Hospital Birmingham, Birmingham, United Kingdom

Jerry Polesel
Unit of Cancer Epidemiology, Centro di Riferimento Oncologico di Aviano (CRO) Istituto di Ricovero e Cura a Carattere Scientifico (IRCCS), Aviano, Italy

Enrica Rampazzo
Department of Surgery, Oncology and Gastroenterology, Section of Oncology and Immunology, University of Padova, Padova, Italy

Binbin Li and Weiping Jie
Department of Oral Pathology, Peking University School and Hospital of Stomatology, Beijing, China
Research Unit of Precision Pathologic Diagnosis in Tumors of the Oral and Maxillofacial Regions, Chinese Academy of Medical Sciences, Beijing, China
National Clinical Research Center for Oral Diseases, Peking University School and Hospital of Stomatology, Beijing, China

Huiying He
Department of Pathology, School of Basic Medical Sciences, Third Hospital, Peking University Health Science Center, Beijing, China

Li-Han Lin and Hui-Wen Cheng
Department of Medical Research, MacKay Memorial Hospital, Taipei, Taiwan

Kuo-Wei Chang
Department of Stomatology, Taipei Veterans General Hospital, Taipei, Taiwan
School of Dentistry, Institute of Oral Biology, National Yang-Ming University, Taipei, Taiwan

Chung-Ji Liu
School of Dentistry, Institute of Oral Biology, National Yang-Ming University, Taipei, Taiwan
Department of Oral and Maxillofacial Surgery, Taipei MacKay Memorial Hospital, Taipei, Taiwan

Katharina Lübbers, Mykola Pavlychenko, Theresa Wald, Susanne Wiegand, Andreas Dietz, Veit Zebralla and Gunnar Wichmann
Department of Otorhinolaryngology, Head and Neck Surgery, University Hospital Leipzig, Leipzig, Germany

Po-Chuan Lee and Yi-Chiung Hsu
Department of Biomedical Sciences and Engineering, National Central University, Taoyuan, Taiwan

Yi-Chao Huang
Department of Biomedical Sciences and Engineering, National Central University, Taoyuan, Taiwan
Department of Medical Laboratory, Taoyuan Armed Forces General Hospital, Taoyuan, Taiwan

Jane Jen Wang
The Department of Nursing, School of Nursing, National Taipei University of Nursing and Health Sciences, Taipei, Taiwan

Ruma Dey Ghosh
Tata Translational Cancer Research Center, Tata Medical Center, Kolkata, India

Arun Pattatheyil
Department of Head and Neck Surgical Oncology,Tata Medical Center, Kolkata, India

Susanta Roychoudhury
Saroj Gupta Cancer Centre and Research Institute, Kolkata, India

Erika Naakka, Ahmed Al-Samadi, Katja Korelin and Ilida Suleymanova
Department of Oral and Maxillofacial Diseases, University of Helsinki, Helsinki, Finland
Translational Immunology Research Program (TRIMM), University of Helsinki, Helsinki, Finland

Mateus Camargo Barros-Filho, Fábio Albuquerque Marchi and Hellen Kuasne
Centro Internacional de Pesquisa (CIPE) - A.C.Camargo Cancer Center, São Paulo, Brazil

Shady Adnan-Awad
Translational Immunology Research Program (TRIMM), University of Helsinki, Helsinki, Finland
Hematology Research Unit, Department of Clinical Chemistry and Hematology, University of Helsinki, Helsinki University Hospital Comprehensive Cancer Center, Helsinki, Finland

Amy Louise Brown, Vera Cavalcanti Araújo and Fabricio Passador-Santos
Department of Oral Pathology, Faculdade São Leopoldo Mandic, Campinas, Brazil

Cristovam Scapulatempo-Neto
Molecular Oncology Research Center, Barretos, and Diagno´s ticos da Ame´r ica (DASA), Barueri, Brazil

Silvia Vanessa Lourenço
Department of Pathology, A.C.Camargo Cancer Center, São Paulo, Brazil
Department of General Pathology, Dental School, University of São Paulo, São Paulo, Brazil

Rogério Moraes Castilho
Department of Periodontics and Oral Medicine, University of Michigan School of Dentistry, Ann Arbor, MI, United States

Luiz Paulo Kowalski
Department of Head and Neck Surgery and Otorhinolaryngology, A.C.Camargo Cancer Center, São Paulo, Brazil
Department of Head and Neck Surgery, University of Sao Paulo Medical School, São Paulo, Brazil

Antti Mäkitie
Department of Otorhinolaryngology - Head and Neck Surgery, University of Helsinki and Helsinki University Hospital, Helsinki, Finland
Research Program in Systems Oncology, Faculty of Medicine, University of Helsinki, Helsinki, Finland
Division of Ear, Nose and Throat Diseases, Department of Clinical Sciences, Intervention and Technology, Karolinska Institute and Karolinska Hospital, Stockholm, Sweden

Ilmo Leivo
Institute of Biomedicine, Pathology, University of Turku and Turku University Hospital, Turku, Finland

Silvia Regina Rogatto
Department of Clinical Genetics, University Hospital of Southern Denmark, Vejle, Denmark
Institute of Regional Health Research, University of Southern Denmark, Odense, Denmark

Tuula Salo
Department of Oral and Maxillofacial Diseases, University of Helsinki, Helsinki, Finland
Translational Immunology Research Program (TRIMM), University of Helsinki, Helsinki, Finland
Department of Pathology, Helsinki University Hospital, Helsinki, Finland
Cancer and Translational Medicine Research Unit, University of Oulu, Oulu, Finland
Medical Research Center, Oulu University Hospital, Oulu, Finland

Liyuan Dai, Qigen Fang, Peng Li and Xu Zhang
Department of Head Neck and Thyroid, Affiliated Cancer Hospital of Zhengzhou University, Henan Cancer Hospital, Zhengzhou, China

Fei Liu
Department of Oral Medicine, The First Affiliated Hospital of Zhengzhou University, Henan Cancer Hospital, Zhengzhou, China

Laura Deborah Locati and Stefano Cavalieri
Head and Neck Cancer Medical Oncology Unit, Fondazione Istituto di Ricovero e Cura a Carattere Scientifico (IRCCS) Istituto Nazionale dei Tumori, Milan, Italy

Mara Serena Serafini, Andrea Carenzo and Loris De Cecco
Integrated Biology Platform, Department of Applied Research and Technology Development, Fondazione Istituto di Ricovero e Cura a Carattere Scientifico (IRCCS) Istituto Nazionale dei Tumori, Milan, Italy

Silvana Canevari
Fondazione Istituto di Ricovero e Cura a Carattere Scientifico (IRCCS) Istituto Nazionale dei Tumori, Milan, Italy

Federica Perrone
Pathology Department, Fondazione Istituto di Ricovero e Cura a Carattere Scientifico (IRCCS) Istituto Nazionale dei Tumori, Milan, Italy

Ester Orlandi
Radiation Oncology Clinical Department, National Center of Oncological Hadrontherapy, Pavia, Italy

Serena Delbue
Department of Biomedical, Surgical and Dental Sciences, University of Milan, Milan, Italy

Giulia Berzeri
Department of Brain and Behavioral Sciences, University of Pavia, Pavia, Italy

Anna Pichiecchio
Department of Brain and Behavioral Sciences, University of Pavia, Pavia, Italy
Advanced Imaging and Radiomics Center, Neuroradiology Department, Istituto di Ricovero e Cura a Carattere Scientifico (IRCCS) Mondino Foundation, Pavia, Italy

Lisa Francesca Licitra
Head and Neck Cancer Medical Oncology Unit, Fondazione Istituto di Ricovero e Cura a Carattere Scientifico (IRCCS) Istituto Nazionale dei Tumori, Milan, Italy
Department of Hematology and Oncology, University of Milan, Milan, Italy

Enrico Marchioni
Neuroncology Unit, Istituto di Ricovero e Cura a Carattere Scientifico (IRCCS) Mondino Foundation, Pavia, Italy

Maxime Brunet
Department of Medicine, Institut Bergonié, Bordeaux, France

Emmanuel Khalifa
Department of Tumor Genetics, Institut Bergonié, Bordeaux, France

Antoine Italiano
Department of Medicine, Institut Bergonié, Bordeaux, France
Faculty of Médicine, University of Bordeaux, Bordeaux, France
INSERM, ACTION U1218, Bordeaux, France

Fang Song
Department of Anesthesiology, College of Medicine, The First Affiliated Hospital, Zhejiang University, Hangzhou, China

Jiong Lv
Department of Oral and Maxillofacial Surgery, College of Medicine, The First Affiliated Hospital, Zhejiang University, Hangzhou, China

Cheng Xiao, Yu Long Zheng, Qiang Feng Wang and Nong Xu
Department of Medical Oncology, College of Medicine, The First Affiliated Hospital, Zhejiang University, Hangzhou, China

Hanna Klimza, Piotr Nogal and Małgorzata Wierzbicka
Department of Otolaryngology and Laryngological Oncology, Poznan´ University of Medical Sciences, Poznań , Poland

Wioletta Pietruszewska and Joanna Morawska
Department of Otolaryngology, Head and Neck Oncology, Medical University of Lodz, Lodz, Poland

Oskar Rosiak
Balance Disorder Unit, Department of Otolaryngology, Medical University of Lodz, Lodz, Poland

Tong-Hong Wang
Tissue Bank, Chang Gung Memorial Hospital, Tao-Yuan, Taiwan
Research Center for Chinese Herbal Medicine, Graduate Institute of Health Industry Technology and Research Center for Food and Cosmetic Safety, College of Human Ecology, Chang Gung University of Science and Technology, Tao-Yuan, Taiwan
Department of Hepato-Gastroenterology, Liver Research Center, Chang Gung Memorial Hospital, Tao-Yuan, Taiwan

Yann-Lii Leu
Graduate Institute of Natural Products, Chang Gung University, Tao-Yuan, Taiwan
Chinese Herbal Medicine Research Team, Healthy Aging Research Center, Chang Gung University, Tao-Yuan, Taiwan
Center for Traditional Chinese Medicine, Chang Gung Memorial Hospital, Tao-Yuan, Taiwan

Tzong-Ming Shieh
Department of Dental Hygiene, China Medical University, Taichung, Taiwan

Jang-Hau Lian
Genomic Medicine Core Laboratory, Chang Gung Memorial Hospital, Tao-Yuan, Taiwan

Chi-Yuan Chen
Tissue Bank, Chang Gung Memorial Hospital, Tao-Yuan, Taiwan
Research Center for Chinese Herbal Medicine, Graduate Institute of Health Industry Technology and Research Center for Food and Cosmetic Safety, College of Human Ecology, Chang Gung University of Science and Technology, Tao-Yuan, Taiwan

Chin-Chuan Chen
Tissue Bank, Chang Gung Memorial Hospital, Tao-Yuan, Taiwan
Graduate Institute of Natural Products, Chang Gung University, Tao-Yuan, Taiwan

Lisa Lorenz and Joscha von Rappard
Department of Internal Medicine, Hirslanden Klinik St. Anna, Lucerne, Switzerland

Walter Arnold
Department of Pathology, Cantonal Hospital Lucerne, Lucerne, Switzerland

Nicole Mutter
Department of Oncology, Hirslanden Klinik St. Anna, Lucerne, Switzerland

Udo Schirp
Institute of Radiology and Nuclear Medicine, Hirslanden Klinik St. Anna, Lucerne, Switzerland

Andreas Scherr
Department of Pneumology, Hirslanden Klinik St. Anna, Lucerne, Switzerland

Andreas Werner Jehle
Department of Internal Medicine, Hirslanden Klinik St. Anna, Lucerne, Switzerland
Transplantation Immunology and Nephrology, University Hospital Basel, Basel, Switzerland

Hélène Carinato, Martin Demarchi, Mickaël Burgy, Cathie Fischbach, Michal Kalish, Thierry Petit and Christian Borel
Institut de Cancérologie Strasbourg Europe, Department of Medical Oncology, Strasbourg, France

Régine Ferry
Centre Paul Strauss, Department of Medical Oncology, Strasbourg, France

Sébastien Guihard and Youssef Brahimi
Institut de Cancérologie Strasbourg Europe, Department of Radiation Oncology, Strasbourg, France

Henri Flesch and Guy Bronner
Clinique Sainte Barbe, Head and Neck Surgery Unit, Strasbourg, France

Philippe Schultz
Hôpitaux Universitaires de Strasbourg, Department of Otorhinolaryngology and Head and Neck Surgery, Strasbourg, France

Véronique Frasie
Institut de Cancérologie Strasbourg Europe, Supportive Care Unit, Strasbourg, France

Alicia Thiéry
Institut de Cancérologie Strasbourg Europe, Department of Biostatistics, Strasbourg, France

Alain C. Jung
Institut de Cancérologie Strasbourg Europe, Laboratoire de Biologie Tumorale, Strasbourg, France
Universitéde Strasbourg, Inserm, UMR_S1113, Strasbourg, France

Pierre Wagner
Centre Paul Strauss, Department of Radiology, Strasbourg, France

Pierre Coliat
Institut de Cancérologie Strasbourg Europe, Pharmacy Department, Strasbourg, France

Xuanchen Zhou, Yiqing Liu, Zhaoyang Cui, Zhiyong Yue and Ling Ding
Department of Otorhinolaryngology Head and Neck Surgery, Shandong Provincial Hospital Affiliated to Shandong First Medical University, Jinan, China

Jie Han and Shuai Xu
Department of Otorhinolaryngology Head and Neck Surgery, Shandong Provincial Hospital Affiliated to Shandong University, Jinan, China

Xiaoyue Zhen
Minimally Invasive Urology Center, Shandong Provincial Hospital Affiliated to Shandong First Medical University, Jinan, China

Wei-long Zhang, Zhuo-li Zhu, Mei-chang Huang, Yaling Tang and Xin-hua Liang
State Key Laboratory of Oral Diseases, National Clinical Research Center for Oral Diseases, West China Hospital of Stomatology, Sichuan University, Chengdu, China

Ya-Jie Tang
State Key Laboratory of Microbial Technology, Shandong University, Qingdao, China

Fengjie Zhu and Kai Ba
Department of Oral Medicine, The First Affiliated Hospital of Zhengzhou University, Zhengzhou, China

Shuhan Sun
Department of Oral Medicine, The Third Affiliated Hospital of Zhengzhou University, Zhengzhou, China

Virginia Arrazubi
Oncology, Complejo Hospitalario de Navarra, Pamplona, Spain

Gerardo Cajaraville
Hospital Pharmacy, Fundación Onkologikoa, San Sebastián, Spain

David Cantero
Quality and Innovation, Organización Sanitaria Integrada (Integrated Health Organisation) (OSI) Barrualde Galdakao, Galdakao, Spain

Jordi Giralt
Radiation Oncology, Hospital Universitari Vall d´Hebrón, Barcelona, Spain

Florencio Monje
Oral and Maxillofacial Surgery, Hospital Universitario de Badajoz, Badajoz, Spain

Antonio Rueda
Oncology, Hospital Regional Universitario de Málaga, Málaga, Spain

Alexander Sistiaga
Otolaryngology, Hospital Universitario Donostia, San Sebastián, Spain

Jorge Suarez and Alejandro Mut
Bristol Myers Squibb, Madrid, Spain

Marta Comellas
Outcomes'10, Castellón de la Plana, Spain

Luis Lizán
Outcomes'10, Castellón de la Plana, Spain
Medicine Department, Jaume I University, Castellón de la Plana, Spain

Hui-Ching Wang
Graduate Institute of Clinical Medicine, College of Medicine, Kaohsiung Medical University, Kaohsiung, Taiwan
Division of Hematology and Oncology, Department of Internal Medicine, Kaohsiung Medical University Hospital, Kaohsiung Medical University, Kaohsiung, Taiwan

Leong-Perng Chan
Graduate Institute of Clinical Medicine, College of Medicine, Kaohsiung Medical University, Kaohsiung, Taiwan
Department of Otolaryngology-Head and Neck Surgery, Kaohsiung Medical University Hospital, Kaohsiung Medical University, Kaohsiung, Taiwan

Index

www.ingramcontent.com/pod-product-compliance
Lightning Source LLC
LaVergne TN
LVHW082141200926
848484LV00008B/2091